Innate Immunity

Infectious Disease

SERIES EDITOR: *Vassil St. Georgiev*

National Institute of Allergy and Infectious Diseases
National Institutes of Health

Infectious Disease

Innate Immunity

Edited by

R. Alan B. Ezekowitz

MB ChB, DPhil, FAAP

Laboratory of Developmental Immunology, Massachusetts General Hospital;
Department of Pediatrics, Harvard Medical School, Boston, MA

Jules A. Hoffmann, PhD

Institute of Molecular and Cellular Biology, CNRS, Strasbourg, France

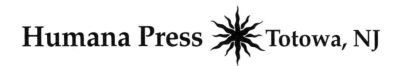

Humana Press ⚹ Totowa, NJ

Cover design by Patricia F. Cleary.

For additional copies, pricing for bulk purchases, and/or information about other Humana titles, contact Humana at the above address or at any of the following numbers: Tel: 973-256-1699; Fax: 973-256-8341; E-mail: humana@humanapr.com, or visit our Website: http://humanapress.com

Printed in the United States of America. 10 9 8 7 6 5 4 3 2 1

Library of Congress Cataloging in Publication Data

Innate immunity / edited by R. Alan B. Ezekowitz, Jules A. Hoffmann
    p. : cm. -- (Infectious disease)
  Includes bibliographical references and index.
  ISBN 1-58829-046-8 (alk. paper); 1-59259-320-8 (e-book)
  1. Natural immunity. 2. Immunology, Comparative. I. Ezekowitz, R. Alan B. II. Hoffman, Jules A. III. Infectious disease (Totowa, N.J.)
  [DNLM: 1. Immunity, Natural--physiology. QW 541 I58 2003]
QR185.2.I487 2003
571.9'6--dc21
                                         2002024204

Preface

The concept of innate immunity refers to the first-line host defense that serves to limit infection in the early hours after exposure to microorganisms. Recent data have highlighted similarities between pathogen recognition, signaling pathways, and effector mechanisms of innate immunity in *Drosophila* and mammals, pointing to a common ancestry of these defenses. In addition to its role in the early phase of defense, innate immunity in mammals appears to play a key role in stimulating the subsequent clonal response of adaptive immunity.

Recent exciting information has determined that the templates that are laid down in primitive life forms, like flowering plants and insects, form the basic principles of first-line host defense that are conserved in mammalian systems. The next frontier in the field is to understand the dynamic adaptive changes that occur as a result of the interplay between host defenses and infectious agents. One emerging theme is that microorganisms are constantly seeking ways to co-opt host defenses. On the other hand, host defense to infection is mediated by the coordinate action of pattern recognition molecules and receptors that, in mammals, are important and probably necessary antecedents to the development of an adaptive immune response. *Innate Immunity* aims to explore the intersection between host pathogen interactions across an evolutionary spectrum that will inform our understanding of the dynamic interplay between infectious agents and host defense in man.

Innate Immunity is divided into four sections that focus on a combination of plant, insect, and vertebrate systems to elucidate the origins of the human system of defense against infection. We hope this book will further our understanding of the development and functioning of the innate immune system.

R. Alan B. Ezekowitz, MB ChB, DPhil, FAAP
Jules A. Hoffmann, PhD

Contents

Contributors

SHIZUO AKIRA, MD, PhD • *Professor, Department of Host Defense, Research Institute for Microbial Diseases, Osaka University, Suita City, Osaka, Japan*

K. FRANK AUSTEN, MD • *Director, Inflammation and Allergic Diseases Research Section, Division of Rheumatology, Immunology, and Allergy, Brigham and Women's Hospital; Astrazeneca Professor of Respiratory and Inflammatory Diseases, Department of Medicine, Harvard Medical School, Boston, MA*

FREDERICK M. AUSUBEL, PhD • *Department of Molecular Biology, Massachusetts General Hospital; Professor, Department of Genetics, Harvard University, Boston, MA*

KATI BAKSA, PhD • *Laboratory of Developmental Immunology, Massachusetts General Hospital; Research Fellow in Pediatrics, Harvard Medical School, Boston, MA*

STÉPHANIE BLANDIN • *European Molecular Biology Laboratory, Heidelberg, Germany*

JOSHUA A. BOYCE, MD • *Inflammation and Allergic Diseases Research Section, Division of Rheumatology, Immunology, and Allergy, Brigham and Women's Hospital; Assistant Professor, Department of Medicine, Harvard Medical School, Boston, MA*

PHILIPPE BULET, PhD • *Institut de Biologie Moléculaire et Cellulaire (IBMC), UPR 9022 du CNRS, Strasbourg Cedex, France*

MICHAEL C. CARROLL, PhD • *Center for Blood Research, Professor of Pediatrics (Pathology), Harvard Medical School, Boston, MA*

MAURICE CHARLET, PhD • *Institut de Biologie Moléculaire et Cellulaire (IBMC), UPR 9022 du CNRS, Strasbourg Cedex, France*

JONATHAN COHN, PhD • *Boyce Thompson Institute for Plant Research, Cornell University, Ithaca, NY*

ERIKA C. CROUCH, MD, PhD • *Professor of Pathology and Immunology, George Washington University School of Medicine; Barnes Jewish Hospital, St. Louis, MO*

ERIC H. DAVIDSON, PhD • *Norman Chandler Professor of Cell Biology, Division of Biology, California Institute of Technology, Pasadena, CA*

JEFFREY G. ELLIS, PhD • *Commonwealth Scientific and Industrial Research Organisation–Plant Industry, Canberra ACT, Australia*

DOMINIQUE FERRANDON, PhD • *Institut de Biologie Moléculaire et Cellulaire (IBMC), UPR 9022 du CNRS, Strasbourg Cedex, France*

MIHAELA GADJEVA, PhD • *Center for Blood Research, Department of Pediatrics, Harvard Medical School, Boston, MA*

TOMAS GANZ, MD, PhD • *Professor of Medicine and Pathology, UCLA School of Medicine, Los Angeles, CA*

SIAMON GORDON, MB, ChB, PhD • *GlaxoWellcome Professor of Cellular Pathology, Sir William Dunn School of Pathology, University of Oxford, Oxford, United Kingdom*

DJILALI HAMMACHE, PhD • *Department of Cell Biology and Physiology, George Washington University School of Medicine, George Washington University Medical Center, St. Louis, MO*

ASHA HARIKRISHNAN, PhD • *Laboratory of Developmental Immunology, Massachusetts General Hospital; Research Fellow in Pediatrics, Harvard Medical School, Boston, MA*

MICHÈLE C. HEATH, PhD, FRSC • *Professor, Department of Botany, University of Toronto, Toronto, Ontario, Canada*

CHARLES HETRU, PhD • *Institut de Biologie Moléculaire et Cellulaire (IBMC), UPR 9022 du CNRS, Strasbourg Cedex, France*

CORY M. HOGABOAM, PhD • *Department of Pathology, University of Michigan Medical School, Ann Arbor, MI*

SADAAKI IWANAGA, PhD • *Professor Emeritus, Department of Biology, Faculty of Sciences, Kyushu University, Fukuoka, Japan*

DAVID A. JONES, PhD • *Research School of Biological Sciences, Australian National University, Canberra ACT, Australia*

FOTIS C. KAFATOS, PhD • *European Molecular Biology Laboratory, Heidelberg, Germany*

TSUNEYASU KAISHO, MD, PhD • *Research Institute for Microbial Diseases; Associate Professor, Department of Host Defense, Osaka University, Suita City, Osaka; Riken Research Center for Allergy and Immunology, Kanagawa, Japan*

SHUN-ICHIRO KAWABATA, PhD • *Associate Professor, Department of Biology, Faculty of Sciences, Kyushu University, Fukuoka, Japan*

STEVEN L. KUNKEL, PhD • *Professor, Department of Pathology, University of Michigan Medical School, Ann Arbor, Michigan*

MARIE LAGUEUX, PhD • *Institut de Biologie Moléculaire et Cellulaire (IBMC), UPR 9022 du CNRS, Strasbourg Cedex, France*

MYKOL LARVIE, MD, PhD • *Laboratory of Developmental Immunology, Massachusetts General Hospital; Harvard Medical School, Boston; Harvard–MIT Division of Health Sciences and Technology, Cambridge, MA*

ROBERT I. LEHRER, MD • *Department of Medicine/Infectious Diseases, UCLA School of Medicine, UCLA Center for the Health Sciences, Los Angeles, CA*

ELENA A. LEVASHINA, PhD • *European Molecular Biology Laboratory, Heidelberg, Germany*

GREGORY B. MARTIN, PhD • *Scientist, Boyce Thompson Institute for Plant Research; Professor, Department of Plant Pathology, Cornell University, Ithaca, NY*

MARIE MEISTER, PhD • *Institut de Biologie Moléculaire et Cellulaire (IBMC), UPR 9022 du CNRS, Strasbourg Cedex, France*

LUIS F. MOITA, MD • *European Molecular Biology Laboratory, Heidelberg, Germany*

D. Branch Moody, MD • *Division of Rheumatology, Immunology, and Allergy, Brigham and Women's Hospital; Assistant Professor, Department of Medicine, Harvard Medical School, Boston, MA*

Tsukasa Osaki • *Graduate Student, Department of Molecular Biology, Graduate School of Medical Sciences, Kyushu University, Fukuoka, Japan*

Alan Pearson, PhD • *Laboratory of Developmental Immunology, Massachusetts General Hospital; Research Fellow in Pediatrics, Harvard Medical School, Boston, MA*

Mika Rämet, MD, PhD • *Laboratory of Developmental Immunology, Massachusetts General Hospital; Research Fellow in Pediatrics, Harvard Medical School, Boston, MA*

Thiruvamoor P. Ramkumar, PhD • *Department of Cell Biology and Physiology, George Washington University School of Medicine, George Washington University Medical Center, St. Louis, MO*

Jean-Marc Reichhart, PhD • *Institut de Biologie Moléculaire et Cellulaire (IBMC), UPR 9022 du CNRS; Professor, Louis Pasteur University; Strasbourg Cedex, France*

Ellen V. Rothenberg, PhD • *Division of Biology, California Institute of Technology, Pasadena, CA*

Julien Royet, PhD • *Institut de Biologie Moléculaire et Cellulaire (IBMC), UPR A9022 du CNRS, Strasbourg Cedex, France*

Philip D. Stahl, PhD • *Chair, Department of Cell Biology and Physiology, George Washington University School of Medicine, George Washington University Medical Center, St. Louis, MO*

Thilo Stehle, PhD • *Laboratory of Developmental Immunology, Massachusetts General Hospital; Assistant Professor of Pediatrics, Harvard Medical School, Boston, MA*

Peter S. Tobias, PhD • *Department of Immunology, Scripps Research Institute, La Jolla, CA*

David M. Underhill, PhD • *The Institute for Systems Biology, Seattle, WA*

Admar Verschoor, MSc • *Center for Blood Research, Department of Pathology, Harvard Medical School, Boston, MA*

Jeffrey A. Whitsett, MD • *Divisions of Neonatology and Pulmonary Biology, The Children's Hospital Research Foundation, Children's Hospital Medical Center, Cincinnati, OH*

Wayne M. Yokoyama, MD • *Sam J. and Audrey Loew Levin Professor of Rheumatology, Department of Medicine and Department of Pathology and Immunology; Investigator, Howard Hughes Medical Institute, George Washington University School of Medicine and Barnes Jewish Hospital, St. Louis, MO*

Section I
Plant Immunity
Section Editor: Frederick M. Ausubel

In the context of *Innate Immunity*, the most relevant question concerning the plant defense response to pathogen attack is the evolutionary relationship between innate immune responses in plants and animals. In comparing insects and mammals, clear similarities in innate immunity are apparent, including most prominently the conservation of Toll-like receptors (TLRs) and the downstream signaling cascades leading to the activation of Rel-family transcription factors. Plants have neither proteins that are directly homologous to TLRs nor Rel transcription factors. Despite these differences, innate immune responses in plants and animals share a variety of common features. Both animals and plants are able to respond to microbial pathogen-associated molecular patterns (PAMPs) that distinguish pathogen from host cells. For example, plant cells respond to Gram-negative lipopolysaccharide (LPS), eubacterial flagella, and to a variety of fungal cell wall components including glycoproteins and carbohydrates. However, different plant species may recognize different pathogen-derived PAMPs to greater or lesser extents, whereas at least mammals as a group all recognize the same set of PAMPs and have a limited number of TLRs corresponding to these PAMPs.

An important distinction between two different aspects of the plant innate immune response may not have a direct parallel in insect and mammalian innate immunity. Most plants are resistant to most phyto (plant) pathogens; susceptibility is uncommon. For example, the inability of a wheat pathogen to cause disease on rice is generally referred to as *non-host* resistance, because rice is not a host for the wheat pathogen. The expression of non-host resistance is a multigenic phenomenon, the molecular basis of which is poorly understood. On the other hand, many pathogens of a particular plant species are able to cause disease on some cultivars of that species but not on other cultivars. This latter type of resistance is referred to as *gene-for-gene* resistance

From: *Infectious Disease: Innate Immunity*
Edited by: R. A. B. Ezekowitz and J. A. Hoffmann © Humana Press Inc., Totowa, NJ

because the difference in resistance between resistant and susceptible cultivars is usually determined by a single gene difference.

The molecular basis of gene-for-gene resistance has been the subject of extensive investigation during the past decade and has been shown to be mediated by highly conserved multigene families of so-called resistance proteins, all characterized by the presence of a leucine-rich repeat (LRR) motif. The largest of these resistance gene families, containing over 100 members in *Arabidopsis*, is also characterized by a nucleotide binding site (NBS). Interestingly, a subset of these NBS-LRR resistance proteins also contains a so-called TIR (Toll-interleukin-1 receptor) domain present in TLRs in insects and in mammals. It appears likely that plant resistance proteins function as receptors for pathogen-associated molecules, but not for highly conserved PAMPs such as LPS or flagellin. Instead, the NBS-LRR proteins studied to date function as receptors for pathogen-derived virulence factors (also referred to as effector proteins) that are translocated directly in host cells, for example, by the Type III secretory system in bacterial pathogens.

Instead of serving solely as recognition receptors for pathogen effector proteins, an intriguing possibility is that NBS-LRR receptors form multiprotein complexes with their corresponding effector proteins and the intracellular targets of the effector proteins. In this latter scenario, the NBS-LRR proteins are hypothesized to "guard" these cellular targets from attack by particular pathogen effector proteins. Interestingly, recently identified mammalian proteins that appear to function as intracellular LPS receptors are homologs of NBS-LRR plant resistance proteins. It is unlikely, however, that NBS-LRR proteins also function as LPS receptors in plants because plant bacterial pathogens are almost exclusively extracellular.

Given these aspects of the plant immune response, one can envision the evolution of plant immunity along the following lines. An ancient common ancestor of plants and animals evolved the ability to recognize a variety of PAMPs, thereby affording broad-range resistance against a variety of microbial pathogens. During plant evolution, particular pathogens evolved to circumvent the host defense response of particular host species, in part by the elaboration of effector proteins that targeted the plant defense response. In turn, plants evolved resistance proteins corresponding to particular effectors (virulence factors). An unresolved question is whether cultivar-specific and non-host resistance share a variety of common molecular features. Both types of resistance involve the activation of similar sets of host defense responses. In support of a common mechanism underlying cultivar-specfic and non-host resistance, recent results suggest that molecular components first identified as part of the cultivar-specific resistance response also function in non-host resistance. Thus non-host resistance is most likely a consequence of the recognition of PAMPs as well as the recognition of specific pathogen effector proteins. Chapters by Cohn and by Martin, Ellis, and Jones, and by Heath in this section of *Innate Immunity* explore each of these issues in detail.

Frederick M. Ausubel

1
Pathogen Recognition and Signal Transduction in Plant Immunity

Jonathan Cohn and Gregory B. Martin

1. INTRODUCTION

In natural environments, plants must defend themselves against attack from a variety of organisms, including bacteria, viruses, fungi, invertebrates, and, in some instances, other plants. However, we generally pay little attention to plant diseases in nature because spread is usually limited to small populations and is often restricted to small areas of tissue on individual plants. Uncontrolled spread of disease does occur however, in agricultural settings, often as a result of growing large fields of genetically uniform crops. This practice, known as monoculture, can promote the spread of a particular pathogen, which may result in greatly reduced yields and diminished product quality. Our current understanding of how plants defend themselves against pathogen ingress has provided some clues as to how plants might be engineered for increased disease resistance. These plants will help prevent disease epidemics and be an important component of more sustainable agricultural systems *(1)*.

Disease resistance in plants is largely dependent on the ability of plants to respond quickly to external stimuli, including pathogens. Recognition of a potential pathogen leads to the rapid activation of defense systems that limit colonization and spread. The genotype's of both the invading microbe and the host plant are key components of this recognition event. It has become clear that only a limited number of microbes can cause disease on a particular plant species. One of the most intriguing questions, then, is what allows a plant to distinguish a pathogen from a nonpathogen.

One of the ways in which plants are able to sense pathogen attack very early during an infection is by recognition of signal molecules known as elicitors. Elicitors can be host cell wall components released by degradation, but they are often compounds produced by the invading microbe. A variety of compounds have been shown to be elicitors, including polysaccharides, lipids, and proteins. In many cases, minute quantities of pure elicitors are sufficient to induce a series of host defense responses. Therefore, it has been proposed that these molecules interact with specific plant receptors *(2)*.

Protein elicitors are often the products of pathogen-encoded avirulence *(avr)* genes, also referred to as effectors. It is generally accepted that the protein products of specific plant resistance *(R)* genes play a critical role in the perception of these *avr* effectors

From: *Infectious Disease: Innate Immunity*
Edited by: R. A. B. Ezekowitz and J. A. Hoffmann © Humana Press Inc., Totowa, NJ

(3). One model of plant disease resistance signaling, the gene-for-gene hypothesis, predicts that plant resistance often occurs when a plant possesses a dominant *R* gene and the pathogen possesses a complementary *avr* gene *(4)*. In this review, we will highlight relevant findings that have furthered our understanding of the involvement of *R* genes in the perception of pathogen-derived signals. We will also discuss the events downstream of signal recognition that lead to the induction of plant defense responses.

2. COMMON PLANT DEFENSE RESPONSES

Upon pathogen recognition, resistant plants respond rapidly (i.e., within minutes) by activating a battery of defense responses. In many instances, pathogen invasion of a resistant plant results in macroscopic necrotic lesions that form as the result of rapid localized cell death *(3,5)*. This response has been termed the hypersensitive response (HR) and is believed to benefit the plant by limiting pathogen growth and proliferation throughout healthy tissue. Several physiologic changes are associated with the HR, including the production of reactive oxygen species (ROS), cell wall fortifications, callose deposition, transient opening of ion channels, alkalinization of growth media, transcriptional activation of pathogenesis-related (PR) genes, production of antimicrobial phytoalexins, and changes in protein phosphorylation. There are several excellent reviews that describe events associated with the HR *(3,5,–9)*. In addition to these physiologic changes, secondary signaling molecules are generated that might be involved in long-distance signaling of plant defense responses and increased resistance to further pathogen attack (*see* refs. *10–12*, and references therein).

2.1. Oxidative Burst

One of the earliest host responses to pathogen attack is the production of ROS *(13)*. Production of ROS, referred to as the *oxidative burst,* is triggered within just minutes after infection and involves a series of signaling events that involve guanosine Triphosphate (GTP)-binding proteins, changes in protein phosphorylation, Ca^{2+} flux, and H^+/K^+ ion exchange, resulting in intracellular acidification. The production of ROS, such as H_2O_2, and superoxide ($\cdot O_2^-$) radicals results in cellular damage to both the plant and the invading microbe. H_2O_2 probably also contributes to cell wall reinforcement. For example, H_2O_2 has been demonstrated to be essential to lignification of cell walls *(14)*. Cell wall strengthening around the site of pathogen ingress might serve to limit microbial spread to uninfected plant tissues. ROS have also been suggested to be critical components of defense signaling. Indeed, ROS were shown to induce a variety of defense-related genes *(7,15,16)*. Exogenous application of H_2O_2 to transgenic tobacco plants deficient in catalase production was found to activate PR gene expression. Possibly owing to increased production of ROS, the plants also displayed enhanced resistance to the plant pathogen *Pseudomonas syringae* pv. *syringae (16)*. H_2O_2 has also been shown to activate the induction of defense genes in response to wounding *(17)*.

Recent evidence suggests that the oxidative burst in plants is similar to the oxidative burst described in mammalian neutrophils, which employs a reduced nicotinamide adenine dinucleotide phosphate (NADPH)-oxidase dependent system *(18,19,3)*. This idea is supported by the identification and cloning of plant homologs of two NADPH-oxidase components; gp91[phox] and Rac *(20,21)*. Studies using transgenic plants that constitutively overexpress Rac, or dominant negative variants of Rac, suggest that this protein plays a role in regulating cell death *(21)*. Plant gp91[phox] genes are members of a multigene family, so they might serve a variety of roles in plant metabolism, or they may be functionally redundant. Other than their similarity to the mammalian proteins, there is no evidence yet that plant gp91[phox] genes are involved in plant defense, although it is likely that they will be shown to be. Although it is not clear how the plant NADPH oxidase complex is regulated or what proteins constitute it, chemical inhibitors of the enzyme complex found in mammalian cells have been demonstrated to inhibit pathogen, and elicitor-induced accumulation of H_2O_2 produced from the plant oxidative burst *(15,22–24)*.

2.2. Production of Antimicrobial Compounds

One of the most significant quantitative changes in protein composition that occurs during the HR is the accumulation of PR proteins *(9)*. Several of the PR proteins, which have been classified into at least 11 families, act as general antibacterial or antifungal molecules. For example, PR-1 and PR-5 family members interact with the plasma membrane of fungal pathogens *(25,26)*. PR-5 proteins might create transmembrane pores, and one family member from tobacco, osmotin, was shown to be active against several fungal pathogens *(26)*. Several *PR* genes have been shown to encode chitinases and β-1,3-glucanases that actively attack fungal cell walls. Chitinases can also act as antibacterial enzymes, in that they have lysozyme activity and thus possess the ability to hydrolyze bacterial cell walls *(9)*. Interestingly, chitinase and β-1,3-glucanase action on fungal cell walls can result in the production of small oligosaccharidic fragments that act as elicitors *(27)*. Therefore, these enzymes can amplify a plant defense response as well as attack invading microbes directly. In addition to PR proteins, another class of peptides referred to as defensins are induced upon pathogen infection. Plant defensins share similarities to mammalian and insect defensins and are potent inhibitors of microbial growth *(28)*.

Phytoalexins are another class of compounds that accumulate around sites of pathogen infection and also in response to a variety of elicitor compounds. Phytoalexins are low molecular weight, lipophilic compounds that have been shown to have antimicrobial activity *(3)*. Several different phytoalexins have been analyzed, but it is still not clear whether these molecules are directly involved in defense responses mediated by *avr/R* gene interaction. Interestingly, plant mutants have been isolated that are deficient in phytoalexin production (PAD). These mutant plant lines display an enhanced susceptibility to a number of different pathogens *(29)*. In addition, several of the *PAD* genes have been shown to be required for resistance to the eukaryotic biotroph *Peronospora parasitica*.

Some of the elicitors that induce phytoalexin production are the β-1,3-glucans and chitin fragments released from fungal cell walls by the enzymatic products of *PR* genes, which are transcriptionally induced rapidly after primary pathogen infection. It is likely that these cell wall breakdown products stimulate phytoalexin production, which might help the plant prevent secondary infections *(30)*.

2.3. Secondary Signaling Molecules Involved in Plant Defense

2.3.1. Systemic Acquired Resistance

It has become apparent that plants employ multiple signaling pathways to defend themselves against pathogen attack. Studies over the years have shed some light on how plants respond to individual pathogens, but in natural environments, plants must protect themselves from a variety of invading microbes. Subsequent to an initial pathogen infection, plants often develop a heightened and sustained resistance to a broad spectrum of pathogens at sites distant from the point of infection. This immune response of plants is referred to as systemic acquired resistance (SAR) *(10)*. One of the physiologic indicators that has been used to distinguish SAR is the induction of a number of *PR* genes. Many *PR* genes that have been characterized are widely distributed throughout the plant kingdom. It is likely that a number of different PR proteins act in concert to maintain SAR.

2.3.2. Salicylic Acid

Accumulating evidence suggests that salicylic acid (SA) plays a critical role in both disease resistance and SAR signaling *(31)*. Some of the most compelling evidence supporting this idea has come from studies showing that transgenic plants expressing the bacterial *nahG* gene, which encodes an SA-degrading enzyme (salicylate hydroxylase), were incapable of inducing an SAR in response to microbial pathogens *(10)*. Normally, plants responding to pathogen attack accumulate significantly higher levels of SA than uninfected plants. In several studies, transgenic plants expressing *nahG* did not accumulate SA after exposure to pathogens. In addition, these plants were more susceptible to pathogen attack, indicating that SA is required for SAR (e.g., refs. *32–34*). For example, expression of the *nahG* gene in *Arabidopsis thaliana* led to a loss of gene-for-gene resistance and a loss of a detectable SAR response. Inoculation of *Arabidopsis* lines expressing NahG with the pathogens *P. parasitica* or *P. syringae* led to the development of severe disease symptoms. Interestingly, addition of exogenous SA has been shown in several plant species to result in the transcriptional activation of PR genes, which are normally induced by pathogen inoculation *(31,35,36)*.

Further evidence that SA plays a role in the induction of *PR* genes comes from studies of *Arabidopsis* mutants, such as the *npr1* (nonexpressor of *PR* genes), also known as *nim1* (noninducible immunity) mutant. These plants are unable to induce the expression of many *PR* gene transcripts when challenged with pathogens. These plants also displayed enhanced disease susceptibility, despite exogenous treatment with SA *(37,38)*. In fact, elevated levels of SA in growth media were toxic to these mutants, whereas similar levels of SA had no effect on wild-type plants *(39)*. It appears that failure to activate defense responses in these mutant lines is owing to a defect in the plant's response to SA, not in metabolism of SA. Endogenous SA levels in the mutant plants were actually shown to increase in response to pathogen infection *(38)*.

2.3.3. Jasmonate and Ethylene

Two other known regulators of defense signaling in plants are ethylene and jasmonic acid (JA). A great deal is known about the role of JA in response to mechanical wounding, such as damage that occurs as a result of insect attack *(11)*. Wounding induces the octadecanoid pathway which is responsible for the synthesis of JA, which is in turn involved in the transcriptional regulation of proteinase inhibitor genes *(40,41)*. A wealth of knowledge also exists about the role of the phytohormone ethylene, although its role in plant defense responses is still unclear. Ethylene has long been known to play a role in fruit ripening and is also produced in many plants in response to mechanical wounding or stress *(42)*. It is likely that JA and ethylene signaling pathways act synergistically, as inhibition of ethylene production via mutation, reverse genetics, or chemical inhibition has been demonstrated to affect the JA pathway negatively *(11,42)*. A recent study reported global changes in gene expression patterns in *Arabidopsis* in response to pathogen inoculation or treatment with SA, methyl jasmonate (an active form of JA), or ethylene *(43)*. Microarray analysis indicated that there was a high degree of overlap in genes upregulated in response to the different chemical treatments or inoculation with the fungal pathogen *Alternaria brassicicola*. The results of this study indicated that different defense pathways regulated by these signaling molecules are highly coordinated. These data are quite interesting, since SA and JA pathways were previously thought to act antagonistically *(44)*. A similar study, which used microarray analysis to study changes in gene expression in *Arabidopsis* in response to 14 different SAR-inducing or-repressing conditions, also found that similar patterns of gene expression were induced by different stimuli *(45)*. Clustering analysis was used to identify regulons, or groups of genes that responded in a similar fashion to the same stimuli. Interestingly, a common promoter element, which binds members of a plant transcription factor family, was found in a regulon that contained several *PR* genes, including *PR-1*.

2.3.4. Nitric Oxide

Nitric oxide (NO), a well-studied molecule involved in secondary signaling in mammalian systems, has been demonstrated to play a role in defense signaling in plants. In fact, it was demonstrated that NO is a key player in plant defense responses *(46,47)*. NO is sufficient to activate the expression of PR proteins and is necessary for induction of ROS-dependent cell death. NO probably acts in a synergistic manner with both ROS and SA. However, the role of NO in cell death is not well understood. It has been suggested that SA enhances redox signaling of NO and ROS via a feedback loop mechanism *(12)*.

SAR is very likely to be regulated by a diffusible, mobile element, and NO, possibly bound to nitrosylated glutathione, has been proposed to be this long-distance signal *(12)*. SA was originally proposed to be the systemically mobile element responsible for mediating SAR; however this is probably not the case *(10,48)*. Interestingly, another candidate for a long-distance signal is ROS, such as H_2O_2. In support of this idea, *Arabidopsis* plants inoculated with *P. syringae* were shown to form secondary oxidative bursts in leaves positioned distally from the site of inoculation *(22)*. Establishment of SAR was correlated with these "microbursts," which were dependent on an initial oxidative burst at the site of infection.

3. WHAT TRIGGERS THE PLANT DEFENSE RESPONSE? *R*-GENE-MEDIATED RESISTANCE

The HR is often triggered by a gene-for-gene interaction that involves a pathogen *avr* gene and a dominant *R* gene in the plant *(4)*. If either the pathogen *avr* gene or the corresponding plant *R* gene is missing, then the interaction results in disease and thus is referred to as a compatible interaction. In the instance of an incompatible interaction, the products of *avr* genes, delivered either intercellularly or intracellularly to the plant cell, interact in some fashion with the products of *R* genes. Proteins encoded by *R* genes are either transmembrane or intracellular proteins that are presumed to initiate signal transduction cascades upon ligand binding. To date, over 20 plant *R* genes have been identified and grouped into five classes according to their structural characteristics *(see* Table 1; *1,6).* Many *R* gene products share structural motifs, indicating that resistance to diverse pathogens may be controlled by similar pathways. The five different classes of R proteins include: (1) a cytoplasmic protein kinase; (2) transmembrane receptor-like proteins with extracellular *l*eucine-*r*ich *r*epeats (LRRs) and cytoplasmic protein kinase domains; (3) intracellular receptor-like proteins with LRR domains and nucleotide binding sites (NBS); (4) intracellular receptor-like proteins with LRR domains, NBS domains, and a region of homology to the Toll family of receptors from *Drosophila* and mammals, including the human interleukin-1 receptor, thus known as the *T*oll/*i*nter-leukin-1 *r*eceptor (TIR) domain; and (5) transmembrane receptor-like proteins with extracellular LRR domains.

It is possible that additional types of R proteins might exist that do not contain any of these structural characteristics. Indeed, an *R* gene locus conferring broad-spectrum resistance to mildew pathogens was recently cloned from *Arabidopsis* and found to have little homology to any known *R* genes *(49).* This locus was found to contain two genes, *RPW8.1* and *RPW8.2.* These genes are similar to known *R* genes, in that they are both dominant genes that exist in a cluster and induce defense responses associated with the HR. However, it is not clear whether *RPW8.1* and *RPW8.2* act as classic *R* genes, as the RPW8 locus does not conform to the gene-for-gene model of disease resistance. Another example is the *mlo* gene from barley, which is involved in resistance to powdery mildew *(50).* The product of the *mlo* gene is putatively a seven trans-membrane protein; thus it resembles G-protein-coupled receptors *(51).* Unlike the well-characterized dominant *R* genes, the *mlo* gene is recessive and confers broad-spectrum resistance to several powdery mildew isolates. It is likely that Mlo negatively regulates defense responses, leading to cell death: multiple *mlo* alleles form spontaneous legions even when grown axenically *(52).*

3.1. Pathogen Effector Proteins: Virulence and Avirulence Determinants

Many pathogen effector proteins were originally identified as genetic determinants of incompatibility toward specific plant genotypes and thus were referred to as avirulence (Avr) proteins. Clearly, the presence of the proper *avr* gene can limit the capacity of a particular pathogen to grow on its host plant, with no disease symptoms resulting. It seems counterintuitive that microbial pathogens would produce proteins that allow a possible plant host to recognize them and subsequently mount a defense response. Therefore, it was not surprising that several proteins originally characterized as Avr effectors have also been found to enhance the virulence of pathogens on plant hosts lacking a corresponding *R* gene *(53,–59).* It is likely that these effector proteins originally served as virulence determinants, and plant R proteins evolved to recognize these molecules specifically.

Avr proteins and other pathogenic effector proteins probably interact with specific plant targets to disrupt cellular processes and thus allow increased pathogen proliferation and enhanced disease development. One recent hypothesis suggests that plants may have evolved R proteins to recognize specifically the physical association of pathogen-encoded effector proteins with their plant cellular targets *(60).* Interaction of R proteins with this complex might then initiate plant defense responses associated with the incompatible interaction, such as the HR. This *guard hypothesis* may explain

Table 1
Classes of Plant Resistance Genes

R Gene	Class	Plant	Cloned *avr* gene	Pathogen	Protein motifs	Reference
Pto	**1**	Tomato	*avrPto*	*Pseudomonas syringae* pv. *tomato*	PK	88
Xa21	**2**	Rice	Unknown	*Xanthomonas oryzae* pv. *oryzae*	xLRR TM-PK	66
Prf	**3**	Tomato	*avrPto*	*P. syringae* pv. *tomato*	NBS-LRR	84
12C-1	**3**	Tomato	Unknown	*Fusarium oxysporum*	NBS-LRR	134, 135
Mi	**3**	Tomato	Unknown	*Meloidogyne incognita*	NBS-LRR	86, 87
Rp1-D	**3**	Maize	*avrRp1D*	*Puccinia sorghi*	NBS-LRR	136
Xa1	**3**	Rice	Unknown	*X. oryzae* pv. *oryzae*	NBS-LRR	137
Pi-ta	**3**	Rice	*AVR-Pita*	*Magnaporthe grisea*	NBS-LRR	64
RPS2	**3**	Arabidopsis	*avrRpt2*	*P. syringae* pv. *tomato*	LZ-NBS-LRR	138
RPS5	**3**	Arabidopsis	*avrPphB*	*P. syringae* pv. *maculicola*	LZ-NBS-LRR	139
RPM1	**3**	Arabidopsis	*avrRpml, avrB*	*P. syringae* pv. *maculicola*	LZ-NBS-LRR	140
RPP8	**3**	Arabidopsis	Unknown	*Peronospora parasitica*	LZ-NBS-LRR	141
HRT	**3**	Arabidopsis	*TCV-CP*	Turnip crinkle virus	LZ-NBS-LRR	142
Rx	**3**	Potato	*CP*	Potato virus X	LZ-NBS-LRR	143
Gpa2	**3**	Potato	Unknown	*Globodera palllida*	LZ-NBS-LRR	144
N	**4**	Tobacco	Replicase	Tobacco mosaic virus	TIR-NBS-LRR	145
L6	**4**	Flax	Unknown	*Melampsora lini*	TIR-NBS-LRR	146
M	**4**	Flax	Unknown	*M. lini*	TIR-NBS-LRR	147
RPS4	**4**	Arabidopsis	*avrRps4*	*P. syringae* pv. *tomato*	TIR-NBS-LRR	148
RPP5	**4**	Arabidopsis	Unknown	*Peronospora parasitica*	TIR-NBS-LRR	149
RPP1	**4**	Arabidopsis	Unknown	*P. parasitica*	TIR-NBS-LRR	150
Cf-2	**5**	Tomato	*Avr2*	*Cladosporium fulvum*	xLRR-TM-LRR	151
Cf-4	**5**	Tomato	*Avr4*	*C. fulvum*	xLRR-TM-LRR	152
Cf-5	**5**	Tomato	*Avr5*	*C. fulvum*	xLRR-TM-LRR	153
Cf-9	**5**	Tomato	*Avr9*	*C. fulvum*	xLRR-TM-LRR	154
mlo		Barley	Unknown	*Erysiphe graminis* f.sp. *hordeᵃ*	7 TM-G-protein-coupled receptor	50
RPW8		Arabidopsis	Unknown	*E cruciferarum, E. cichoracearumᵃ*	Unclear; TM-(sig. peptide?) CC	49
Hml		Maize	None	*Cochliobolus carbonum*, race 1	Toxin reductase	155
Hs1pro1		Sugar beet	Unknown	*Heterodera schachtii*	Unclear	156

Abbreviations: TM, transmembrane; PK, protein kinase; x, extracellular; LRR, leucine-rich repeat; NBS, possible nucleotide binding site; LZ, leucine zipper; TIR, Toll/interleukin 1-receptor; CP, coat protein; CC, coiled coll.
ᵃ Broad-spectrum resistance.

some of the unknown details of *R* gene-mediated defense signaling. However, there is evidence that argues against this hypothesis, as will be discussed in more detail in subsequent sections.

3.1. Pathogen Recognition: Gene-for-Gene Interaction

3.1.1. Direct Evidence of Interaction of Avr/R Proteins

The gene-for-gene model states that complementary pairs of dominant genes in the plant and pathogen are required for disease resistance. One possible mechanism underlying this model is that Avr proteins are ligands for R protein receptors that initiate signal transduction cascades upon ligand binding *(61)*. Experimental evidence has suggested that this model of gene-for-gene interaction in plant disease resistance is probably correct. The first direct evidence came from two separate studies of the *P. syringae avrPto* gene and the *Pto* gene of tomato. *Agrobacterium*-mediated transient expression of *avrPto* inside tomato leaf cells induced a Pto-dependent HR *(62,63)*, and AvrPto and Pto were shown to interact in a yeast two-hybrid system *(62,63)*. A similar study was recently performed with the *AVRPita* gene from the rice blast fungus *Magnaporthe grisea* and the product of the *R* gene, *Pi-ta*, from rice *(64)*. These two proteins were shown to interact using a yeast two-hybrid system and also by using an in vitro binding assay. Although these data provided strong evidence of protein/protein interaction, they did not clearly demonstrate that Avr and R proteins interact in the plant cell.

The first demonstration of in vivo interaction between an Avr protein and an R protein came from a study of the *Arabidopsis* RPS2 and *P. syringae* AvrRpt2 proteins *(65)*. Using a transient assay in which the genes encoding the RPS2 and AvrRpt2 proteins were expressed in leaf mesophyll protoplasts, the authors demonstrated that the two proteins co-immunoprecipitated along with at least one additional plant protein of approx 75 kDa. These data are not contradictory to the guard hypothesis, in that it is possible that this other protein is a cellular target of the AvrRpt2 effector protein. This might explain why the authors found that another *P. syringae* effector protein, AvrB, immunoprecipitated with RPS2, using the same system. An alternative explanation, however, is that the 75-kDa protein is necessary for complex formation between AvrRpt2 and RPS2. Although unlikely, it is also possible that the protein is an artifact of the immunoprecipitation procedure used in the assay system. There has been no previous indication that AvrB and RPS2 interact. In fact, AvrB is believed to interact with a distinct R protein, RPM1, from *Arabidopsis*.

3.1.2. Indirect Evidence for Interaction of Avr/R Proteins

The Xa21 protein from rice contains an extracytoplasmic LRR, a single transmembrane region, and an intracellular serine/threonine kinase domain *(66)*. Xa21 confers resistance to *Xanthomonas oryzae* pv. *oryzae*, but the *avr* gene that might interact with this R protein has not yet been characterized. Xa21 is a member of the growing class of plant receptor-like kinases (RLKs) *(67)*. A recent report suggested that RLKs possessing a LRR region share a general signaling mechanism *(68)*. In this study, the extracellular LRR region and transmembrane domain of the *Arabidopsis* BR11 RLK was fused to the intracellular Ser/Thr kinase domain of Xa21. BR11 has been implicated in brassinosteroid signaling in *Arabidopsis* *(69)*. The fusion construct, transfected into rice cells, was able to elicit defense responses upon stimulation with brassinosteroids. This study indicated that RLKs are indeed receptors that can initiate signal transduction cascades and provided further evidence that R proteins act as receptor molecules.

Recent studies have provided clues as to how RLK proteins interact with their ligands and how this interaction might lead to the initiation of signaling cascades. Mutations at three loci in *Arabidopsis* (CLV1, CLV2, and CLV3) resulted in plants with enlarged shoot meristems and aberrant floral development. CLV1 encodes an LRR-RLK, similar to the *R* gene *Xa21* from rice *(70)*. CLV2 encodes a LRR-RLK similar to CLV1; however, it has only a short cytoplasmic tail *(71)*. CLV3 encodes a small, secreted polypetide that probably acts as a diffusible ligand *(72)*. CLV3 was demonstrated to co-immunoprecipitate with a CLV1/CLV2 receptor complex in vivo *(73)*. Additionally, CLV3 from plant extracts was demonstrated to bind to yeast cells expressing CLV1 and CLV2 *(73)*. Interestingly, results of this same study indicated that CLV3 was not able to bind to a kinase-inactive form of CLV1. These results were confirmed in a separate study also showing that the CLV signaling complex is controlled by CLV3 via a feedback loop mechanism *(74)*. Previous studies had indicated that CLV1 is present in two distinct protein complexes and that the larger of these complexes contains a kinase-associated protein phosphatase (KAPP) and a Rho-type GTPase, which might be involved in CLV3-dependent downstream signaling *(75)*.

Recently, a unique gene in *Arabidopsis,* FLS2, was cloned and demonstrated to be similar to the LRR-RLK class of *R* genes; it contains a membrane-spanning region *(76)*. This is quite interesting, because this gene is involved in the perception of the most conserved region of bacterial flagellin, the flg22 elicitor, indicating that this protein may be involved in the general recognition of phyotopathogenic bacteria. This is in contrast to most *R* genes identified thus far, which are believed to be specific receptors for individual effector proteins, thus providing the specificity observed in disease resistance. Biochemical analyses of the flg22 elicitor, the proposed ligand for FLS2, found that this peptide bound specifically, saturably, and with high affinity to receptor sites in membrane preparations from tomato *(77)*. At this point, however, it has not been demonstrated that this binding site in tomato corresponds to the *Arabidopsis* FLS2 protein.

3.2. Cellular Localization of Avr/R Proteins

3.2.1. Type III Secretion of Avr Proteins

As mentioned above many characterized *R* genes encode putative cytoplasmic proteins, indicating that interaction with their Avr effector ligands probably occurs intracellularly. Therefore, many pathogenic effector proteins are likely to be delivered inside the plant cell. Clearly, there is a great deal of evidence that Avr proteins are active inside the plant cell. Avr proteins can elicit an HR following expression of the *avr* gene inside the plant cell from plant transcriptional control signals (*see* ref. *78* and references therein). Further evidence comes from the recent demonstration that the AvrRpt2 effector protein is processed by a plant protease *(79,80)*.

The phenotypes of many Avr proteins have been shown to be dependent on the functional expression of the pathogen hypersensitive response and pathogenicity *(hrp)* genes, which code for proteins of the type III secretion pathway *(81)*. The type III secretion system was originally characterized in bacterial pathogens of animals, such as *Yersinia* and *Salmonella* spp. (*see* ref. 82 for a recent review), which inject pathogenic effector proteins into host cells via the type III system. Several Avr proteins are believed to be delivered to the plant cell by the type III secretion system; however, researchers are just beginning to learn about the fate of these proteins once they are inside the plant cell.

Some Avr proteins have been shown to possess eukaryotic nuclear localization-like sequences and to interact with host nuclear factors, which might affect host defense gene transcription (*83*). Several Avr proteins (e.g., AvrPto) have predicted N-terminal myristylation motifs. One study demonstrated that acylation of Avr proteins inside the plant cell mediated translocation to the plasma membrane. This translocation was also reported to enhance their functionality (*58*). Consistent with this study, Shan et al. (*56*) demonstrated that the AvrPto protein of *P. syringae* is localized to the plasma membrane of plant cells. Mutation of a putatively critical myristylation motif of AvrPto completely abolished the avirulence activity of this protein in two host plants, tomato and tobacco (*56*). These studies indicate that plant recognition of several Avr proteins likely occurs on the plasma membrane.

3.2.2. The Guard Hypothesis

The guard hypothesis was originally formulated based on the Pto-mediated defense response in tomato (*60*). In this model, R proteins have evolved to recognize complexes between Avr proteins and host virulence target proteins. As mentioned earlier, the effector protein AvrPto from *P. syringae* pv. *tomato* has been shown to interact in a yeast two-hybrid system with Pto (*62,63*). As these two proteins are both required for resistance to bacterial speck disease in tomato, following the gene-for-gene hypothesis, it is assumed that Pto is a receptor for AvrPto that mediates disease resistance. However, another protein, Prf is required for resistance to bacterial speck and for the development of an HR caused by transient expression of AvrPto (*57,84*). The predicted protein product of the *Prf* gene is an R protein of the NBS-LRR class, the class with the most members identified thus far (*84*). As this class of R proteins is so prevalent, it has been proposed that Prf might actually be a key recognition component involved in the incompatible interaction of AvrPto and Pto (*60*). It has been suggested that the virulence target of AvrPto might be Pto. Prf may have evolved to recognize a complex between AvrPto and Pto. This could explain why Prf is also necessary for the HR-like response initiated by the organophosphorous insecticide fenthion, which requires the presence of another Pto family member, the Fen kinase (*85*). That is, Prf might also recognize an activated Fen:fenthion complex. There have been reports of dual recognition specificity for other NBS-LRR proteins (*6,86,87*). The observation that an unknown protein, p75, co-immunoprecipitates with RPS2 (an LZ-NBS-LRR R protein) and AvrRpt2 in vivo, possibly forming a complex, provides further evidence that R proteins may have evolved to recognize interaction between virulence factors and their intracellular targets (*65*).

Although the guard hypothesis is an attractive molecular explanation for gene-for-gene based plant disease resistance, there is experimental evidence against this hypothesis. Resistance mediated by the Pto pathway can be activated in an effector-independent manner. Overexpression of Pto in transgenic plants provides increased, broad spectrum resistance that requires the presence of Prf (*90*). Likewise, overexpression of Prf also leads to increased resistance, yet is Pto dependent. Furthermore, transient expression of

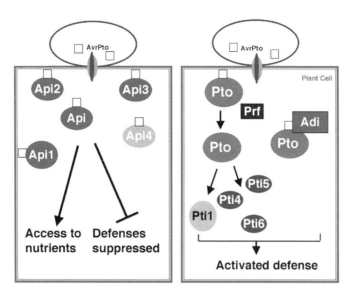

Fig. 1. Models for the virulence and avirulence activities of AvrPto. AvrPto is probably intro-duced into the plant cell via a bacterial type III secretion mechanism. If the plant possesses the R protein Pto **(right),** then AvrPto is recognized and interacts with Pto. This interaction might be part of a complex with the NBS-LRR protein Prf, which is necessary for Pto-mediated signaling events. The complex of AvrPto and Pto may also interact with additional proteins, the Adis, which may play a role in signaling. Pto is known to phosphorylate the kinase Ptil, and this phos-phorylation event might be necessary for additional signaling events downstream. Pto has also been shown to interact directly with the transcription factors Pti4/5/6, which are involved in the transcriptional activation of PR genes. AvrPto is also a known virulence factor **(left),** and has been demonstrated to interact with Api proteins, which might be targets when Pto is not present in the plant cell. Interaction of AvrPto with these proteins might inhibit plant defense responses and lead to disease development.

a constitutively active mutant, Pto (Y207D), causes an HR in the absence of AvrPto that is Prf dependent. Taken together, these data indicate that Pto and Prf can activate resistance in an AvrPto-independent manner, thus arguing that Prf does not necessarily recognize an AvrPto/Pto complex.

Another argument against the guard hypothesis is the lack of evidence that Pto is a virulence target. Clearly, AvrPto acts as a virulence factor when Pto is not present in the host plant, allowing for greater bacterial proliferation and increased disease symptoms *(57,90a).* In addition, specific mutations in AvrPto that interfere with its ability to inter-act with Pto do not affect its virulence function. Furthermore, AvrPto has been shown to interact with intracellular tomato proteins distinct from Pto *(92).* These Api proteins (AvrPto interactors) have been postulated to be virulence targets of AvrPto (Fig. 1). Additionally, yeast three-hybrid experiments using AvrPto and Pto as bait were success-ful in identifying interacting proteins, yet to date, they have failed to identify Prf as an AvrPto-dependent, Pto-interacting protein (Adi) *(91).* Although this result may be owing to the absence of a functional Prf in the library screened, it clearly demonstrates that pro-teins distinct from Prf interact with Pto in an AvrPto-dependent manner. These results suggest that AvrPto, when acting as a virulence factor, might indeed seek out specific intracellular proteins, yet it is unlikely that Pto itself is one of these pathogenicity targets.

4. SIGNAL TRANSDUCTION IN PLANT DISEASE RESISTANCE

We are just beginning to understand the signaling mechanisms involved in plant disease resistance. Even though several *R* genes and *Avr* genes have been cloned, relatively little is known about the downstream events that occur after recognition between these two partners. What is known is that reversible phosphorylation cascades probably play a critical role in defense signaling in plants. For example, two *R* genes, *Pto* and *Xa21*, encode Serine/Threonine kinase domains *(66,88)*. Additionally, one of the *R* gene classes shares a region of homology with the Toll family of receptors, such as the interleukin-1 receptor (IL-1R) from humans, and the Toll receptor from *Drosophila*, the so-called TIR domain *(1,6)*. Further evidence is emerging that phosphorylation events regulate plant defense signaling, including the characterization of kinases that are activated in an *R* gene-dependent manner *(92)*. Evidence is also emerging that *R* gene-mediated signaling cascades specifically activate transcription factors that are necessary for induction of PR genes.

4.1. Ancient Mechanism of Defense Signaling in Plants, Insects, and Mammals?

The discovery that *R* gene products share similarities with the Toll family of receptors was one of the first clues that some components of defense signaling in plants are similar to those involved in innate immunity in animals. The wealth of information about Toll-mediated signaling pathways has provided several clues about defense signaling pathways of plants.

IL-1R is a human Toll-like receptor (TLR) that is known to play a critical role in immunity and inflammation responses of mammals by initiating a signaling cascade upon binding its cognate ligand, the cytokine IL-1. One of the immediate responses to ligand binding, in this case, is the activation of the transcription factor NF-κB. Binding of IL-1 is known to stimulate recruitment of members of a protein complex. The adaptor molecule MyD88, which has been shown to be a member of this complex, binds to the receptor and interacts with the protein kinase IL-1R-associated kinase (IRAK) via a conserved "death domain," originally defined in proteins involved in apoptosis. IRAK has been demonstrated to recruit the adaptor protein TRAF-6, which subsequently interacts with NF-κB-inducing kinase (NIK), resulting in phosphorylation of I-κB kinase (IKK), an inhibitor of NF-κB. Upon phosphorylation, IKK dissociates from NF-κB, which is translocated to the nucleus, where it stimulates gene transcription. Several excellent reviews are available that elaborate further on IL-1 signaling pathways *(93–97)*.

A very similar pathway has been appreciated for some time in *Drosophila*. The Toll pathway is involved both in dorsoventral patterning and in the production of antimicrobial signals. Upon binding a proteolytically cleaved form of its ligand, Spätzle, the Toll receptor initiates a signaling cascade that requires the proteins Tube and Pelle, which are homologous to MyD88 and IRAK. Signaling from Toll results in degradation of Cactus, a *Drosophila* I-κB homolog, which is complexed with Dorsal, a transcription factor related to the Rel/NF-κB family of transcription factors. Interestingly, Tube and Pelle have been shown to be required for production of both the antifungal compound drosomycin and antibacterial toxins in response to infection *(98)*. Over 10 TLRs have currently been identified in humans, and at least 2 of the family members, TLR2 and TLR4, have been shown to mediate responses to multiple bacterial cell wall components including lipopolysaccharide (LPS) *(99–101)*.

A recently described human protein, Nod1/Card 4, which is related to the apoptosis regulator Apaf-1, shares significant homology to R proteins from plants *(102,103)*. Nod1 is similar to the most abundant class of R proteins, the NBS-LRR class *(6)*. Interestingly, signaling from Nod1 results in the induction of NF-κB activation, similar to IL-IR-dependent signaling *(96,103)*. It is possible that Nod1 and other family members are receptors for cellular pathogen components, such as LPS. Indeed, Nod1 has been shown to have LPS binding capacity and to mediate transcriptional activation of the transcription factor NF-κB by LPS *(104)*. The similarity of TLR proteins and plant *R* genes has led to the proposal that certain components of the innate immune response of plants and animals might share a common evolutionary origin *(105)*.

4.2. Phosphorylation Events Involved in Defense Signaling

Because protein phosphorylation is critical to signaling events in yeast and animal systems, it was not surprising to find that phosphorylation events play an important role in plant defense signaling. Protein phosphorylation was implicated in defense signaling in plants when researchers demonstrated that treatment of cell suspension cultures with elicitors such as oligosaccharides and chitin fragments caused rapid changes in protein phosphorylation profiles *(106–108)*. The isolation of the first *R* gene, the *Pto* gene from tomato, provided further evidence that kinases are involved in defense signaling, as Pto is a serine/threonine kinase *(88)*.

4.2.2. Tomato Pto Kinase Signaling

The signal transduction cascade controlled by Pto is an excellent model of defense signaling in plants *(109)*. Pto-controlled resistance conforms to the gene-for-gene model. That is, resistance to *P. syringae* pv. *tomato* only occurs when the plant expresses *Pto* and the bacterium expresses the corresponding *avrPto* effector gene. Moreover, Pto has been shown to activate defense responses constitutively and to confer broad resistance to a variety of pathogens when overexpressed in transgenic plants *(89)*.

As mentioned previously, AvrPto and Pto were the first Avr/R proteins demonstrated to interact directly, thus providing a molecular explanation for the gene-for-gene model of plant defense *(62,63)*. Although these two proteins have not been demonstrated to interact in vivo, there is a great deal of evidence that this interaction is critical for defense signaling in tomato. For example, the interaction that was detected in the yeast two-hybrid system strictly correlated to the activation of defense responses in the plant. Analysis of mutated forms of AvrPto indicated that the ability to interact with Pto in yeast also affected the ability of the protein, expressed transiently via *Agrobacterium*, to induce a defense response *in planta (63)*.

Domain swapping between Pto and the closely related Fen protein kinase, also from tomato, resulted in the identification of regions required for specific recognition of AvrPto *(62,63)*. Within this region, a conserved threonine residue, Thr204 was demonstrated to be required for interaction with AvrPto and for elicitation of the HR *(110)*. Additionally, introduction of this threonine residue into the Fen kinase protein conferred the ability to interact with AvrPto in yeast and to elicit an HR in plants when introduced transiently along with AvrPto *(110)*. The wild-type Fen protein is a functional ser/thr protein kinase that does not interact with AvrPto *(85,111)*. Interestingly, the *Fen* gene is one of five Pto family members that are tightly clustered on chromosome five of tomato and is required for sensitivity to the insecticide fenthion, which produces an HR-like reaction on tomato plants *(85)*. Thr204 might be a target for autophosphorylation of Pto, or phosphorylation by another kinases. Interestingly, several protein kinases related to Pto have a conserved threonine residue corresponding to Thr204, including the R protein Xa21 from rice, the RLK5 protein in *Arabidopsis,* the *Drosophila* Pelle protein, and the human IRAK *(92)*. This is significant, since Pelle and IRAK are involved in signaling downstream of the IL-1R and Toll receptors, respectively, which, as stated previously, share significant homology with a family of plant R proteins *(6,93)*.

It is very likely that physical interaction between Avr proteins and the products of some *R* genes results in the activation of downstream signaling components (Fig. 1). However, no direct evidence for this has yet been demonstrated in vivo. One possible mechanism for R protein activation is that interaction results in a conformational change in the activation domains of critical enzymatic components, such as kinases. In support of this hypothesis, there is evidence that Pto undergoes a change in conformation upon binding AvrPto. An activation domain mutant of Pto that replaced tyrosine 207 with aspartate, Y207D, was able to elicit an HR in the absence of AvrPto *(90)*. It is important to note that this "constitutive" mutant of Pto is only active when the *Prf* gene is present. As mentioned, the *Prf* gene is a member of the NBS-LRR class of cytoplasmic *R* genes and is required both for tomato resistance to *P. syringae* pv. *tomato* and for sensitivity to fenthion *(84)*.

Autophosphorylation of Pto is a likely mechanism of Pto activation. It has been clearly demonstrated that Pto autophosphorylates in vitro via an intramolecular mechanism. There is precedent for this mechanism, as the activation domain of several well-characterized ser/thr kinases is regulated by autophosphorylation *(112)*. It is possible that AvrPto binding causes a conformational change in Pto, resulting in autophosphorylation and subsequent induction of kinase activity. Interestingly, a mutation in the Pto autophosphorylation site, Ser-198, interfered with the elicitation of a HR. However interaction with AvrPto was not affected by this mutation *(113)*.

Another possibility for Pto activation via interaction with AvrPto is that the two proteins are part of a larger protein complex. This might explain why the *Prf* gene is necessary for activation of defense responses, such as development of the HR, in response to AvrPto/Pto-initiated signaling. In support of this model, the predicted protein product of *Prf* contains an LRR, which has been shown to mediate protein/protein interaction in other proteins *(84)*.

Autophosphorylation may also be required for the interaction of Pto with downstream signaling components. Indeed, Pto has been shown to interact with several tomato proteins that might be downstream targets of a signaling cascade. Yeast two-hybrid screens using Pto as bait and tomato cDNA as prey identified several interacting proteins, including Pto-interacting kinase (Pti1), and three transcription factors, Pti4, Pti5 and Pti6 *(114,115)*. Interestingly, mutation of the autophosphorylation site Ser198 also alters the interaction of Pto with Pti1 and two other proteins that remain to be functionally characterized, Pti3 and Pti10 *(113)*.

Pti1 is a functional serine/threonine protein kinase that is probably localized in the cytoplasm; however, its substrate has not been identified *(114)*. Overexpression of *Pti1* in transgenic tobacco was shown to enhance the HR in leaves inoculated with *P. syringae* pv. *tabaci* expressing the *avrPto* gene. Pti1 was demonstrated to autophosphorylate via an intramole]cular mechanism in vitro and to be a substrate for Pto phosphorylation *(113,114,116)*. A detailed biochemical analysis of Pto and Pti1 identified several serine and threonine residues of both proteins that were critical to their ability to interact in yeast *(113,116)*. However, the physiologic significance of Pti1 phosphorylation by Pto is not known, and similar studies have yet to be performed *in planta*.

4.2.3. Kinases Downstream of R Proteins

In vivo phosphorylation experiments and studies using specific substrates and enzymatic inhibitors have demonstrated that protein kinases and phosphatase are critical for activation of plant defense responses *(1)*. For example, mitogen-activated protein kinases (MAPKs) have been shown to be involved in plant defense signaling *(92)*. MAPKs in mammalian systems and yeast are critical components of signal transduction cascades triggered by extracellular ligands *(117,118)*. Several MAPKs have been found in plants that are activated in response to pathogen inoculation and wounding *(92,119–121)*. One of the kinases that is activated by wounding is the wound-induced protein kinase WIPK *(122)*. Initially found to be both transcriptionally and posttranscriptionally activated in response to wounding, the WIPK MAPK was recently shown to be activated by resistance gene-mediated pathways *(120)*. The kinase activity of WIPK was induced by tobacco mosaic virus infection and was dependent on the tobacco *R* gene *N*. Furthermore, increases in WIPK activity were demonstrated in tobacco plants expressing the tomato *Cf-9 R* gene when the plants were inoculated with *Cladosporium fulvum* strains expressing the *avr9* gene *(123)*. The *Cf-9 R* gene confers on tomato resistance to strains of *C. fulvum* expressing the *avr9* gene *(6)*. Another MAPK that has been associated with defense response is the tobacco salicylic acid-induced protein kinase (SIPK) *(124)*. SIPK has been shown to be activated by both SA treatment and in response to a variety of biotic and abiotic stresses. Similar to WIPK, SIPK activity is activated by tobacco mosaic virus infection in an *N*-gene dependent manner and also by Avr9 in a *Cf-9*-dependent manner *(121,123,124)*. However, in the case of SIPK, no increase in mRNA or protein levels was detected, as was the case for WIPK. The fact that both of these MAPKs were activated by a wide variety of inducers suggests that these proteins might represent a connection point between defense signaling pathways initiated from different *R* genes.

A phenotype was recently described for a MAPK in *Arabidopsis* that was inactivated by transposon mutagenesis *(125)*. The mutant line containing the transposon-inactivated form of MAPK MPK4, exhibited constitutive SAR elevated levels of SA, as well as enhanced disease resistance to pathogens. Microarray analysis of genes expressed in either wild-type seedlings or seedlings of the *mpk4* mutant line indicated that PR genes are constitutively expressed in the *mpk4* mutant.

The enhanced disease resistance *(edr1)* mutation confers resistance to powdery mildew caused by the fungus *Erysiphe cichoracearum*. The *EDR1* gene of *Arabidopsis* was recently identified by positional cloning and was found to encode a putative

MAPK kinase *(126)*. EDR1 shares a high degree of sequence similarity with the *CTR1* protein which is involved in the negative regulation of ethylene responses in *Arabidopsis*. The phenotype of the mutation indicates that EDR1 negatively regulates defense responses. This is a surprising finding, because several other MAPKs are activated by plant defense responses, as mentioned above.

Romeis et al. *(127)* reported the identification of a calcium-dependent protein kinase (CDPK), one of a class of serine/threonine kinases that are unique to plants (and some protists); this CDPK is specifically activated by interaction of the Avr9 protein from *C. fulvum* with the Cf-9 R protein from tomato. In addition, the phosphorylation-dependent activation of the CDPK was accompanied by an increase in enzymatic activity. CDPKs are believed to be analogous to protein kinase C isomers characterized in animal systems. Interestingly, protein kinase C activity is required for induction of the defense-activated oxidative burst in macrophages *(128)*.

4.4. Transcriptional Activation of PR Genes

One of the major changes associated with *R* gene-mediated plant defense responses is transcriptional activation of PR proteins. Even though *PR* genes are believed to play critical roles in plant defense, relatively little is known about their transcriptional regulation. One mechanism by which these genes might be activated is the specific regulation of transcription factors such as Pti4, Pti5, and Pti6 (Fig. 1). The tomato Pti4/5/6 genes were originally isolated as proteins that interacted with Pto in a yeast two-hybrid screen *(115)*. Using gel shift assays, Pti4/5/6 were shown to bind to a *cis*-acting element required for ethylene responsiveness that is present in promoters of *PR* genes: the GCC box *(115,129)*. In addition, mRNA transcript levels of *Pti4* and *Pti5* increased in response to inoculation of tomato by the pathogen *P. syringae (130)*. Interestingly, gel shift analysis indicated that Pti4 binding to a GCC box element was enhanced by phosphorylation of Pti4 by Pto *(129)*. These data suggest that Pto might directly activate these transcription factors via phosphorylation; however, it is not presently clear what role phosphorylation of Pti4/5/6 might play.

The NPR1, or NIM1, protein of *Arabidopsis* is known to play a critical role in SAR *(37)*. The NPR1 protein has been demonstrated to be necessary for the transcriptional activation of PR proteins such as PR-1, via SA-mediated signaling pathways. The NPR1 protein shares a sequence with I-κB, a mammalian transcriptional regulator, and possesses an ankyrin-like repeat domain known to mediate protein-protein interaction *(39)*. I-κB negatively regulates the major target of IL-1R signaling, the transcription factor NF-κB *(96)*. In three separate yeast two-hybrid screens, NPR1 was shown to interact with members of the TGA family of transcription factors in *Arabidopsis (131–133)*. TGA proteins are members of the basic region/leucine zipper (bZIP) family of transcription factors and are known to recognize promoter elements of *PR* genes. At least one of these genes, *PR-1*, is thought to be involved in the SA response pathway leading to SAR. Each of the three studies showed that NPR1 was able to enhance the ability of TGA factors to bind to promoter elements present in *PR* genes. The results of these studies suggest that NPR1 is directly involved in the transcriptional activation of SA-induced PR proteins via interaction with TGA transcription factors. It is not clear whether NPR1 negatively regulates TGA factors via a mechanism analogous to mammalian I-κB, as has been proposed *(132)*. On the contrary, most of the data on NPR1 action suggest that it positively regulates defense responses.

5. FUTURE DIRECTIONS

Research during the past decade has provided an incredible amount of information about how plants recognize pathogens and respond to attack. The cloning and characterization of *R* genes and pathogen effectors have provided a molecular model for gene-for-gene based resistance in plants. This information can now be used in new research that is sure to lead to a greater understanding of the initial events involved in pathogen recognition. This will require intensive studies of the structure of both plant R proteins and pathogen effectors, as well as analysis of complexes that form between these proteins. In addition, a greater emphasis on cell biology will be needed to elucidate the localization of plant and pathogen proteins, as well as basic biochemical analyses to determine the factors effecting R-protein activation. We are just beginning to understand the signaling events that occur downstream of R proteins. A better understanding of these events will require forward and reverse genetics to define new gene loci: cell biology, biochemistry, and proteomics technologies including yeast two-hybrid systems to learn more about how the signaling components work. Additionally, the mechanisms of plant defense responses and their relative importance need to be addressed in greater detail. This information will probably come from newly emerging gene expression profiling technologies such as microarray analysis and functional genomics technologies including gene silencing and mutational studies.

REFERENCES

1. Martin GB. Functional analysis of plant disease resistance genes and their downstream effectors. Curr Opin Plant Biol 1999;2:273–279.
2. Benhamou N. Elicitor-induced plant defence pathways. Trends Plant Sci 1996;1:233–240.
3. Hammond-Kosack KE, Jones JDG. Resistance gene-dependent plant defense responses. Plant Cell 1996;8:1773–1791.
4. Flor H. Current status of the gene-for-gene concept. Annu Rev Phytopathol 1971;9:275–296.
5. Dangl JL, Dietrich RA, Richberg MH. Death don't have no mercy: cell death programs in plant-microbe interactions. Plant Cell 1996;8:1793–1807.
6. Hammond-Kosack K, Jones JDG. Plant disease resistance genes. Annu Rev Plant Physiol Plant Mol Biol 1997;48:575–607.
7. Lamb C, Dixon RA. The oxidative burst in plant disease resistance. Annu Rev Plant Physiol Plant Mol Biol 1997;48:251–275.
8. Yang Y, Shah J, Klessig DF. Signal perception and transduction in plant defense responses. Genes Dev 1997;11:1621–1639.
9. Fritig B, Heitz T, Legrand M. Antimicrobial proteins in induced plant defense. Curr Opin Immunol 1998;10:16–22.
10. Ryals JA, Neuenschwander HU, Willits MG, et al. Systemic acquired resistance. Plant Cell 1996;8:1809–1819.
11. Dong X. SA, JA, ethylene, and disease resistance in plants. Curr Opin Plant Biol 1998;1:316–323.
12. Durner J, Klessig DF. Nitric oxide as a signal in plants. Curr Opin Plant Biol 1999;2:369–374.
13. Bolwell GP. Role of active oxygen species and NO in plant defence responses. Curr Opin Plant Biol 2000;2:287–294.

14. Bradley D, Kjellbom P, Lamb CJ. Elicitor- and wound-induced oxidative cross-linking of a pro-line-rich plant cell wall protein: a novel, rapid defense response. Cell 1992;70:21–30.

15. Levine A, Tenhaken R, Dixon RA, Lamb CJ. H_2O_2 from the oxidative burst orchestrates the plant hypersensitive response. Cell 1994;79:583–593.

16. Chamnongpol S, Willekens H, Moeder W, et al. Defense activation and enhanced pathogen tolerance induced by H_2O_2 in transgenic tobacco. Proc Natl Acad Sci USA 1998;95: 5818–5823.

17. Orozco-Cárdenas ML, Narváez-Vásquez J, Ryan CA. Hydrogen peroxide acts as a second messenger for the induction of defense genes in tomato plants in response to wounding, systemin, and methyl jasmonate. Plant Cell 2001;13:179–191.

18. Dwyer SC, Legender L, Heinstein PF, Low PS, Leto TL. Plant and humann neutrophil oxidative burst complexes contain immunologically related proteins. Biochim Biophys Acta 1996;1289:231–237.

19. Groom QJ, Torres MA, Fordham-Skelton AP, et al. *rbohA,* a rice homologue of the mammalian gp91phox respiratory burst oxidase gene. Plant J 1996;10:515–522.

20. Keller T, Damude HG, Werner D, et al. A plant homolog of the neutrophil NADPH oxidase gp91phox subunit gene encodes a plasma membrane protein with Ca^{2+} binding motifs. Plant Cell 1998;10:255–266.

21. Kawasaki T, Henmi K, Ono E, et al. The small GTP-binding protein rac is a regulator of cell death in plants. Proc Natl Acad Sci USA 1999;96:10922–10926.

22. Alvarez ME, Pennell RI, Meijer P-J. Reactive oxygen intermediates mediate a systemic signal network in the establishment of plant immunity. Cell 1998;92:773–784.

23. Piedras P, Hammond-Kossak KE, Harrison K, Jones JDG. A rapid Cf-9 and Avr9-dependent production of active oxygen species in tobacco suspension cultures. Mol Plant Microbe Interact 1998;11:1155–1166.

24. Orozco-Cárdenas ML, Ryan CA. Hydrogen peroxide is generated systemically in plant leaves by wounding and systemin via the octadecanoid pathway. Proc Natl Acad Sci USA 1999;96:6553–6557.

25. Niderman T, Genetet I, Bruyere T, et al. Pathogenesis-related PR-1 proteins are antifungal. Plant Physiol 1995;108:17–27.

26. Abad LR, D'Urzo MP, Liu D, et al. Antifungal activity of tobacco osmotin has specificity and involves plasma membrane permeabilization. Plant Sci 1996;118:11–23.

27. Hahn MG. Microbial elicitors and their receptors in plants. Annu Rev Phytopathol 1996;34:387–412.

28. Broekaert WF, Terras FRG, Cammue BPA, Osborn RW. Plant defensins: novel antimicrobial peptides as components of the host defense system. Plant Physiol 1995;108:1353–1358.

29. Glazebrook J, Zook M, Mert F, et al. Phytoalexin-deficient mutants of *Arabidopsis* reveal that PAD4 encodes a regulatory factor and that four PAD genes contribute to downy mildew resistance. Genetics 1997;146:381–392.

30. Brunner F, Stintzi A, Fritig B, Legrand M. Substrate specificities of tobacco chitinases. Plant J 1998;14:225–234.

31. Dempsey D, Shah J, Klessig DF. Salicylic acid and disease resistance in plants. Crit Rev Plant Sci 1999;18:547–575.

32. Gaffney T, Friedrich L, Vernooij B, et al. Requirement of salicylic acid for the induction of systemic acquired resistance. Science 1993;261:754–756.

33. Delaney TP, Uknes S, Vernooij B, et al. A central role of salicylic acid in plant disease resistance. Science 1994;266:1247–1250.

34. Lawton K, Weymann K, Fridrich L, et al. Systemic acquired resistance in *Arabidopsis* requires salicylic acid but not ethylene. Mol Plant Microbe Interact 1995;8:863–870.

35. Ward ER, Uknes SJ, Williams SC, et al. Coordinate gene activity in response to agents that induce systemic acquired resistance. Plant Cell 1991;3:1085–1094.

36. Malamy J, Klessig DF. Salicylic acid and plant disease resistance. Plant J 1992;2:643–654.

37. Cao H, Bowling S, Gordon A, Dong X. Characterization of an *Arabidopsis* mutant that is nonresponsive to inducers of systemic acquired resistance. Plant Cell 1994;6:1583–1592.

38. Delaney TP, Friedrich L, Ryals JA. *Arabidopsis* signal transduction mutant defective in chemically and biologically induced disease resistance. Proc Natl Acad Sci USA 1995;92:6602–6606.

39. Cao H, Glazebrook J, Clarke JD, Volko S, Dong X. The *Arabidopsis* NPR1 gene that controls systemic acquired resistance encodes a novel protein containing ankyrin repeats. Cell 1997;88:57–63.

40. Pearce G, Strydom D, Johnson S, Ryan C. A polypeptide from tomato leaves induces wound-inducible proteinase inhibitor proteins. Science 1991;25:895–898.

41. Farmer EE, Ryan CA. Octadecanoid precursors of jasmonic acid activate the synthesis of would-inducible proteinase inhibitors. Plant Cell 1992;4:129–134.

42. O'Donnell PJ, Calvert G, Atzorn R, et al. Ethylene as a signal mediating the wound response of tomato plants. Science 1996;274:1914–1917.

43. Schenk PM, Kazan K, Wilson I, et al. Coordinated plant defense responses in *Arabidopsis* revealed by microarray analysis. Proc Natl Acad Sci USA 2000;97:11655–11660.

44. Doares SH, Narvaez-Vasquez J, Conconi A, Ryan CA. Salicylic acid inhibits synthesis of proteinase inhibitors in tomato leaves induced by systemin and jasmonic acid. Plant Physiol 1995;108:1741–1746.

45. Maleck K, Levine A, Eulgem T, et al. The transcriptome of *Arabidopsis thaliana* during systemic acquired resistance. Nat Genets 2000;26:403–410.

46. Durner J, Wendehenne D, Klessig DF. Defense gene induction in tobacco by nitric oxide, cyclic GMP and cyclic ADP-ribose. Proc Natl Acad Sci USA 1998;95:10328–10333.

47. Delledonne M, Xia Y, Dixon RA, Lamb C. Nitric oxide signal functions in plant disease resistance. Nature 1998;394:585–588.

48. Vernooji B, Friedrich L, Morse A, et al. Salicylic acid is not the translocated signal responsible for inducing systemic acquired resistance but is required in signal transduction. Plant Cell 1994;959–965.

49. Xiao S, Ellwood S, Calis O, et al. Broad-spectrum mildew resistance in *Arabidopsis thaliana* mediated by RPW8. Science 2001;291:118–120.

50. Buschges R, Hollricher K, Panstruga R, et al. The barley Mlo gene: a novel control element of plant pathogen resistance. Cell 1997;88:695–705.

51. Devoto A, Piffanelli P, Nilsson I, et al. *Schulze-Lefert, P.* Topology, subcellular localization, and sequence diversity of the Mlo family in plants. J Biol Chem 1999;274:34993–35004.

52. Wolter M, Hollricher K, Salamini F, Schulze-Lefert P. The *mlo* resistance to powdery mildew infection in barley triggers a developmentally controlled defence mimic phenotype. Mol Gen Genet 1993;239:122–128.

53. Kearney B, Staskawicz BJ. Widespread distribution and fitness contribution of *Xanthomonas campestris* avirulence gene *avrBs2*. Nature 1990;346:385–386.

54. Lorang JM, Shen H, Kobayashi D, Cooksey D, Keen NT. *avrA* and *avrE* in *Pseudomonas syringae* pv. *tomato* PT23 play a role in virulence on tomato plants. Mol Plant Microbe Interact 1994;7:508–515.

55. Ritter C, Dangl JL. The *avrRpm1* gene of *Pseudomonas syringae* pv. *maculicola* is required for virulence on *Arabidopsis*. Mol Plant Microbe Interact 1995;8:444–453.

56. Shan L, Thara VK, Martin GB, Zhou JM, Tang X. The *Pseudomonas* AvrPto protein is differentially recognized by tomato and tobacco and is localized to the plant plasma membrane. Plant Cell 2000;12:2323–2328.

57. Chang JH, Rathjen JP, Bernal AJ, Staskawicz BJ, Michelmore RW. avrPto enhances growth and necrosis caused by *Pseudomonas syringae* pv. *tomato* in tomato lines lacking Pto or Prf. Mol Plant Microbe Interact 2000;13:568–571.

58. Nimchuk Z, Marois E, Kjemtrup S, et al. Eukaryotic fatty acylation drives plasma membrane targeting and enhances function of several type III effector proteins from *Pseudomonas syringae*. Cell 2000;101:353–363.

59. Chen ZK, AP, Boch J, Katagiri F, Kunkel BN. The *Pseudomonas syringae avrRpt2* gene product promotes pathogen virulence from inside the plant cells. Mol Plant Microbe Interact 2000;13:1312–1321.

60. Van der Biezen EA, Jones JD. Plant disease-resistance proteins and the gene-for-gene concept. Trends Biochem Sci 1998;23:454–456.

61. Gabriel DW, Rolfe BG. Working models of specific recognition in plant-microbe interactions. Annul Rev Phytopathol 1990;28:365–391.

62. Scofield SR, Tobias CM, Rathjen JP, et al. Molecular basis of gene-for-gene specificity in bacterial speck disease of tomato. Science 1996;274:2063–2065.

63. Tang X, Frederick RD, Zhou J, et al. Initiation of plant disease resistance by physical interaction of AvrPto and Pto kinase. Science 1996;274:2060–2063.

64. Jia Y, McAdams SA, Brya GT, Hershey HP, Valent B. Direct interaction of resistance gene and avirulence gene products confers rice blast resistance. EMBO J. 2000;19:4004–4014.

65. Leister RT, Katagiri F. A resistance gene product of the nucleotide binding site-leucine rich repeats class can form a complex with bacterial avirulence proteins *in vivo*. Plant J 2000;22:345–354.

66. Song W-Y, Wang G-L, Chen L-L, et al. A receptor kinase-like protein encoded by the rice disease resistance gene, *Xa21*. Science 1995;270:1804–1806.

67. Lease K, Inhgam E, Walker JC. Challenges in understanding RLK function. Curr Opin Plant Biol 1998;1:388–392.

68. He Z, Wang Z-Y, Li J, et al. Perception of brassinosteroids by the extracellular domain of the receptor kinase BRl1. Science 2000;288:2360–2363.

69. Li J, Chory J. A putative leucine-rich repeat receptor kinase involved in brassinosteroid signal transduction. Cell 1997;90:929–938.

70. Clark SE, Williams RW, Meyerowitz EM. The CLAVATA1 gene encodes a putative receptor kinase that controls shoot and floral meristem size in *Arabidopsis*. Cell 1997;89:575–585.

71. Jeong S, Trotochaud A, Clark S. The *Arabidopsis* CLAVATA2 gene encodes a receptor-like protein required for the stability of the CLAVATA1 receptor-like kinase. Plant Cell 1999;11:925–1933.

72. Fletcher JC, Brand U, Running MP, Simon R, Meyerowitz EM. Signaling of cell fate decisions by CLAVATA3 in *Arabidopsis* shoot meristems. Science 1999;283:1911–1914.

73. Trotochaud AE, Jeong S, Clark SE. CLAVATA3, a multimeric ligand for the CLAVATA1 receptor-kinase. Science 2000;289:613–617.

74. Brand U, Fletcher JC, Hobe M, Meyerowitz EM, Simon R. Dependence of stem cell fate in *Arabidopsis* on a feedback loop regulated by CLV3 activity. Science 2000;289:617–619.

75. Trotochaud AE, Hao T, Wui G, Yang Z, Clark SE. The CLAVATA1 receptor-like kinase requires CLAVATA3 for its assembly into a signaling complex that includes KAPP and a Rho-related protein. Plant Cell 1999;11:393–406.

76. Gómez-Gómez L, Boller T. FLS2: an LRR receptor-like kinase involved in the perception of the bacterial elicitor flagellin in *Arabidopsis*. Mol Cell 2000;5:1003–1011.

77. Meindl T, Boller T, Felix G. The bacterial elicitor flagellin activates its receptor in tomato cells according to the address-message concept. Plant Cell 2000;12:1783–1794.

78. Mudgett MB, Staskawicz BJ. Protein signaling via type III secretion pathways in phytopathogenic bacteria. Curr Opin Microbiol 1998;1:109–114.

79. McNellis TW, Mudgett MB, Li K, et al. Glucocorticoid-inducible expression of a bacterial avirulence gene in transgenic *Arabidopsis* induces hypersensitive cell death. Plant J 1998;14:247–257.

80. Mudgett MB, Staskawicz BJ. Characterization of the *Pseudomonas syringae* pv. *tomato* Avr-Rpt2 protein: demonstration of secretion and processing during bacterial pathogenesis. Mol Microbiol 1999;32:927–941.

81. Alfano JR, Collmer A. The type III (Hrp) secretion pathway of plant pathogenic bacteria: trafficking harpins, Avr proteins, and death. J. Bacteriol. 1997;179:5655–5662.

82. Galan JE, Collmer A. Type III secretion machines: bacterial devices for protein delivery into host cells. Science 1999;284:1322–1328.

83. Zhu W, Yang B, Kurata N, Johnson LB, White FF. The C terminus of AvrXa10 can be replaced by the transcriptional activation domain of VP16 from the herpes simplex virus. Plant Cell 1999;11:1665–1674.

84. Salmeron JM, Oldroyd GED, Rommens CMT, et al. Tomato *Prf* is a member of the leucine-rich repeat class of plant disease resistance genes and lies embedded within the *Pto* kinase gene cluster. Cell 1996;86:123–133.

85. Martin GB, Frary A, Wu T, et al. A member of the tomato Pto gene family confers sensitivity to fenthion resulting in rapid cell death. Plant Cell 1994;6:1543–1552.

86. Rossi M, Goggin FL, Milligan SB, et al. The nematode resistance gene *Mi* of tomato confers resistance against the potato aphid. Proc Natl Acad Sci USA 1998;95:9750–9754.

87. Milligan SB, Bodeau J, Yaghoobi J, et al. The root knot nematode resistance gene *Mi* from tomato is a member of the leucine zipper, nucleotide binding, leucine-rich repeat family of plant genes. Plant Cell 1998;10:1307–1319.

88. Martin GB, Brommonschenkel S, Chunwongse J, et al. Map-based cloning of a protein kinase gene conferring disease resistance in tomato. Science 1993;262:1432–1436.

89. Tang X, Xie M, Kim JJ, et al. Overexpression of *Pto* activates defense responses and confers broad resistance. Plant Cell 1999;11:15–29.

90. Rathjen JP, Chang JH, Staskawicz BJ, Michelmore RW. Constitutively active Pto induces a Prf-dependent hypersensitive response in the absence of AvrPto. EMBO J 1999;18:3232–3240.

90a. Shan L, He P, Zhou JM, Tang X. A cluster of mutations disrupt the avirulence but not the virulence function of AvrPto. Mol Plant Microbe Interact 2000;13:592–598.

91. Bogdanove AJ, Martin GB. AvrPto-dependent Pto-interacting proteins and AvrPto-interacting proteins in tomato. Proc Natl Acad Sci USA 2000;97:8836–8840.

92. Sessa G, Martin GB. Protein kinases in the plant defense response. In: Kreis M, Walker JC (ed.) Advances in Botanical Research (incorporating Advances in Plant Pathology), vol. 32. London: Academic Press, 2000, pp. 379–398.

93. Aderem A, Ulevitch RJ. Toll-like receptors in the induction of the innate immune response. Nature 2000;406:782–787.

94. Bowie A, O'Neill LA. The interleukin-1 receptor/Toll-like receptor superfamily: signal generators for pro-inflamatory interleukins and microbial products. J Leukoc Biol 2000;67:508–514.

95. Medzhitov R, Janeway C. Innate immunity. N Engl J Med 2000;343:338–344.

96. Hatada EN, Krappmann D, Scheidereit C. NF-κB and the innate immune response. Curr Opin Immunol 2000;12:52–58.

97. Hoffmann JA, Kafatos FC, Janeway CA, Ezekowitz RAB. Phylogenetic perspectives in innate immunity. Science 1999;284:1313–1318.

98. Williams MJ, Rodriguez A, Kimbrell DA, Eldon ED. The 18-wheeler mutation reveals complex antibacterial gene regulation in *Drosophila* host defense. EMBO J 1997;16:6120–6130.

99. Yang RB, Mark MR, Gray A, et al. Toll-like receptor-2 mediates lipopolysaccharide-induced cellular signalling. Nature 1998;395:284–288.

100. Poltorak A, He X, Smironova I, et al. Defective LPS signaling in C3H/HeJ and C57BL/10ScCr mice: mutations in Tlr4 gene. Science 1998;282:2085–2088.

101. Aliprantis AO, Yang RB, Mark MR, et al. Cell activation and apoptosis by bacterial lipoproteins through toll-like receptor-2. Science 1999;285:738–739.

102. Zou H, Henzel WJ, Liu X, Lutschg A, Wang X. Apaf-1, a human protein homologous to *C. elegans* CED-4, participates in cytochrome c-dependent activation of caspase-3. Cell 1997;20:405–413.

103. Inohara N, Koseki T, del Peso L, et al. Nodq, and Apaf-1-like activator of Caspase-9 and nuclear factor kappa B. J Biol Chem 1999;274:14560–14567.

104. Inohara N, Ogura Y, Chen FF, Muto A, Nunez. Human Nod1 confers responsiveness to bacterial lipopolysaccharides. J Biol Chem 2001;276:2551–2554.

105. Cohn J, Sessa G, and Martin GB. Innate immunity in plants. Curr Opin Immunol 2001;13:55–62.

106. Grab D, Feger M, Ebel J. An endogenous factor from soybean (*Glycine max* L.) cell cultures activates phosphorylation of a protein which is dephosphorylated in vivo in elicitor-challenged cells. Planta 1989;179:340–348.

107. Dietrich A, Mayer JE, Hahlbrock K. Fungal elicitor triggers rapid, transient, and specific protein phosphorylation in parsley cell suspension cultures. J Biol Chem 1990;265:6360–6368.

108. Felix G, Grosskopf DG, Regenass M, Boller T. Rapid changes of protein phosphorylation are involved in transduction of the elicitor signal in plant cells. Proc Natl Acad Sci USA 1991;88:8831–8834.

109. Sessa G, Martin GB. Signal recognition and transduction mediated by the tomato Pto kinase: a paradigm of innate immunity in plants. Microbes Infect 2000;2:1591–1597.

110. Frederick RD, Thilmony RL, Sessa G, Martin GB. Recognition specificity for the bacterial avirulence protein AvrPto is determined by Thr-204 in the activation loop of the tomato Pto kinase. Mol Cell 1998;2:241–245.

111. Loh Y-T, Martin GB. The *Pto* bacterial resistance gene and the *Fen* insecticide sensitivity gene encode functional protein kinases with serine/threonine specificity. Plant Physiol 1995;108:1735–1739.

112. Johnson LN, Noble MEM, Owen DJ. Active and inactive protein kinases: structural basis for regulation. Cell 1996;85:149–158.

113. Sessa G, D'Ascenzo M, Martin GB. Thr-38 and Ser-198 are Pto autophosphorylation sites required for the AvrPto-Pto mediated hypersensitive response. EMBO J 2000;19:2257–2269.

114. Zhou J, Loh Y-T, Bressan RA, Martin GB. The tomato gene *Pti1* encodes a serine/threonine kinase that is phophorylated by Pto and is involved in the plant hypersensitive response. Cell 1995;83:925–935.

115. Zhou J, Tang X, Martin GB. The Pto kinase confering resistance to tomato bacterial speck disease interacts with proteins that bind a *cis*-element of pathogenesis-related genes. EMBO J 1997;16:3207–3218.

116. Sessa G, D'Ascenzo M, Loh Y-T, Martin GB. Biochemical properties of two protein kinases involved in disease resistance signaling in tomato. J Biol Chem 1998;273:15860–15865.

117. Herskowitz I. MAP kinase pathways in yeast: for mating and more. Cell 1995;80:187–197.

118. Seger R, Krebs EG. The MAPK signaling cascade. FASEB J 1995;9:726–735.

119. Ligterink W, Kroj T, zur Nieden U, Hirt H, Scheel D. Receptor-mediated activation of a MAP kinase in pathogen defense of plants. Science 1997;276:2054–2057.

120. Zhang S, Klessig DF. N resistance gene-mediated de novo synthesis and activation of a tobacco MAP kinase by TMV infection. Proc Natl Acad Sci USA 1998;95:7433–7438.

121. Zhang S, Du H, Klessig DF. Activation of the tobacco SIP kinase by both a cell wall-derived carbohydrate elicitor and purified proteinaceous elicitins from *Phytophthora* spp. The Plant Cell 1998;10:435–449.

122. Seo S, Okamoto M, Seto H, et al. Tobacco MAP kinase: a possible mediator in wound signal transduction pathways. Science 1995;270:1988–1992.

123. Romeis T, Piedras P, Zhang S, et al. Rapid *avr 9-* and *Cf-9*-dependent activation of MAP kinases in tobacco cell cultures and leaves: convergence of resistance gene, elicitor, wound, and salicylate responses. Plant Cell 1999;11:273–288.

124. Zhang S, Klessig DF. Salycylic acid activates a 48-kD kinase in tobacco. Plant Cell 1997;9:809–824.

125. Petersen M, Brodersen P, Naested H, et al. *Arabidopsis* MAP kinase 4 negatively regulates systemic acquired resistance. Cell 2000;103:1111–1120.

126. Frye CA, Tang D, Innes RW. Negative regulation of defense reponses in plants by a conserved MAPKK kinase. Proc Natl Acad Sci USA 2001;98:373–378.

127. Romeis T, Piedras P, Jones JDG. Resistance gene-dependent activation of a calcium-dependent protein kinase in the plant defense response. Plant Cell 2000;12:803–815.

128. Perkins RS, Lidsay MA, Barnes PJ, Giembycz MA. Early signaling events implicated in leukotriene B4-induced activation of the NADPH oxidase in eosinophils: role of Ca^{2+}, protein kinase C and phopholipases C and D. Biochem J 1995;310:795–806.

129. Gu Y-QY, Thara VK, Zhou J, Martin GB. The *Pti4* gene is regulated by ethylene and salicylic acid and its product is phophorylated by the Pto kinase. Plant Cell 2000;12:771–785.

130. Thara VK, Tang X, Gu YQ, Martin GB, Zhou J-M. *Pseudomonas syringae* pv. *tomato* induces the expression of tomato EREBP-like genes *Pti4* and *Pti5* independent of ethylene, salicylate, and jasmonate. Plant J 1999;20:475–483.

131. Zhang Y, Fan W, Kinkema M, Li X, and Dong X. Interaction of NPR1 with basic leucine zipper protein transcription factors that bind sequences required for salicylic acid induction of the *PR-1* gene. Proc Natl Acad Sci USA 1999;96:6523–6528.

132. Despres C, DeLong C, Glaze S, Liu E, Fobert PR. The *Arabidopsis* NPR1/NIM1 protein enhances the DNA binding activity of a subgroup of the TGA family of bZIP transcription factors. Plant Cell 2000;12:279–290.

133. Zhou J-M, Trifa Y, Silva H, et al. NPR1 differentially interacts with members of the TGA/OBF family of transcription factors that bind an element of the *PR-1* gene required for induction by salicylic acid. Mol Plant Microbe Interact 2000;13:191–202.

134. Ori N, Tanksley SD, Zamir D, et al. The 12C family from the wilt disease resistance locus 12 belongs to the nucleotide binding leucine-rich repeat superfamily of plant resistance genes. Plant Cell 1997;9:521–532.

135. Simons G, Groenendijk J, Wijbrandi J, et al. Dissection of the fusarium 12 gene cluster in tomato reveals six homologs and one active gene copy. Plant Cell 1998;10:1055–1068.

136. Collins N, Drake J, Ayliffe M, et al. Molecular characterization of the maize Rp1-D rust resistance haplotype and its mutants. Plant Cell 1999;11:1365–1376.

137. Yoshimura S, Yamanouchi U, Katayose Y, et al. Expression of Xa1, a bacterial blight-resistance gene in rice, is induced by bacterial inoculation. Proc Natl Acad Sci USA 1998;95:1663–1668.

138. Bent AF, Kunkel BN, Dahlbeck DJ, et al. *RPS2* of *Arabidopsis thaliana:* a leucine-rich repeat class of plant disease resistance genes. Science 1994;265:1856–1860.

139. Warren RF, Henk A, Mowery P, Holub E, Innes RW. A mutation within the leucine-rich repeat domain of the *Arabidopsis* disease resistance gene RPS5 partially suppresses multiple bacterial and downy mildew resistance genes. Plant Cell 1998;10:1439–1452.

140. Grant MR, Godiar L, Straube E, et al. Structure of the *Arabidopsis RPM1* gene enabling dual specificity disease resistance. Science 1995;269:843–846.

141. McDowell JM, Dhandaydham M, Long TA, et al. Intragenic recombination and diversifying selection contribute to the evolution of downy mildew resistance at the RPP8 locus of *Arabidopsis.* Plant Cell 1998;10:1861–1874.

142. Cooley MB, Pathirana S, Wu HJ, Kachroo P, Klessig DF. Members of the *Arabidopsis* HRT/RPP8 family of resistance genes confer resistance to both viral and oomycete pathogens. Plant Cell 2000;12:663–676.

143. Bendahamane A, Kanyuka K, Baulcombe DC. The *Rx* gene from potato controls separate virus resistance and cell death responses. Plant Cell 1999;11:781–791.

144. van der Vossen EA, van der Voort JN, Kanyuka K, et al. Homologues of a single resistance-gene cluster in potato confer resistance to distinct pathogens: a virus and a nematode. Plant J 2000;23:567–576.

145. Whitham S, Dinesh-Kumar SP, Choi D, et al. The product of the tobacco mosaic virus resistance gene *N:* similarity to Toll and the interleukin-1 receptor. Cell 1994;78:1011–1015.

146. Lawrence GJ, Ellis JG, Finnegan EJ. Cloning a rust-resistance gene in flax. In: 7th ISMPM I—Advances in Molecular Genetics of Plant-Microbe Interactions, vol III, 1995.

147. Anderson PA, Lawrence GJ, Ellis JG, et al. Inactivation of the flax rust resistance gene M associated with loss of a repeated unit within the leucine-rich repeat coding region. Plant Cell 1997;9:641–651.

148. Gassmann W, Hinsch ME, Staskawicz BJ. The *Arabidopsis* RPS4 bacterial-resistance gene is a member of the TIR-NBS-LRR family of disease-resistance genes. Plant J 1999;20:265–277.

149. Parker JE, Coleman MJ, Dean C, et al. The *Arabidopsis* downy mildew resistance gene RPP5 shares similarity to the Toll and interleukin-1 receptors with N and L6. Plant Cell 1997;9:879–894.

150. Botella MA, Parker JE, Frost LN, et al. Three genes of the *Arabidopsis* RPP1 complex resistance locus recognize distinct *Peronospora parasitica* avirulence determinants. Plant Cell 1998;10:1847–1860.

151. Dixon MS, Jones DA, Keddie JS, et al. The tomato Cf-2 disease resistance locus comprises two functional genes encoding leucine-rich repeat proteins. Cell 1996;84:451–459.

152. Thomas CM, Jones DA, Parniske M, et al. Characterisation of the tomato Cf-4 gene for resistance to *Cladosporium fulvum* identifies sequences which determine recognitional specificity in Cf-4 and Cf-9. Plant Cell 1997;9:1–17.

153. Dixon MS, Hatzixanthis K, Jones DA, Harrison K, Jones JD. The tomato Cf-5 disease resistance gene and six homologs show pronounced allelic variation in leucine-rich repeat copy number. Plant Cell 1998;10:1915–1925.

154. Jones DA, Thomas CM, Hammond-Kosack KE, Balint-Kurti PJ, Jones JDG. Isolation of the tomato *Cf-9* gene for resistance to *Cladosporium fulvum* by transposon tagging. Science 1994;266:789–793.

155. Johal GS, Briggs SP. Reductase activity encoded by the *HM1* disease resistance gene in maize. Science 1992;258:958–987.

156. Cai D, Kleine M, Kifle S, et al. Positional cloning of a gene for nematode resistance in sugar beet. Science 1997;275:832–834.

2

Plant Disease Resistance Genes

Jeffrey G. Ellis and David A. Jones

1. INTRODUCTION

No adaptive immune system equivalent to the highly effective vertebrate immune system has been detected in plants. Nevertheless, the very existence of plants in the presence of many pathogens bears witness to the presence of highly effective systems for defense against pathogen invasion and disease. One system is based on disease resistance genes, which allow plants to detect pathogen infection and mount effective defense responses. These genes were first identified in the early years of the 20th century and were cloned and characterized more than 90 years later in the last decade of the century (see refs. 1 and 2 for reviews). Intense studies of these genes are now taking place in the present century to discern how their products function and how this knowledge can be applied to problems of disease resistance and food security.

2. RESISTANCE AND SUSCEPTIBILITY IN PLANTS

It is interesting to contemplate which of the two, plant diseases or human diseases, is the greater potential threat to human health. The human immune system, as effective as it is, cannot meet the challenge of plant disease-induced famine. Significant diseases of plants in agriculture are caused by diverse pathogens, including viruses, bacteria, fungi, and nematodes. These diseases cause various visible symptoms, and some result in death of the infected plant, but all important diseases result in reduced crop yields and quality and in some instances complete regional crop failures. In contrast to susceptibility, plant disease resistance is characterized by either partial or complete suppression of pathogen growth or replication at the site of infection. One of the most dramatic visible phenotypes that is frequently (but not always) associated with plant resistance is rapid localized cell death, the *hypersensitive response* (HR), at the site of infection, which is often compared with animal programmed cell death. This is an especially effective process in limiting pathogens that require living host cells. Other resistance responses include (but are not limited to) activation of defense gene expression, leading to production of antimicrobial proteins or low molecular weight antibiotics. In this respect, plant disease resistance has been likened to the innate immunity systems that have been described in insects and vertebrates. Most of the major plant pathogens mentioned above, with the exception of viruses, cause disease from the outside of plant cells. This includes patho-

From: *Infectious Disease: Innate Immunity*
Edited by: R. A. B. Ezekowitz and J. A. Hoffmann © Humana Press Inc., Totowa, NJ

genic bacteria whose extracellular life styles in plants are in contrast to the intracellular life styles of many mammalian bacterial pathogens.

3. GENETIC STUDIES OF HOST PLANT RESISTANCE AND PATHOGEN VIRULENCE

When a single isolate of a plant pathogen species (e.g., the wheat rust fungus) is inoculated onto a collection of host (e.g., wheat) genotypes, it is common to find that some genotypes are resistant and others are susceptible to the pathogen. Thus the pathogen isolate distinguishes host plant variation that is manifested as clear differences in disease reaction. Furthermore, if several isolates of the rust fungus are inoculated separately onto a set of different wheat genotypes, the different rust isolates are frequently distinguished by their ability to infect different host genotypes. For example, rust isolate 1 may infect host genotype 1 but not host genotype 2, while rust isolate 2 infects wheat 2 but not wheat 1. These sorts of observations are general for many different host-pathogen interactions. The ability of the pathogen to infect and cause disease in its host plant is referred to as *virulence;* the inability of a pathogen isolate to infect a resistant genotype of its normal host is called *avirulence.* In these ways, pathogen isolates can be used to distinguish host genotypes and, conversely, host plant genotypes can be used to distinguish isolates of the pathogen.

The existence of polymorphism for resistance/susceptibility in the host plant and for virulence/avirulence in a pathogen was initially found in crop plant species and their pathogens and more recently in wild plant species such as the "model" plant *Arabidopsis thaliana* and its pathogens. These polymorphisms provide the opportunity to carry out simultaneous genetic analysis of the inheritance of resistance and susceptibility in host species and inheritance of virulence and avirulence in the pathogen species. The most extensive classical genetic analyses were carried out on the flax plant, a crop plant grown for linseed oil and linen fiber production, and the fungal pathogen, flax rust *(3).* This fungus grows at the expense of living plant tissue and produces masses of orange spores over the leaf surfaces of susceptible plants. These genetic experiments involved the analysis of sexual crosses between resistant and susceptible flax genotypes and also sexual crosses between different rust isolates that differed in their ability to infect the host genotypes. Particular rust strains were used to follow the segregation of resistance/susceptibility in the host plant and particular flax genotypes were used as hosts to follow the segregation of avirulence/virulence in the pathogen. The following points summarize the results of these experiments with flax and flax rust and with other host-pathogen systems, which have provided a genetic description of plant-pathogen interactions.

1. Resistance to a pathogen isolate can be determined by a single gene difference between the resistant and susceptible host genotype. This gene is referred to as a *resistance gene.*
2. Resistance is most commonly dominant to susceptibility.
3. Multiple resistance genes can occur in a single species. Each resistance gene frequently encodes resistance to some but not all isolates of a pathogen species. The resistance gene's ability or inability to determine resistance to different pathogen isolates can distinguish one resistance gene from another. This difference between resistance genes is referred to as *resistance gene specificity.* For example, 30 different rust resistance specificities have been identified in the flax genome.

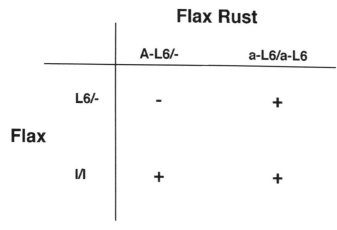

Fig. 1. Growth (+) or no growth (–) of the flax rust fungus on its host plant flax is determined by matching gene pairs at the host resistance locus and the pathogen avirulence locus. No growth (host resistance) occurs when the host carries one or more copies of the dominant resistance gene *L6* and the rust carries one or more copies of the corresponding avirulence gene *A-L6*.

4. Different resistance genes against a particular pathogen species can occur at several different loci in plant genomes, and in addition multiple resistance specificities often map to each genetic locus. In flax, for example, 30 rust resistance genes map to 5 loci with 11 specificities at the *L* locus.
5. Plant species are frequently highly polymorphic for resistance. Populations often contain individuals with different resistance specificities.

The results of the genetic analysis of pathogenicity of flax rust and other pathogens are summarized as follows:

1. Inability of a pathogen isolate to infect a resistant plant (referred to as *avirulence*) can be determined by a single gene difference between the virulent and avirulent isolate.
2. Avirulence is most commonly dominant to virulence.
3. Pathogen species often carry multiple avirulence genes and are often highly polymorphic for these genes.

The joint analysis of genetic segregation data for resistance of the host on one hand and rust avirulence on the other demonstrated that for each resistance gene specificity that is identified in the flax plant, a single corresponding avirulence gene is identified in the rust. For instance, flax plants carrying only the *L6* rust resistance gene are resistant to rusts carrying the *A-L6* avirulence gene but are susceptible to those strains without this avirulence gene (Fig. 1). This one-for-one or gene-for-gene relationship has been observed in many different host-pathogen interactions and has been used to propose a receptor-ligand model (see below). Under this model, it is postulated that the resistance gene encodes a receptor that perceives the direct (protein) or indirect (enzymatic) product of the corresponding avirulence gene in the pathogen. The cloning of host resistance genes and corresponding plant pathogen avirulence genes is beginning to provide the opportunity to test this model directly. As will be seen later, physical proof of a simple receptor-ligand pair in general has been difficult to obtain and (as discussed below), this model, based on genetic data, may be an oversimplification.

4. MOLECULAR NATURE OF AVIRULENCE GENES

Avirulence genes in pathogens are those genes that confer the ability to be recognized by a resistant host plant. This concept is one that is often problematic to animal pathologists. The simplest analogy is probably with genes encoding antigens in animal pathogens that are recognized by the mammalian immune system. Clearly, the principal function of these sorts of pathogen genes is not to trigger recognition by the host resistance mechanism. However, ultimately, in the presence of the appropriate host receptor, they are determinants of avirulence.

A number of avirulence genes have been cloned from plant pathogens, particularly viral and bacterial avirulence genes *(4)*. Viral avirulence genes encode a range of functions including capsid proteins and replicase proteins. Comparisons of the gene products of bacterial avirulence genes show that they are mostly unrelated and their function is largely unknown. There is now evidence that the bacterial avirulence gene products are introduced into plant cells by a type III secretion mechanism *(5)*. Further evidence suggests that these gene products are involved in enhancement of bacterial virulence (in the absence of the corresponding host resistance gene) and so are analogous to the virulence effector proteins delivered to animal cells by mammalian bacterial pathogens *(6)*. Only a few fungal avirulence genes have been cloned owing to the more complex genomes of fungi. The products of these genes include small, secreted proteins of unknown function *(4)*. In one case, a fungal avirulence protein from the rice blast fungus has similarity to a zinc protease *(7)*.

5. MOLECULAR NATURE OF RESISTANCE GENES

A growing number of resistance genes that recognize viral, bacterial, fungal, nematode, and insect pathogens have been cloned from both crop plants and the model plant *Arabidopsis*. Most of these genes are predicted to encode proteins with at least three core domains, a C-terminal leucine-rich repeat (LRR) domain, a central nucleotide binding site (NBS) domain, and an N-terminal domain that either contains homology to cytosolic domains of the *Drosophila* Toll or animal interleukin-1 receptors (TIR) or a potential coiled-coil (CC) domain (TIR-NBS-LRR or CC-NBS-LRR) *(8)* (Fig. 2). Two subclasses of CC domains have been described *(8)*, but there are probably at least three subclasses of CC domains in the CC-NBS-LRR class of resistance proteins. The tripartite structure of the NBS-LRR resistance proteins resembles the tripartite structure of CARD-NBS-WD40 [caspase recruitment domain-NBS-tryptophan aspartic acid (WD) repeat, with a periodicity of approx. 40 amino acids], CARD-NBS-LRR, AT-NBS-LRR (acetyl transferase-NBS-LRR), and BIR-NBS-LRR (baculovirus inhibition of apoptosis repeat-NBS-LRR) proteins controlling either apoptosis or the activation of cellular defenses or both in animals.

Simplistically, in NBS-LRR plant resistance proteins, the C-terminal domain is thought to be a receptor domain involved primarily in recognition of the avirulence ligand, the central NBS domain a regulatory domain, and the N-terminal TIR or CC domain an effector domain; however, biochemical evidence is still lacking. Similarly, in the human apoptotic protease-activating factor-1 (Apaf-1) CARD-NBS-WD40 apoptosis protein, the C-terminal WD40 domain is thought to be involved in the recognition of cytochrome *c* released from the mitochondria following an apoptotic stimulus, the central NBS domain in the regulatory binding of ATP or dATP,

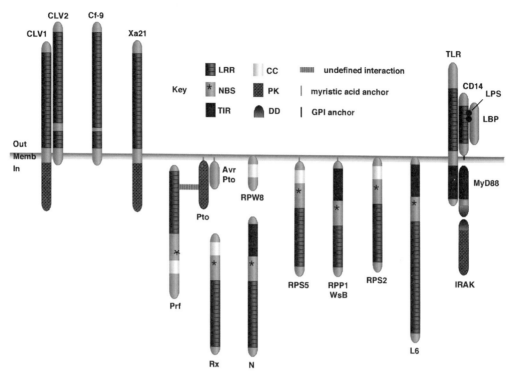

Fig. 2. Domain structures and predicted membrane topology of representative plant disease resistance proteins in comparison with one another and with similar proteins involved in plant development or animal innate immunity. All plant proteins have been described in the text apart from Rx, which is a potato gene for resistance to potato virus X *(27)*. CD14 is a glycophosphoinositol (GPI)-anchored LRR protein, and LBP is a lipopolysaccharide binding protein that form part of the TLR complex recognizing bacterial lipopolysaccharides. MyD88 is an adaptor protein with TIR and DD domains that link signal transduction from the TLR complex to the serine/threonine protein kinase IRAK. The nature and function of these and other protein components involved in TLR signaling are described elsewhere in this book. The horizontal bar depicts a cell membrane with the cytosol below. All proteins except Prf are shown with the N terminus at the top. *Abbreviations:* LRR, leucine-rich repeat; PM, plasma membrane; NBS, nucleotide binding site; TIR, Toll/interleukin-1 receptor domain; CC, coiled-coil; PK, serine/threonine protein kinase; DD, death domain; TLR, Toll-like receptor; LPS, lipopolysaccharide; IRAK, interleukin-1 receptor-associated kinase. (Adapted from ref. *8*.)

and the N-terminal CARD in the triggering of the caspase cascade that effects apoptosis *(9–11)*.

Initially, the NBS domain was defined in plant resistance proteins by the presence of kinase 1a (P-loop), kinase 2, and kinase 3a motifs likely to be involved in ATP/GTP or dATP/dGTP binding. As more resistance genes were cloned, at least five additional motifs were recognized, not only among resistance proteins, but also among the animal Apaf-1 *(10)*, CED-4 (*Caenorhabditis elegans* death-regulating CARD-NBS protein) *(12)*, and Ark (*Drosophila* Apaf-1-related killer CARD-NBS-WD-40 protein) *(13)* apoptosis proteins *(8,14,15)* (Fig. 3), leading to the redesignation of the NBS domain as an NB-ARC domain (nucleotide binding domain shared by Apaf-1, plant resistance proteins, and CED-4) *(15)*. The additional motifs present in the NB-ARC domain do

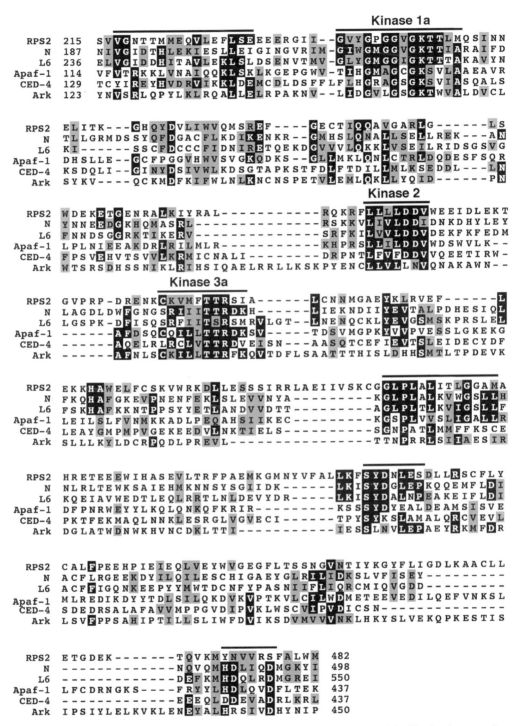

Fig. 3. Conserved motis in the NBS regions of the *Arabidopsis* RPS2 (Genbank accession U14158), tobacco N (U15605), and flax L6 (U27081) disease resistance proteins and the human Apaf-1 (AF013263), *Caenorhabditis elegans* CED-4 (X69016), and *Drosophila* Ark (AAF57916) apoptosis-activating proteins. Blocks of conserved motifs were aligned using Macaw *(71)*. Amino acid identities are highlighted with black boxes and similarities with gray boxes. Conserved motifs are overlined, and the kinase 1a, 2, and 3a motifs of the NBS are indicated.

not seem to be present in the NBS domains of the human CIITA (MHC class II transcriptional activator) AT-NBS-LRR protein *(16,17)*, Nod1 *(18,19)*, Nod2 *(20)*, and DEFCAP (death effector filament-forming CED-4-like apoptosis protein) *(21)*, CARD-NBS-LRR proteins, or the BIR-NBS-LRR protein NIAP (neuronal apoptosis inhibitor protein) *(22,23)*.

Superficially, the latter proteins resemble plant resistance proteins more than Apaf-1, CED-4, or Ark, because they share both NBS and LRR domains, but the resemblance is misleading because only the motifs directly involved in nucleotide binding are shared between the two types of NBS domain. This finding suggests that any other interactions mediated or regulated by the two types of NBS domain may differ. However, despite this difference, the proteins carrying this kind of NBS domain appear to be functionally more similar to plant disease resistance genes. Apaf-1, CED-4, and Ark are only involved in regulation of apoptosis, whereas CIITA, Nod1, Nod2, DEFCAP, and NIAP are involved in the regulation of apoptosis and/or cellular defenses *(16,19,20,21,24)*. The latter function is more similar to that of plant disease resistance proteins, which regulate both cell death and pathogen-response protein expression, and in some cases plant disease resistance can be effected without cell death *(25–27)*.

The remainder of the cloned resistance genes have been found in only one or a few kinds of plant-pathogen interactions. These comprise the rice *Xa-21* gene encoding an extracytosolic LRR receptor domain connected by a single transmembrane domain to a cytosolic serine/threonine protein kinase (LRR-TM-PK) and conferring resistance to the bacterial blight bacterium *Xanthomonas oryzae* pv. *oryzae (28)*; the tomato *Pto* gene encoding a serine/threonine protein kinase (PK) and conferring resistance to the bacterial speck bacterium *Pseudomonas syringae* pv. *tomato (29)*; the tomato *Cf-2, Cf-4, Cf-5, Cf-9,* and *Cf-ECP2* genes on the one hand and the tomato *Ve1* and *Ve2* genes on the other, encoding extracytosolic LRR receptor domains connected by a single transmembrane domain to a short cytosolic tail (LRR-TM) and conferring resistance to the leaf mold fungus *Cladosporium fulvum* or the vascular wilt fungus *Verticillium dahliae,* respectively *(30–35)*; the *Arabidopsis RPW8.1* and *RPW8.2* genes encoding CC proteins conferring broad resistance to the powdery mildew fungi *Erysiphe cruciferarum* and *E. cichoracearum (36)*; and the sugar beet *Hs1-pro* gene (possibly based on an incomplete clone) encoding a novel protein conferring resistance to the cyst nematode *Heterodera schachtii (37)*.

LRR domains are common to both the NBS-LRR resistance proteins and a number of the non-NBS resistance proteins. However, the LRR domains of NBS-LRR proteins are predicted to be cytosolic and have slightly different and highly degenerate repeat motifs in terms of length and composition compared with the LRR domains of the LRR-TM or LRR-TM-PK proteins, which are predicted to be extracytosolic and have very regular and well-conserved repeat motifs *(38)*. In fact, the LRRs of the NBS-LRR proteins are often difficult to discern, and assignments of LRRs are sometimes rather arbitrary as a consequence. A useful way to determine the presence of LRRs in a protein is to carry out similarity searches against the very large array of LRR proteins present in publicly available sequence databases. Such searches do not, for example, substantiate the original claim that Hs1-pro is an LRR protein. Despite the structural diversity of LRRs, their role as determinants of recognitional specificity in plant pathogen interactions is now well established (see below).

Besides LRR domains, the non-NBS-LRR proteins also show other intriguing relationships to one another, to NBS-LRR proteins, and to proteins involved in development and innate immunity in both plants and animals. The Xa-21 LRR-TM-PK protein bears an obvious resemblance to the Cf and Ve LRR-TM proteins and the Pto PK protein (Fig. 2), and it is not uncommon to find interacting protein domains that are separate in some organisms joined together in others *(39)*. The Xa-21 protein is also structurally similar to a number of *Arabidopsis* LRR-TM-PK proteins including developmental proteins such as the CLV1 protein involved in shoot meristem development *(40)* (Fig. 2), the hormone receptor BRI protein involved in brassinosteriod perception *(41)*, and the innate-immunity FLS2 protein involved in the sensing of bacterial flagellin and triggering of defense responses similar to those triggered by disease resistance proteins *(42)*. Moreover, the CLV1 protein requires and interacts with CLV2, a LRR-TM protein structurally similar to the Cf and Ve proteins *(43)* (Fig. 2). The FLS2 protein is functionally analogous to the animal innate immunity Toll and Toll-like receptor (TLR) proteins involved in detection of pathogen-associated molecular profiles (PAMPs), such as bacterial lipopolysaccharides and proteoglycans (as described in detail elsewhere in this book).

One might therefore predict that animal cells will recognize and respond to flagellins, perhaps via a TLR protein and, *vice versa,* that plant cells will respond to the PAMPs detected by Toll and the TLR proteins, perhaps by other as yet uncharacterized LRR-TM-PK proteins. Interestingly, Toll performs a dual function in both development and innate immunity, controlling development of the dorsal-ventral axis in the *Drosophila* embryo and innate immunity in the adult fly. Moreover, at least one TLR protein has been shown to have a role in the activation of apoptosis as well as cellular defenses *(44,45)*. However, in addition to functional similarities, there are also structural similarities between the non-NBS-LRR plant disease resistance proteins and the Toll and TLR proteins besides that already noted for the TIR-NBS-LRR proteins. The Toll and TLR proteins are LRR-TM-TIR proteins with structural similarity to the LRR-TM domains of the Xa-21, Cf, and Ve proteins (Fig. 2). Moreover, the TIR domains of Toll, the interleukin-1 receptor, and the TLR proteins interact with serine/threonine protein kinases Pelle and interleukin-1 receptor-associated kinase (IRAK), which are similar to the PK domains of Xa-21 and Pto (Fig. 2). Nor does the web of intrigue end here. For functioning, Pto requires Prf, a CC-NBS-LRR protein *(46,47)*, and the RPW8 proteins are similar to the amino-terminal CC domain of a subclass of CC-NBS-LRR proteins *(36)*, suggesting a possible homotypic interaction.

Thus, there would seem to be at least two functional connections between the NBS-LRR and the non-NBS-LRR resistance proteins. A similar connection has also been made in animal cells with innate immunity to bacteria determined by both extracellular TLR4-mediated and intracellular Nod1-mediated recognition of bacterial lipopolysaccharides feeding into the same signaling pathway *(48)*. However, owing to the extracellular life style of plant bacterial pathogens, it is unlikely that cytoplasmic plant NBS-LRR proteins would be involved in the recognition of the PAMPs associated with innate immunity in animals.

Proximity to cell membranes is another potential similarity between NBS-LRR proteins and other resistance proteins that needs to be explored. The LRR-TM and LRR-TM-PK proteins have obvious membrane associations. Pto has an N-terminal myristoylation site that is dispensable for Pto function *(49)*, but its presence nevertheless suggests that Pto is membrane-associated. Furthermore, Fen, another member of the Pto family *(50,51)*, and AvrPto, the bacterial avirulence ligand recognized by Pto *(52)*, both have functionally-indispensable N-terminal myristoylation sites *(51,53)*, with that of Avr-Pto processed in the plant, strengthening the argument that Pto functions at a membrane. RPW8.1 and RPW8.2 are predicted to be type Ib membrane proteins, i.e., anchored to the cytosolic face of the cell membrane by an N-terminal hydrophobic signal anchor domain that remains uncleaved *(36,* and our own analysis). The flax L6 *(54)*, flax M *(55)*, and *Arabidopsis* RPS2 *(56,57)* resistance proteins have N-terminal hydrophobic regions predicted to be potential translocation signal peptides *(54,* and our own analysis), but in light of the cytosolic composition of their LRR domains are more likely to function as type Ib signal anchors. Like RPW8, the tomato I2 *(58)*, tomato Mi *(59,60)*, lettuce Dm3 *(61,62)*, and *Arabidopsis* RPP1-WsA *(63)* resistance proteins are also predicted to have N-terminal hydrophobic signal anchor domains that remain uncleaved *(63,* and our own analysis).

A number of other NBS LRR resistance proteins are not predicted to have translocation signal peptides or signal anchors at their N termini. The *Arabidopsis* RPM1 protein *(64)* is one of these, but nevertheless it has been shown experimentally to behave as a peripheral membrane protein *(65)*. The *Arabidopsis* RPP1-WsB, RPP1-WsC *(66)*, and RPS5 *(63)* NBS-LRR resistance proteins are also not predicted to have translocation signal peptides or signal anchors, but instead have predicted N-terminal myristoylation sites (our own analysis) and are therefore possibly associated with a cell membrane. Moreover, the bacterial avrB *(67)* and avrRpm1 *(68)* avirulence ligands recognized by RPM1 and the bacterial avrPphB *(69)* avirulence ligand recognized by RPS5 also have functionally indispensable plant-processed N-terminal myristoylation sites (revealed after removal of a propeptide in the case of AvrPphB), suggesting targeting to the host membrane *(70)*.

Collectively, these examples might tend to point toward membrane association for the NBS-LRR proteins as a whole, however, it is possible that resistance proteins may be targeted to the same location as their cognate avirulence ligands, so only a subset of NBS-LRR resistance proteins recognizing membrane targeted avirulence ligands may themselves be membrane-associated. Thus, NBS-LRR proteins recognizing cytosolic viral or nuclear-targeted bacterial components may not have any functional association with membranes. Although perhaps indicative, type Ib membrane anchors and N-terminal myristoylation may be insufficient by themselves to ensure membrane localization, and other proteins may be required to stabilize any membrane associations. Moreover, it is possible that membrane associations provided by other proteins in a resistance complex could render those of the resistance protein redundant under some circumstances, as may be the case for Pto.

Large numbers of NBS-LRR, LRR-TM-PK, and LRR-TM genes have been revealed in the sequence of the *Arabidopsis* genome. There are at least 135 NBS-LRR genes distributed somewhat unevenly over the five *Arabidopsis* chromosomes and at least 208 LRR-TM-PK genes distributed more evenly (Table 1), although genes of both types show a degree of clustering within each chromosome. Despite the large numbers of NBS-LRR sequences, of which several have been shown to function as disease resistance genes, none as yet have been shown to be involved in any other function, whereas LRR-TM-PK and LRR-TM genes have been shown to be involved in a number of other

Table 1
Number and Chromosomal Distribution of NBS-LRR
and LRR-TM-PK Genes in the *Arabidopsis* Genome[a]

Chromosome	NBS-LRRs	LRR-TM-PKs
1	33	66
5	55	53
3	15	33
2	4	34
4	28	22
Total	135	208

[a] Chromosomes are listed in descending size.
Adapted from http://www.niblrrs.ucdavis.edu, May 2001.

functions including development, disease resistance, and innate immunity. It would therefore seem that NBS-LRR genes are dedicated plant disease resistance genes, whereas the LRR-TM-PK and LRR-TM genes seem able to diversify, and part of this diversification may be recruited into or from a disease resistance function.

6. COMPLEX AND SIMPLE GENETIC LOCI

Different disease resistance specificities often map to tightly linked regions of plant genomes, referred to as complex loci. Recent molecular analysis of these loci show that they consist of several genes closely related in DNA sequence (called *paralogs*) that occur as tandem direct repeats *(71–74)*. Any particular complex locus can differ between genotypes of particular plant species in the absolute number of genes, the DNA sequence of the genes, and the resistance specificities encoded. A particular complement of related resistance genes at a complex locus in an individual genotype is referred to as a resistance gene *haplotype*. For example, 14 different resistance specificities (*Rp1-A, -B,* and so on) for common maize rust that map to the *Rp1* locus of maize have been identified in the maize gene pool, and these occur in different resistance gene haplotypes *(75)*. The *Rp1* haplotype contains a family of nine CC-NBS-LRR genes, five of which are transcribed and only one of which encodes an identified resistance specificity (the Rp1-D specificity) *(75)*. In contrast, only a single gene occurs in the naturally occurring Rp1-D haplotype of the maize line A188, and this gene encodes no known resistance specificity (A. Pryor, personal communication).

Locus expansion and contraction probably occur by unequal crossing over events at meiosis. In *Arabidopsis,* extensive genome sequence data provide further insight into the molecular complexity of resistance gene haplotypes. For example, nine TIR-NBS-LRR genes occur at the RPP5 locus of the *Landsberg erecta* ecotype *(73)*. One of these genes encodes the RPP5 resistance specificity (resistance to *Peronospora parasitica*), whereas the eight other genes in this haplotype contain stop codons or insertions of transposable elements in their coding regions. Two further well-studied complex resistance gene loci are *Cf-4/Cf-9 (72)* and *Cf-2/Cf-5 (31,32),* which occur on tomato chromosomes 1 and 6, respectively. These loci contain genes for resistance to the fungus *Cladosporium fulvum.* The occurrence of multiple repeated related genes at these loci indicates several episodes of gene duplication during their evolution.

Resistance genes can also occur in simple loci apparently containing only a single gene. Multiple resistance specificities can be encoded by different allelic variants of a single gene. For example, 11 rust resistance specificities map to the *L* locus in flax, which contains a single TIR-NBS-LRR gene *(76)*.

7. MOLECULAR BASIS FOR RESISTANCE GENE SPECIFICITY

The receptor-ligand model postulates that specificity differences are caused by different ligand recognition capacities. The most informative analyses of the molecular basis of gene-for-gene specificity have been generated using sequence information from either multiple alleles of a simple locus or several closely related resistance genes from a single complex locus. Examples of these situations are the 11 alleles at the *L* locus of flax *(76)*, the 30 specificities (two cloned; *77,78*) at the *Mla* locus in barley and the 2 specificities at each of the *Cf-4/Cf-9 (30,33)* and *Cf-2/Cf-5 (31,32)* loci in tomato. The experimental approach has been to compare the sequences of closely related genes and their protein products and attempt to correlate sequence differences with specificity differences. The correlations can then be tested by making in vitro exchanges between genes encoding different specificities and testing the function and specificity of the recombinant genes in transgenic plants using discriminating isolates of the appropriate pathogen species. The most extensive studies have been carried out using the multiple allelic resistance specificities at the flax *L* locus *(76)* and two resistance specificities at the tomato *Cf-4/Cf-9* locus *(79,80)*.

The common structural domain in several different classes of plant disease resistance proteins, and originally proposed as a specificity determinant, is the leucine-rich repeat (LRR). Although no crystal structure of the LRR region of a plant disease resistance protein has been reported, structures are known for the human and porcine ribonuclease LRR proteins either alone or in complex with their ligands *(81)*. These proteins adopt nonglobular, horseshoe-shaped, α/β-helical structures. Each repeat unit includes a short β-strand/β-turn region with consensus xxLxLxx (where x is any amino acid and L is a leucine or other aliphatic residue buried in the hydrophobic core of the protein helix; Fig. 4A); most of the ligand contact points involve the variable x residues in this motif. Among products of resistance gene alleles or paralogs from complex loci, extremely high levels of polymorphism frequently occur in the LRR sequences, and particularly in the analogous xxLxLxx motif (Fig. 4B). This motif, which is found in many proteins, is involved in protein-protein interactions.

The role of the LRR regions in resistance protein specificity has now been demonstrated experimentally *(76)*, and the importance of variation in the β-strand region has now also been confirmed *(82)*. For example, the alleles of the flax rust resistance gene *L,* encoding closely related, polymorphic TIR-NBS-LRR resistance proteins, control distinct rust resistance specificities. In most cases, the corresponding avirulence genes in the flax rust fungus map to unlinked loci. Comparison of 11 L protein sequences indicated that although sequence differences occur in all domains of the protein, the most polymorphic domain is indeed the LRR region. The importance of the LRR region in specificity is indicated by comparison of the L6 and L11 proteins. L6 and L11 are identical in the TIR and NBS domains and differ at 33 positions in the LRR region (Fig. 4B). Therefore one or more of these polymorphisms must differentiate L6 and L11 specificities. These LRR polymorphisms in the products of the *L* alleles occur pre-

A

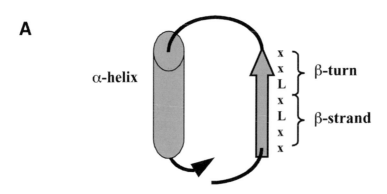

B

```
L6    601  FLNLSELRYLHAREAMLTGDFNNLLPNLKWLELPFYKHGEDDPPLTNYTMKNLIIVILEH  660
L11   601  ...........S..............................F............  660

L6    661  SHITADDWGGWRHMMKMAERLKVVRLASNYSLYGRRVRLSDCWRFPKSIEVLSMTAIEMD  720
L11   661  ....................................................  720

L6    721  EVDIGELKKLKTLVLKFCPIQKISGGTFGMLKGLRELCLEFNWGTNLREVVADIGQLSSL  780
L11   721  ..................L.................................  780

L6    781  KVLKTTGAKEVEINEFPLGLKELSTSSRIPNLSQLLDLEVLKVYDCKDGFDMPPASPSED  840
L11   781  .........................................A..........  840

L6    841  ESSVWWKVSKLKSLQLEKTRINVNVVDDASSGGHLPRYLLPTSLTYLKIYQCTEPTWLPG  900
L11   841  ....................................................  900

L6    901  IENLENLTSLEVNDIFQTLGGDLDGLQGLRSLEILRIRKVNGLARIKGLKDLLCSSTCKL  960
L11   901  ...........K........................................  960

L6    961  RKFYITECPDLIELLPCELGGQTVVVPSMAELTIRDCPRLEVGPMIRSLPKFPMLKKLDL 1020
L11   961  ..L..R...........R.........D........................ 1020

L6   1021  AVANITKEEDLDAIGSLEELVSLELELDDTSSGIERIVSSSKLQKLTTLVVKVPSLREIE 1080
L11  1021  ...........................K...........L............ 1080

L6   1081  GLEELKSLQDLYLEGCTSLGRLPLEKLKELDIGGCPDLTELVQTVVAVPSLRGLTIRDCP 1140
L11  1081  ........R.F.V.............................VE...W.... 1140

L6   1141  RLEVGPMIQSLPKFPMLNELTLSMVNITKEDELEVLGSLEELDSLELTLDDTCSSIERIS 1200
L11  1141  ...........N................A...........V.K......... 1200

L6   1201  FLSKLQKLTTLIVEVPSLREIEGLAELKSLRILYLEGCTSLERLWPDQQQLGSLKNLNVL 1260
L11  1201  S.......R.K.................YE...Q.................E...EI 1260

L6   1261  DIQGCKSLSVDHLSALKTTLPPRARITWPDQPYR 1294
L11  1261  N.R................P.............. 1294
```

Fig. 4. (A) The LRR structural unit. L, leucine or another aliphatic amino acid; x, any amino acid. **(B)** Amino acid alignment of the LRR region of the flax rust resistance proteins L6 and L11. (Identical residues are indicated by dots.) These proteins are identical in the TIR and NBS regions (residues 1–600) and differ at 33 positions in the LRR region, principally in or close to the xxLxLxx motif (overlined) of the LRR units.

dominantly in the predicted solvent-exposed xxLxLxx motifs in several of the individual LRR units (Fig. 4B). Analysis of TIR-NBS-LRR flax rust resistance proteins encoded at the flax *P* locus was also informative. The difference between *P* and *P2* specificity is owing to at most six amino acid differences between the two proteins and these differences occur exclusively in the xxLxLxx motifs of four LRR units *(82)*.

Other sequence comparisons and domain swaps indicate that specificity differences are not solely determined by the LRR. The N-terminal domain TIR domain can also affect specificity. For example, the L6 and L7 proteins, which have distinct resistance specificities, are identical in the NBS-LRR region and differ at 11 residues in the TIR region *(76)*. Domain swaps implicate at most three polymorphisms as being sufficient for the specificity differences *(83)*. Whether these residues, together with the LRR region, are involved in the postulated interactions with pathogen ligands is unknown.

Extensive analysis of the molecular basis of specificity has also been carried out with the TM-LRR resistance proteins Cf-4 and Cf-9, from tomato. More than 50% of the single-amino acid substitution polymorphisms between the two proteins occur in the nonleucine residues of the xxLxLxx motif. Domain swap and gene shuffling experiments between *Cf-4* and *Cf-9* have further refined the definition of critical polymorphisms and have shown that the Cf-4 protein can be converted to *Cf-9* specificity (and *vice versa*) by a limited number of sequence changes *(79,80)*. It is important to stress that these sorts of sequence comparisons and domain swaps can only identify the regions that contribute to the *differences* in specificity between the genes under comparison. Conserved residues can also contribute to binding and thus to the overall specificity of recognition.

8. EVOLUTION OF DISEASE RESISTANCE SPECIFICITIES

When extensive comparisons have been made between closely related resistance genes from a single locus, it is evident that variation is generated by standard evolutionary processes, including point mutation, small deletions, insertions, and meiotic recombination. No evidence has been uncovered suggesting that specialized processes accelerate the evolution of resistance genes, such as site-directed recombination or mutation mechanisms. Although point mutations provide the source of new sequence variation in resistance gene evolution, much of the variability among resistance gene families appears to result from recombination, which shuffles polymorphic sites between individual genes. Patchworks of sequence similarities shared between alleles of a single gene and also between members of complex resistance gene haplotypes are frequently observed and provide evidence for past exchanges of blocks of sequence variation by recombination. There is also evidence from sequence comparisons that unequal exchanges can occur after mispairing of complex resistance loci; however, the extent of this sort of exchange appears to decrease as the sequence similarly diverges.

Intragenic unequal sequence exchanges between repeated sequences within LRR-encoding regions also appear to be an important source of variation between resistance gene homologs. Unequal exchange can delete and duplicate sequence information that could form new ligand binding surfaces and alter spatial arrangements between critical residues involved in ligand binding. These events could alter or optimize specific ligand interactions. Examples of this type of variation are found among the *L* alleles of flax, which contain one, two or four copies of a 450-bp DNA sequence encoding six

LRR units (where one unit is approx 24 residues) *(76)*. A second example is provided by the *RPP5* locus of *Arabidopsis*. *RPP5* homologs, with variable numbers of direct DNA repeats, encode proteins with 13, 17, 21, or 25 LRR units *(74)*. Homologs from the *Cf-2/Cf-5* locus of tomato also differ widely in the number of LRR units, which result from deletion/duplication of individual LRR units *(32)*.

When the individual LRR units of a resistance protein are aligned with those of its homologs or allelic variants, it is apparent that the leucine or other hydrophobic residues that form the backbone of the repeats are highly conserved, whereas the intervening residues are more variable *(72,76)*. Variation is particularly evident in the x residues of the xxLxLxx motif within each repeat. Analysis of DNA sequence variation using approaches pioneered for the analysis of variation in the human MHC genes *(84)* has been applied to studies of plant disease resistance gene variation *(62,72,82,85)*. Analysis of the rates of synonymous (non-amino acid altering) and nonsynonymous (amino acid altering) nucleotide substitution rates (Ks and Ka, respectively) in closely related resistance gene sequences has been particularly informative.

Most genes are subject to conservative selection because most amino acid changes to proteins are deleterious, or at best neutral, and hence allelic gene comparisons find Ka < Ks. However, in resistance genes it has generally been found that Ka < Ks for non-LRR coding regions, the LRR coding regions showing Ka > Ks. This is particularly evident in the codons for the x residues in the xxLxLxx motif. The result indicates that selection favors amino acid variation at these sites, presumably because such changes can introduce new or more efficacious recognition specificities. These molecular evolutionary analyses further support the view that this region is involved in binding pathogen-derived ligands and thus specificity of recognition. Similarly, diversifying selection has been detected in the TIR-encoding region of *L* alleles of flax, which also contributes to the specificity of these resistance proteins *(83)*.

9. THE RECEPTOR-LIGAND MODEL AND THE GUARD HYPOTHESIS

Although direct interaction between a resistance protein receptor and the corresponding avirulence gene product has been predicted on the basis of gene-for-gene interactions, little direct evidence exits from biochemical analysis. Furthermore, apart from viruses, the other major groups of plant pathogens are extracellular, and the largest class of resistance proteins, the NBS-LRR group, is probably located in the cytoplasm. Bacterial avirulence proteins and resistance proteins are probably brought together via the bacterial type III secretion system *(5)*, and although no evidence has yet been reported, uptake of proteins secreted by pathogenic fungi at the host-pathogen interface is also likely. Direct interaction in a yeast two-hybrid system has been demonstrated between the cytoplasmic serine/threonine protein kinase Pto (a resistance protein from tomato) and AvrPto (the corresponding bacterial avirulence protein) *(86,87)*. Although there is a strong correlation between the ability of mutant forms of Pto to bind AvrPto in the yeast test system and the ability to function as a resistance protein in vivo, no direct evidence for in vivo binding has been reported. Direct interaction between the NBS-LRR resistance protein Pi-ta and its corresponding avr protein has been reported from in vitro but not in vivo experiments *(88)*. Failure to detect direct interaction between several other resistance proteins and their corresponding Avr proteins has also been reported in meetings, but not published. Although these negative

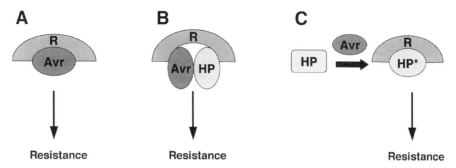

Fig. 5. The guard model. (**A**) Data supporting the simple direct binary interaction of resistance proteins (R) and avirulence proteins (Avr) have been difficult to obtain, and no demonstration of in vivo interactions is reported. (**B**) Higher order interactions have been proposed whereby the interaction between Avr and one or more host proteins (HP), potentially involved in enhancing virulence in susceptible plants, is detected in resistant plants by the resistance protein. (**C**) Alternatively, the HP may be enzymatically modified to HP* by Avr, for instance for repression of a defense activity, and the HP* may act as a ligand for R. (Reprint with permission from Trends in Plant Science vol 9, 2000 p. 373–379. Ellis J, Dodds P, and Pryor T. The generation of plant disease resistance gene specifications.)

data may reflect technical difficulties and/or low affinity between the receptor-ligand pairs, the possibility that simple binary interactions may not generally occur is now being seriously considered. Recently, the first documentation of resistance proteins and Avr proteins being involved in higher order complexes has been reported *(89)*. Furthermore, mutation experiments have identified other plant genes necessary for activity of specific resistance genes *(46,47)*. A new scenario is therefore being considered and examined in experimental systems. Avirulence proteins are postulated to have a primary role as virulence determinants through interaction with host proteins, similar to the type III effector proteins of bacterial pathogens of animals. Resistance proteins, it is further postulated, have a role in guarding host cellular proteins from recruitment by pathogen avirulence proteins *(90)*. Models for this so-called guard hypothesis are presented in Fig. 5.

REFERENCES

1. Ellis J, Jones D. Structure and function of proteins controlling strain-specific pathogen resistance in plants. Curr Opin Plant Biol 1998;1:288–293.
2. Ellis J, Dodds P, Pryor T. Structure, function and evolution of plant disease resistance genes. Curr Opin Plant Biol 2000;3:278–284.
3. Flor HH. Current status of the gene-for-gene concept. Annu Rev Phytopathol 1971;9:278–296.
4. Lauge R, De Wit PJ. Fungal avirulence genes: structure and possible functions. Fungal Genet Biol 1998;24:285–297.
5. Mudgett MB, Staskawicz BJ. Protein signaling via type III secretion pathways in phytopathogenic bacteria. Curr Opin Microbiol 1998;1:109–114.
6. Chen Z, Kloek AP, Boch J, Katagiri F, Kunkel BN. The *Pseudomonas syringae* avrRpt2 gene product promotes pathogen virulence from inside plant cells. Mol Plant Microbe Interact 2000;13:1312–1321.
7. Bryan GT, Wu K-S, Farrall L, et al. A single amino acid difference distinguishes resistant and susceptible alleles of the rice blast resistance gene *Pi-ta*. Plant Cell 2000;12:2033–2046.

8. Jones DA. Resistance genes and resistance protein function. In: Dickinson M, Beynon J (eds.). Molecular Plant Pathology, Annual Plant Reviews, vol. 4. Sheffield: Sheffield Academic Press, 2000, pp. 108–143.
9. Li P, Nijhawan D, Budihardjo J, et al. Cytochrome *c* and dATP-dependent formation of Apaf-1/caspase-9 complex initiates an apoptotic protease cascade. Cell 1997;91:479–489.
10. Zou H, Henzel WJ, Liu X, Lutschg A, Wang X. Apaf-1, a human protein homologous to *C. elegans* CED-4, participates in cytochrome *c*-dependent activation of caspase-3. Cell 1997;90:405–413.
11. Zou H, Li Y, Liu X, Wang X. An Apaf-1-cytochrome *c* multimeric complex is a functional apoptosome that activates procaspase-9. J Biol Chem 1999;274:11549–11556.
12. Yuan J, Horvitz HR. The *Caenorhabditis elegans* cell death gene *CED-4* encodes a novel protein and is expressed during the period of extensive programmed cell death. Development 1992;116:309–320.
13. White K. Cell death: Drosophila Apaf-1—no longer in the (d)Ark. Curr Biol 2000;10:R167–R169.
14. Chinnaiyan AM, Chaudhary D, O'Rourke K, Koonin EV, Dixit VM. Role of CED-4 in the activation of CED-3. Nature 1997;388:728–729.
15. van der Biezen EA, Jones JDG. The NB-ARC domain: a novel signaling motif shared by plant resistance gene products and regulators of cell death in animals. Curr Biol 1998;8:R226–R227.
16. Steimle V, Otten LA, Zufferey M, Mach B. Complmentation cloning of an MHC class-II transactivator mutated in hereditary MHC class-II deficiency (or bare lymphocyte syndrome). Cell 1993;75:135–146.
17. Raval A, Howcroft TK, Weissman JD, et al. Transcriptional coactivator, CIITA, is an acetyltransferase that bypasses a promoter requirement for TAF(II)250. Mol Cell 2001;7:105–115.
18. Bertin J, Nir W-J, Fischer CM, et al. Human CARD4 protein is a novel CED-4/Apaf-1 cell death family member that activates NF-κB. J Biol Chem 1999;274:12955–12958.
19. Inohara N, Koseki T, del Peso L, et al. Nod1, and Apaf-1-like activator of caspase-9 and nuclear factor-κB. J Biol Chem 1999;274:14560–14567. Erratum ibid. 18675.
20. Ogura Y, Inohara N, Benito A, Chen FF, Yamaoka S, Nunez G. Nod2, a Nod1/Apaf-1 family member that is restricted to monocytes and activates NFκB. J Biol Chem 2001; online.
21. Hlaing T, Guo RF, Dilley KA, et al. Molecular cloning and characterization of DEFCAP-L and -S, two isoforms of a novel member of the mammalian Ced-4 family of apoptosis proteins. J Biol Chem 2001;276:9230–9238.
22. Roy N, Mahadevan MS, McLean M, et al. The gene for neuronal apoptosis inhibitory protein is partially deleted in individuals with spinal muscular atrophy. Cell 1995;80:167–178.
23. Chen QF, Baird SD, Mahadevan M, et al. Sequence of a 131-kb region of 5q13.1 containing the spinal muscular atrophy candidate genes SMN and NAIP. Genomics 1998;48:121–127.
24. Liston P, Roy N, Tamai K, et al. Suppression of apoptosis in mammalian cells by NAIP and a related family of IAP genes. Nature 1996;379:349–353.
25. Hammond-Kosack KE, Jones JDG. Incomplete dominance of tomato *Cf* genes for resistance to *Cladosporium fulvum*. Mol Plant Microbe Interact 1994;7:58–70.
26. Yu I-C, Parker J, Bent AF. Gene-for-gene disease resistance without the hypersensitive response in *Arabidopsis dnd1* mutant. Proc Natl Acad Sci USA 1998;95:7819–7824.
27. Bendahmane A, Kanyuka K, Baulcombe DC. The *Rx* gene from potato controls separate virus resistance and cell death responses. Plant Cell 1999;11:781–791.
28. Song Wy, Wang GL, Chen LL, et al. A receptor kinase-like protein encoded by the rice disease resistance gene, *Xa21*. Science 1995;270:1804–1806.
29. Martin GB, Brommonschenkel SH, Chunwongse J, et al. Map-based cloning of a protein kinase gene conferring disease resistance in tomato. Science 1993;262:1432–1436.
30. Jones DA, Thomas CM, Hammond-Kosack KE, Balint-Kurti PJ, Jones JDG. Isolation of the tomato *Cf-9* gene for resistance to *Cladosporium fulvum* by transposon tagging. Science 1994;266:789–793.

31. Dixon MS, Jones DA, Keddie JS, et al. The tomato *Cf-2* disease resistance locus comprises two functional genes encoding leucine-rich repeat proteins. Cell 1996;84:451–459.

32. Dixon MS, Hatzixanthis K, Jones Da, Harrison K, Jones JDG. The tomato *Cf-5* disease resistance gene and six homologs show pronounced allelic variation in leucine-rich repeat copy number. Plant Cell 1998;10:1915–1925.

33. Thomas CM, Jones DA, Parniske M, et al. Characterization of the tomato *Cf-4* gene for resistance to *Cladosporium fulvum* identifies sequences that determine recognitional specificity of *Cf-4* and *Cf-9*. Plant Cell 1997;9:2209–2224.

34. Lauge R, Joosten MHAJ, Haanstra JPW, et al. Successful search for a resistance gene in tomato targeted against a virulence factor of a fungal pathogen. Proc Natl Acad Sci USA 1998;95:9014–9018.

35. Kawchuk LM, Hachey J, Lynch DR, et al. Tomato *Ve* disease resistance genes encode cell surface-like receptors. Proc Natl Acad Sci USA 2001; online.

36. Xiao SY, Ellwood S, Calis O, et al. Broad-spectrum mildew resistance in *Arabidopsis thaliana* mediated by *RPW8*. Science 2001;291:118–120.

37. Cai DG, Kleine M, Kifle S, et al. Positional cloning of a gene for nematode resistance in sugar beet. Science 1997;275:832–834.

38. Jones DA, Jones JDG. The role of leucine-rich repeat proteins in plant defenses. Adv Bot Res 1997;24:89–167.

39. Marcotte EM. Computational genetics: finding protein function by nonhomology methods. Curr Opinion Struct Biol 2000;10:359–365.

40. Clark SE, Williams RW, Meyerowitz EM. The *CLAVATA1* gene encodes a putative receptor kinase that controls shoot and floral meristem size in *Arabidopsis*. Cell 1997;89:575–585.

41. Li JM, Chory J. A putative leucine-rich repeat receptor kinase involved in brassinosteroid signal transduction. Cell 1997;90:929–938.

42. Gómez-Gómez L, Boller T. FLS2: an LRR receptor-like kinase involved in the perception of the bacterial elicitor flagellin in *Arabidopsis*. Mol Cell 2000;5:1003–1011.

43. Jeong S, Trotochaud AE, Clark SE. The *Arabidopsis CLAVATA2* gene encodes a receptor-like protein required for the stability of the CLAVATA1 receptor-like kinase. Plant Cell 1999;11:1925–1933.

44. Aliprantis AO, Yang RB, Weiss DS, Godowski P, Zychlinsky A. The apoptotic signaling pathway activated by Toll-like receptor-2. EMBO J 2000;19:3325–3336.

45. Aliprantis AO, Yang RB, Mark MR, et al. Cell activation and apoptosis by bacterial lipoproteins through Toll-like receptor-2. Science 1999;285:736–739.

46. Salmeron JM, Barker SJ, Carland FM, Mehta AY, Staskawicz BJ. Tomato mutants altered in bacterial disease resistance provide evidence for a new locus controlling pathogen recognition. Plant Cell 1994;6:511–520.

47. Salmeron JM, Oldroyd GE, Rommens CM, et al. Tomato *Prf* is a member of the leucine-rich repeat class of plant disease resistance genes and lies embedded within the *Pto* kinase gene cluster. Cell 1996;86:123–133.

48. Inohara N, Ogura Y, Chen FF, Muto A, Nuñez G. Human Nod1 confers responsiveness to bacterial lipopolysaccharides. J Biol Chem 2001;276:2551–2554.

49. Loh YT, Zhou JM, Martin GB. The myristylation motif of Pto is not required for disease resistance. Mol Plant Microbe Interact 1998;11:572–576.

50. Loh YT, Martin GB. The disease-resistance gene *Pto* and the fenthion-sensitivity gene *Fen* encode closely related functional protein kinases. Proc Natl Acad Sci USA 1995;92:181–4184.

51. Rommens CMT, Salmeron JM, Baulcombe DC, Staskawicz BJ. Use of a gene expression system based on potato virus X to rapidly identify and characterize a tomato *Pto* homolog that controls fenthion sensitivity. Plant Cell 1995;7:249–257.

52. Salmeron JM, Staskawicz BJ. Molecular characterization and *hrp* dependence of the avirulence gene *avrPto* from *Pseudomonas syringae* pv. *tomato*. Mol Gen Genet 1993;239:6–16.

53. Shan LB, Thara VK, Martin GB, Zhou JM, Tang XY. The *Pseudomonas* AvrPto protein is differentially recognized by tomato and tobacco and is localized to the plant plasma membrane. Plant Cell 2000;12:2323–2337.

54. Lawrence GJ, Finnegan EJ, Ayliffe MA, Ellis JG. The *L6* gene for flax rust resistance is related to the *Arabidopsis* bacterial resistance gene *RPS2* and the tobacco viral resistance gene *N*. Plant Cell 1995;7:1195–1206.

55. Anderson PA, Lawrence GJ, Morrish BC, et al. Inactivation of the flax rust resistance gene *M* associated with loss of a repeated unit within the leucine-rich repeat coding region. Plant Cell 1997;9:641–651.

56. Bent AF, Kunkel BN, Dahlbeck D, et al. *RPS2* of *Arabidopsis thaliana:* a leucine-rich repeat class of disease resistance genes. Science 1994;265:1856–1860.

57. Mindrinos M, Katagiri F, Yu GL, Ausubel FM. The *A. thaliana* disease resistance gene *RPS2* encodes a protein containing a nucleotide-binding site and leucine-rich repeats. Cell 1994;78:1089–1099.

58. Simons G, Groenendijk J, Wijbrandi J, et al. Dissection of the *Fusarium I2* gene cluster in tomato reveals six homologs and one active gene copy. Plant Cell 1998;10:1055–1068.

59. Milligan SB, Bodeau J, Yaghoobi J, et al. The root knot nematode resistance gene *Mi* from tomato is a member of the leucine zipper, nucleotide binding, leucine-rich repeat family of plant genes. Plant Cell 1998;10:1307–1319.

60. Vos P, Simons G, Jesse T, et al. The tomato *Mi-1* gene confers resistance to both root-knot nematodes and potato aphids. Nature Biotechnol 1998;16:1365–1369.

61. Meyers BC, Chin DB, Shen KA, et al. The major resistance gene cluster in lettuce is highly duplicated and spans several megabases. Plant Cell 1998;10:1817–1832.

62. Meyers BC, Shen KA, Rohani P, Gaut B, Michelmore RW. Receptor-like genes in the major resistance locus of lettuce are subject to divergent selection. Plant Cell 1998;10:1833–1846.

63. Botella MA, Parker JE, Frost LN, et al. Three gene of the *Arabidopsis RPP1* complex resistance locus recognize distinct *Peronospora parasitica* avirulence determinants. Plant Cell 1998;10:1847–1860.

64. Grant MR, Godiard L, Straube E, et al. Structure of the *Arabidopsis RPM1* gene enabling dual specificity disease resistance. Science 1995;269:843–846.

65. Boyes DC, Nam J, Dangl JL. The *Arabidopsis thaliana RPM1* disease resistance gene product is a peripheral plasma membrane protein that is degraded coincident with the hypersensitive response. Proc Natl Acad Sci USA 1998;95:15849–15854.

66. Warren RF, Henk A, Mowery P, Holub E, Innes RW. A mutation within the leucine-rich repeat domain of the *Arabidopsis* disease resistance gene *RPS5* partially suppresses multiple bacterial and downy mildew resistance genes. Plant Cell 1998;10:1439–1452.

67. Tamaki S, Dahlbeck D, Staskawicz B, Keen NT. Characterization and expression of two avirulence genes cloned from *Pseudomonas syringae* pv. *glycinea*. J Bacteriol 1988;170:4846–4854.

68. Dangl JL, Ritter C, Gibbon MJ, et al. Functional homologs of the *Arabidopsis RPM1* disease resistance gene in bean and pea. Plant Cell 1992;4:1359–1369.

69. Jenner C, Hitchin E, Mansfield J, et al. Gene-for-gene interactions between *Pseudomonas syringae* pv. *phaseolicola* and *Phaseolus*. Mol Plant Microbe Interact 1991;4:553–562.

70. Nimchuk Z, Marois E, Kjemtrup S, et al. Eukaryotic fatty acylation drives plasma membrane targeting and enhances function of several type III effector proteins from *Pseudomonas syringae*. Cell 2000;101:353–363.

71. Schuler GD, Altschul SF, Lipman DJ. A workbench for multiple alignment construction and analysis. Protein Struct Funct Genet 1991;9:180–190.

72. Parniske M, Hammond-Kosack Ke, Goldstein C et al. Novel disease resistance specificities result from sequence exchange between tandemly repeated genes at the *Cf-4/9* locus of tomato. Cell 1997;91:821–832.

73. Noel L, Moores TL, van der Biezen EA, Pronounced intraspecific haplotype divergence at the *RPP5* complex disease resistance locus of *Arabidopsis*. Plant Cell 1999;11:2099–2112.

74. Collins N, Drake J, Ayliffe M, et al. Molecular characterisation of the maize *Rp1-D* rust resistance haplotype and its mutants. Plant Cell 1999;111:1365–1376.

75. Sun Q, Collins N, Ayliffe M, et al. Recombination between paralogues at the *Rp1* rust resistance locus in maize. Genetics 2001;158:423–438.

76. Ellis JG, Lawrence GJ, Luck JE, Dodds PN. Identification of regions in alleles of the flax rust resistance gene *L* that determine differences in gene-for-gene specificity. Plant Cell 1999;11:495–506.

77. Zhou F, Kurth J, Wei F, et al. Cell-autonomous expression of barley Mla1 confers race-specific resistance to the powdery mildew fungus via a rar1-independent signaling pathway. Plant Cell 2001;13:337–350.

78. Halterman D, Zhou F, Wei F, Wise RP, Schulze-Lefert P. The MLA6 coiled-coil, NBS-LRR protein confers AvrMla6-dependent resistance specificity to *BLumeria graminis* f. sp. *hordei* in barley and wheat. Plant J 2001;25:335–348.

79. Van der Hoorn RAL, Roth R, De Wit PJGM. Identification of distinct specificity determinants in resistance protein *cf-4* allows construction of a cf-9 mutant that confers recognition of avirulence protein avr4. Plant Cell 2001;13:273–285.

80. Wulff BBH, Thomas CM, Smoker M, Grant M, Jones JDG. Domain swapping and gene shuffling identify sequences required for induction of an avr-dependent hypersensitive response by the tomato cf-4 and cf-9 proteins. Plant Cell 2001;13:255–272.

81. Kobe B, Diesenhofer J. The leucine-rich repeat: a versatile binding motif. Trends Biol Sci 1994;19:415–421.

82. Dodds PN, Lawrence GJ, Ellis JG. Six amino acid changes confined to the leucine-rich repeat β-strand/β-turn motif determine the difference between the *P* and *P2* rust resistance specificities n flax. Plant Cell 2001;13:163–178.

83. Luck JE, Lawrence GJ, Dodds PN, Shepherd KW, Ellis JG. Regions outside of the leucine-rich repeats of flax rust resistance proteins have a role in specificity determination. Plant Cell 2000;12:1367–1378.

84. Hughes AL. Origin and evolution of HLA class-I pseudogenes. Mol Biol Evol 1995;12:247–258.

85. Dodds PN, Lawrence G, Pryor T, Ellis J. Genetic analysis and evolution of plant disease resistance genes. In: Dickinson M, Beynon J (eds.). Molecular Plant Pathology. Sheffield: Sheffield Academic Press, 2000, pp. 88–107.

86. Scofield SR, Tobias CM, Rathgen JP, et al. Molecular basis of gene-for-gene specificity on bacterial speck disease of tomato. Science 1996;274:2063–2065.

87. Tang X, Frederick RD, Zhou J, et al. Initiation of plant disease resistance by physical interaction of AvrPto and Pto kinase. Science 1996;274:2060–2063.

88. Jia Y, McAdams SA, Bryan GT, Hershey HP, Valent B. Direct interaction of resistance gene and avirulence gene products confers rice blast resistance. EMBO J 2000;19:4004–4014.

89. Leister RT, Katagiri F. A resistance gene product of the nucleotide binding site—leucine rich repeats class can form a complex with bacterial avirulence proteins *in vivo*. Plant J 2000;22:345–354.

90. van der Biezen EA, Jones JD. Plant disease-resistance proteins and the gene-for-gene concept. Trends Biochem Sci 1998;23:454–456.

3

Nonhost Resistance in Plants to Microbial Pathogens

Michèle C. Heath

1. INTRODUCTION

Like microbial parasites in general, microorganisms that cause disease in plants exhibit host specificity. Indeed, resistance to disease is the norm in plants, as any single microbial pathogen successfully infects only a small fraction of the approx 250,000 extant species of flowering plants. Disease resistance to a single pathogen may be exhibited by a complete plant species, in which case the species is considered a nonhost, or may be shown by only certain genotypes within what is otherwise considered a host species. This latter resistance is called host resistance and, as discussed below, how much it differs from nonhost resistance depends on which specific plant-pathogen combinations are being compared. For the purpose of this chapter, "pathogen" is used as a general term for a microorganism capable of causing a disease in at least one plant species.

In some cases, nonhost resistance to disease may involve features or life history characteristics that, in themselves, are not antimicrobial. However, such phenomena rarely totally account for the nonhost status of a plant species, and additional, antimicrobial, features are usually involved. Plants have a multitude of antimicrobial features, both constitutive and inducible, that could potentially confer disease resistance. Although there are common themes of defense among all plants, there are also differences between species, and sometimes between genotypes within species, in the structure, biochemical nature, and (for inducible defenses), the eliciting features of these defenses.

Pathogens are similarly diverse in their mode of infection and in the type of interaction that they have with their hosts. Fungal pathogens, which tend to predominate in terms of economically important diseases of crop plants, usually have a filamentous growth habit that gives them autonomous invasive capabilities lacking in bacteria or viruses. Bacteria, however, have the ability to inject materials directly into plant cells by type III secretion systems (1) and to exchange genetic material, (including pathogenicity factors) with each other relatively readily. Viruses, in contrast, are unlike either type of cellular pathogen in their need to commandeer the metabolic machinery of the host and in the common linkage of host range with the plant specificity of their vectors. These differences between pathogens makes it very likely that different plant defenses will be differentially effective against different types of

From: *Infectious Disease: Innate Immunity*
Edited by: R. A. B. Ezekowitz and J. A. Hoffmann © Humana Press Inc., Totowa, NJ

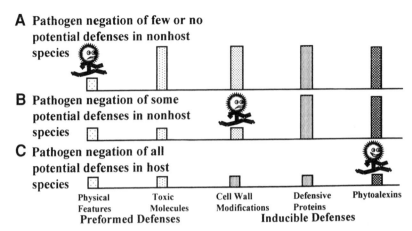

Fig. 1. Cartoon illustrating that a nonhost plant may have many (**A**) or few (**B**) effective defenses against a microbial pathogen, depending on how many defensive features in the plant the microorganism can overcome. In its host species (**C**), the pathogen can negate all potential defenses that it may encounter or elicit.

pathogens even though defensive plant responses are not generally "tailor-made" for a particular microorganism.

Given the ubiquity and multiplicity of antimicrobial features in plants, a successful pathogen must not only be adapted to obtain nutrients from its host species, but must also be able to overcome the multiple defensive "hurdles" that it would normally encounter or elicit (2,3) (Fig. 1C). The corollary of this is that a nonhost plant may have a number of effective defenses against a particular pathogen so that eliminating only one of them may not appreciably affect resistance. In a nonhost species for which a pathogen has few or no successful pathogenicity factors, the number of effective defenses may be large (4) (Fig. 1A). However, one can envisage situations in which the pathogen may be adapted to defensive features shared by both by host and nonhost species, so that the number of effective defenses left in the nonhost is small (4) (Fig. 1B) and more easily investigated.

This is probably the case for many of the examples of nonhost resistance in which single defensive features, or single eliciting molecules, have been identified. Such may be the case in the interaction between an oomycete potato pathogen and one particular nonhost species in which nonhost resistance is lost if the pathogen does not produce a single cell death-eliciting protein (5). However, the interpretation of this particular example is complicated by the fact that, in some plant-pathogen interactions, resistance is governed by plant resistance genes involved in the recognition of molecules from specific pathogens. Such recognition leads to the activation of the same inducible defenses that can be elicited nonspecifically by a variety of stresses and pathogen activities. This type of recognition (governed by *gene-for-gene interactions* involving *matching* of an avirulence gene in the pathogen with a resistance gene in the plant) is most common in host resistance (*see* Chapters 1 and 2), but evidence is accumulating that it may also be involved in some forms of nonhost resistance.

Whether the potato pathogen-nonhost interaction mentioned above involves a gene-for-gene interaction remains to be determined, but demonstrated gene-for-gene interactions resulting in visible and localized plant cell death (the hypersensitive response)

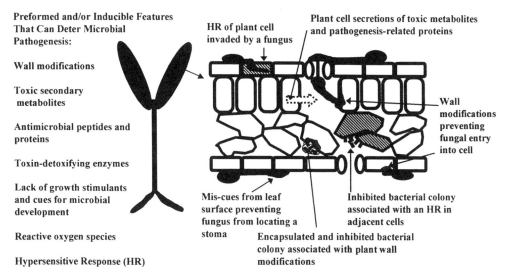

Preformed and/or Inducible Features That Can Deter Microbial Pathogenesis:

Wall modifications

Toxic secondary metabolites

Antimicrobial peptides and proteins

Toxin-detoxifying enzymes

Lack of growth stimulants and cues for microbial development

Reactive oxygen species

Hypersensitive Response (HR)

HR of plant cell invaded by a fungus

Plant cell secretions of toxic metabolites and pathogenesis-related proteins

Wall modifications preventing fungal entry into cell

Mis-cues from leaf surface preventing fungus from locating a stoma

Encapsulated and inhibited bacterial colony associated with plant wall modifications

Inhibited bacterial colony associated with an HR in adjacent cells

Fig. 2. Summary of preformed and/or inducible features in plants that can potentially play a role in defense against microorganism-induced disease. How some of these features interact with a pathogen on a cellular level is shown in the diagrammatic cross-section of a leaf shown on the right.

seem particularly common in nonhost-bacteria interactions *(6,7)*. However, it has been pointed out that the abolition of this recognition and the hypersensitive response often does not abolish nonhost resistance *(8,9)* indicating either that this recognition is a non-functional evolutionary legacy of avirulences genes inherited from the pathogen's ancestors or that it controls only one of several effective nonhost defenses.

This review focuses on the types of nonhost resistance that probably do not involve specific parasite recognition. However, it must be pointed out that in most examples of nonhost resistance in which inducible defenses are involved, there is little or no hard evidence to indicate whether or not these defenses are the result of nonspecific elicitation, or the result of a specific recognition event controlled by a parasite-specific resistance gene. It also has been difficult to determine which of the many defenses elicited during host or nonhost resistance are actually responsible for the restriction of pathogen growth. Only recently have studies using plants genetically compromised in specific types of defenses begun to unequivocally reveal their role in particular plant-pathogen interactions *(10–12)*. Figure 2 is a simplified diagrammatic summary of some of the features that may contribute to nonhost resistance and that are discussed below.

2. PREFORMED DEFENSES INVOLVED IN NONHOST RESISTANCE

2.1. Defensive Plant Features That Are Not Inherently Antimicrobial

Plants otherwise susceptible to certain fungal diseases can avoid them by, for example, changes in flowering times *(13)* or the presence of physical barriers to infection such as bud scales *(14)*. How prevalent such phenomena are in determining nonhost resistance in plants is unknown, but one might expect such features to be the first of several defensive features that face a nonadapted pathogen. It has been well documented that some species of rust fungi respond to topographic cues from their host species in order to locate the stomatal pores through which they enter the leaf *(15)*. On nonhost species with significantly different surface topographies, incorrect responses of the fungus can result in very few fungal individuals gaining entry into the nonhost tissue, and these then succumb to successful inducible defenses *(15)*. For bacteria and fungi that lack the capability of breaching outer epidermal cells walls and normally enter through wounds, the mere presence of an intact epidermal cell surface in both host or nonhost plants can be an effective defense irrespective of whether or not the pathogen can overcome defenses encountered within the plant.

2.2. Plant Features That Are Potentially Antimicrobial

Plants contain a number of constitutive components that are potentially toxic or inhibitory to microbes or herbivores, and such antimicrobial compounds are known as phytoanticipins *(16)*. Seeds tend to be particularly well endowed with physical barriers (hard seed coat impregnated with substances resistant to microbial degradation), toxic secondary metabolites *(17)*, and proteinaceous compounds such as lectins *(18)*, cysteine-rich antimicrobial peptides resembling defensins found in insects and mammals *(19,20)*, antifungal lipid-transfer proteins *(21)*, and proteinase inhibitors *(22)* that can interfere with pathogen growth. Constitutive antimicrobial materials in other plant parts include potentially antiviral proteins *(23)*, antifungal lipid transfer proteins *(24)*, proteinaceous inhibitors of pathogen enzymes *(25)*, and secondary metabolites, such as alkaloids, cyanogenic glycosides, sesquiterpenes, and isoflavonoids *(17)*. Some secondary metabolites require the action of plant hydrolytic enzymes to release the antimicrobial agent from an inactive conjugate and often they, or the hydrolytic enzymes, are stored in the plant vacuole so that they are not released until the plant cell is damaged *(17)*. Others impregnate cell walls and may inhibit fungal penetration into the cell *(26)*. Interestingly, most phytoanticipins, including peptide defensins *(19)*, tend to have a greater effect on fungi than on bacteria. An exception is a recently discovered antimicrobial compound in strawberry with a particularly high antibacterial activity *(27)*.

Although it is reasonable to assume that these antimicrobial compounds play a role in the nonhost resistance of plants to microbial pathogens, unequivocal proof is rare. Evidence suggesting that secondary metabolites contribute to plant defense include the enhanced disease susceptibility of maize mutants defective in the ability to synthesize 2,4-dihydroxy-1,4-benzoxazin-3-one *(28)* and of tobacco plants with reduced accumulations of phenypropanoids *(10)*. Perhaps the best example of a clear role of preformed toxic metabolites in nonhost resistance comes from the study of saponin-deficient mutants in oats. These mutants are susceptible to a fungal pathogen that is normally a pathogen of wheat roots *(12)*. Significantly, saponin deficiency does not increase susceptibility to a leaf-infecting nonpathogen of oat, illustrating the need for experimental evidence to reveal which of a plant's battery of defensive features are effective in a given example of nonhost resistance.

2.3. Lack of Growth Stimulants or Nutrients

The concept that disease susceptibility is correlated with the presence of plant compounds that fulfill some nutrient requirement for the pathogen has generally not been supported by experimental evidence, not even for obligately parasitic fungi that cannot be grown away from the living plant *(15)*. However, the notable exception is the case of the susceptibility of wheat anthers to the fungus *Fusarium graminearum,* which correlates with the presence of choline and betaine in this tissue *(29)*. Presumably, resistance to this fungus in other parts of the wheat plant, and in nonhost plant species, is at least partly owing to the absence of these substances.

2.4. Enzymes That Detoxify Pathogen Toxins

The successful pathogenicity of a number of bacterial and fungal pathogens depends, in part, on the killing the plant tissue with toxins. There are at least two known examples in which the nonhost resistance of plants to toxin-producing fungi seems associated with the ability of the plant species to detoxify the toxin enzymatically. Cereals other than maize have been suggested to owe part of their resistance to a corn pathogen to the presence of a toxin-detoxifying enzyme *(30)*, and resistance of a white mustard to a pathogen of rapeseed has similarly been associated with the rapid metabolism of the toxin to a less toxic product *(31)*. However, insensitivity to microbial toxins cannot account for all examples of nonhost resistance to toxin-producing pathogens, as there are examples of nonhost species that are sensitive to fungal toxins but are still nonhosts to the pathogens that produces them *(32)*

3. INDUCIBLE DEFENSIVE RESPONSES IN PLANTS

Plants are extraordinarily sensitive to their environment and have a large battery of potentially defensive responses that can be triggered by abiotic and biotic stresses. Different stresses may trigger different subsets of these responses, but there can be considerable overlap between responses to stresses (such as drought, wounding, or herbivory damage) and responses to pathogens. Unlike the situation in insects, in which a given class of pathogen results in the preferential elicitation of appropriate antimicrobial peptides *(33)*, there is little evidence to suggest that plants modify their responses to make them more applicable to the invading microorganism. Pathogen components such as peptides, glycoproteins, unsaturated fatty acids, or oligosaccharides may trigger defensive responses *(34)*, as may plant molecules that are released during the pathogen invasion *(35)*. These "nonspecific" elicitors are commonly active in a wide range of plant species irrespective of whether the plant is a host or nonhost of the pathogen, and they trigger a wide array of defensive responses. It seems reasonable to assume that this nonspecific elicitation of defenses plays a role in many examples of nonhost resistance and that being able to suppress, detoxify, or otherwise negate these defenses in its host is an important component of the pathogenicity factors of a pathogen. The rest of this section describes the main categories of inducible defensive responses that have so far been documented in plants.

3.1. Defensive Responses Associated with the Plant Wall

Rapid and localized responses associated with plant cell walls are a common response to nonspecific elicitors, the introduction of bacteria into the intracellular spaces of a plant, and attempts by fungi to breach the wall physically. These responses include the generation of reactive oxygen species via a plasma membrane-located reduced nicotinamide adeninedinucleotide phosphate (NADPH) oxidase system analogous to that of mammalian phagocytes, or via enzymes such as peroxidases or amine oxidases within the plant wall *(36)*. Other wall-associated responses include the "toughening" of the wall through the crosslinking of structural proteins *(37)* and the impregnation of the wall with potentially antimicrobial phenolic compounds *(38)* and/or impermeable and degradation-resistant compounds such as lignin *(38)* and silica *(39)*. Localized changes within the wall are usually accompanied by the deposition of the wound-response carbohydrate callose between the wall and the plasma membrane to form a hemispherical papilla that usually becomes impregnated with other compounds such as phenolics or silica *(39,40)*.

The role of such wall-associated responses in nonhost resistance has been best studied for fungal pathogens that attempt, and fail, to penetrate epidermal cell walls. Papillae have been associated with this penetration failure in grasses inoculated with a variety of pathogens for which they are nonhosts, but the components within them that stop fungal growth have not been identified *(26)*. Papillae and wall modifications may also be induced in cells other than epidermal cells if the pathogen enters the intercellular spaces of the plant, and one example of nonhost resistance has been attributed to silica deposits in walls adjacent to the extracellular fungus that prevent the formation of intracellular fungal feeding structures *(39)*. However, wall modifications adjacent to bacterial colonies in the plant's intercellular spaces may not have a role in nonhost resistance as the bacteria do not try to breach the plant wall and resistance may be related to the encapsulation of the bacteria in an extracellular matrix *(40)*. Phenolic compounds within modified walls and papillae are widely assumed to have defensive roles, but in vitro studies show that their antifungal and antibacterial activities differ for different compounds *(41)*, and in at least one situation, their primary role may be to foster the precipitation of silica *(39)*. Hydrogen peroxide generation has recently been implicated in the inhibition of fungal growth within the plant wall in nonhost interactions involving rust and powdery mildew fungi *(42)*,

3.2. Antimicrobial Secondary Metabolites

Every flowering plant appears to be able to accumulate low molecular weight, antimicrobial compounds locally at the sites of attempted pathogen invasion. These *phytoalexins* tend to fall within the same chemical class within plant families, but a wide range of compounds including phenylpropanoid derivatives, sesquiterpenes, and polyketides, involving several biosynthetic pathways, can be found among various plant groups *(43)*. In addition to phytoalexins, which by definition are generally not detectable in uninfected plants, some preformed antimicrobial secondary metabolites also increase in concentration following infection. Phytoalexin accumulation is typically elicited by nonspecific elicitors *(35)*, and it seems reasonable to assume that they play a role in at least some examples of nonhost resistance, particularly when the pathogen cannot detoxify or otherwise tolerate the compounds. Nevertheless, a role may not be universal, as a phytoalexin-deficient mutant of the weed *Arabidopsis* does not become more susceptible to a rust fungus for which it is a nonhost (Mellersh and Heath, unpublished data) or other bacterial or fungal pathogens for which the plant is either a nonhost or resistant host *(44)*.

3.3. Pathogenesis-Related Peptides and Proteins

In plants resistant to a particular pathogen, a variety of novel proteins and peptides are synthesized after infection that are collectively known as *pathogenesis-related pro-*

teins (PRs). Generally these not only accumulate at the infection site but are also induced systemically in association with increased resistance of uninfected parts of the plant to further microbial attack. A large number of classes are recognized that include the peptide plant defensins and lipid transfer proteins, proteinase inhibitors, and enzymes such as glucanases, chitinases, and peroxidases *(45)*. It has recently become apparent that PRs play diverse roles in plant that may not be restricted to plant defense. Some occur constitutively, often in the plant vacuole and in specific cell types or organs, some seem essential for morphogenesis, and others accumulate extracellularly and exhibit antifreeze activity. Commonly those PRs that are induced by pathogen infection are secreted into the cell wall or extracellular spaces of the tissue *(45)*. Although antimicrobial activity has been demonstrated for many PRs *(45)*, a clear role in nonhost resistance has not yet been proved. Nevertheless, the fact that their induction seems to be the culmination of signaling pathways (discussed below) involved in inducible plant responses makes it likely that they play a significant role in at least some forms of nonhost resistance.

3.4. The Hypersensitive Response

A common expression of host resistance controlled by gene-for-gene interactions is the rapid and localized death of plant cells in association with the restriction of pathogen growth, a phenomenon known as the *hypersensitive response* (HR). As cell death, in itself, is not a defense mechanism against most microbial pathogens, the restriction of pathogen growth is usually attributed to the antimicrobial environment that develops within and around the dead cells through the accumulation of phytoalexins and other inducible antimicrobial compounds *(46)*. The HR appears to be a form of programmed cell death that has some similarity to mammalian apoptosis, although many of the genes critical to this process in mammals have no homology in plants *(46)*.

The role of the HR in nonhost resistance is more equivocal than it is in host resistance. Although there is good evidence that an HR is responsible for nonhost resistance in one plant-pathogen combination *(5)*, nonhost resistance to fungi often does not involve an HR unless the fungus penetrates plant cells *(47)*. An HR more commonly accompanies nonhost resistance to bacteria *(48)*, but in some situations the HR may be eliminated without compromising this resistance (*see* Introduction). The elicitation of defense responses in the absence of an HR has been demonstrated for mutant bacterial pathogens and for nonphytopathogenic bacteria, suggesting that these, rather than (or as well as) the HR, may be important in nonhost resistance to bacteria *(49)*

4. SIGNAL TRANSDUCTION INVOLVED IN INDUCIBLE DEFENSES

As discussed above, inducible defenses in nonhost plants are likely to be triggered by nonspecific elicitors released either from the pathogen or from the plant as a result of pathogen activities. In general, the putative receptors that have been isolated for such nonspecific elicitors are located in membranes, most likely the plasma membrane *(34,35,50)*. Binding of an elicitor to a receptor does not, however, always lead to a plant response, as there is one example of a proteinaceous elicitor that only induces cell death in tobacco, although binding sites have also been found in plant species in which the elicitor seems inactive *(51)*. This plasma membrane location of receptors of nonspecific elicitors contrasts with the common cytoplasmic location of host resistance gene products involved in the perception of specific avirulence gene products of a pathogen *(52)*. There may be some overlap in the type of receptors involved in host and nonhost resistance, however, as the perception of flagellin, a bacterial nonspecific elicitor, involves a leucine rich repeat receptor-like kinase similar to one type of resistance gene product involved in gene-for-gene recognition *(53)*. In an evolutionary context, it is interesting that other host resistance genes in plants code for proteins with a Toll/interleukin-1 receptor domain *(52)* resembling that of *Drosophila* Toll proteins and related receptors in mammals *(33)* that are central to nonspecific defense against bacteria and fungi.

Perhaps not surprisingly, given the fact that host and nonhost resistance are accompanied by the same types of inducible responses, similar signaling systems are activated by nonspecific elicitors or the avirulence gene products ("specific elicitors") that trigger resistance controlled by host resistance genes. These appear to involve ion fluxes similarly across the plasma membrane *(35)* and to trigger signal cascades involving protein kinases, elements of the mitogen-activated protein kinase pathway and protein phosphatases *(54)*.

Recent genetic analysis of plant mutants impaired in exhibiting host resistance has revealed a number of interconnecting signaling pathways involving small signaling molecules such as salicylic acid, jasmonic acid, and ethylene *(55,56)*. Despite some crosstalk, each pathway is associated with certain types of inducible defenses, although phytoalexin accumulation in *Arabidopsis* seems to involve none of these pathways *(11)*. As yet, these signaling pathway mutants have not been exploited much for studies of nonhost resistance, but the available data suggest that the salicylic acid pathway is involved in at least some examples (e.g., ref. 9) and ethylene production in others *(57)*. Consistent with the idea that host and nonhost resistance share signaling pathways and inducible defenses, a gene that is required for both host and nonhost resistance to *Pseudomonas* bacteria has recently been identified in *Arabidopsis (9)*.

5. GENE SILENCING

The resistance of totally symptomless nonhost plants to plant pathogenic viruses has rarely been studied directly and, therefore, the mechanisms of resistance are generally unknown. However, a plant feature that has been suggested to be an effective defense against virus infection is an RNA-mediated defense resembling the posttranscriptional gene silencing that is commonly seen in transgenic plants *(58)* and that has phenomenologic similarities in fungi and animals. Suppression of this gene silencing has been suggested to be a widespread strategy for pathogenicity among plant viruses, and it is possible that nonhost species are those for which this suppression by a particular virus is ineffective *(58)*. In support of this hypothesis, mutations in genes that control gene silencing in *Arabidopsis* enhance susceptibility to virus infection *(59)*.

6. CONCLUSIONS

Nonhost resistance in plants to microbial pathogens has been difficult to study because it is frequently multicomponent and multigenically controlled. An additional problem is that effective defenses vary with the pathogen and the plant, and it has been difficult to pick out effective defensive features from the ineffective ones that the plant may be expressing at the same time. Mutational studies, particularly with the model plant, *Arabidopsis,* have now made it possible to explore signaling pathways involved in inducible defensive features and have started to provide unequivocal information on which features are responsible for the cessation of pathogen growth in a given situation. Although studies of nonhost resistance have lagged behind host resistance, the fact that nonhost resistance is the most ubiquitous and most stable form of disease resistance in plants makes it important to understand so that its principles may be applied to future disease control in crop plants *(8).*

REFERENCES

1. He SY. Type III protein secretion systems in plant and animal pathogenic bacteria. Annu Rev Phytopathol 1998;36:363–392.
2. Heath MC. Evolution of plant resistance and susceptibility to fungal parasites. In: Carroll G, Tudzynski P (eds.). The Mycota, vol V. Plant Relationships. New York: Springer, 1997, pp. 257–276.
3. Heath MC. A generalised concept of host-parasite specificity. Phytopathology 1981;71:1121–1123.
4. Heath MC. Implications of non-host resistance for understanding host-parasite interactions. In: Groth JV, Bushnell WR (eds). Genetic Basis of Biochemical Mechanisms of Disease. St Paul, MN: APS Press, 1985, pp. 25–42.
5. Kamoun S, van West P, Vleeshouwers VGAA, de Groot KE, Govers F. Resistance of *Nicotiana benthamiana* to *Phytophthora infestans* is mediated by the recognition of the elicitor protein INF1. Plant Cell 1998;10:1413–1425.
6. Whalen MC, Stall RE, Staskawicz BJ. Characterization of a gene from a tomato pathogen determining hypersensitive resistance in non-host species and genetic analysis of this resistance in bean. Proc Natl Acad Sci USA 1988;85:6743–6747.
7. Kobayashi DY, Tamaki SJ, Keen NT. Cloned avirulence genes from the tomato pathogen *Pseudomonas syringae* pv. *tomato* confer cultivar specificity on soybean. Proc Natl Acad Sci USA 1990;86:157–161.
8. Heath MC. Non-host resistance to plant pathogens: nonspecific defense or the result of specific recognition events? Physiol Mol Plant Pathol 2001;58:53–54.
9. Lu M, Tang X, Zhou J-M. Arabidopsis *NHO1* is required for general resistance against *Pseudomonas* bacteria. Plant Cell 2001;13:437–447.
10. Maher EA, Bate NJ, Ki W, et al. Increased disease susceptibility of transgenic tobacco plants with suppressed levels of preformed phenylpropanoid products. Proc Natl Acad Sci USA 1994;91:7802–7806.
11. Thomma BPHJ, Nelissen I, Eggermont K, Broekaert WF. Deficiency in phytoalexin production causes enhanced susceptibility of *Arabidopsis thaliana* to the fungus *Alternaria brassicicola.* Plant J 1999;19:163–171.
12. Papadopoulou K, Melton RE, Leggett M, Daniels MJ, Osbourn AE. Compromised disease resistance in saponin-deficient plants. Proc Natl Acad Sci USA 1999;96:12923–12928.
13. Alexander HM, Thrall PH, Antonovics J, Jarosz AM, Oudemans PV. Population dynamics and genetics of plant disease: a case study of anther-smut disease. Ecology 1996;77:990–996.
14. Parker MA. 1988. Genetic uniformity and disease resistance in a clonal plant. Am Nat 1988;132:538–549.
15. Heath MC. Signal exchange between higher plants and rust fungi. Can J Bot 1995;73(suppl. 1):S616–S623.
16. Van Etten HD, Mansfield JW, Bailey JA, Farmer EE. Letter to the editor. Two classes of plant antibiotics: phytoalexins versus "phytoanticipins." Plant Cell 1994;6:1191–1192.
17. Osbourn AE. Preformed antimicrobial compounds and plant defense against fungal attack. Plant Cell 1996;8:1821–1831.

18. Gomes VM, Mosqueda M-I, Blanco-Labra A, et al. Vicilin storage proteins from *Vigna unguiculata* (legume) seeds inhibit fungal growth. J Agric Food Chem 1997;45:4110–4115.

19. Broekaert WF, Terras FRG, Cammune BPA, Osborn RW. Plant defensins: novel antimicrobial peptides as components of the host defense system. Plant Physiol 1995;108:1353–1358.

20. Almeida MS, Cabral KMS, Zingali RB, Kurtenbach E. Characterization of two novel defense peptides from pea *(Psium sativum)* seeds. Arch Biochem Biphys 2000;378:278–286.

21. Regente MC, de la Canal L. Purification, characterization and antifungal properties of a lipid-transfer protein from sunflower *(Helianthus annuus)* seeds. Physiol Plant 2000;110:158–163.

22. Joshi BN, Sainani MN, Bastawade KB, Gupta VS, Ranjekar PK. Cysteine protease inhibitor from pearl millet: a new class of antifungal protein. Biochem Biophys Res Commun 1998;246:382–387.

23. Wang P, Zoubenko O, Tumer NE. 1998. Reduced toxicity and broad spectrum resistance to viral and fungal infection in transgenic plants expressing pokeweed antiviral protein II. Plant Mol Biol 1998;38:957–964.

24. Kristensen AK, Brunstedt J, Nielsen KK, Roepstorff P, Mikkelsen JD. Characterization of a new antifungal non-specific lipid transfer protein (nsLTP) from sugar beet leaves. Plant Science 2000;155:31–40.

25. Stotz HU, Bishop JG, Bergmann CW, et al. Identification of target amino acids that affect interactions of fungal polygalacturonases and their plant inhibitors. Physiol Mol Plant Pathol 2000;56:117–130.

26. Sherwood RT, Vance CP. Resistance to fungal penetration in Gramineae. Phytopathology 1980;70:273–279.

27. Filippone MP, Ricci JD, de Marchese AM, Farias RN, Castagnaro A. Isolation and purification of a 316 Da preformed compound from strawberry *(Fragaria ananassa)* leaves active against plant pathogens. FEBS Lett 1999;459:115–118.

28. Frey M, Chomet P, Glawischnig E, et al. Analysis of a chemical plant defense mechanism in grasses. Science 1997;277:696.

29. Strange RN, Majer JR, Smith H. The isolation and identification of choline and betaine as the two major components in anthers and wheat germ that stimulate *Fusarium graminearum* in vitro. Physiol Plant Pathol 1974;4:277–290.

30. Meeley RB, Johal GS, Briggs SP, Walton JD. A biochemical phenotype of a disease resistance gene of maize. Plant Cell 1992;4:71–77.

31. Pedras MSC, Zaharia IL, Gai Y, Zhou Y, Ward DE. 2001. *In planta* sequential hydroxylation and glycosylation of a fungal phytotoxin: avoiding cell death and overcoming the fungal invader. Proc Natl Acad Sci USA 2001;98:747–752.

32. Brandwagt BF, Kneppers TJA, Van der Weerden GM, Nijkamp HJJ, Hille J. Most AAL toxin-sensitive *Nicotiana* species are resistant to the tomato fungal pathogen *Alternaria alternata* f. sp. *lycopersici.* Mol Plant Microbe Interact 2001;4:460–470.

33. Janeway CA Jr, Medzhitov R. Innate immunity: lipoproteins take their Toll on the host. Curr Biol 1999;9:R879–R882.

34. Hahn MG. Microbial elicitors and their receptors in plants. Annu Rev Phytopathol 1996;34:387–412.

35. Ebel J, Cosio EG. Elicitors of plant defense responses. Int Rev Cytol 1994;148:1–36.

36. Bolwell GP, Wojtaszek P. Mechanisms for the generation of reactive oxygen species in plant defence—a broad perspective. Physiol Mol Plant Pathol 1997;51:347–366.

37. Brisson LF, Tenhaken R, Lamb C. Function of oxidative cross-linking of cell wall structural proteins in plant disease resistance. Plant Cell 1994;6:1703–1712.

38. Nicholson RL, Hammerschmidt R. Phenolic compounds and their role in disease resistance. Annu Rev Phytopathol 1992;30:369–389.

39. Perumalla CJ, Heath MC. The effect of inhibitors of various cellular processes on the wall modifications induced in bean leaves by the cowpea rust fungus. Physiol Mol Plant Pathol 1991;38:293–300.

40. Brown I, Trethowan J, Kerry M, Mansfield JM, Bolwell GP. Localization of components of the oxidative cross-linking of glycoproteins and of callose synthesis in papillae formed during the interaction between non-pathogenic strains of *Xanthomonas campestris* and French bean mesophyll cells. Plant 1998;15:333–343.

41. Barber MS, McConnell VS, DeCaux BS. Antimicrobial intermediates of the general phenylpropanoid and lignin specific pathways. Phytochemistry 2000;54:53–56.

42. Mellersh DG, Foulds IV, Higgins VJ, Heath MC. H_2O_2 plays different roles in determining penetration failure in three diverse plant-fungal interactions. Plant J 2002;29:257–268.

43. Hammerschmidt R. Phytoalexins: what have we learned after 60 years? Annu Rev Phytopathol 1999;37:285–306.

44. Glazebrook J, Zook M, Mert F, et al. Phytoalexin-deficient mutants of *Arabidopsis* reveal that PAD4 encodes a regulatory factor and that four PAD genes contribute to downy mildew resistance. Genetics 1997;46:381–392.

45. van Loon LC, van Strien EA. The families of pathogenesis-related proteins, their activities, and comparative analysis of PR-1 type proteins. Physiol Mol Plant Pathol 1999;55:85–97.

46. Heath MC. Hypersensitive response-related death. Plant Mol Biol 2000;44:321–334.

47. Fernandez MR, Heath MC. Cytological responses induced by five phytopathogenic fungi in a nonhost plant *Phaseolus vulgaris*. Can J Bot 1986;64:648–657.

48. Goodman RN, Novacky AJ. The hypersensitive reaction in plants to pathogens. St Paul, MN: APS Press, 1994.

49. Lindgren PB. The role of *hrp* genes during plant-bacterial interactions. Annu Rev Phytopathol 1997;35:129–152.

50. Meindl T, Boller T, Felix G. The bacterial elicitor flagellin activates its receptor in tomato cells according to the address-message concept. Plant Cell 2000;12:1783–1794.

51. Bourque S, Binet M-N, Ponchet M, Pugin A, Lebrun-Garcia A. Characterization of the cryptogein binding sites on plant plasma membranes. J Biol Chem 1999;274:34699–34705.

52. Staskawicz BJ. Genetics of plant-pathogen interactions specifying plant disease resistance. Plant Physiol 2001;125:73–76.

53. Gómez-Gómez L, Boller T. FLS2: an LRR receptor-like kinase involved in the perception of the bacterial elicitor flagellin in *Arabidopsis*. Mol Cell 2000;5:1003–1011.

54. Heath MC. Nonhost resistance and nonspecific plant defenses. Curr Opin Plant Biol 2000;3:315–319.

55. Freys BJ, Parker JE. Interplay of signaling pathways in plant disease resistance. Trends Genet 2000;16:449–455.

56. Thomma BPHJ, Penninckx IAMA, Broekaert WF, Cammune BPA. The complexity of disease signaling in *Arabidopsis*. Curr Opin Immunol 2001;13:63–68.

57. Knoester M, van Loon LC, van den Heuvel J, et al. Ethylene-insensitive tobacco lacks nonhost resistance against soil-borne fungi. Proc Natl Acad Sci USA 1998;95:1933–1937.

58. Voinnet O, Pinto YM, Baulcombe DC. Suppression of gene silencing: a general strategy used by diverse DNA and RNA viruses of plants. Proc Natl Acad Sci USA 1999;96:14147–14152.

59. Mourrain P, Béclin C, Elmayan T, et al. *Arabidopsis SGS2* and *SGS3* genes are required for post-transcriptional gene silencing and natural virus resistance. Cell 2000;101:533–542.

Section II
Invertebrate Host Defense Immunity
Section Editor: Jean-Marc Reichhart

O
ver the last ten years, our understanding of the innate immune system has changed so rapidly that we need to pause in order to integrate the wealth of data appearing on an almost daily basis. *Innate Immunity* gives us an excellent opportunity to review the findings of the last few years before continuing with this adventure.

The adaptive immune system arose in the chordate assemblage of the Deuterostomes with the appearance, in the first jawed Vertebrates, of *RAG* genes allowing for somatic recombination in B and T lymphocytes and leading to antigen–dependent immune memory. The adaptive immune system exists in Vertebrates, entangled in a complex network of interactions with the innate immune system. In all other Metazoans, the defense mechanisms are purely innate. Chapter 4 of this section by Rothenberg and Davidson delineates the origins and frontiers of these two systems, shedding light on the defense mechanisms in one of the earliest emerging groups of Deuterostomes, the echinoderms. As this immune system is cellular, the reader will have a transcription factor-based evolutionary description of the development of the different cell types in the adaptive and innate immune systems.

The knowledge that we have on the protostoman immune systems is restricted to the ecdysozoan arthropods. More precisely, we have information on two systems: the holometabolous dipteran insects *Drosophila* and *Anopheles* and the cheliceratan merostomata, *Tachypleus*. Chapter 6 is a review of the wonderful work conducted over the last 20 years by Iwanaga and his group, which has led to the almost complete dissection of the cellular immune response of the horseshoe crab. For the dipteran insects, several laboratories have been working on their humoral response. This began with the purification and cloning of the effector molecules of the humoral response, the antimicrobial peptides, which are reviewed in Chapter 5 by Bulet et al. These peptides are

From: *Infectious Disease: Innate Immunity*
Edited by: R. A. B. Ezekowitz and J. A. Hoffmann © Humana Press Inc., Totowa, NJ

mainly synthesized in the insect fat body. This work followed the elucidation of the control of expression of the genes encoding these peptides as reviewed in Chapter 8 by Royet et al.

The pathways leading to the induction of the antimicrobial peptide genes are themselves activated by a recognition process. This process takes place outside the fat body effector cells and is mediated by Pattern Recognition Receptors (PRR) binding to microbial molecular patterns. Rämet et al. discuss the possible PRRs in *Drosophila* in Chapter 7. As a sign of the speed with which new information becomes available, four important publications have appeared since this chapter was written. It is shown that the Gram-negative bacteria perception process requires a specific peptidoglycan recognition protein *(1,2,3)* that is different from the molecule needed to recognize Gram-positive bacteria *(4)*. However, fungal recognition still awaits its receptor.

In insects, we know much less about the cellular arm of host defense. However, the recent discovery of a prototypical innate immune component related to the complement system, has led Levashina et al. to write on the Thio-ester containing proteins secreted by the *Anopheles* and *Drosophila* hemocytes in Chapter 9.

The data reviewed in this section shows that we have made tremendous progress, but also that we still lack crucial information on antimicrobial responses in a major group of Metazoans, the Lophotrochozoa. With the knowledge of the immune system in annelids or molluscs, we should be able to reconstruct an image of the ancestral defense mechanism through comparison of extant innate immune systems and careful evaluation of their possible homologous characters. Only then, will we be able to understand how this system evolved independently in each of these different groups and thus be able to give us the present complex picture. In conclusion, I would like to paraphrase the sentence of J. Monod by saying that "What is true for arthropods is true for elephants, only more so".

Jean-Marc Reichhart

1. Rämet M, Manfruelli P, Pearson A, Mathey-Prevot B, Ezekowitz, RA. Functional genomic analysis of phagocytosis and identification of a *Drosophila* receptor for *E. coli*. Nature 2002; 416:644-8.
2. Gottar M,. Gobert V, Michel T, et al. The *Drosophila* immune response against Gram-negative bacteria is mediated by a peptidoglycan recognition protein. Nature 2002; 416:640-4.
3. Choe KM, Werner T, Stoven S, Hultmark D, Anderson KV. Requirement for a peptidoglycan recognition protein (PGRP) in Relish activation and antibacterial immune responses in *Drosophila*. Science 2002; 296:359-62.
4. Michel T, Reichhart JM, Hoffmann JA, Royet J. *Drosophila* Toll is activated by Gram-positive bacteria through a circulating peptidoglycan recognition protein. Nature 2001;414:756-9.

4

Regulatory Co-options in the Evolution of Deuterostome Immune Systems

Ellen V. Rothenberg and Eric H. Davidson

1. INTRODUCTION

Nowhere can Archimedes' famous dictum, that to move the Earth one would need only a foot of ground somewhere else to stand on, be more aptly cited than in evolutionary bioscience. To understand where our own working systems come from, we must examine equivalent systems in animals that are not ourselves but that are of known evolutionary relationship to us. If the other species are wisely chosen, and if we know enough, then by logic the characteristics of the ancestral states will fall out, and at least the main steps in the evolutionary construction of our own divergence from these ancestors can be understood. As yet we clearly do not know nearly enough to do this for the evolution of innate immune systems in the deuterostomes, the subject of this chapter. However, it is possible to make a start: several recent observations on the workings of the innate immune system in a distantly related deuterostome animal, the sea urchin, prove immensely interesting when viewed comparatively with respect to the innate immune systems of vertebrates. In this chapter we have focused on the evolution of the gene regulatory foundations on which the very different innate immune systems of these different animals are built. Everything in this argument rests on the phylogeny of the deuterostomes, which determines the topography of the tree that organizes the currently extant deuterostomes in respect to their similarities and differences, and from which their ancestral relations are deduced. So it is with a brief reprise of deuterostome phylogeny that we begin.

2. PHYLOGENY

2.1. Molecular Phylogeny

The concept of the deuterostome clade was put forward in 1908 by Grobben, on the basis of perceived anatomic homologies between the embryos of "lower" deuterostomes. The most important feature in the classical analysis was the developmental fate of the embryonic blastopore, which in invertebrate deuterostomes can be seen to give rise to the anus of the completed embryo, whereas in (some) protostomes it becomes the mouth, or is at least situated near the site of the mouth. A number of other striking homologies

From: *Infectious Disease: Innate Immunity*
Edited by: R. A. B. Ezekowitz and J. A. Hoffmann © Humana Press Inc., Totowa, NJ

among deuterostomes were noted by comparative embryologists, of which the most obvious is the embryologic origin of the coelomic mesoderm. For instance, in echinoderms, hemichordates, and the invertebrate chordate amphioxus, the major mesodermal constituents can be seen to arise as an outpocketing or delamination from the invaginated gut. [The anatomic arguments are summarized in Brusca and Brusca *(1)*.] The developmental homologies among deuterostomes are convincing, and the reality of the deuterostome clade was accepted by some long before molecular evidence became available *(2–4)*, despite the completely disparate adult body plans that the deuterostome assemblage includes. However, for others, it was hard to swallow the conclusion that the vertebrate and invertebrate chordates and urochordates share a common ancestor with the radially symmetric echinoderms, which display such peculiar features as a calcite endoskeleton and a water vascular system; or with the vermiform hemichordates, some of which have tentacles on their heads, and which are characterized by an enormous anterior proboscis and both dorsal and ventral nerve cords.

Molecular phylogenetics has very recently brought about a major revolution on our image of evolutionary relationships within the Bilateria. Many aspects of the phylogenetic trees found in all except the very newest textbooks were about as wrong as could be. Not so the concept of the deuterostomes, however: molecular phylogenetics has confirmed the reality of the deuterostome assemblage in an exceptionally robust way *(5)*. This result has fully justified the (unspoken) conviction of classical morphologists that the characters they felt to be important are so deeply embedded in the developmental process that they must have a fundamental genealogic significance. The main support comes from ribosomal RNA phylogenies, but that is not all. Even before contemporary rRNA phylogenetics were available, it was noticed that intron positions in actin genes constitute a set of shared, deuterostome-specific characters *(6–8)*. Furthermore, the molecular phylogeny of *hox* cluster genes independently demonstrates the existence of the deuterostome clade. What this means essentially is that the deuterostomes indeed descend from a common ancestor and that they are all more closely related to one another and to their ancestor than any of them is to any other, non-deuterostome bilaterian animal.

A strong point that was not so clear earlier, and that is especially important for our purposes, has emerged from rRNA phylogeny. This concerns the internal phylogenetic organization of the deuterostome clade, as illustrated in Fig. 1 *(9–11)*. It can be seen that the deuterostomes consist of two large assemblages, the chordates, and a sister group that includes the echinoderms and the hemichordates. The echinoderm-hemichordate sister grouping is supported not only by rRNA phylogenetics *(9–11)* but also by mitochondrial sequence organization *(12)*. It too was very strongly suggested earlier, by the remarkably similar morphologic organization of the larvae of indirectly developing echinoderms and hemichordates (for review, *see* ref. *13*). It follows from the phylogeny shown in Fig. 1 that characters of the innate immune system shared between echinoderms and chordates are very likely to be characters also possessed by the deuterostome common ancestor and therefore the "starting point" characters for innate immunity throughout the deuterostomes. Whether these are deuterostome-specific characters (synapomorphies of the deuterostomes) or primitive characters (plesiomorphies) also present in the remote common ancestor of all bilaterians will depend on whether they are also shared with protostomes (such as *Drosophila*).

A

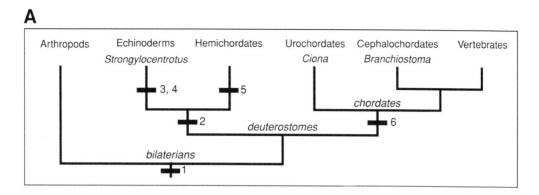

B

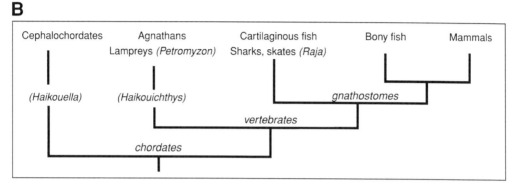

Fig. 1. Phylogeny. **(A)** Deuterostome phylogeny. The tree is based on molecular evidence, mainly rRNA phylogeny (see text for references); arthropods are shown as an outgroup. Numbers represent the morphologic character shared by all organisms belonging to groups situated on the chart above the numbered mark: 1, bilateral organization of the body plan; 2, paired tripartite larval coeloms; 3, fivefold radially symmetric adult body plan; 4, calcite endoskeleton; 5, proboscis; 6, notochord. **(B)** Vertebrate phylogeny featuring organisms mentioned in this chapter. Cephalochordates are shown as the outgroup (*cf.* A): agnathans, jawless fish; gnathostomes, jawed vertebrates; *Haikouella* and *Haikouichthys,* the Lower Cambrian fossil forms shown in Fig. 2. (From Davidson EH, San Diego, CA: Academic, 2001, pp. 158–202. With permission from Academic Press.)

2.2. The Antiquity of the Deuterostome Divergence

The only unequivocal way to determine the (minimal) age of a clade of animals is by its fossil record. Discoveries made in just the last few years in a fine-grained deposit from the Lower Cambrian of Yunnan, China have now begun to fill out the real-time fossil record of the deuterostomes. Three different groups of echinoderms that appear in the Lower Cambrian (eocrinoids, helicoplacoids, and edrioasteroids; *14*), and a suspected cephalochordate-like Middle Cambrian animal called Pikaia, which seemed to resemble amphioxus, were known before *(15)*, but the evidence is now greatly expanded. Some relevant recent fossils from the Lower Cambrian of Yunnan are reproduced in Fig. 2. In Fig. 2A we see an exceptionally well-preserved animal of cephalochordate grade, in which classic chordate features such as notochord, segmented trunk, and branchial arches can be seen *(16)*. Figure 2B shows a fish-like true chordate of

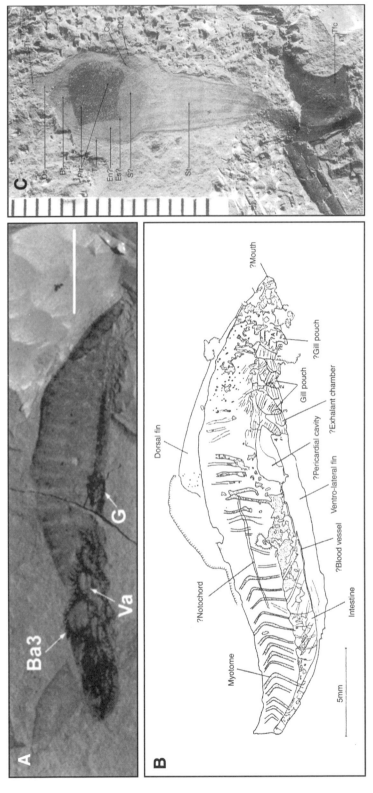

Fig. 2. Lower Cambrian chordate fossils recently discovered in Yunnan, China. (**A**) *Haikouella*, a cephalochordate grade animal, anterior left. This animal apparently had a more extensively developed brain than does the modern amphioxus, with which it otherwise shares many structures such as a series of branchial arches (Ba), heart, aorta (Va, ventral aorta), gonad (G), bucal cavity, segmented trunk muscles, postanal tail, and so forth. (**B**) Reconstruction of *Haikouichthys*, a vertebrate of agnathan grade, anterior right. This animal displays many characters of jawless fish, as indicated. (**C**) Probable tunicate (urochordate). The scale bar on left is calibrated in millimeters. The animal is structured similarly to the modern ascidian genus *Styela*. St, stem; S, Es, En, possibly stomach, esophagus, and endostyle, respectively; T, tunic; Ph, pharynx, Bt, buccal region; Os and Cs, oral and cloacal siphons, respectively. (From Chen J-y, Huang D-\Y, Li C-W. Nature 1999;402:518–522; © 1999 Macmillan Magazines Inc., Shu D-G, Chen L, Han J, Zhang X-L. Nature 1999;411:427–473; © Shu D-G, Chen L, Han J, Zhang X-L. Nature 2001;411:472–473. © 2001 Macmillan Magazines Ltd.)

64

agnathan grade, which had a cartilaginous skull, dorsal fin, and other vertebrate structures *(17,18)*. Figure 2C, from the same Lower Cambrian deposit, shows a beautifully preserved adult ascidian form *(19)*.

What these fossils demonstrate is that divergence of the major deuterostome clades had already occured by about 530 million years ago, i.e., only a few million years after the Lower Cambrian boundary. Therefore in real time all the evolutionary divergences represented by branch points in the diagram of Fig. 1A had occured well before this. It is an inescapable conclusion that the common deuterostome ancestor (let alone the last common protostome-deuterostome ancestor) lived in Precambrian time, and this sets the real-time antiquity of regulatory features that are held in common between echinoderms and chordates.

3. INNATE IMMUNITY IN AN ECHINODERM: *A WINDOW ON ANCESTRAL REGULATORY ASSIGNMENTS*

There is a long history of more or less casual phenomenologic observations on the innate immune functions executed by sea urchin coelomocytes. These are the immunocytes of the echinoderm, a free-wandering population of cells that inhabit the coelomic cavity. They are also present in large numbers within certain organs, such as the late season ovary, where their function is phagocytosis of unused oocytes. In the sea urchin *Strongylocentrotus purpuratus,* the California purple sea urchin, on which most modern experiments have been carried out, there are about 7.5×10^6 coelomocytes per ml of coelomic fluid. Coelomocytes chemotactically accumulate at sites of injury, they generate cellular clots, they are extremely active in phagocytic encapsulation of bacteria or particles, and they carry out secretory activities as well (for reviews, *see* refs. *20,* and *21*). They participate in graft rejection *(22,23)*, but these animals have no immunologic memory: they reject second grafts with equal alacrity irrespective of their source (for review, *see* ref. *24*). There are at least four kinds of coelomocytes, the major phagocytic class (or petaliferous amebocytes), red spherule cells, colorless spherule cells, and vibratile cells. The red cells and the phagocytes form inflammatory infiltrates at infections and injuries; and the phagocytic cells are capable of clearing relatively enormous amounts of bacteria injected into the coelomic cavity within hours. Beyond this sort of information, however, very little is known of how the coelomocytes really work at the cellular level, or what they actually do in terms of individual cellular function to provide the animal with immune protection. That they work well, and that the innate immune systems of sea urchins confer extremely effective defenses against pathogens, there can be no doubt. These are long-lived animals (the record so far for *S. purpuratus* is a 16-year-old individual bred and cultured in our marine laboratory facility). We have often observed the remarkable ability of *S. purpuratus* to recover from apparently global epidermal infections or severe, obviously infected wounds.

3.1. Effectors of Coelomocyte Immune Function

Molecular biology has revealed three classes of immune effector proteins that are expressed by sea urchin coelomocytes. Qualitatively, these are all familiar from the innate immune systems of mammals: they are complement proteins; scavenger receptor cysteine-rich repeat (SRCR) proteins; and Toll-class receptors. It is possible that at least the latter two gene families are functionally elaborated in sea urchins to a much greater extent than in mammals. Conversely, there is no sign in sea urchins of immunoglobulin-based immune effector proteins, nor of any but an innate system of immunity.

A C3-type complement component was discovered in a coelomocyte expressed sequence tag (EST) project in 1996 *(25)*. Further work revealed that the mRNA encodes a 186-kDa protein that gives rise to α- and β-chains that display the major features of C3-class complement proteins of vertebrates, from hagfish to human *(26)*. The gene is single copy and is expressed specifically in coelomocytes. A second complement gene was soon discovered as well, also expressed specifically by coelomocytes, encoding a factor B (Bf; or C2-like) protein. This 91-kDa protein contains five "consensus repeats" similar to the three commonly found in vertebrate Bf/C2 proteins, as well as several other sequence features that are also common to the mammalian proteins *(27)*. Phylogenetic analysis places both the C3 and Bf proteins of *S purpuratus* in basal positions with respect to the vertebrate complement proteins. Their joint presence, and their particular sequence features suggest that sea urchin coelomocytes express an "alternative pathway" opsonization function, which is deployed to assist the phagocytes in cleaning up incident bacteria (for review, *see* ref. *28*). Similar proteins are apparently utilized for opsonization in the lamprey *(29,30)*. Furthermore, these complement genes could represent a true deuterostome synapomorphy *(27)*; the closest known protostome relatives of C3 *(31)* are more closely related to the α$_2$-macroglobulins of deuterostomes than to C3 itself. It is particularly interesting to note that the C3 and Bf genes are linked in *S. purpuratus,* having been recovered on a single 140-kb bacterial artificial chromosome (BAC) recombinant *(32)*; they are also linked within the MHC class III region in mammals.

The second class of immune effector genes expressed in coelomocytes that have been discovered in the sea urchin encodes SRCR proteins. The SRCR proteins constitute a pan-metazoan superfamily, having been found in sponges, nematodes, flies, tunicates, lampreys, and mammals *(33)*. Several of these proteins function in the development of the immune system and in regulation of the immune response in mammals, e.g., the WC1 and TC9 families of T-cell surface receptors in pigs and sheep *(34–38)*. Macrophage SRCR proteins in mammals are involved in binding and phagocytosis of bacteria, entocytosis, and regulation of opsonization functions *(39–46)*. In the sea urchin the SRCR genes are likely to be major players in the immune functions mediated by coelomocytes, although unfortunately the only information that so far exists is descriptive and correlative. However, along these lines, some remarkable features have emerged *(33,47)*.

The *S. purpuratus* genome contains well over 100 of these genes (and possibly a much larger number). This follows from the isolation from a coelomocyte cDNA library of representatives of a number of different SRCR subfamilies, as well as results obtained when these probes were used to screen a genomic BAC library, and also from sequence comparisons with a set of about 80,000 BAC-end sequences that have been obtained for this genome *(48)*. There are an average of up to seven SRCR domains per gene, and the genes themselves are clustered in those BACs that have been mapped *(33)*. The current estimate is that the *S. purpuratus* genome contains a total of about 22,000 ± 5000 genes *(49)*, so the SRCR genes family may account for at least a half of a percent of all the genes, perhaps more. The SRCR genes are expressed in coelomocytes in sets, which vary from animal to animal and which thereby distinguish each individual sea urchin from each other individual. A correlation analysis shows that many factors contribute to these individual patterns of expression, which are of transcriptional origin (all the animals appear to possess similar complements of SRCR genes): some SRCR proteins are preferentially expressed on immune challenge (injection of bacteria or injury); expression of others is modulated over time, for unknown reasons *(33)*. There are also correlations with the origin (i.e., individual past history) of the experimental animals, and with their genetic constitutions, as displayed at least preliminarily in experiments on inbred *S. purpuratus* (Z. Pancer and E. Davidson, unpublished data). Judging from their sequence features, some of the encoded SRCR proteins are secreted, but others are apparently mounted in the coelomocyte membranes *(47)* and could serve as receptors or co-receptors. The importance for immune function of at least some SRCR genes is directly suggested by the observation that the transcriptional expression of these genes is sharply upregulated after immune challenge *(33)*.

The third class of coelomocyte genes that also form part of the genetic armamentarium for innate immunity in mammals is the Toll-like receptors (Z. Pancer and E. Davidson, unpublished data). Their presence in sea urchin immune effector cells and their likely functional role are clearly plesiomorphies: Toll-class receptors serve as recognition elements for immune responses to bacterial and fungal substances from *Drosophila* to mammals *(50–53)*. Several cDNAs encoding Toll-class receptors have been cloned from *S. purpuratus* coelomocytes. Both genome blots and the prevalence of sequences quite similar to the cloned Toll-class receptors in the BAC-end sequence collection indicate that this genome contains many genes encoding similar proteins.

Sketchy as it is, this glimpse of the repertoire of immune effector genes utilized by sea urchin coelomocytes suggests some of the ways they do business. They secrete or mount on their surfaces a tremendous variety of proteins containing SRCR domains, which might bind to different components produced by pathogens. Since these are encoded by prevalent mRNAs, they are likely to be end products of the defense apparatus, although there is no direct evidence to this effect. Synthesis of the SRCR proteins is transcriptionally controlled. It is a reasonable speculation that the variety in the set of SRCR proteins expressed individual to individual reflects the past immunologic experience of the animal, implying some receptor mechanism that relates the nature of the incident challenge to the set of genes activated. The existence of many Toll-class receptors suggests that the coelomocytes have a complex repertoire of recognition capabilities. The most prominent and easy to observe feature of coelomocytes is their avid phagocytic activity, and the discovery that they produce Bf and C3 complement proteins indicates the role of opsonization in a major aspect of their function.

3.2. Transcriptional Regulation of Coelomocyte Immune Responses

The first indication of transcriptional responses to immune challenge on the part of sea urchin coelomocytes came from experiments of Smith et al. *(24,54)* on expression of the gene encoding profilin. These measurements showed that the level of transcripts of this cytoskeletal protein, which is involved in actin mobilization, is sharply increased on injection of bacteria into the coelomic cavity. Responses were measured after one to several days, and similar results were obtained on injection of lipopolysaccharide (LPS; at the same low levels as are effective on mammalian immunocytes), instead of bacteria. The expression of the gene encoding the C3 complement protein is also upregulated by LPS injection, and responses were observed as early as 1 hour post injection *(55)*.

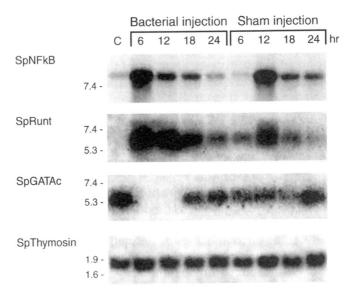

Fig. 3. Changes in level of expression of three transcriptional regulatory genes in sea urchin coelomocytes following immune challenge. Bacteria isolated from the skin of sea urchins were cultured, and 1 mL of this culture ($OD_{600} = 0.5$) was injected into the coelom of each of five animals per time point. Total coelomocytes were extracted at the indicated times and pooled. Coelomocytes from three control animals were similarly pooled. Sham injection indicates samples from sets of animals in which 1 mL of sea water was injected rather than bacterial culture; these samples were otherwise similarly treated. The figure shows an RNA gel blot hybridization in which 10 µg of total RNA was loaded in each lane. The thymosin transcript, always present in coelomocytes irrespective of treatment, served as a loading control. Probes were obtained by PCR from cDNA clones. Each of the five probes was reacted in turn with the same blot. Numerals indicate the positions of size markers (in kb). (From Pancer Z, Rast JP, Davidson EH. Immunogenetics 1999;49:773–786. © Springer-Verlag.)

Genes encoding three transcription factors expressed in coelomocytes are now known to respond to introduction of bacteria within hours *(47)*. The responses measured, as reproduced in Fig.3, consist of large changes in transcript level, i.e., they are most likely the result of changes in expression of these regulatory genes. The least surprising, given the above, is the response of a gene encoding a rel domain regulator similar to NF-κB (SpNF-κB in Fig. 3). Within 2-hours after injection of bacteria into the coelom of a sea urchin, the NF-κB response peaks. (The earliest point shown in Fig. 3 is at 16-hours.) The puncture needle wound in itself suffices to produce a response on the part of this gene, although a much slower one (this could be caused by inadvertent introduction and replication of surface bacteria with the needle). Note that in these experiments the whole coelomocyte population is being sampled. The second tier of Fig. 3 shows the even more dramatic response of a gene encoding a Runt-class transcription factor. This mRNA is present at very low levels in coelomocytes from healthy unchallenged animals (Fig. 3C) but quickly becomes fairly prevalent on injection of bacteria. Figure 3 shows that the opposite happens with *gata-c* gene transcripts. The *S. purpuratus gata-c* gene is expressed in embryonic mesoderm cells and is later constitutively transcribed in adult coelomocytes (unpublished data). On introduction of bacteria, *gata-c* transcripts abruptly disappear (Fig. 3, tier 3), but within about half a day the cells recover (or are replaced).

The sharp dynamics of the responses shown in Fig. 3 provide several inferences: they implicate all three regulatory genes in the dedicated control system underlying coelomocyte immune functions; they imply that all three genes are somehow hooked up to a cellular recognition apparatus that detects the presence of bacteria; and they suggest that this is mediated by response to diffusible substances; otherwise, i.e., unless a large fraction of the coelomocytes are involved, it is unlikely that responses of this magnitude could have been observed. For instance, one can see in Fig. 3 that virtually all the coelomocytes normally expressing the *gata-c* gene turn it off (or degrade its mRNA) on introduction of bacteria.

There is an evolutionary as well as a mechanistic significance to the discovery that these transcriptional regulatory genes are involved in the innate immune system of sea urchins *(32)*. The same regulators are expressed during the development and operation of the innate immune systems of mammals, and also in their adaptive immune systems. In the innate and adaptive immune systems of mammals, however, many of the downstream genes they control are likely to be different. What this tells us of the pathways of regulatory immune system evolution is now to be our subject, but first it is important to focus on regulatory synapomorphies of vertebrates that underlie the special features of their innate immune systems.

4. REGULATORS THAT CONTROL GENES OF THE VERTEBRATE IMMUNE SYSTEM(S)

The adaptive immune system, with its B- and T-lymphocytes, antigen-dependent clonal selection mechanisms, and antigen-specific immunologic memory, is found only in vertebrates within the chordate assemblage of deuterostomes *(56–60)*. Supplementing the innate immune system, this results in a layered system of innate and adaptive responses, interconnected and cemented by many potent regulatory links between the two kinds of response *(61)*. In evolutionary terms, lymphocytes presumably arose by the modification of developmental pathways, leading to more basal hematopoietic cell types. In this section, we consider the relationships between the innovations required for the adaptive immune system and the underlying regulatory structures of deuterostome innate immunity.

4.1. Immune System Innovations of Jawed Vertebrates

Two innovations are conspicuous in this comparison. One, of course, is the elaborate recombinase system, which rearranges antigen receptor gene segments in vertebrates to assemble the transcription units that encode immunoglobulins and T-cell receptors. This first innovation is made possible by the presence of the *RAG-1* and *RAG-2* genes in the genome and their regulated expression in the differentiation of specialized immune cells. The other innovation is the development of the distinctive lymphocyte cell type. Lymphocytes are not only distinguished by their use of the RAG-mediated DNA rearrangement process, but also by their long lives and antigen-dependent control of proliferation and death. They combine sophisticated, differentiated effector functions with a self-renewal potential that is second only to that of stem cells within the hematopoietic series. The origins of adaptive immunity in a deuterostome ancestor depend on the origins of the *RAG* genes and the origins of the lymphocyte cell type.

4.2. Potential Evolutionary Bridges Between Innate
and Adaptive System Components

RAG gene homologs are not evident in any animals thus far studied except jawed vertebrates *(57–62)*. Sequence data for agnathans and invertebrate deuterostomes are admittedly scarce, and there might be *RAG* homologs waiting to be discovered in such animals. However, there is also no trace of *RAG* homologs in protostomes, giving reason to suspect that the discontinuity is real. The *RAG-1* and *RAG-2* genes could have entered the genomes of vertebrate ancestors only after the split between agnathans and gnathostomes, perhaps by horizontal transfer of a transposable element with its transposase gene from a prokaryotic source *(63)*. A true discontinuity of this kind would give little indication of what characteristics to look for in cells of agnathans and invertebrates that might be functional counterparts of the ancestors of vertebrate lymphocytes.

In contrast, the differentiation pathways of lymphocytes do suggest traces of a continuum with other hematopoietic lineages. Evidence for such a continuum emerges from the detailed studies that have been performed in recent years on mammalian lymphocyte precursors. Lymphocytes differentiate continuously from the same hematopoietic stem cells that give rise to phagocytic and nonimmune blood cell types. Intermediates in this process retain certain subsets of developmental potentials after having lost others. It has long been assumed that lymphocyte development branches off from the development of all erythroid and myeloid blood cell types at an early stage. There are descriptions of a "common lymphoid progenitor," with the ability to give rise to all classes of lymphocytes but not to other hematopoietic cell types *(64,65)*, and of a complementary "common myeloid progenitor" with the opposite potentials *(66)*. The existence of such partially restricted precursors has been taken to suggest a profound early split. However, it appears that a common lymphoid precursor is not the only intermediate through which lymphocytes can be made.

In fetal life, especially, mouse T- and B-cells arise from precursors that may also give rise to macrophages, although not to other blood cell types *(67,68)*. Many fetal T-cell precursors can still give rise to mixed T/myeloid clones even though they cannot give rise to B-cells, and the reverse is true for B-cell precursors *(69)*. There are numerous cases of cell lines that appear to be immortalized B/macrophage precursors, and recently a naturally occurring cell population in the bone marrow that expresses many B-lineage properties has been shown to be able to generate macrophages or dendritic cells, which play key sentinel roles in the innate immune system *(70,71)*. Mouse and human T-cell precursors after birth similarly retain the ability to differentiate into dendritic cells until they start undergoing antigen receptor gene rearrangement *(72–75)*. Yet another fate as an innate immune system effector is available to T-cell precursors as well: that of becoming a natural killer (NK) cell. These branch points in B- and T-cell development are shown in Fig. 4. Most strikingly, even cells that appear to be committed "common lymphoid progenitors" turn out to retain the ability to differentiate into macrophages and neutrophilic granulocytes, after all, provided they are given an appropriate growth factor receptor signal *(76)*. Thus, the division between the developmental programs leading to adaptive and innate immune function is not so deep. Right up to the first stages of their receptor gene rearrangement events, mammalian lymphoid precursors preserve the developmental alternative of becoming a macrophage or dendritic cell, as shown in Fig. 4.

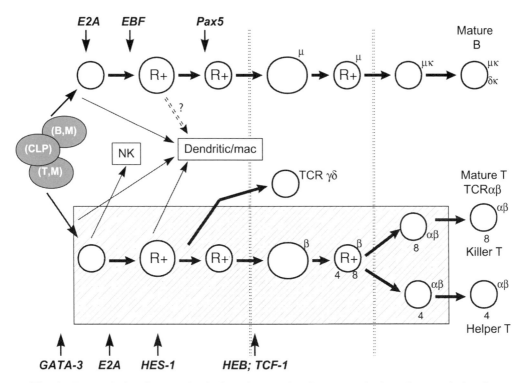

Fig. 4. Transcription factor roles in lymphocyte development. Timing of transcription factor action relative to developmental branch points and checkpoints in B- and T-cell development. For details and evidence, see the reviews cited in the text. The relevant stages of lymphocyte development appear to be the same whether the cells are differentiating from a panlymphoid common lymphoid progenitor (CLP) or from a B/myeloid (B, M) or T/myeloid (T, M) precursor, so all three types of potential precursors are shown at the left. The timing of activity of E2A, EBF, and Pax5 in B-cell development and of GATA-3, E2A, HES-1, HEB, and TCF-1 in T-cell development are based on the stages at which homozygous knockouts of these genes cause the most severe phenotype. Arrows leading to alternative fates (NK, or Dendritic/mac) show the latest stages at which individual precursor cells can give rise to both T-or B-lymphocytes and the indicated alternative. Bold arrows, major developmental pathways; thin arrows, confirmed minor pathways; broken arrow, conditional pathway. Stages when RAG-1/2-mediated recombination is active are indicated as R+. Stages at which further developmental progression becomes dependent on successful rearrangement events (checkpoints) are indicated for B- and T-cells by vertical dotted double lines. Important cell surface molecules are shown: for B-cells, immunoglobulin chains μ and/or δ and κ; for T-cells, CD4, CD8, the T-cell receptor chains α and β, and the alternative class of T-cell receptors TCR$\gamma\delta$.

A corollary is that the difference between lymphoid and myeloid developmental programs should be attributable to specific regulatory changes that occur in lymphoid precursors when these two programs diverge. Cells that do not undergo these events should develop by default into macrophages, dendritic cells, or NK cells. The key regulatory molecules at these points are thus the first candidates we consider as effectors or targets of evolutionary innovations that may have made lymphocyte development possible.

4.3. Critical Regulators of B-Cell Specification

Three transcription factors play key roles in driving B-cells to differentiate from precursors that initially retain the ability to give rise to macrophages (reviewed in refs. *77–80*). These factors appear to act in a mutually reinforcing cascade. The first one required for B-lineage specification is a class A basic helix-loop-helix (bHLH) factor encoded by the *E2A* gene. (differential splicing products E47 and E12 are both active.) The second is the HLH factor early B cell factor (EBF) (Olf-1, COE1), which collaborates closely with E2A to turn on B-cell genes. Even if these two factors have initiated a B-lineage gene expression program, specification is not stabilized into commitment until a third factor, Pax5, is also activated. Pax5 participates in both the positive regulation of B-cell genes and the negative regulation of alternative fates and the genes associated with them *(79)*. The stages at which these factors are required to act are shown in Fig. 4 (upper part).

As probes for the events leading to evolutionary change, these transcription factors are illuminating, although perhaps in an unexpected way. None of them is a vertebrate innovation, or even a deuterostome innovation, in terms of its structure or DNA binding specificity. All three are members of small multigene families of extremely ancient provenance, with close relatives in protostomes as well as deuterostomes. *E2A* is a homolog of *daughterless* in *Drosophila (81)* with a close relative in the sea urchin (J.P. Rast, personal communication); EBF has homologs in the *Drosophila* Collier protein and CeO/E in *Caenorhabditis elegans (82)*; and *Pax5* is a member of the pan-bilaterian *Pax2/5/8* gene family *(83)*. Furthermore, all these transcription factors have important functions outside the immune system, functions that are conserved from mammals to protostomes. Both EBF and Pax5 are used in the mammalian nervous system, D-Pax2 is used for external sensory organogenesis in *Drosophila,* and the EBF homolog CeO/E is used in neuronal differentiation in *C. elegans (84)*. The evolutionary innovations that gave these factors roles in B-cell development must have been primarily regulatory, i.e., changes that gave EBF and Pax5 a new domain of expression within the hematopoietic system.

The case of *E2A* is particularly striking, for the products of this gene are not generally restricted to any particular cell type at all. Mammalian E47 and E12, like *Drosophila* Daughterless, are expressed ubiquitously. They are used as developmentally neutral dimerization partners of other bHLH transcription factors that enable the heterodimers to carry out various tissue-specific differentiative functions. The only respect in which the B-cell use of E47 is distinct from that of muscle or nerve cells is that B-cells lack any other dimerization partners, and instead employ E47 as a homodimer. It is what the B-lineage cells lack, not what they express, that gives the E2A product(s) their unique roles in B-cells. Thus, in all three cases, the transcription factors that establish the unique B-cell identity in developing hematopoietic cells have been "seconded" to this task from other assignments of greater antiquity.

4.4. Regulators of T-Cell Specification

The initial events leading to specification of T-cells from multilineage or bipotent precursors are not yet as well understood as those for B-cells (reviewed in refs. *75,85, and 86*). Still, mutational and expression analysis in mice suggests that at least four kinds of transcription factors are needed specifically in T-cell differentiation (Fig. 4, lower part). The zinc finger factor GATA-3 is required cell autonomously from a very early stage *(87,88)*. The bHLH repressor HES-1 (a target of activation by Notch signaling) is also required in immature T-cells, particularly for proliferative expansion *(89)*. Class A bHLH proteins are essential for T-cell development in general: inhibition of these transcription factors can be sufficient to drive the earliest precursor cells into an NK developmental pathway *(90)*. The class A bHLH activator Hela E-box binding protein (HEB) and the high mobility group (HMG box) factor T-cell factor-1 (TCF-1; a target of Wnt pathway signaling) are also needed later, for transition through the first T-cell receptor-dependent checkpoint *(91,92)*. Precursor cells in older adult mice require TCF-1 even earlier in the T-cell differentiation pathway, perhaps as early as they require GATA-3 *(93)*. By analysis of the *cis*-regulatory elements of T-cell-specific genes, it is evident that additional classes of factors, e.g., Ets, Runx, and Myb, are also essential *(75,86,94)*, but individually these do not reveal T-cell-specific effects either because of the presence of multiple, partially redundant family members (for Ets: ref. 95), or because they are needed in hematopoietic precursors generally.

Like the transcription factors that orchestrate B-lineage specification, the T-cell differentiation factors are members of pan-bilaterian families that are used in diverse developmental programs. HEB is another member of the same small bHLH factor family as the E2A gene products, and there is extensive overlap between the functions of HEB and E2A even in mammalian lymphocyte development *(96)*. Like the E2A products, HEB is a homolog of Daughterless in *Drosophila*. The bHLH repressor, HES-1, is closely related to *Drosophila* Hairy and the products of the various Enhancer of split complex genes. TCF-1 and its close vertebrate relative Lef-1 have a sea urchin homolog *(97)* and are members of the same family as *Drosophila* Pangolin. GATA-3 and its close vertebrate relative GATA-2 are similarly closely related to *Drosophila* dGATAc, as well as to sea urchin SpGATAc.

There are broad similarities in the ways that these transcription factors are utilized throughout the bilaterian radiation. As for the B-cell factors, all the T-cell transcription factors are used in other tissues as well as in lymphocytes, and it is these nonlymphoid sites of action that are conserved. GATA-3 (and dGATAc) and the bHLH activators and repressors all play prominent roles in neurogenesis, in both vertebrates and flies *(98,99)*. TCF/Lef factors in vertebrates and in sea urchins mediate signals from the Wnt pathway *(97,100–102);* similarly, Pangolin mediates Wg signals throughout the fly embryo *(103)*. Among the T-cell factors, only GATA-3 appears to have an additional, specific role in hematopoiesis that may be shared with animals that do not have lymphocytes. GATA-3 and its close relative GATA-2 are used in vertebrate hematopoietic stem cells *(104,105)*, and we have already seen how SpGATAc, a GATA-2/3 homolog, is used by sea urchin coelomocytes. Even *Drosophila* hemocytes express a kind of GATA factor, Serpent, although this is not an ortholog of deuterostome hematopoietic GATA factors *(106,107)*. Such instances of hematopoietic use cannot be simply interpreted as evidence that the invertebrates have T-lymphocyte-like cells *per se,* however, because the nonlymphoid sites of function of each of these factors and their close relatives are so diverse. The conclusion is evident that the T-cell developmental program, as far as it is understood, is again a new application for old regulators.

4.5. Regulators of Lymphomyeloid Precursor Generation

To find evidence for regulatory molecules that might contribute novel functions for lymphocyte development, perhaps surprisingly, we must look at the factors that control

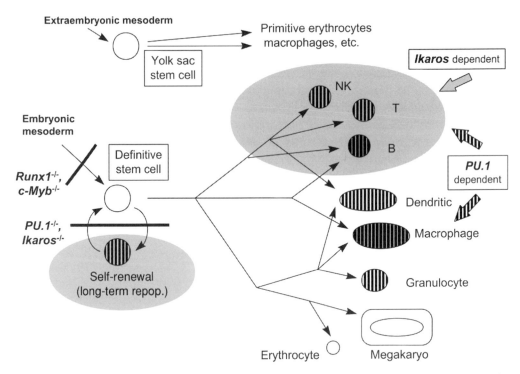

Fig. 5. Timing of transcription factor activities in hematopoiesis. The figure emphasizes the roles of *Ikaros* and *PU.1* in definitive fetal hematopoiesis and in the differentiation of various hematopoietic cell types. Primitive, extraembryonic yolk sac hematopoiesis does not depend on either of these transcription factors, nor on *Runx1* or *c-Myb*. Definitive intraembryonic stem cell generation, in contrast, depends acutely on *Runx1* and *c-Myb*. Two kinds of derivatives of definitive stem cells show further dependence on *PU.1* and *Ikaros:* these are the special long-term repopulating set of definitive stem cells (lower left) and the lymphocytes (NK, T, B). Myeloid cells also depend for their development on *PU.1* to greater (macrophages) or lesser (granulocytes) extents, but they do not depend on *Ikaros*. In the figure, cell types that are *Ikaros*-dependent are shown in gray. Cell types that are at least partially *PU.1*-dependent are shown vertically striped. Heavy vertical stripes in B-cells and macrophages indicate the complete absence of cells of these lineages in *PU.1*$^{-/-}$ mice. Megakaryo, megakaryocyte.

the development of uncommitted lymphomyeloid precursors. It has become increasingly clear in the past decade that the long-term self-renewing hematopoietic stem cells of adult vertebrates are not a "primitive" cell type, but rather the product of a regulated developmental program that maintains their pluripotentiality *(108)*. Several additional transcription factors are involved in the generation of these definitive (post-yolk sac) hematopoietic precursors that can later continue to play essential roles in gene expression throughout lymphocyte differentiation, linking the stem cell and lymphocyte regulatory states. Differentiation programs for which these factors are required are shown in Fig. 5. In mice, these factors include the Runt class transcription factor Runx1 (AML1, CBFα2, PEBP2αB), the Myb class transcription factor c-Myb, the zinc finger transcription factor Ikaros, and the divergent Ets subfamily member PU.1 (Spi-1). There is nothing lymphocyte-specific about these transcription factors, and yet, as we shall see, it is PU.1 that provides our best current evidence for a factor that is a verte-brate lymphohematopoietic innovation.

These transcription factors regulate lymphocyte and stem cell development via sets of target genes that may overlap but are certainly not the same. In mammals, c-Myb and Runx1 are essential for the establishment of definitive hematopoietic stem cells *(109–111)* (Fig. 5). Runx is also essential for the expression of T-cell receptor α, β, γ, and δ genes, and c-Myb is used by T-cells not only to drive their cell cycle progression in response to stimulation by antigen *(112),* but also for expression of the T-cell recep-tor γ and δ genes (data not shown). Ikaros *(113)* and PU.1 *(114)* are important for establishing the pool of definitive long-term repopulating stem cells in the bone mar-row prior to birth (Fig. 5). Even in the fetal stages at which other blood cell types can develop without them, though, these two transcription factors still turn out to be essen-tial for any lymphocyte development whatsoever (Fig. 5).

Both the Myb and the Runx/Runt family are extremely ancient, at least predating the protostome/deuterostome split. The cases of Ikaros and PU.1 (or the PU.1 subfamily of Ets factors) are a little different, as described in the next section.

Both Ikaros and PU.1 have particularly complex functions that include inhibitory as well as stimulatory effects on particular target genes. Recent studies imply that one of the major roles of Ikaros may be as a repressor of subset-specific lymphoid genes that are inappropriate for the current differentiation state *(115);* it also appears to keep lym-phocytes from responding too easily to subthreshold activation signals *(116).* PU.1 is intimately involved in positive regulation of B-cell cytokine receptor and antigen receptor genes *(117,118).* However, in its most general role, PU.1 is a potent positive regulator of the differentiation and growth of macrophages and granulocytes, cells of the innate immune system *(119)* (Fig. 5). Whereas at moderate levels of expression it is needed for early events in both T- and B-lymphocyte lineages *(120,121),* at higher lev-els, PU.1 can actually block lymphocyte development *(122,123).* The fact that lympho-cytes depend on the activity of a myeloid transcription factor for their initial development is an additional feature linking the lymphocyte lineages with the phago-cytic lineages. The compatibility between the regulators needed to initiate lymphoid and phagocytic differentiation programs in jawed vertebrates is consistent with the pos-sibility that the lymphocyte developmental program evolved as a modification of a phagocytic cell program.

5. A REGULATORY DIVIDE BETWEEN AGNATHANS AND GNATHOSTOMES

In the case of the adaptive immune system, several critical innovations appear to have occured only after the divergence of the ancestors of jawed and jawless verte-brates, as already noted. Among these changes are alterations and expansions of the repertoires of transcription factors available to direct lymphocyte differentiation pro-grams. There are numerous examples of transcription factors encoded by a single gene in invertebrates up to cephalochordates, but by a family of three or four members in bony vertebrates (reviewed in ref. *124*). The expansion of these gene families and the evolutionary specialization of their expression patterns and "downstream" functions greatly enhances the potential regulatory sophistication in vertebrates. PU.1, and possi-bly Ikaros as well, are members of families that underwent threefold expansion well after the origin of vertebrates, between the divergence of agnathan and gnathostome vertebrates and the divergence of bony and cartilaginous fish.

5.1. PU.1/Spi-1 Origins

PU.1 is a valuable probe for evolutionary shifts in transcription factor function because of its relation to the rest of the Ets family and because of its well-mapped domain structure. The PU.1/Spi (spleen focus-forming virus preferential integration site) subfamily of Ets factors uses an easily recognizable Ets domain to bind to DNA, but this version of the Ets domain sequence is distinctive enough to define one of the five major subdivisions of Ets factors *(125)*. In PU.1 itself there are additional discrete, well-mapped "activation" domains carrying out separate functions. The region N-terminal to the Ets domain contains acidic and glutamine-rich transactivation domains and a PEST domain, each of which carries out interactions with different transcriptional partners in a modular fashion *(117,118)*. As a positive regulator, PU.1 uses these interaction domains to synergize powerfully with other developmentally regulated factors for activation of different batteries of cell type-specific target genes. PU.1 can also act as an important negative regulator, for example, by a mutually inhibitory protein/protein interaction with hematopoietic GATA factors *(126–129)*. GATA/PU.1 competition is thought to help regulate erythroid *vs.* myeloid specification of pluripotent precursors and could conceivably play a role in T-cell development as well *(123,130)*. Thus, the complex and central function of PU.1 in the hematopoietic system depends on more than its DNA-binding Ets domain. Conservation of the structure of each of its non-Ets domains may be an indicator of conservation of PU.1 activity in a different regulatory context.

The PU.1 Ets domain is conserved throughout the vertebrate radiation. There is an indisputable PU.1/Spi family member even in the agnathan lamprey *(Petromyzon marinus) (131)*. Cartilaginous fish have a whole family of three PU.1/Spi members, like mammals *(123)*. By contrast, the PU.1 Ets domain cannot be detected in any invertebrate to date. No member of this subfamily of Ets factors is encoded in the *Drosophila* or *C. elegans* genome sequences, and even deuterostome invertebrates seem to lack such genes. Multiple attempts to detect a family member in sea urchin genomic DNA or cDNA have been unseccessful (M.K. Anderson, X. Sun, R. Pant, and E.V.R., unpublished data). Thus, the divergence of this PU.1/Spi subfamily from other Ets factor genes is probably a vertebrate-specific innovation.

Phylogenetic comparison yields another interesting result, namely, evidence for a further discontinuity, occuring after the origin of the PU.1/Spi Ets domain. The sequence of the transcription factor gene itself provides structural evidence for an evolutionary shift in function. The protein-interaction domains of lamprey Spi do not maintain the organization of any other PU.1/Spi family member *(123,131)* (Fig. 6, middle and bottom). However, in the cartilaginous fish *Raja eglanteria,* there is a PU.1 ortholog with a sequence that meticulously corresponds to the mammalian, avian, and teleost fish versions in every domain (Fig. 6, top), and another *Raja* family member that resembles, throughout its length, both PU.1 and the closely related factor, SpiB *(132)*. This implies that the transcription factor interaction circuits in which PU.1 (and SpiB) take part are older than the chondrichthyan divergence, about 450 Mya, but that for the most part they arose since the divergence between the agnathans and gnathostomes

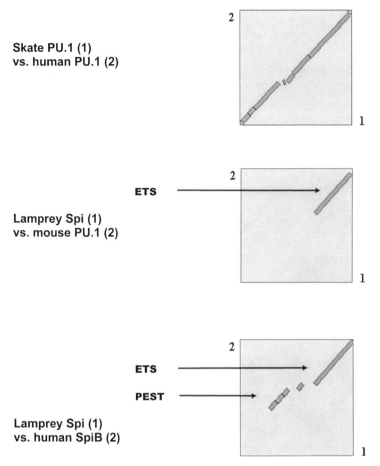

**Skate PU.1 (1)
vs. human PU.1 (2)**

**Lamprey Spi (1)
vs. mouse PU.1 (2)**

ETS

**Lamprey Spi (1)
vs. human SpiB (2)**

ETS

PEST

Fig. 6. A discontinuity in conservation of PU.1/Spi structural domains between lampreys and cartilaginous fish. Sequences are from refs. *131* and *132*. **(Top)** Alignment of skate PU.1 (sequence 1, gi:11245498) with human PU.1 (sequence 2, gi:36561). The same results are obtained using murine instead of human PU.1. **(Middle)** Alignment of lamprey PU.1 (sequence 1, gi:8748404) with mouse PU.1 (sequence 2, gi: 111187). Only the Ets domain is detectably similar. **(Bottom)** Alignment of lamprey PU.1 (sequence 1) with human SpiB (sequence 2, gi:36563). Some similarity is detectable in the PEST domain as well as the Ets domain. Alignments were done by BLASTP 2.1.2 using the BLOSUM62 matrix with penalties of 11 for gap opening and 1 for gap extension, a wordsize of 3, x_dropoff of 50 and "expect" value of 300.

approx. 50–100 My earlier. As already seen, this is the same phylogenetic interval in which the components of the adaptive immune system became established in vertebrates.

5.2. PU.1 and the Agnathan/Gnathostome Divide in Immune System Function

Cartilaginous fish have all the components of an adaptive immune system that have been examined so far. Not only do they have *RAG* genes, immunoglobulins, T-cell receptors, and MHC molecules, but they also have well-organized lymphoid organs, including a thymus that is homologous to that of bony vertebrates *(133)*. Consistent with a conserved developmental role for PU.1, they have a well-differentiated PU.1/Spi transcription factor family, and this is expressed, as in mammals, in the tissues that harbor B-cell and macrophage cell types.

In contrast, agnathans still have not revealed any molecular traces of an adaptive immune system, although cell morphologies and tissues suggest some links to gnathostome counterparts. Searches for genes encoding adaptive immune system receptors, histocompatibility antigens, and recombinases in the lamprey have remained uniformly unsuccessful even with recent technologies *(57)*. The lamprey does have round hematopoietic cells that have been referred to as possible lymphocytes, but there is no molecular evidence to distinguish them from any other kind of small, nongranular circulating cell *(134)*.

The single, highly divergent PU.1/Spi family member in the lamprey could be associated with the lymphocyte-like cells *(131)*, but the identities of any target genes are a complete mystery. A critical question is whether these cells share anything other than the expression of a PU.1/Spi family factor with mammalian lymphocytes; it seems unlikely from its structure that lamprey Spi can participate in most of the transcription factor interaction circuits that give mammalian hematopoietic cells their identities. There is some weak similarity between the lamprey Spi and mammalian *SpiB* within the PEST domain of the latter (Fig. 6, bottom). This is the domain in which interferon regulatory factors (IRF4 or interferon consensus sequence binding protein [ICSBP]) interact with PU.1 (or SpiB) to turn on common target genes. Initially, this kind of interaction was defined as important for immunoglobulin light chain gene expression in later stages of B-cell development *(135)*, but more recently it has been shown to play an important role in macrophage gene expression as well *(136,137)*. If this PEST domain interaction is significant, it could indicate that IRFs are the most ancient interaction partners of PU.1/Spi family transcription factors.

5.3. Use and Modification of Other Transcription Factor Innovations

Ikaros is another gene that is needed for early T-cell development in the mammalian fetus, and for all B-cell (and NK-cell) development. Although it is dispensable for myeloid and erythroid cell development, and thus is distinct from *PU.1*, its role in establishing a normal stem cell pool *(113)* implies that lymphocytes require some overlapping or common function(s) shared with stem cells. *Ikaros*, like *PU.1*, is a member of a small family of related genes, all members of which are found in vertebrates from mammals to cartilaginous fish *(138,139)* In all these animals, *Ikaros* family members appear to have homologous sites of expression, suggesting a linkage to hematopoietic cell development throughout jawed vertebrates. Only a single member of the family has been found to date in lamprey *(139)*. Here the lamprey *"Ikaros"* sequence is much more similar to those of members of the family seen in jawed vertebrates than is the case for the lamprey *Spi*, suggesting that the function of *Ikaros* should be conserved in the lamprey even if the lack of related genes with overlapping functions limits the complexity of the regulatory patterns. As in the case of *PU.1*, however, no *Ikaros* family member has been found yet in sea urchins (J.P. Rast, personal communication), and only the sequences encoding individual hunchback-type zinc finger domains can be recognized in the genome sequences of flies or nematodes. Thus it may be that the functions mediated by this transcription factor family are also vertebrate innovations.

6. TRANSCRIPTIONAL HISTORY OF DEUTEROSTOME IMMUNITY

This chapter has sketched out three kinds of mechanisms that have contributed to the layered evolution of deuterostome immune systems: continuity, co-option, and innovation. Establishing much of the bedrock of innate immunity are the profoundly conserved functions of regulators like Runt/Runx, NF-κB/Rel, and GATAc (GATA-2/3), which work in innate immunity throughout the deuterostomes and have close relatives in protostomes. At the opposite extreme, we have suggested that other hematopoietic regulators, such as PU.1, may have been "invented" and further specialized only after the beginning of the vertebrate radiation. Between these two extremes lie the transcription factors and target genes that are used for much of the immune cell-specific differentiation. These genes are used at least throughout the deuterostomes, but the way they are used, their relationships to other regulators and target genes, and the sites in which they are expressed have undergone functionally important changes to work in vertebrate immunity.

6.1. Continuity and Co-option in the Generation of Functional Novelty

Much of this volume concerns the conservation of whole regulatory circuits of innate immune function over long evolutionary times. In such a conserved circuit, not only individual gene products but the connectivity between them are retained, for example, the ability of an ancient receptor (e.g., Toll/Toll-like receptor) to trigger activation of an ancient transcription factor (e.g., NF-κB/Rel), which will turn on an ancient target gene (e.g., a defensin). This kind of conservation does not preclude individual transcription factors from expanding their range of target genes, however. The use of NF-κB to drive expression of the immunoglobulin light chain genes in vertebrates is an obvious case of this kind of target set expansion.

Expansion of a family of target genes, with subsequent diversification, provides another way that the gene family can acquire novel patterns of expression. The scavenger receptor (SRCR) genes of sea urchins, discussed earlier in this chapter, is an example of such a family that is highly expanded and diversified in a particular clade. In sea urchins the polymorphism and incorporation of different C-terminal structures may give this receptor family multiple effector functions as well as multiple recognition specificities. We do not know yet which coelomocyte transcription factors primarily regulate the complex expression of SRCR genes, but it is likely that some stress-inducible family members will be found to have acquired binding sites for inducible transcription factors such as NF-κB or SpRunt.

The appropriation of old transcription factors for new cell types is a clear example of co-option. This is most vividly illustrated by the case of a factor like EBF, which has a highly specific developmental role in protostomes and deuterostomes and then appears to have acquired a discrete new site of action within the developing B-cells of the gnathostome immune system. There is no developmental continuity between the various cell types—olfactory epithelium, adipose cells, early B-cells—in which EBF is expressed in mammals (and in cartilaginous fish: Anderson et al., in preparation). It thus appears that in the jawed vertebrates, the *EBF* gene has become co-opted into the B-cell developmental regulatory program, presumably by acquiring a *cis*-regulatory element, or module, that responds to pro-B-cell regulatory cues. *EBF* is a particularly likely case of regulatory element acquisition because there is remarkable conservation of domain structure among its small family of genes, and the other members of the family remain confined to their neuronal differentiation roles *(82)*. In the case of the T-cell factors, such as GATA-3, the picture is complicated by the pan-deuterostome roles in many kinds of blood cells of the hematopoietic GATA family as a whole. Still, the distinction between GATA-2, mostly expressed in stem cells, and GATA-3, which is upregulated in T-cell development, could also have arisen from the modification or acquisition of a new regulatory element by GATA-3 (e.g., responsive to HEB/E2A; *140*).

6.2. Innovations

PU.1 (and perhaps Ikaros) may indeed be a vertebrate innovation, but it is worth considering what functional innovations they may have made possible. From a lymphocentric perspective, the lack of PU.1 in invertebrates could simply be connected to the lack of recognizable lymphocytes in all these animals. However, from another perspective, the recent provenance of PU.1 is surprising. By far the most prominent role of PU.1 in mammals is that of a positive regulator of myeloid cell development, yet these cell types, as this volume shows in detail, have apparent homologs throughout deuterostomes and equivalents throughout bilateria. Focusing on these PU.1-dependent cells, one would imagine that PU.1 function would be as ancient and universal as that of the NF-κB/Rel family genes. It is not, however. This is most vividly seen in the case of particular effector genes, e.g., the use of macrophage scavenger receptor-class genes by sea urchin coelomocytes. In vertebrates, genes encoding scavenger receptors are PU.1-dependent for their expression *(141)*, yet, so far, it appears that sea urchins express these genes without using any PU.1/Spi family member. Thus, the developmental program of phagocytes, including the expression of scavenger receptors, is older than the use of PU.1 to "control" that program. We can interpret this in two ways. One possibility is that phagocytes in invertebrates are completely nonhomologous with those in vertebrates, in spite of the sharing of parts of their gene expression programs. The other interpretation is that, in jawed vertebrates, PU.1 has been intercalated into the regulatory cascade that controls phagocyte gene expression and development *(142)*. Intercalation is a powerful mechanism for altering the spectrum of activities of a differentiation cascade without risking loss of activity of the differentiated cells.

There is indeed some evidence that mammals themselves retain some ability to develop phagocytic cells in the absence of PU.1: this is in the primitive hematopoiesis in the earliest embryos. PU.1, like c-Myb, has a more essential role in definitive hematopoietic than in primitive hematopoiesis, and it turns out to be dispensable for expression of macrophage-like characteristics in cells from extraembryonic blood islands in the yolk sac *(143,144)*. What, then, is the function that might be contributed to the phagocytic cells and pluripotent precursors through the addition of PU.1 activity? A hallmark of earliest yolk sac hematopoiesis is that cells proceed directly to effector differentiation with little or no generation of long-term proliferating precursors or stem cells *(108)*. The complex transcription factor interactions that PU.1 mediates could balance the developmental progress of the cells with controlled proliferative expansion. Thus, in spite of its many effects on target genes of differentiated macrophages, PU.1 may be most uniquely important for the generation of long-term, proliferating macrophage progenitors. Such cells could provide a necessary precondition for development of lymphocytes as well. In this context, the repression and activation-damping roles of another potential vertebrate innovation, Ikaros, could also be important to prevent premature differentiation.

Enormous gaps in our of knowledge need to be filled in, but one element of a pattern will have emerged: the transcription factors that appear most likely to be new in vertebrates are factors that are vital for the generation of particular kinds of multipotent progenitors, and/or stem cells capable of long-term self renewal, as well as for the generation of lymphocytes. By contrast, the transcription factors known to turn on definitive lymphocyte differentiation genes, such as the E2A products GATA-3, TCF-1, EBF, and Pax5, appear to be co-opted without major structural alteration from roles in nervous system development and elsewhere. This is a reminder that although the lymphocyte gene rearrangement program is the showiest of the distinctive properties of these cells, these cells may also incorporate profound regulatory innovations in the form of properties they share with stem cells. We do not know whether true long-term repopulating hematopoietic stem cells exist in invertebrates at all. Conceivably the radical uncoupling of proliferation from differentiation, in both stem cells and lymphocytes, is the feature that requires innovative regulatory mechanisms.

ACKNOWLEDGMENTS

E.H.D. gratefully acknowledges support from the Lucille P. Markey Charitable Trust. Work from the laboratory of E.V.R. was supported by a grant from NASA (NAG 2-1370). E.V.R. would also like to thank Dr. Michele K. Anderson for critical reading of this manuscript, for many insights into lower vertebrate immunity, and for her essential role in developing many of the ideas that are discussed here (*see* ref. *124*).

REFERENCES

1. Brusca RC, Brusca GJ. Invertebrates. Sunderland, MA: Sinauer, 1990.
2. Davidson EH. Gene Activity in Early Development. New York: Academic, 1968.
3. Davidson EH. Gene Activity in Early Development, 2nd ed. New York: Academic, 1976.
4. Davidson EH. Spatial mechanisms of gene regulation in metazoan embryos. Development 1991;113:1–26.
5. Adoutte A, Balavoine G, Lartillot N, et al. The new animal phylogeny: reliability and implications. Proc Natl Acad Sci USA 2000;97:4453–4456.
6. Davidson EH, Thomas TL, Scheller RH, Britten RJ. The sea urchin actin genes and a speculation on the evolutionary significance of small gene families. In: Dover GA, Flavell RB (eds.). Genome Evolution. London: Academic, 1982, pp. 177–191.
7. Cooper AD, Crain WR Jr. Complete nucleotide sequence of a sea urchin actin gene. Nucleic Acids Res 1982;10:4081–4092.
8. Kusakabe T, Araki I, Satoh N, Jeffery WR. Evolution of chordate actin genes: evidence from genomic organization and amino acid sequences. J Mol Evol 1997;44:289–298.
9. Turbeville JM, Schultz JR, Raff RA. Deuterostome phylogeny and the sister group of the chordates: evidence from molecules and morphology. Mol Biol Evol 1994;11:648–655.
10. Wada H, Satoh N Details of the evolutionary history from invertebrates to vertebrates, as deduced from the sequences of 18S rDNA. Proc Natl Acad Sci USA 1994;91:1801–1804.
11. Cameron CB, Garey JR, Swalla BJ. Evolution of the chordate body plan: new insights from phylogenetic analyses of deuterostome phyla. Proc Natl Acad Sci USA 2000;97:4469–4474.
12. Castresana J, Feldmaier-Fuchs G, Yokobori S, Satoh N, Paabo S. The mitochondrial genome of the hemichordate *Balanoglossus carnosus* and the evolution of deuterostome mitochondria. Genetics 1998;150:1115–1123.
13. Peterson KJ, Cameron RA, Davidson EH. Set-aside cells in maximal indirect development: evolutionary and developmental significance. Bioessays 1997;19:623–631.

14. Sprinkle J. Phylum echinodermata. In: Boardman RS, Cheetham AH, Rowell AJ (eds.). Fossil Invertebrates. Cambridge, MA: Blackwell Science, 1987, pp. 550–611.

15. Conway Morris S, Whittington HB. The animals of the Burgess Shale. Sci Am 1979;241:122–133.

16. Chen J-y, Huang D-Y, Li C-W. In early Cambrian craniate-like chordate.

17. Shu D-G, Chen L, Han J, Zhang X-L. An early Cambrian tunicate from China. Nature 1999;411:427–473.

18. Janvier P. Catching the first fish. Nature 1999;402:21–22.

19. Shu D-G, Chen L, Han J, Zhang X-L. An Early Cambrian tunicate from China. Nature 2001;411:472–473.

20. Smith LC, Davidson EH. The echinoderm immune system: characters shared with vertebrate immune systems, and characters arising later in deuterostome phylogeny. NY Acad Sci 1994;712:213–226.

21. Gross PS, Al-Sharif WZ, Clow LA, Smith LC. Echinoderm immunity and the evolution of complement system. Dev Comp Immunol 1999;23:429–442.

22. Coffaro KA, Hinegardner RT. Immune response in the sea urchin *Lytechinus pictus*. Science 1977;197:1389–1390.

23. Coffaro KA. Transplantation immunity in the sea urchin. Doctoral dissertation, University of California, Santa Cruz, CA, 1979.

24. Smith LC, Davidson EH. The echinoid immune system and the phylogenetic occurrence of immune mechanisms in deuterostomes. Immunol-Today 1992;13:356–362.

25. Smith LC, Chang L, Britten RJ, Davidson EH. Sea urchin genes expressed in activated coelomocytes are identified by expressed sequence tags. J Immunol 1996;156:593–602.

26. Al-Sharif WZ, Sunyer JO, Lambris JD, Smith LC. Sea urchin coelomocytes specifically express a homologue of the complement component C3. J Immunol 1998;160:2983–2997.

27. Smith LC, Shih C-S, Dachenhausen SG. Coelomocytes express SpBf, a homologue of factor B, the second component in the sea urchin complement system. J Immunol 1998;161:6784–6793.

28. Smith L C., Azumi K Nonaka M. Complement systems in invertebrates: the ancient alternative and lectin pathways. Immunopharmacology 1999;42:107–120.

29. Nonaka M, Takahashi K. Complete complementary of lamprey. Implication for the evolution of thioester containing proteins. J Immunol 1992;148:3290–3295.

30. Nonaka M, Takahashi M, Sasaki M. Molecular cloning of a lamprey homologue of the mammalian MHS class III gene, complement factor B. J Immunol 1994;152:2263–2269.

31. Lagueux M, Perrodou E, Levashina EA, Capovilla M, Hoffmann JA. Constitutive expression of a complement-like protein in Toll and JAK gain-of-function mutants of *Drosophila*. Proc Natl Acad Sci USA 2000;97:11427–11432.

32. Rast JP, Oliveri P, Davidson EH. Conserved linkage among sea urchin homologs of genes encoded in the vertebrate MHC region. In: Kasahard M (ed.). Major Histocompatibility Complex. Tokyo: Springer, 2000, pp. 66–74.

33. Pancer Z. Dynamic expression of multiple scavenger receptor cysteine-rich genes in coelomocytes of the purple sea urchin. Proc Natl Acad Sci USA 2000;97:13156–13161.

34. Wijngaard PLJ, Metzelaar MJ, MacHugh ND, Morrison WI, Clevers HC. Molecular characterization of the WC1 antigen expressed specifically on bovine CD4⁻CD8⁻ γδ T lymphocytes. J Immunol 1992;149:3273–3277.

35. Walker ID, Glew MD, O'Keefe MA, et al. A novel multi-gene family of sheep γδ cells. Immunology 1994;83:517–523.

36. Kanan JHC, Nayeem N, Binns RM, Chain BM. Mechanisms for variability in a member of the scavenger-receptor cysteine-rich superfamily. Immunogenetics 1997;46:276–282.

37. Kirkham PA, Takamatsu H-H, Parkhouse RME. Growth arrest of γδ T cells induced by monoclonal antibody against WC1 correlates with activation of multiple tyrosine phosphatases and dephosphorylation of MAP kinase erk2. Eur J Immunol 1997;27:717–725.

38. O'Keeffe MA, Metcalfe SA, Cunningham CP, Walker ID. Sheep CD4+ αβ T cells express novel members of the *T19* multigene family. Immunogenetics 1999;49:45–55.

39. Freeman M, Ashkenas J, Rees DJG, et al. An ancient, highly conserved family of cysteine-rich protein domains revealed by cloning type I and type II murine macrophage scavenger receptors. Proc Natl Acad Sci USA 1990;87:8810–8814.

40. Dunne DW, Resnick D, Greenberg J, Krieger M, Joiner KA. The type I macrophage scavenger receptor binds to Gram-positive bacteria and recognizes lipoteichoic acid. Proc Natl Acad Sci USA 1994;91:1863–1867.

41. Elomaa O, Kangas M, Sahlberg C, et al. Cloning of a novel bacteria-binding receptor structurally related to scavenger receptors and expressed in a subset of macrophages. Cell 1995;80:603–609.

42. Greenberg JW, Fischer W, Joiner KA. Influence of lipoteichoic acid structure on recognition by the macrophage scavenger receptor. Infect Immun 1996;64:3318–3325.

43. Holmskov U, Mollenhauer J, Madsen J, et al. Cloning of gp-340, a putative opsonin receptor for lung surfactant protein D. Proc Natl Acad Sci USA 1999;96:10794–10799.

44. Trahey M, Weissman IL. Cyclophilin C-associated protein: a normal secreted glycoprotein that down-modulates endotoxin and proinflammatory responses *in vivo*. Proc Natl Acad Sci USA 1999;96:3006–3011.

45. Van der Laan LJW, Dôpp EA, Haworth R, et al. Regulatin and functional involvement of macrophage scavenger receptor MARCO in clearance of bacteria in vivo. J Immunol 1999;62:939–947.

46. Thomas CA, Li Y, Kodama T, et al. Protection from lethal Gram-positive infection by macrophage scavenger receptor-dependent phagocytosis. J Exp Med 2000;191:147–155.

47. Pancer Z, Rast JP, Davidson EH. Origins of immunity: transcription factors and homologues of effector genes of the vertebrate immune system expressed in sea urchin coelomocytes. Immunogenetics 1999;49:773–786.

48. Cameron RA, Mahairas G, Rast JP, et al. A sea urchin genome project: sequence scan, virtual map, and additional resources. Proc Natl Acad Sci USA 2000;97:9514–9518.

49. Cameron RA, Oliveri P, Wyllie J, Davidson EH. *Cis*-regulatory activity of randomly chosen genomic fragments from the sea urchin. Submitted.

50. Ozinsky A, Underhill DM, Fontenot JD, et al. The repertoire for pattern recognition of pathogens by the innate immune system is defined by cooperation between toll-like receptors. Proc Natl Acad Sci USA 2000;97:13766–13771.

51. Imler JL, Hoffmann JA. Toll and Toll-like proteins: an ancient family of receptors signaling infection. Rev Immunogenet 2000;2:294–304.

52. Anderson KV. Toll signaling pathways in the innate immune response. Curr Opin Immunol 2000;12:13–19.

53. Kimbrell DA, Beutler B. The evolution and genetics of innate immunity. Nat Rev Genet 2001;2:256–267.

54. Smith LC, Britten RJ, Davidson EH. Lipopolysaccharide activates the sea urchin immune system. Dev Comp Immun 1995;19:217–224.

55. Chow LA, Gross PS, Shih C-S, Smith LC. Expression of SpC3, the sea urchin complement component, in response to lipopolysaccharide. Immunogenetics 2000;51:1021–1033.

56. Laird DJ, De Tomaso AW, Cooper MD, Weissman IL. 50 million years of chordate evolution: seeking the origins of adaptive immunity. Proc Natl Acad Sci USA 2000;97:6924–6926.

57. Hansen JD, McBlane JF. Recombination-activating genes, transposition, and the lymphoid-specific combinatorial immune system: a common evolutionary connection. Curr Top Microbiol Immunol 2000;248:111–135.

58. Schluter SF, Bernstein RM, Bernstein H, Marchalonis JJ. 'Big Bang' emergence of the combinatorial immune system. Dev Comp Immunol. 1999;23:107–111.

59. Flajnik MF, Ohta Y, Namikawa-Yamada C, Nonaka M. Insight into the primordial MHC from studies in ectothermic vertebrates. Immunol Rev 1999;167:59–67.

60. Rast JP, Litman GW. Towards understanding the evolutionary origins and early diversification of rearranging antigen receptors. Immunol Rev 1998;166:79–86.

61. Medzhitov R, Janeway CA Jr. Innate immune recognition and control of adaptive immune responses. Semin Immunol 1998;10:351–353.

62. Litman GW, Anderson MK, Rast JP. Evolution of antigen binding receptors. Annu Rev Immunol 1999;17:109–147.

63. Bernstein RM, Schluter SF, Bernstein H, Marchalonis JJ. Primordial emergence of the recombination activating gene 1 (RAG1): sequence of the complete shark gene indicates homology to microbial integrases. Proc Natl Acad Sci USA 1996;93:9454–9459.

64. Wu L, Antica M, Johnson GR, Scollay R, Shortman K. Developmental potential of the earliest precursor cells from the adult mouse thymus. J Exp Med 1991;174:1617–1627.

65. Kondo M, Weissman IL, Akashi K. Identification of clonogenic common lymphoid progenitors in mouse bone marrow. Cell 1997;91:661–672.

66. Akashi K, Traver D, Miyamoto T, Weissman IL. A clonogenic common myeloid progenitor that gives rise to all myeloid lineages. Nature 2000;404:193–197.

67. Cumano A, Paige CJ, Iscove NN, Brady G. Bipotential precursors of B cells and macrophages in murine fetal liver. Nature 1992;356:612–615.

68. Lacaud G, Carlsson L, Keller G. Identification of a fetal hematopoietic precursor with B cell, T cell, and macrophage potential. Immunity 1998;9:827–838.

69. Katsura Y, Kawamoto H. Stepwise lineage restriction of progenitors in lympho-myelopoiesis. Int Rev Immunol 2001;20:1–20.

70. Hunte BE, Capone M, Zlotnik A, Rennick D, Moore TA. Acquisition of CD24 expression by Lin−CD43+B220lowckithi cells coincides with commitment to the B cell lineage. Eur J Immunol 1998;28:3850–3856.

71. Montecino-Rodriguez E, Leathers H, Dorshkind K. Bipotential B-macrophage progenitors are present in adult bone marrow. Nat Immunol 2001;2:83–88.

72. Ardavin C, Wu L, Li CL, Shortman K. Thymic dendritic cells and T cells develop simultaneously in the thymus from a common precursor population. Nature 1993;362:761–763.

73. Lucas K, Vremec D, Wu L, Shortman K. A linkage between dendritic cell and T-cell development in the mouse thymus: the capacity of sequential T-cell precursors to form dendritic cells in culture. Dev Comp Immunol 1998;22:339–349.

74. Res PCM, Couwenberg F, Vyth-Dreese FA, Spits H. Expression of a pTα mRNA in a committed dendritic cell precursor in the human thymus. Blood 1999;94:2647–2657.

75. Rothenberg EV, Telfer JC, Anderson MK. Transcriptional regulation of lymphocyte lineage commitment. Bioessays 1999;21:726–742.

76. Kondo M, Scherer DC, Miyamoto T, et al. Cell-fate conversion of lymphoid-committed progenitors by instructive actions of cytokines. Nature 2000;407:383–386.

77. Reya T, Grosschedl R. Transcriptional regulation of B-cell differentiation. Curr Opin Immunol 1998;10:158–165.

78. Liberg D, Sigvardsson M. Transcriptional regulation in B cell differentiation. Crit Rev Immunol 1999;19:127–153.

79. Busslinger M, Nutt SL, Rolink AG. Lineage commitment in lymphopoiesis. Curr Opin Immunol 2000;12:151–158.

80. Kee BL, Murre C. Transcription factor regulation of B lineage commitment. Curr Opin Immunol 2001;13:180–185.

81. Atchley WR, Fitch WM. A natural classification of the basic helix-loop-helix class of transcription factors. Proc Natl Acad Sci USA 1997;94:5172–5176.

82. Wang SS, Tsai RYL, Reed RR. The characterization of the Olf-1/EBF-like HLH transcription factor family: implications in olfactory gene regulation and neuronal development. J Neurosci 1997;17:4149–4158.

83. Czerny T, Bouchard M, Kozmik Z, Busslinger M. The characterization of novel Pax genes of the sea urchin and Drosophila reveal an ancient evolutionary origin of the Pax2/5/8 subfamily. Mech Dev 1997;67:179–192.

84. Prasad BC, Ye B, Zackhary R, et al. *unc-3,* a gene required for axonal guidance in *Caenorhabditis elegans,* encodes a member of the O/E family of transcription factors. Development 1998;125:1561–1568.

85. Bain G, Murre C. The role of E-proteins in B- and T-lymphocyte development. Semin Immunol 1998;10:143–153.

86. Kuo CT, Leiden JM. Transcriptional regulation of T lymphocyte development and function. Annu Rev immunol 1999;17:149–187.

87. Ting C-N, Olson MC, Barton KP, Leiden JM. Transcription factor GATA-3 is required for development of the T-cell lineage. Nature 1996;384:474–478.

88. Hendriks RW, Nawijn MC, Engel JD, et al. Expression of the transcription factor GATA-3 is required for the development of the earliest T cell progenitors and correlates with stages of cellular proliferation in the thymus. Eur J Immunol 1999;29:1912–1918.

89. Tomita K, Hattori M, Nakamura E, et al. The bHLH gene *Hes1* is essential for expansion of early T cell precursors. Genes Dev. 1999;13:1203–1210.

90. Heemskerk MHM, Blom B, Nolan G, et al. Inhibition of T cell and promotion of natural killer cell development by the dominant negative helix loop helix factor Id3. J Exp Med 1997;186:1597–1602.

91. Barndt R, Dai MF, Zhang Y. A novel role for HEB downstream or parallel to the pre-TCR signaling pathway during αβ thymopoiesis. J Immunol 1999;163:3331–3343.

92. Okamura RM, Sigvardsson M, Galceran J, et al. Redundant regulation of T cell differentiation and TCRα gene expression by the transcription factors LEF-1 and TCF-1. Immunity 1998;8:11–20.

93. Verbeek S, Izon D, Hofhuis F, et al. An HMG-box-containing T-cell factor required for thymocyte differentiation. Nature 1995;374:70–74.

94. Clevers HC, Grosschedl R. Transcriptional control of lymphoid development: lessons from gene targeting. Immunol Today 1996;17:336–343.

95. Anderson MK, Hernandez-Hoyos G, Diamond RA, Rothenberg EV. Precise developmental regulation of Ets family transcription factors during specification and commitment to the T cell lineage. Development 1999;126:3131–3148.

96. Zhuang Y, Cheng P, Weintraub H. B-lymphocyte development is regulated by the combined dosage of three basic helix-loop-helix genes, *E2A, E2-2,* and *HEB.* Mol Cell Biol 1996;16:2898–2905.

97. Huang L, Li X, El-Hodiri HM, et al. Involvement of Tcf/Lef in establishing cell types along the animal-vegetal axis of sea urchins. Dev Genes Evol 2000;210:73–81.

98. Lin WH, Huang LH, Yeh JY, et al. Expression of a *Drosophila* GATA transcription factor in multiple tissues in the developing embryos. Identification of homozygous lethal mutants with P-element insertion at the promoter region. J Biol Chem 1995;270:25150–25158.

99. Pandolfi PP, Roth ME, Karis A, et al. Targeted disruption of the *GATA3* gene causes severe abnormalities in the nervous system and in fetal liver haematopoiesis. Nat Genet 1995;11:40–44.

100. Staal FJT, Meelidijk J, Moerer P, et al. Wnt signaling is required for thymocyte development and activates Tcf-1 mediated transcription. Eur J Immunol 2001;31:285–293.

101. Reya T, O'Riordan M, Okamura R, et al. Wnt signaling regulates B lymphocyte proliferation through a LEF-1 dependent mechanism. Immunity 2000;13:15–24.

102. Roose J, Clevers H. TCF transcription factors: molecular switches in carcinogenesis. Biochim Biophys Acta 1999;1424:M23–M37

103. Brunner E, Peter O, Schweitzer L, Basler K. *pangolin* encodes a Lef-1 homologue that acts downstream of *Armadillo* to transduce the *Wingless* signal in *Drosophila*. Nature 1997;385:829–833.

104. Manaia A, Lemarchandel V, Klaine M, et al. Lmo2 and GATA-3 associated expression in intraembryonic hemogenic sites. Development 2000;127:643–653.

105. Labastie M-C, Cortes F, Romeo P-H, Dulac C, Péault B. Molecular identity of hematopoietic precursor cells emerging in the human embryo. Blood 1998;92:3624–3635.

106. Petersen U-M, Kadalayil L, Rehorn K-P, et al. Serpent regulates *Drosophila* immunity genes in the larval fat body through an essential GATA motif. EMBO J 1999;18:4013–4022.

107. Lowry JA, Atchley WR. Molecular evolution of the GATA family of transcription factors: conservation within the DNA-binding domain. J Mol Evol 2000;50:103–115.

108. Dzierzak E, Medvinsky A, de Bruijn M. Qualitative and quantitative aspects of haematopoietic cell development in the mammalian embryo. Immunol Today 1998;19:228–236.

109. North T, Gu T-L, Stacy T, et al. *Cbfa2* is required for the formation of intra-aortic hematopoietic clusters. Development 1999;126:2563–2575.

110. Mukouyama Y, Chiba N, Hara T, et al. The AML1 transcription factor functions to develop and maintain hematogenic precursor cells in the embryonic aorta-gonad-mesonephros region. Dev Biol 2000;220:27–36.

111. Cai Z, de Bruijn M, Ma X, et al. Haploinsufficiency of AML1 affects the temporal and spatial generation of hematopoietic stem cells in the mouse embryo. Immunity 2000;13:423–431.

112. Gewirtz AM, Anfossi G, Venturelli D, et al. G_1/S transition in normal human T-lymphocytes requires the nuclear protein encoded by *c-myb*. Science 1989;245:180–183.

113. Nichogiannopoulou A, Trevisan M, Neben S, Friedrich C, Georgopoulos K. Defects in hemopoietic stem cell activity in Ikaros mutant mice. J Exp Med 1999;190:1201–1214.

114. Scott EW, Fisher RC, Olson MC, et al. PU.1 functions in a cell-autonomous manner to control the differentiation of multipotential lymphoid-myeloid progenitors. Immunity 1997;6:437–447.

115. Brown KE, Guest SS, Smale ST, et al. Association of transcriptionally silent genes with Ikaros complexes at centromeric heterochromatin. Cell 1997;91:845–854.

116. Winandy S, Wu L, Wang J-H, Georgopoulos K. Pre-T cell receptor (TCR) and TCR-controlled checkpoints in T cell differentiation are set by Ikaros. J Exp Med 1999;190:1039–1048.

117. Lloberas J, Soler C, Celada A. The key role of PU.1/SPI-1 in B cells, myeloid cells and macrophages. Immunol Today 1999;20:184–189.

118. Fisher RC, Scott EW. Role of PU.1 in hematopoiesis. Stem Cells 1998;16:25–37.

119. Nerlov C, Graf T. PU.1 induces myeloid lineage commitment in multipotent hematopoietic progenitors. Genes Dev 1998;12:2403–2412.

120. Singh H, DeKoter RP, Walsh JC. PU.1, a shared transcriptional regulator of lymphoid and myeloid cell fates. Cold Spring Harbor Symp Quant Biol 1999;64:13–20.

121. Spain LM, Guerriero A, Kunjibettu S, Scott EW. T cell development in PU.1-deficient mice. J Immunol 1999;163:2681–2687.

122. DeKoter RP, Singh H. Regulation of B lymphocyte and macrophage development by graded expression of PU.1. Science 2000;288:1439–1441.

123. Anderson MK, Weiss A, Hernandez-Hoyos G, et al. Constitutive expression of PU.1 in fetal hematopoietic progenitors blocks T-cell development at the pro-T stage. Immunity 2002;16:285–296.

124. Anderson MK, Rothenberg EV. Transcription factor expression in lymphocyte development: clues to the evolutionary origins of lymphoid cell lineages? Curr Top Microbiol Immunol 2000;248:137–155.

125. Laudet V, Hanni C, Stéhelin D, Duterque-Coquillaud M. Molecular phylogeny of the ETS gene family. Oncogene 1999;18:1351–1359.

126. Zhang P, Behre G, Pan J, et al. Negative cross-talk between hematopoietic regulators: GATA proteins repress PU.1. Proc Natl Acad Sci USA 1999;96:8705–8710.

127. Rekhtman N, Radparvar F, Evans T, Skoultchi A. Direct interaction of hematopoietic transcription factors PU.1 and GATA-1: functional antagonism in erythroid cells. Genes Dev 1999;13:1398–1411.

128. Nerlov C, Querfurth E, Kulessa H, Graf T. GATA-1 interacts with the myeloid PU.1 transcription factor and represses PU.1-dependent transcription. Blood 2000;95:2543–2551.

129. Matsumura I, Kawasaki A, Tanaka H, et al. Biologic significance of GATA-1 activities in Ras-mediated megakaryocytic differentiation of hematopoietic cell lines. Blood 2000;96:2440–2450.

130. Hernandez-Hoyos G, Anderson MK, Rothenberg EV. Distinct actions of GATA-3 in three phases of thymocyte development: specification, β-selection, and CD4/CD8 differentiation. Submitted.

131. Shintani S, Terzic J, Saraga-Babic M, et al. Do lampreys have lymphocytes? The Spi evidence. Proc Natl Acad Sci USA 2000;97:7417–7422.

132. Anderson MK, Sun X, Miracle AL, Litman GW, Rothenberg EV. Evolution of hematopoiesis: three members of the PU.1 transcription factor family in a cartilaginous fish, *Raja eglanteria*. Proc Natl Acad Sci USA 2001;98:553–558.

133. Miracle AL, Anderson MK, Litman RT, et al. Complex expression patterns of lymphocyte-specific genes during the development of cartilaginous fish implicate unique lymphoid tissues in generating an immune repertoire. Int Immunol 2001;13:567–580.

134. Zapata A, Amemiya CT. Phylogeny of lower vertebrates and their immunological structures. Curr Top Microbiol Immunol 2000;248:67–107.

135. Brass AL, Kehrli E, Eisenbeis CF, Storb U, Singh H. Pip, a lymphoid-restricted IRF, contains a regulatory domain that is important for autoinhibition and ternary complex formation with the Ets factor PU.1. Genes Dev 1996;10:2335–2347.

136. Marecki S, Fenton MJ. PU.1 interferon regulatory factor interactions: mechanisms of transcriptional regulation. Cell Biochem Biophys 2000;33:127–148.

137. Tamura T, Nagamura-Inoue T, Shmeltzer Z, Kuwata T, Ozato K. ICSBP directs bipotential myeloid progenitor cells to differentiate into mature macrophages. Immunity 2000;13:155–165.

138. Hansen JD, Strassburger P, Du Pasquier L. Conservation of a master hematopoietic switch gene during vertebrate evolution: isolation and characterization of *Ikaros* from teleost and amphibian species. Eur J Immunol 1997;27:3049–3058.

139. Haire RN, Miracle AL, Rast JP, Litman GW. Members of the Ikaros gene family are present in early representative vertebrates. J Immunol 2000;165:306–312.

140. Grégoire J-M, Roméo P-H. T-cell expression of the human *GATA-3* gene is regulated by a non-lineage specific silencer. J Biol Chem 1999;274:6567–6578.

141. Moulton KS, Semple K, Wu H, Glass CK. Cell-specific expression of the macrophage scavenger receptor gene is dependent on PU.1 and a composite AP-1/ets motif. Mol Cell Biol 1994;14:4408–4418.

142. Davidson EH. Changes that make new forms: gene regulatory systems and the evolution of body parts. In: Genomic Regulatory Systems, 1st ed.

143. Olson MC, Scott EW, Hack AA, et al. PU.1 is not essential for early myeloid gene expression but is required for terminal myeloid differentiation. Immunity 1995;3:703–714.

144. Lichanska AM, Browne CM, Henkel GW, et al. Differentiation of the mononuclear phagocyte system during mouse embryogenesis: the role of transcription factor PU.1. Blood 1999;94:127–138.

5

Antimicrobial Peptides in Insect Immunity

Philippe Bulet, Maurice Charlet, and Charles Hetru

1. INTRODUCTION

With around one million named species and probably 8–10 times that number unnamed, insects account for the great majority of animal species on earth. Insects can be found in almost all terrestrial and freshwater habitats, from the driest deserts to freshwater ponds, from the canopy of a tropical rainforest (where their diversity is unbelievably great) to the arctic wastes. They are a tremendously successful group. They are a fundamental part of our ecosystem. They are responsible for the pollination of many plants; the decomposition of organic materials, facilitating the recycling of carbon, nitrogen, and other essential nutrients; the control of populations of harmful invertebrate species (including other insects); the direct production of certain foods (honey, for example); and the manufacture of useful products such as silk. However, they are often considered as negative, mainly because they are important vectors of animal and human diseases.

Important features of their success are their short life cycle and their ability to evolve rapidly to colonize new niches and to mount rapid and efficient immune defenses against pathogens. The response of insects to infection can be divided into three main mechanisms (for review, *see* ref. *1*). First, when the size of the foreign body is small enough, particular hemocytes (blood cells) can internalize these foreign bodies by phagocytosis (for review, *see* ref. 2). A second aspect, initiated upon contact of the foreign bodies with the internal cavity of the insect, is the rapid activation of proteolytic cascades leading to (1) melanization and encapsulation of the foreign material within an envelope of highly flattened cells, which become pigmented (melanized); (2) localized clotting of wound; and (3) opsonization. Finally, holometabolous insects respond to infection by a transient transcription of antimicrobial peptides (AMPs) by the fat body tissue (analogous to the mammalian liver). The AMPs are then secreted into the hemolymph (blood), where they accumulate to high concentrations and diffuse throughout the body. Interestingly, local expression of genes coding the AMPs is also observed in various surface epithelia at the site of infection; for an example, see the work of Tzou and co-workers *(3)* on the tissue-specific expression of AMP genes in *Drosophila melanogaster* epithelia. However, in insects that undergo an incomplete metamorphosis (heterometabolous), AMPs are produced constitutively by the hemocytes and secreted during infection *(4)*.

From: *Infectious Disease: Innate Immunity*
Edited by: R. A. B. Ezekowitz and J. A. Hoffmann © Humana Press Inc., Totowa, NJ

Name	Concentration	Gene	Activity	3D structure
α-helical				
Cecropins	20 μM	4 genes 99E4, 3R	G-> G+> F	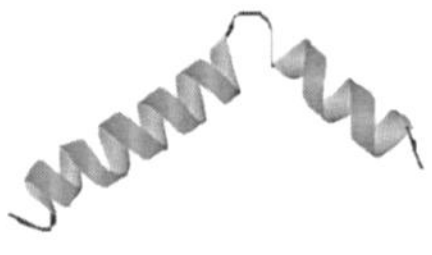
Open-ended cyclic				
Defensin	<1 μM	1 gene 46D7, 2R	G+> G-> F	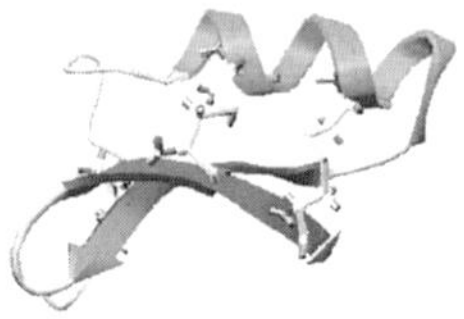
Drosomycins	>100 μM	7 genes 63D, 3L 63C5, 3L	F	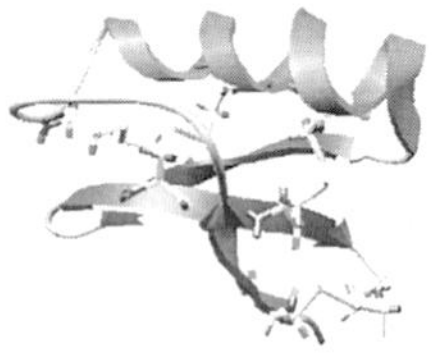
Proline-rich				
Drosocin (O-glycosylated)	40 μM	1 gene 51C2, 2R	G-	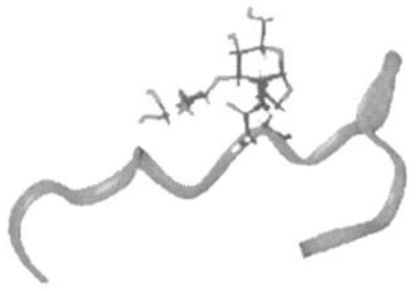
Metchnikowin	40 μM	1 gene 52A, 2R	F	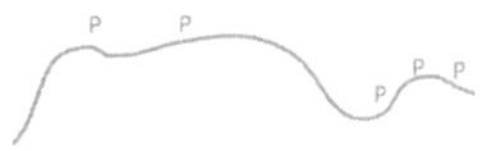
Glycine-rich				
Diptericins (O-glycosylated)	<1 μM	2 genes 55F5, 2R	G-	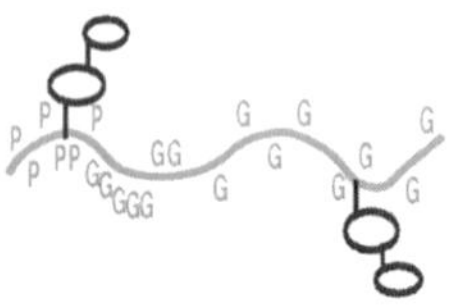
Attacins	not defined	4 genes 51C2, 2R 50A8, 2R 46D7, 2R 90B6, 3R	G-	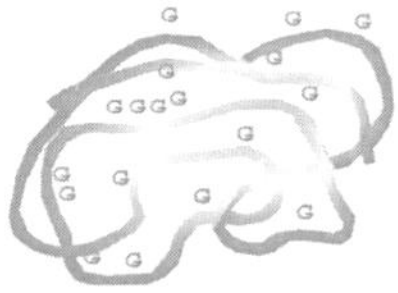

Fig. 1. Features of the seven *Drosophila* antimicrobial peptide families produced following a septic injury in adult insect. Peptides are listed on the basis of sequence and structural characteristics: *(1)* linear peptide devoid of cysteine residues and forming α-helices, *i.e.,* cecropins; *(2)* open-ended cyclic peptides containing cysteine residues with a Csαβ motif, *i.e.,* defensin and drosomycins; *(3)* peptides with an high content of one amino acid, as proline, *i.e.,* drosocin and metchnikowin, or glycine, *i.e.,* diptericins and attacins. Hemolymph concentrations are given in μ*M*. G+ and G– antibacterial activity against Gram-positive and Gram-negative bacteria, respectively; F, antifungal activity. Three-dimensional structures of defensin, drosomycin, drosocin, and cecropin are based on information from the Brookhaven Protein Data Bank and are designed using a Swiss PDBviewer. Diptericin, metchnikowin, and attacin are schematically represented.

Since the first report by Hans Boman and co-workers *(5)* in 1981 of AMPs from the moth *Hyalophora cecropia (5),* several hundreds of these molecules have been isolated from immune-challenged insects (for reviews, *see* refs. *6* and *7*). AMPs are not only part of the insect immune response; they are also found in microorganisms, various invertebrates, mammals, and plants (for review, *see* ref. *8*).

Insect AMPs enclose a wide variety of primary structures that can be arbitrarily classified, according to their amino acid composition and three-dimensional structure, into three main classes: (1) linear peptides forming amphipathic and hydrophobic α-helices; (2) open-ended cyclic peptides with one or more cysteine bonds that form β-sheet or α-helix/β-sheet structures; and (3) AMPs with an overrepresentation of particular amino acids such as proline and/or glycine residues. Most of these AMPs are amphipathic, with a net positive charge at physiologic pH. They can be particularly abundant, in terms of concentration and diversity. For example, after a septic injury, *Drosophila* produces at least seven distinct AMP families (Fig. 1), peptides forming α-helices (cecropins), open-ended cyclic peptides (defensin and drosomycins), and molecules with unique amino acid compositions, such as proline-rich peptides (drosocins and metchnikowin), as well as glycine-rich molecules such as attacins and diptericins (for review, *see* ref. *9*). Their total concentration estimated in the hemolymph of infected *Drosophila* reaches a value around 200 μM (Fig. 1).

We will discuss in this review what is known about the structure, activity, and mechanism of action of the different groups of AMPs from insects, with special reference to the α-helical peptides and the open-ended cyclic molecules, including AMPs from spiders and scorpions. Special mention is made of AMP gene organization in *Drosophila.*

2. α-HELICAL PEPTIDES: CECROPINS

2.1. Primary Structure

The cecropin family is perhaps the one of the largest and best studied classes of AMPs (Fig. 2). In insects, the AMPs forming α-helical structures are, for the most part, cecropins. Cecropins were initially discovered in the hemolymph of bacteria-challenged diapausing pupae of the giant silk moth *Hyalophora cecropia (5)*. To date, more than 40 cecropins and cecropin-like molecules have been isolated from invertebrates. Cecropins were isolated from several phylogenetically higher insect species belonging to the orders of Diptera *(Drosophila* spp., *Sarcophaga peregrina, Aedes* spp., *Anopheles gambiae,* and *Ceratitis capitata)* and Lepidoptera *(Hyalophora cecropia, Antheraea pernyi, Manduca sexta, Bombyx mori, Heliothis virescens, Agrius convolvuli, Estigmene acraea,* and *Hyphantria cunea)*. Recently, a new group of cecropin-like molecules were isolated from the venom glands of a third order of insects (Hymenoptera), the ant *Pachycondylas goeldii (10)*. Interestingly, cecropin homologs were found in pig intestine *(11)* and more recently in a simple marine invertebrate, the solitary tunicate *Styela clava, (12,13)*. All these molecules have been identified either by biochemical characterization or by cloning studies. Similarity studies revealed that dipteran cecropins fit into a homogenous group, with more than 70% identical amino acids. The sequence of *Drosophila melanogaster* cecropin A is identical to cecropin IA from *Sarcophaga peregrina* (named sarcotoxin IA). In contrast to the dipteran cecropins, the lepidopteran cecropins present more variations in their amino acid sequence (for review, *see* ref. *14*).

1 and 2D structures

3D structure of
H. cecropia cecropin A

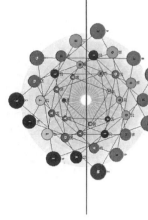

Lepidopteran cecropins

Hyalophora cecropia
cecropin A(3 variants) KWKLFKKIEKVGQNIRDGIIKAGPAVAVVGQATQIAK*

Bombyx mori
cecropin A (3 variants) RWKLFKKIEKVGRNVRDGLIKAGPAIAVIGQAKSL*
cecropin D GNFFKDLEKMGQRVRDAVISAAPAVDTLAKAKALGQ*

Dipteran cecropins

Drosophila melanogaster
cecropin A (3 variants) GWLKKIGKKIERVGQHTRDATIQGLGIAQQAANVAATAR*

Aedes aegypti
cecropin A GGLKKLGKKLEGAGKRVFNAAEKALPVVAGAKALRK

Aedes albopictus
cecropin A (3 variants) GGLKKLGKKLEGVGKRVFKASEKALPVAVGIKALG

Anopheles gambiae
cecropin A GRLKKLGKKIEGAGKRVFKAAEKALPVVAGVKAL*

Helical wheel projection of
D. melanogaster cecropin A

hydrophobic face

hydrophilic face

Hymenopteran ponericins

Pachycondyla goeldii
ponericin G1 (7 variants) GWKDWAKKAGGWLKKKGPGMAKAALKAAMQ
ponericin W1 (6 variants) WLGSALKIGAKLLPSVVGLFKKKQ
ponericin L1 (2 variants) LLKELWTKMKGAGKAVLGKIKGLL*

Fig. 2. Features of selected cecropins (α-helical peptides) from insects. In the primary (1D) and secondary (2D) structures, the characteristic tryptophan residue is noted in bold; the underlined sequences indicate the hinge regions between the amphipatic α-helix and the hydrophobic α-helix, and the * indicates a C-terminal amidation. The 3D structure of cecropin A from the lepidopteran *Hyalophora cecropia* has been determined by 2D NMR and designed using a Swiss PDBviewer. In the Schiffer-Edmundson wheel projection of *Drosophila* cecropin, the numbering corresponds to the amino acid sequence. Additional data from insect ceropins (alignments and phylogenetic relationships) are given in ref. *18*. For complementary information on the ponericins from the ant *Pachycondyla goeldii, see ref. 10.*

The cecropins from dipteran and lepidopteran insects consist of 31–39 amino acid residues and have two characteristics (1) the presence of a tryptophan residue at position 1 or 2; and (2) the amidation of the C-terminal residue. There are a few exceptions: the cecropin D from *Bombyx mori (15)*, the cecropin A from *Aedes aegypti (16,17)* and the cecropin from *Aedes albopictus (16)* have no C-terminal amidation. In addition, neither cecropin D from *Bombyx mori* nor the cecropins from mosquitoes have a tryptophan residue (for review, *see* ref. *18*). Investigations on the importance of the tryptophan residues and the C-terminal amidation tend to indicate that these structural characters contribute to better stability of the cecropins and efficacy against bacteria. Interestingly, *Anopheles* cecropin A (lacking the tryptophan residue) was found to be efficient against yeast and a larger number of Gram-positive bacterial strains compared with *Drosophila* cecropin A, bearing the tryptophan signature *(19)*.

Recently, a new group of cecropin-like molecules, the ponericins, was isolated from venom glands of the predatory ant *Pachycondylas goeldii (10)*. Fifteen ponericins, have been identified and classified into three different families, ponericins G, W, and L. Ponericins G have almost 60% similarity with cecropins, whereas ponericins W share about 70% similarity with the major toxic component of the honey bee venom, the antimicrobial and hemolytic melittin. Most of the ponericins have a tryptophan residue between positions 1 and 3, but only a few are C-terminally amidated.

2.2. Secondary Structure

The structure of insect cecropins consists of a basic N-terminal region and a long hydrophobic C-terminal half. Helical well projection of cecropins and ponericin relatives allows clear visualization of an amphipathic α-helix. Circular dichroism (CD) spectroscopy reveals that all these molecules have unordered structure in aqueous solutions. However, analysis in hydrophobic environments (presence of organic solvents or liposomes) shows a stabilized α-helical conformation. Studies by nuclear magnetic resonance (NMR) on *Hyalophora* cecropin demonstrated organization in the motif helix-bend-helix, with an amphipatic α-helical N-terminus linked to a C-terminal hydrophobic α-helix through a glycine-proline bend. In this model, the hinge region that separates the two helices consists of a triplet, alanine-glycine-proline. This structure in the α-helix has been demonstrated to be important for maintaining the antibacterial activity of these molecules (for review, *see* ref. *20*).

2.3. Biological Activity

In vitro experiments, performed in various media (agar or liquid growth diffusion assays) and at different incubation temperatures (from 25° to 37°C), established that Gram-negative bacteria are generally more sensitive to cecropins than Gram-positive bacteria. Often an exposure period of less than 30 minutes is sufficient to inhibit bacterial growth. Cecropins were initially reported to have no cytotoxic effects against fungi and other eucaryotic cells. However, recent reports revealed that the cecropins from *Hyalophora cecropia (21)*, *Drosophila melanogaster, (17,19,21)*, *Aedes aegypti (17)*, and *Anopheles gambiae (19)* have antifungal properties against different classes of higher fungi including plant pathogens and several *Fusarium* and *Aspergillus* species. None of the cecropins are active against the entomopathogen *Beauveria bassiana*. Interestingly, only the cecropins from the mosquitoes *Aedes aegypti* and *Anopheles gambiae* are effective against some yeast strains *(18,19),* whereas neither *Drosophila* cecropins nor *Hyalophora* cecropins affect the growth of yeast. This difference in biologic efficacy against yeast cells may be linked to the absence of the tryptophan residue (see above). To date, experiments producing the expression of cecropins or analogs into the intercellular compartment of tobacco leaves have failed to enhance the plant resistance to bacterial or fungal infections. This absence of resistance acquisition is owing to a rapid clearance of the cecropin by degradative activity of proteases present in the intercellular fluid *(22),* an observation that will help in the design of protease-resistant cecropin-derived peptides that can enhance plant resistance.

Cecropins have no hemolytic activity, but they can affect the development of viruses and parasites causing malaria and Chagas disease. Surprisingly, in addition to antibacterial activity, ponericins (the cecropin-like molecules from ant venom; see above) are lethal to erythrocytes and are strong insecticides *(10).*

2.4. The Drosophila *Cecropin Gene Family*

Cecropin genetics are particularly well known in *Drosophila melanogaster.* In this model, the first AMP genes to be characterized were a compact cecropin gene cluster localized at position 99E4–99E4 on chromosome 3R with three expressed cecropin genes and two pseudogenes. Two of these genes, *Cec*A1 and *Cec*A2, encode identical peptides, the cecropin A having a deduced amino acid sequence identical to that of sarcotoxin IA, the *Sarcophaga peregrina* cecropin. The two other genes in the cluster code cecropins B and C, which differ from cecropin A in five and three amino acids, respectively. The *Cec*A1 and *Cec*A2 genes are mainly expressed in larvae and adults, whereas *Cec*B and *Cec*C genes are predominantly expressed during metamorphosis. Each of these four genes contains a short intron and codes a prepropeptide of 63 residues. The promoter regions of the cecropin genes contain a number of motifs analogous to mammalian *cis*-regulatory elements involved in the regulation of acute-phase response genes (for review, *see* ref. *23*).

3. OPEN-ENDED CYCLIC ANTIMICROBIAL PEPTIDES

AMPs with an even number of cysteine residues intralinked by disulfide bridges (1–8) are produced in many plants and animals. Here we summarize the information on these molecules from insects, scorpions, and spiders. The cysteine-containing AMPs from these invertebrates can be classified into two subgroups according to their secondary structure: (1) the peptides with an α-helix/β-sheet structure, for example, the insect antibacterial defensins and the antifungal defensins (drosomycin, heliomycin, and termicin); and (2) the AMPs forming a hairpin-like β-sheet structure, such as thanatin, androctonin, and gomesin.

3.1. Insect defensins

Insect defensins were first described almost simultaneously from cell cultures of *Sarcophaga peregrina (24)* and from experimentally infected larvae of the black blowfly *Phormia terranovae (25).* Since then, more than 40 defensins have been reported from a wide range of insect orders including primitive insects, such as the dragonfly (Odonata), and phylogenetically recent orders (for review, *see* ref. *6*). In fact, the family of defensins is certainly the most widespread group of AMPs, as they are present not only in all the insect species investigated so far but also in mussels, scorpions, ticks, and nematodes (Fig. 3).

3.1.1. Primary Structure

According to their main target, insect defensins can be subdivided into two groups: the antibacterial defensins mainly active against bacteria *(Phormia* and *Sarcophaga* defensins as prototypes), and the antifungal defensins, with drosomycin as the first representative.

3.1.1.1. ANTIBACTERIAL DEFENSINS

All insect defensins have three internal disulfide bridges with the same cysteine pairing (Cys1-Cys4, Cys2-Cys5, and Cys3-Cys6), except drosomycin, which has four disulfide bridges (Cys1-Cys8, Cys2-Cys5, Cys3-Cys6, and Cys4-Cys7) *(26)*. Insect defensins are in general 34–46 amino acids long, with three exceptions, the royalisin from royal jelly and two defensins from bees, which have 51 residues (for review, *see* ref. *6*). The shortest defensin (34 residues) is sapecin B from the fleshfly *Sarcophaga peregrina*. Bee defensins have a C-terminal extension of 12 amino acids with an α-helix structure. Interestingly, bee defensins are also the only ones to be C-terminally amidated, a feature often reported for cecropins (see above). No similar large, amidated defensin is found in another well-studied hymenopteran insect, the ant *Formica rufa*. The peptide sequence of defensins is often quite homologous within the same order but considerably different across the orders. Multisequence alignments and phylogenetic analysis of the invertebrate defensins using the six cysteine residues as landmarks revealed salient features. The invertebrate defensins split into two clearly distinct groups (for review, *see* ref. *6*). The dragonfly defensin was similar to the scorpion, and mollusk defensins and to the two recently described acari defensins isolated from the soft tick, *Ornithodoros moubata (27)*. All the other defensins fit into a second compact cluster (for a recent dendrogram, *see* refs. *18* and *27*). Surprisingly, the difference between the defensins from organisms belonging to different phyla such as the dragonfly vs. the mollusk, scorpions, and tick is smaller than that of two closely related dipteran insects, *Drosophila melanogaster* and *Aedes aegypti*.

3.1.1.2. ANTIFUNGAL DEFENSINS

In addition to the production of antibacterial defensins, insects respond to an experimental infection by the synthesis of cysteine-rich peptides with antifungal properties. To date three antifungal defensins have been characterized: (1) drosomycin from *Drosophila melanogaster;* (2) heliomicin from the tobacco budworm *Heliothis virescens;* and (3) termicin from the termite *Pseudacanthotermes spiniger.*

Drosomycin was the first inducible antifungal molecule to be isolated from insects *(28)*. It is a 44-residue peptide with the invariant disulfide array of the insect defensins. However, this AMP has the particularity of an additional disulfide bridge linking the cysteine at position two with the C-terminal cysteine residue. These four disulfide bridges give to the molecule (1) a high stability over a broad pH range and (2) a high resistance to proteolysis. Drosomycin has marked similarities to plant defensins, with only the cysteine residues in common with the antibacterial insect defensins (for review, *see* ref. *29*). The second strictly antifungal peptide isolated from an insect was heliomicin *(30)*. The sequence of heliomicin (44 residues) is evocative of that of antibacterial defensins, in that it shares the cysteine array with these molecules and three glycine residues in its

1 and 2D structures

3D structure

Antibacterial defensins

Diptera

Phormia terranovae (defensin A)
ATC**D**LLSGTGINHSA**C**AAH**C**LLRGNRGGY**C**NGKGV**C**V**C**RN

Sarcophaga peregrina (sapecin B)
LT**C**EIDRSL**C**LLH**C**RLKGYLRAY**C**SQQKV**C**R**C**VQ

Drosophila melanogaster
ATC**D**LLSKWNWNHTA**C**AGH**C**IAKGFKGGY**C**NDKAV**C**V**C**RN

Hymenoptera

Apis mellifera (royalisin)
VT**C**DLLSFKGQVNDSA**C**AAN**C**LSLGKAGGH**C**EKGV**C**I**C**RKTSFKDLWDKYF*

Formica rufa
FT**C**DLLSGAGVDHSA**C**AAH**C**ILRGKTGGR**C**NSDRV**C**V**C**RA

Odonata

Aeschna cyanea
GFG**C**PLDQMQ**C**HRH**C**QTITGRSGGY**C**SGPLKLT**C**T**C**YR

Mollusk

Mytilus galloprovincialis (MGD-1)
GFG**C**PNNYQ**C**HRH**C**KSIPGR**C**GGY**C**GWHRLR**C**T**C**YRCG

Arachnida

Ornithodoros moubata (defensin A)
GYG**C**PFNQYQ**C**HSH**C**SGIRGYKGGY**C**KGTFKQT**C**K**C**Y

Phormia defensin A

Antifungal defensins

Diptera

Drosophila melanogaster (drosomycin)
D**C**LSGRYKGP**C**AVWDNET**C**RRV**C**KEEGRSSGH**C**SPSLK**C**W**C**EG**C**

Lepidoptera

Heliothis virescens (heliomicin)
DKLIGS**C**VWGAVNYTSD**C**NGE**C**KRRGYKGGH**C**GSFANVN**C**W**C**ET

Isoptera

Pseudacanthothermes spiniger (termicin)
ACNFQS**C**WAT**C**QAQHSIYFRRAF**C**DRSQ**C**K**C**VFVRG

drosomycin

heliomicin

Fig. 3. Comparison of defensins (open-ended cyclic peptides) from some insects and two other invertebrates, *Ornithodoros moubata* and *Mytilus galloprovincialis.* The defensins are listed according to their antimicrobial activity assessed *in vitro* using a liquid growth inhibition assay: antibacterial and antifungal. Cysteine residues are marked in bold. Broken lines indicate cysteine bridges in *Phormia terranovae* defensin A (antibacterial peptide with 6 cysteines residues) and drosomycin (antifungal peptide with 8 cysteine residues) from *Drosophila melanogaster.* Underlined sequences indicate the CSαβ motif. Three-dimensional structures are based on information from the Brookhaven Data Bank and are designed using a Swiss PDBviewer.

central part. Heliomicin and drosomycin have in common six cysteine residues and a conserved cluster of four amino acids at the C-terminal part (for details, *see* ref. *30*). The third peptide with antifungal activity was isolated from hemocytes of the termite *Pseudacanthotermes spiniger.* This molecule, named termicin, is rather short, with 36 amino acids, and it has the invariant cysteine array found in the antibacterial defensins drosomycin and heliomycin *(4,6).* However, with the exception of the six cysteine residues, termicin shows little sequence similarity with the other insect defensins (antibacterial or antifungal). The closest sequence similarity for termicin was observed with sapecin B from *Sarcophaga peregrina* (for an alignment, *see* ref. *4*), whereas the activity of termicin is closer to the antifungal drosomycin and heliomicin.

3.1.2. Secondary Structure

The three-dimensional solution (water or methanol) structures of (1) two insect defensins [*Phormia (31)* and *Sarcophaga* defensins *(32)*], (2) Mediterranean mussel defensin-1 (MGD-1; a defensin from mollusk, *33*), and (3) the two antifungal defensins, drosomycin *(34)* and heliomicin *(35),* have been established on recombinant AMPs using ^{1}H-NMR. They mainly consist of an α-helical part and two antiparallel β-strands linked by two disulfide bridges (scaffold αββ). Together, these structural elements give the structure termed the CSαβ motif for cysteine-stabilized α-helix/β-sheet motif. This scaffold refers to the arrangement whereby the tripeptidic motif Cys-Xaa-Cys is present in a strand of a β-sheet and the cysteine residues are attached to two cysteine residues of the pentapeptide Cys-(Xaa)$_3$-Cys (for definition, *see* refs. *36* and *37*). Interestingly, the scaffold for the two antifungal molecules, heliomicin and drosomycin, is βαββ, with an additional short N-terminal β-strand. This βαββ scaffold is identical to the scaffold observed for the plant defensins *(38).* Such a scaffold is not present in mammalian defensins, which are organized exclusively in hairpin-like β-sheet structures with the exception of human β-defensin 2, which has a short α-helical segment next to the N-terminus *(39).* However, the structural organization of human β-defensin 2 does not include the invariant CSαβ motif observed in the insect defensins.

2.1.3. Biologic Activity

Insect antibacterial defensins are active against a large variety of Gram-positive bacteria, whereas few Gram-negative bacteria and filamentous fungal strains are affected by defensins. No inhibitory effect has so far been reported on yeast growth for insect defensins. Interestingly, under low salt concentrations, insect defensins are lytic (within 1 minute) at a low micromolar level (0.1–10 μM) for most of the susceptible

Gram-positive strains. However, this efficacy is rapidly decreased by increasing the salt concentration *(40)*. Such salt sensitivity is also observed for mammalian *(41)* and plant defensins *(42)*. *Phormia* and the dragonfly defensins affect the development of *Plasmodium gallinaceum* sporozoites *in vitro* and cause profound morphologic changes of the *Plasmodium* oocystes in *Aedes (43)*. The *Anopheles gambiae* midgut (initial point of invasion of the mosquito by *Plasmodium*) shows that the parasite invasion is associated with defensin RNA upregulation *(44,45)*. Conceivably, a localized expression of defensin and other AMPs such as cecropin within the gut tissue may help to limit *Plasmodium* parasite infectivity.

In contrast to the antibacterial defensins, heliomicin and drosomycin are potent antifungal compounds. They affect the growth of various filamentous fungi, including plant and human pathogens. Their efficacy was often reported to be below the micromolar range. They have no activity against bacteria and no hemolytic activity even at high concentrations. This is reasonable, considering that these AMPs are secreted in the insect bloodstream and can be in contact with the cytoplasmic membrane of the insect blood cells. Heliomicin is active against some yeast strains, whereas drosomycin has no effect on the same strains. The activity of both AMPs is retained at a high salt concentration, contrasting to the loss of activity of plant defensins in the same conditions. This strongly contrasts to the situation observed for antibacterial defensins but is reminiscent of styelins and clavanins and AMPs from tunicates *(12,13)*. Termicin has the particularity of being active against Gram-positive bacteria, filamentous fungi (including plant and human pathogens), and yeast, but not against Gram-negative bacteria *(4)*.

2.1.4. The Drosophila *Defensin and Drosomycin Genes*

The *Drosophila* defensin (blood titration 1 μM) was first partially characterized from an extract of experimentally infected flies and finally fully characterized following cDNA cloning *(46)*. This 40-residue peptide, of 80% and 82% identity with *Phormia* and *Sarcophaga* defensins, respectively, results from the maturation of a preprodefensin (92 residues), encoded by a single intronless gene mapping at position 46D7-46D7 on chromosome 2R. A local expression of the defensin gene is observed in the female reproductive tract and the labellar glands *(3)*. Such local expression in surface epithelia is also observed in *Anopheles (44,45)* and in *Stomoxys calcitrans (47)*.

Drosomycin (blood titration 100 μM) was first isolated through differential analysis between an extract of experimentally infected and control flies by high-performance liquid chromatography (HPLC) *(28)*. The gene encoding the isoform of drosomycin isolated by biochemical techniques is intronless and maps at position 63D-63D on chromosome 3L. However, in the *Drosophila* genome, seven distinct genes are present, coding seven variants of drosomycin. Only one variant of mature drosomycin has been isolated so far from infected *Drosophila*. The six additional genes are located on chromosome 3L at position 63C5-63C5. The isolated mature drosomycin results from the maturation of a precursor (70 amino acids) with a predomain, the 44-residue sequence of the mature drosomycin but no prosequence *(26)*. This contrasts with what has been observed for the precursors of cecropins and defensin (see above).

3.2. AMPs Forming a Hairpin-Like β-Sheet Structure

Several AMPs with one or two internal disulfide bridges have been isolated from a variety of arthropods including insects, arachnids, and horseshoe crabs. Although AMPs

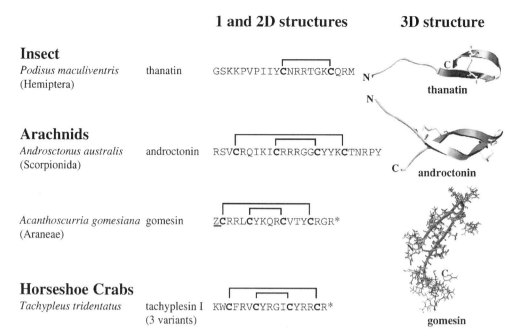

Fig. 4. Features of selected hairpin-like β-sheet structure AMPs from arthropods. Cysteine residues are marked in bold. Broken lines indicate cysteine bridges, the * indicates a C-terminal amidation, and Z stands for pyroglutamic acid, a cyclicized N-terminal amino acid. 3D structures for thanatin and androctonin, determined in solution in water by 2D NMR, are based on information from the Brookhaven Data Bank and designed using a Swiss PDBviewer. For gomesin, the 3D structure is a representation of a superposition of the backbones (in green) and the different side chains of 20 final structures using SYBYL graphic software.

forming a hairpin-like β-sheet structure (Fig. 4) have not been found in *Drosophila,* a similar fold is found for protegrins, AMPs from porcine leukocytes (for review, *see* ref. *48*), and *Ib*-AMP1, a 20-residue AMP from the plant *Impatiens balsamina (49).*

3.2.1. Primary Structure

The first representatives of the invertebrate AMPs with two disulfide bridges were found in the hemocyte granules of horseshoe crabs: the tachyplesins from *Tachypleus tridentatus (50)* and the polyphemusins from *Limulus polyphemus (51).* Since these first reports, two additional AMPs with two disulfide bridges have been reported, namely, androctonin from the scorpion *Androctonus australis (52)* and more recently gomesin from the tarantula spider *Acanthoscurria gomesiana (53).* Only one AMP with a single disulfide bridge has been observed in invertebrates, thanatin from the hemipteran insect, *Podisus maculiventris (54).* All these molecules have been identified following chemical characterization.

In general these AMPs are short, with the number of amino acids being 17–18 residues for the shortest ones, tachyplesins/polyphemusins and gomesin, up to 21 residues for thanatin, and 25 amino acids for the longest, androctonin. These peptides also have a positive net charge (5.5–8) at physiologic pH owing to the presence of a high proportion of arginine and lysine residues (>30%) and an almost identical isoelectric point of around 9.8, with 10.5 for thanatin. Primary sequence alignments between the AMPs with two internal disulfide bridges reveal high similarities between gomesin from the tarantula spider and the peptides from horseshoe crabs *(53)* and limited similarities between gomesin and androctonin.

3.2.2. Secondary Structure

The aqueous solution three-dimensional structures of tachyplesin, thanatin, and androctonin have been established with synthetic molecules using ^{1}H-2D-NMR and molecular modeling. In water, tachyplesin and androctonin adopt a well-defined highly twisted two-stranded-antiparallel β-sheet structure stabilized by their two disulfide bridges *(55,56)*. Tachyplesin has a marked amphipathic character with two clearly distinct faces, whereas the repartition of hydrophobic potentials at the surface of androctonin does not evidence such a dichotomy. In aqueous solution, thanatin also adopts a well-defined two-strand antiparallel β-sheet organization stabilized by the disulfide bridge. However, the N-terminal extension exhibits a large structural variability. Hydrophilic residues are globally situated at the two opposite sides, whereas the central part of thanatin contains mainly hydrophobic residues forming a belt around the core of the molecule *(57)*. The three-dimensional structure of gomesin has also been established in aqueous solution using ^{1}H-2D-NMR and molecular modeling *(58)*. As suspected from its sequence similarities with the AMPs that form a hairpin-like β-sheet structure, described above, gomesin also adopts a β-hairpin-like structure, consisting of a twisted antiparallel β-sheet with a C-terminal extension of two amino acids. The two strands of the β-sheet are associated owing to a turn composed of four residues. The structure of gomesin appears to be perfectly well defined in the β-sheet region stabilized by the two disulfide bridges, whereas one face of its surface is clearly hydrophobic.

3.2.3. Biologic Activity

These short-chain AMPs forming a hairpin-like β-sheet structure are strongly active against both Gram-positive and Gram-negative bacteria (including human pathogens) at a low micromolar level as well as against numerous filamentous fungi and yeasts such as *Candida* spp. Therefore, they are both bactericidal and fungicidal. Although tachyplesins and gomesin have evident hemolytic activity against human erythrocytes, the hemolytic activity of tachyplesins is linearly dependent on the peptide concentration. However, increasing the concentration of gomesin from 1 up to 100 µ*M* does not increase the percentage of hemolysis observed at 1 µ*M (53)*. On the other hand, no hemolytic activity is observed for thanatin and androctonin, even at concentrations up to 150 µ*M*. This difference in hemolytic activity observed for all these AMPs structured in β-hairpins may reflect (1) the difference in the length of their C-terminal tail (five residues in the nonhemolytic androctonin vs. one residue in the highly hemolytic tachyplesins); and (2) the presence of a C-terminal amidated arginine residue in the most hemolytic molecules, tachyplesin and gomesin. Gomesin is more toxic to the protozoan parasite *Leishmania* (L) *amazonensis* at the promastigote stage, with 50% viability in the presence of 2.5 µ*M* of gomesin, than to human erythrocytes. Such an effect on *Leishmania* spp. was also recorded for the cecropin A-melittin hybrid peptide. The presence of a higher percentage of anionic phospholipids in the plasma membrane of this protozoan parasite compared with the plasma membrane of the mammalian cells plus the replacement of the cholesterol by ergosterol may explain such an efficacy on *Leishmania* parasites.

Regarding androctonin, in addition to its effect on bacteria and fungi, this peptide binds to the torpedo nicotinic acetylcholine receptor with an affinity comparable to that of α-conotoxin SII, a small peptide isolated from the venom of the marine mollusk *Conus striatus*, with sequence similarities to androctonin *(52)*. A detailed structure-activity study on an all-D thanatin strongly suggests that more than one mode of action is responsible for killing bacteria or fungi *(54,56)*. *In vitro* antimicrobial experiments combined with structural studies using ¹H-2D-NMR and molecular modeling performed with truncated versions of thanatin outline the necessity to maintain the two-stranded-antiparallel β-sheet structure for maintaining the efficacy of the molecule. Data provided by Mandard and colleagues *(56)* on the three-dimensional structure of thanatin suggest that its activity against Gram-negative bacteria is associated with the positively charged antepenultimate residue (arginine) tightly held to two hydrophobic amino acids (proline and isoleucine) next to the poorly defined N-terminal arm.

4. MODE OF ACTION OF AMPS

Most of AMPs are proposed to act on the bacterial membranes as the primary target. This hypothesis is based on model membrane studies with liposomes showing that the peptides induce efflux of the vesicle contents if the lipids constituting the membrane are negatively charged. Similar studies using living bacteria demonstrate that the peptides cause the efflux of solutes.

The concentration needed to observe such a phenomenon is relatively high, and some calculations indicate that several million AMP molecules are necessary to break liposomes or kill bacteria *(40,59)*. These observations led to the proposal of a mechanism based on accumulation of peptides on the membrane surface: the carpet-like mechanism (Fig. 5) *(60)*. As the AMPs accumulate within the outer leaflet of the bilayer, they insert their hydrophobic residues in the lipid tails and disturb the head groups. The surface area of the outer leaflet becomes larger than the inner, and finally, in some places, accumulation of peptides induces the collapse of the membrane structure, leading to efflux of inner solutes.

This mechanism did not show marked specificity for pathogen compared with animal cells; however, insect AMPs present strong selectivity for prokaryote or pathogen cells compared with those from animals. In the case of AMPs from vertebrates, it has been shown that these molecules are produced by epithelia in specialized structures of some blood cells and that normally the AMPs do not diffuse in the blood or in other body fluids *(61)*. These peptides do, however, present some toxicity for eukaryotic cells *(62,63)*. In contrast, in the case of the systemic immune response in insects, AMPs are produced by the fat body and are secreted into the blood, where they are in direct contact with every cell type. Insect AMPs can reach very high concentrations (up to 100 μ*M*) with no cytotoxicity for the host cells.

Why is the target of most antibacterial substances specifically the outer membrane of such pathogens? There are three main differences between the cellular membranes of eukaryotic and prokaryotic cells in contact with AMPs. In bacteria, the outer leaflet of the bilayer exposed to the external medium is mainly composed of lipids with negatively charged phospholipid headgroups. In contrast, the outer leaflet of the membrane of animal cells is composed essentially of lipids with no net charge, whereas the negatively charged phospholipids are concentrated in the inner leaflet

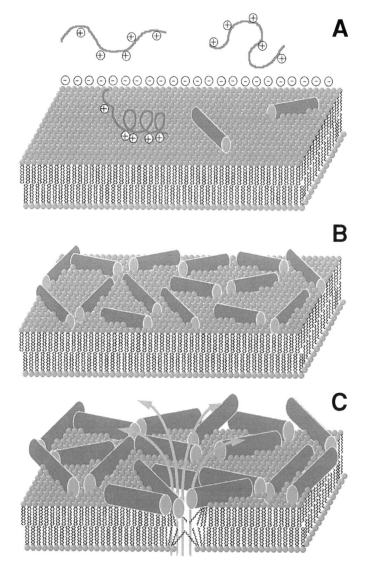

Fig. 5. Carpet mechanism for α-helical amphipathic peptides. (**A**) The cationic peptides in solution have no defined structure. The peptides are attracted through electrostatic interactions to the outer leaflet of bacteria, and the α-helical structure of the peptides is only induced after interaction with the membrane. Amphipathic interactions pull the molecule into the outer leaflet. (**B**) More and more antimicrobial peptides interact with the membrane. (**C**) Punctual aggregation of peptide molecules completely destabilizes the bacterial membrane, inducing permeabilization and efflux of solutes.

that is in contact with the cytoplasm. Thus targeting of AMPs to bacteria results in electrostatic interaction between the cationic peptide and the negatively charged surface of the bacteria, rather than the surface of animal cells.

Another important difference is the high concentration of sterol in eukaryotic membranes; the influence of the presence of this stabilizer is more controversial *(64–66)*.

The third factor that can be crucial for selectivity is the membrane potential, which in eukaryotes is less negative than in prokaryotes. The complexity of these differences makes it difficult to define exactly why some cells are susceptible to cationic peptides and other not. In the case of insect antifungal peptides, which act selectively on eukaryotic fungi, the differences are not as evident.

The initial binding of the cationic peptides to the negatively charged bacterial membrane is a simple electrostatic interaction that must be, in principle, sensitive to charges in the medium, and most of the AMPs are salt-sensitive (for reviews, *see* refs. *67* and *68*). The less sensitive components to the salt effect were found either in marine invertebrates or as a result of synthetic peptide design *(69,70)*. Although most of the insect AMPs are salt-sensitive, some of them, like helimicin, are particularly insensitive to high ionic strength *(30)*. However, this observation does not imply that the peptides are not active under physiologic conditions, as the situation in vivo, where the environment is rich in potentially synergistic compounds, is much more complex than a simple in vitro assay *(71)*.

Besides the membrane active molecules, some antimicrobial peptides have other targets. The proline-rich peptides have long been shown to have specific macromolecular targets. Recently, work on drosocin, pyrrhocoricin, and apidaecin suggested a precise molecular mode of action whereby this type of peptide may bind bacterial DnaK, inhibiting ATPase action and preventing chaperone-assisted protein folding *(72,73)*.

5. CONCLUSIONS

Cationic antimicrobial peptides are paramount and are important and significant actors in the innate immunity of vertebrates, invertebrates, and plants. Since the first report of cecropins from the moth *Hyalophora cecropia,* several hundred AMPs have been isolated from many invertebrate sources. The known diversity in the primary structure of AMPs is increasing with the number of structures elucidated. However, most of the AMPs from the animal and plant kingdom fit into three families, as defined by an arbitrary classification system based on the amino acid composition and/or structural elements. The three families are (1) linear α-helical peptides; (2) open-ended cyclic peptides with a β-sheet structure or the scaffold $\alpha\beta\beta$ or $\beta\alpha\beta\beta$; and (3) AMPs rich in particular amino acids.

Reports on *in vitro* activity of AMPs from invertebrates reveal that these small cationic molecules affect a broad range of microorganisms (bacteria, filamentous fungi, and yeast), often at a physiologic concentration. Their efficacy was reported against human pathogens and phytopathogens. Some of them are also active against protozoan parasites (*Leishmania* spp. and *Plasmodium* spp.), whereas only a few have toxicity to mammalian cells.

In most insects investigated, AMPs are inducible upon an infection (experimental or natural) and are released into the bloodstream (hemolymph), where they can act individually or in concert to kill or inhibit the growth of pathogens. This contrasts to what is observed in vertebrates, in which the AMPs are not normally released in the bloodstream but are stored in the secretory granules of some specific cells.

In addition to a systemic response, studies on the tissue-specific expression of AMPs in invertebrates as well as in vertebrates reveal that AMPs are also involved in a local response, as many surface epithelia can produce AMPs. The presence in insects of

AMPs in the bloodstream and in blood cells or epithelial cells, their low toxicity toward mammalian cells, their efficacy at physiologic salt concentrations, and their resistance to proteases and to pH variations are all in favor of developing these molecules for therapeutic use in a systemic or/and topical approach. Although exact details on the mode of action of these AMPs remain controversial, enough data are now available to orient correctly the design of efficient peptide-antibiotics with enhanced antimicrobial activity and minimal toxicity to mammalian cells.

ACKNOWLEDGMENTS

We thank Dr. Phil Irving for critical reading of the manuscript.

REFERENCES

1. Hoffmann JA, Kafatos FC, Janeway CA Jr, Ezekowitz RAB. Phylogenetic perspectives in innate immunity. Science 1999;284:1313–1318.
2. Ratcliffe NA, Gotz P. Functional studies on insect haemocytes, including non-self recognition. Res Immunol 1990;141:919–923.
3. Tzou P, Ohresser S, Ferrandon D, et al. Tissue-specific inducible expression of antimicrobial peptide genes in *Drosophila* surface epithelia. Immunity 2000;13:737–748.
4. Lamberty M, Zachary D, Lanot R, et al. Constitutive expression of a cysteine-rich antifungal and a linear antibacterial peptide in a termite insect. J Biol Chem 2001;276:4085–4092.
5. Steiner H, Hultmark D, Engström A, Bennich H, Boman HG. Sequence and specificity of two antibacterial proteins involved in insect immunity. Nature 1981;292:246–248.
6. Bulet P, Hetru C, Dimarcq JL, Hoffmann D. Antimicrobial peptides in insects; structure and function. Dev Comp Immuol 1999;23:329–344.
7. Otvos L Jr. Antimicrobial peptides isolated from insects. J Pept Sci 2000;6:497–511.
8. Ganz T, Lehrer RI. Antibiotic peptides from higher eukaryotes: biology and applications. Mol Med Today 1999;5:292–297.
9. Meister M, Hetru C, Hoffmann JA. The antimicrobial host defense of *Drosophila* In: Du Pasquier L, Litman GW (eds.). Springer-Verlag Current Topics in Microbiology and Immunology, vol 248 Origin and Evolution of the Vertebrate Immune System. New York: Springer-Verlag, 2000, pp. 17–36.
10. Orivel J, Redeker V, Le Caer JP, et al. Ponericins, new antibacterial and insecticidal peptides from the venom of the ant *Pachycondyla goeldii*. J Biol Chem 2001;276:17823–17829.
11. Lee JY, Boman A, Sun CX, et al. Antibacterial peptides from pig intestine: isolation of a mammalian cecropin. Proc Natl Acad Sci USA 1989;86:9159–9162.
12. Zhao C, Liaw L, Lee IH, Lehrer RI. cDNA cloning of three cecropin-like antimicrobial peptides (Styelins) from the tunicate, *Styela clava*. FEBS Lett 1997;412:144–148.
13. Lee IH, Zhao C, Cho Y, et al. Clavanins, alpha-helical antimicrobial peptides from tunicate hemocytes. FEBS Lett 1997;400:158–62.
14. Hetru C, Hoffmann D, Bulet P. Antimicrobial peptides from insects. In: Brey PT, Hultmark D (eds.). Molecular Mechanisms of Immune Responses in Insects London: Chapman & Hall, 1998, pp. 40–66.
15. Hara S, Taniai K, Kato Y, Yamakawa M. Isolation and α-amidation of the non-amidated form of cecropin D from *Bombyx mori*. Comp Biochem Physiol 1994;108B:303–308.
16. Sun D, Eccleston ED, Fallon AM. Cloning and expression of three cecropin cDNAs from a mosquito cell line. FEBS Lett 1999;454:147–151.
17. Lowenberger C, Charlet M, Vizioli J, et al. Antimicrobial activity spectrum, cDNA cloning, and mRNA expression of a newly isolated member of the cecropin family from the mosquito vector *Aedes aegypti*. J Biol Chem 1999;274:20092–20097.

18. Lowenberger C. Innate immune response of *Aedes aegypti.* Insect Biochem Mol Biol 2001;31:219–229.

19. Vizioli J, Bulet P, Charlet M, et al. Cloning and analysis of a cecropin gene from the malaria vector mosquito, *Anopheles gambiae.* Insect Mol Biol 2001;9:75–84.

20. Oren Z, Shai Y. Mode of action of linear amphipatic α-helical antimicrobial peptides antibacterial peptides. Biopolymers 1998;47:451–463.

21. Eckengren S, Hultmark D. *Drosophila* cecropin as an antifungal agent Insect Biochem Mol Biol 1999;29:965–972.

22. Florack D, Jonker H, Stiekema W, Bosch D. C-terminal degradation of the antibacterial cecropin B peptide by tobacco. Transgenic Res 1996;4:132–141.

23. Engström Y. Insect immune gene regulation. In: Brey PT, Hultmark D (eds.). Molecular Mechanisms of Immune Responses in Insects. London: Chapman & Hall, 1998, pp. 211–244.

24. Matsuyama K, Natori S. Purification of three antibacterial proteins from the culture medium of NIH Sape-4, an embryonic cell line of *Sarcophaga peregrina.* J Biol Chem 1988;263:17112–17116.

25. Lambert J, Keppi E, Dimarcq JL, et al. Insect immunity: isolation from immune blood of the dipteran *Phormia terranovae* of two insect antibacterial peptides with sequence homology to rabbit lung macrophage bactericidal peptides. Proc Natl Acad Sci USA 1989;86:262–266.

26. Michaut L, Fehlbaum P, Moniatte M, et al. Determination of the disulfide array of the first inducible antifungal peptide from insects: drosomycin from *Drosophila melanogaster.* FEBS Lett 1996;395:6–10.

27. Nakajima Y, van der Goes van Naters-Yasui A, Taylor D, Yamakawa M. Two isoforms of a member of the arthropod defensin family from the soft tick, *Ornithodoros moubata* (Acari: Argasidae). Insect Biochem Mol Biol 2001;31:747–751.

28. Fehlbaum P, Bulet P, Michaut L, et al. Insect immunity: septic injury of *Drosophila* induces the synthesis of a potent antifungal peptide with sequence homology to plant antifungal peptides. J Biol Chem 1994;269:33159–33163.

29. Dimarcq JL, Bulet P, Hetru C, Hoffmann JA. Cysteine-rich antimicrobial peptides in invertebrates. Biopolymers 1998;47:465–477.

30. Lamberty M, Ades S, Uttenweiler-Joseph S, et al. Isolation from the lepidopteran *Heliothis virescens* of a novel insect defensin with potent antifungal activity. J Biol Chem 1999;274:9320–9326.

31. Bonmatin JM, Bonnat JL, Gallet X, et al. Two-dimensional ^{1}H-NMR study of recombinant insect defensin A in water. Resonance assignments, secondary structure and global folding. J Biomol NMR 1992;2:235–256.

32. Hanzawa H, Shimada I, Kuzuhara T, et al. ^{1}H nuclear magnetic resonance study of the solution conformation of an antibacterial protein sapecin. FEBS Lett 1990;269:413–420.

33. Yang YS, Mitta G, Chavanieu A, et al. Solution structure and activity of the synthetic four-disulfide bond Mediterranean mussel defensin (MGD-1). Biochemistry 2000;39:14436–11447.

34. Landon C, Sodano P, Hetru C, Hoffmann JA, Ptak M. Solution structure of drosomycin, the first antifungal protein from insects. Protein Sci 1997;6:1878–1884.

35. Lamberty M, Caille A, Landon C, et al. Solution structures of the antifungal heliomicin and a selected variant with both antibacterial and antifungal activities. Biochemistry 2001;40:11995–2003.

36. Kobayashi Y, Takashima H, Tamaoki H, et al. The cysteine-stabilized α-helix: a common structural motif of ion-channel blocking neurotoxic peptides. Biopolymers 1991;31:1213–1220.

37. Cornet B, Bonmatin JM, Hetru C, et al. Refined three-dimensional solution structure of insect defensin A. Structure 1995;3:435–448.

38. Fant F, Vranken W, Broekaert W, Borresmans, F. Determination of the three-dimensional solution structure of *Raphanus sativus* antifungal protein 1 by ^{1}H-NMR. J Mol Biol 1998;279:257–270.

39. Sawai MV, Jia HP, Liu L, et al. The NMR structure of human beta-defensin-2 reveals a novel alpha-helical segment. Biochemistry 2001;40:3810–3816.

40. Cociancich S, Ghazi A, Hetru C, Hoffmann JA, Letellier L. Insect defensin, an inducible antibacterial peptide, forms voltage-dependent channels in *Micrococcus luteus*. J Biol Chem
1993;268:19239–19245.

41. Ganz T, Weiss J. Antimicrobial peptides of phagocytes and epithelia. Semin Hematol
1997;34:343–354.

42. Broekaert WF, Terras FRG, Cammue BPA, Osborn RW. Plant defensins: novel antimicrobial
peptides as components of the host defense system. Plant Physiol 1995;108:1353–1358.

43. Shahabuddin M, Fields I, Bulet P, Hoffmann JA, Miller L. *Plasmodium gallinaceum:* differential
killing of some mosquito stages of the parasite by insect defensin. Exp Parasitol 1998;89:103–112.

44. Richman AM, Dimopoulos G, Seeley D, Kafatos FC. *Plasmodium* activates the innate immune
response of *Anopheles gambiae* mosquitoes. EMBO J 1997;16:6114–6119.

45. Dimopoulos G, Seeley D, Wolf A, Kafatos FC. Malaria infection of the mosquito *Anopheles
gambiae* activates immune-responsive genes during critical transition stages of the parasite life
cycle. EMBO J 1998;17:6115–6123.

46. Dimarcq JL, Hoffmann D, Meister M, et al. Characterization and transcriptional profiles of a
Drosophila gene encoding an insect defensin. A study in insect immunity. Eur J Biochem
1994;221:201–209.

47. Lehane MJ, Wu D, Lehane SM. Midgut-specific immune molecules are produced by the blood-
sucking insect *Stomoxys calcitrans*. Proc Natl Acad Sci USA 1997;94:11502–11507.

48. Bellm L, Lehrer RI, Ganz T. Protegrins: new antibiotics of mammalian origin. Expert Opin
Investig Drugs 2000;9:1731–1742.

49. Patel SU, Osborn R, Rees S, Thornton JM. Structural studies of *Impatiens balsamina* antimicrobial protein (*Ib*-AMP1). Biochemistry 1998;37:983–990.

50. Nakamura T, Furunaka H, Miyata T, et al. Tachyplesin, a class of antimicrobial peptide from the
hemocytes of the horseshoe crab *(Tachypleus tridentatus)*. Isolation and chemical structure. J
Biol Chem 1988;263:16709–16713.

51. Miyata T, Tokunaga F, Yoneya T, et al. Antimicrobial peptides, isolated from horseshoe crab
hemocytes, tachyplesin II, and polyphemusins I and II: chemical structures and biological activity. J Biochem (Tokyo) 1989;106:663–668.

52. Ehret-Sabatier L, Loew D, Goyffon M, et al. Characterization of novel cysteine-rich antimicrobial peptides from scorpion blood. J Biol Chem 1996;271:29537–29544.

53. Silva PI Jr, Daffre S, Bulet P. Isolation and characterization of gomesin, an 18-residue cysteine-
rich defense peptide from the spider *Acanthoscurria gomesiana* hemocytes with sequence similarities to horseshoe crab antimicrobial peptides of the tachyplesin family. J Biol Chem
2000;275:33464–33470.

54. Fehlbaum P, Bulet P, Chernysh S, et al. Structure-activity analysis of thanatin, a 21-residue
inducible insect defense peptide with sequence homology to frog skin antimicrobial peptides.
Proc Natl Acad Sci USA 1996;93:1221–1225.

55. Tamamura H, Kuroda M, Masuda M, et al. A comparative study of the solution structures of
tachyplesin I and a novel anti-HIV synthetic peptide, T22 ([Tyr5, 12, Lys7]-polyphemusin II),
determined by nuclear magnetic resonance. Biochim Biophys Acta 1993;1163:209–216.

56. Mandard N, Sodano P, Labbe H, et al. Solution structure of thanatin, a potent bactericidal and
fungicidal insect peptide, determined from proton two-dimensional nuclear magnetic resonance
data. Eur J Biochem 1998;256:404–410.

57. Mandard N, Sy D, Maufrais C, et al. Androctonin, a novel antimicrobial peptide from scorpion
Androctonus australis: solution structure and molecular dynamics simulations in the presence of
a lipid monolayer. J Biomol Struct Dyn 1999;17:367–380.

58. Mandard N, Bulet P, Caille A, Daffre S, Vovelle F. The solution structure of gomesin, an antimicrobial cysteine-rich peptide from the spider. Eur J Biochem 2002;269:1190–1198.

59. Hetru C, Letellier L, Oren Z, Hoffmann JA, Shai Y. Androctonin, a hydrophilic disulphidebridged non-haemolytic anti-microbial peptide: a plausible mode of action. Biochem J 2000;345:653–664.
60. Shai Y. Mechanism of the binding, insertion and destabilization of phospholipid bilayer membranes by alpha-helical antimicrobial and cell non-selective membrance-lytic peptides. Biochim Biophys Acta 1999;1462:55–70.
61. Schröder JM. Epithelial antimicrobial peptides: innate local host response elements. Cell Mol Life Sci 1999;56:32–46.
62. Jaynes JM, Burton CA, Barr SB, et al. *In vitro* cytocidal effect of *novel* lytic peptides on *Plasmodium falciparum* and *Trypanosoma cruzi.* FASEB J 1988;2:2878–2883.
63. Zasloff M. in Discussion. Antimicrobial peptides. Ciba Found Sy 1994;186:151–159.
64. De Lucca AJ, Bland JM, Grimm C, et al. Fungicidal properties, sterol binding, and proteolytic resistance of the synthetic peptide D4E1. Can J Microbiol 1998;44:514–520.
65. De Lucca AJ, Bland JM, Jacks TJ, Grimm C, Walsh TJ. Fungicidal and binding properties of the natural peptides cecropin B and dermaseptin. Med Mycol 1998;36:291–298.
66. Matsuzaki K. Why and how are peptide-lipid interactions utilized for self-defense? Magainins and tachyplesins as archetypes. Biochim Biophys Acta 1999;1462:1–10.
67. Lehrer RI, Lichtenstein AK, Ganz T. Defensins: antimicrobial and cytotoxic peptides of mammalian cells. Annu Rev Immunol 1993;11:105–128.
68. Lehrer RI, Ganz T. Antimicrobial peptides in mammalian and insect host defence. Curr Opin Immunol 1999;11:23–27.
69. Lee IH, Cho Y, Lehrer RI. Effects of pH and salinity on the antimicrobial properties of clavanins. Infect Immun 1997;65:2898–2903.
70. Friedrich C, Scott MG, Karunaratne N, Yan H, Hancock RE. Salt-resistant alpha-helical cationic antimicrobial peptides. Antimicrob Agents Chemother. 1999;43:1542–1548.
71. Casteels P, Ampe C, Jacobs F, Tempst P. Functional and chemical characterization of Hymenoptaecin, an antibacterial polypeptide that is infection-inducible in the honeybee *(Apis mellifera).* J Biol Chem 1993;268:7044–7054.
72. Otvos L Jr, Rogers ME, Consolvo PJ, et al. Interaction between heat shock proteins and antimicrobial peptides. Biochemistry 2000;39:14150–14159.
73. Kragol G, Lovas S, Varadi G, et al. The antibacterial peptide pyrrhocoricin inhibits the ATPase actions of DnaK and prevents chaperone-assisted protein folding. Biochemistry 2001;40:3016–3026.

6

Innate Immunity in the Horseshoe Crab

Shun-ichiro Kawabata, Tsukasa Osaki, and Sadaaki Iwanaga

1. INTRODUCTION

Arthropod horseshoe crabs belong to the class Merostomata and are phylogenetically more related to Arachnoidea than Crustacea. Many fossils of horseshoe crabs can be found, primarily in deposits from the Paleozoic era to the Cenozoic era of North America and Europe. However, the distributions of the four extant species, including *Limulus polyphemus, Tachypleus tridentatus, T. gigas,* and *Carcinoscorpius rotundicauda,* are different from those of fossil species. *L. polyphemus* is distributed along the east coast of North America, and the other three species are found in Southeast Asia. In Japan, *T. tridentatus* is distributed along the limited coastal areas of the Inland Sea and the northern part of Kyushu Island. The divergence between *L. polyphemus* and *T. tridentatus* has been calculated to have occurred 135 million years ago during the late Jurassic period of the Mesozoic era, based on mutation distances in a clottable protein, coagulogen: 52.5 million years between *T. gigas* and the two Asian species and 36.3 million years between *T. tridentatus* and *C. rotundicauda (1).*

Innate immune systems in arthopods include hemolymph coagulation, phenoloxidase-mediated melanization, cell agglutination, antimicrobial actions, and phagocytosis *(2).* Despite the absence of acquired immune systems, arthropod hemolymph shows a high degree of specificity against invading pathogens. Hemolymph of *T. tridentatus* contains granular hemocytes, comprising 99% of the total hemocytes *(3).* The granular hemocytes are filled with two types of secretory granules, L-granules and S-granules, which selectively store defense molecules such as coagulation factors, protease inhibitors, lectins, and antimicrobial peptides *(4,5).* The hemocytes are highly sensitive to lipopolysaccharides (LPS) that induce secretion of the defense molecules stored in both types of granules through exocytosis *(6,7).* Here we focus on the molecular mechanisms of hemolymph coagulation, prophenoloxidase activation, and nonself recognition as well as the antimicrobial actions of the horseshoe crab.

2. HEMOLYMPH COAGULATION THROUGH HEAD-TO-TAIL POLYMERIZATION OF COAGULIN

The LPS-mediated coagulation cascade involves four-serine protease zymogens *(5).* Factor C is a biosensor against LPS and is autocatalytically activated to factor $\overline{C}$, which

From: *Infectious Disease: Innate Immunity*
Edited by: R. A. B. Ezekowitz and J. A. Hoffmann © Humana Press Inc., Totowa, NJ

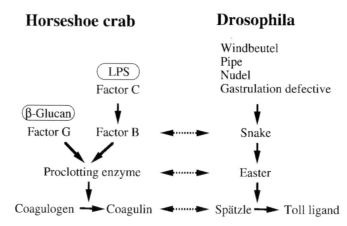

Fig. 1. Comparison of the coagulation cascade in the horseshoe crab with the morphogenetic cascade in *Drosophila*. LPS, lipopolysaccharide.

then activates factor B; in turn, factor $\overline{\text{B}}$ converts the proclotting enzyme to the clotting enzyme. Another biosensor, factor G, is also autocatalytically activated in the presence of β-1,3-glucans to factor $\overline{\text{G}}$, which directly activates the proclotting enzyme (Fig. 1). Another arthropod protease cascade, the morphogenetic cascade for determining embryonic dorsal-ventral polarity in the fly *Drosophila melanogaster*, has been well characterized at the molecular level *(8,9)*. The structural similarity of their target proteins [a clottable protein (coagulogen) of the horseshoe crab and a *Drosophila* Toll ligand (spätzle)], as well as the sequence homology between the serine proteases participating in the two cascades, suggests that these two functionally different cascades may have a common origin *(10,11)*.

It is of interest that the NH_2-terminal L-chains of factor B and proclotting enzyme contain a small compact domain with three disulfide bonds called the *clip domain* *(12,13)*. These clip domains have been found not only in *Drosophila* snake and easter proteases but also in other various insect serine proteases *(14)*. Furthermore, the folding pattern of the three disulfide bridges in the clip domain is identical to those of β-defensins, which are known as strong antimicrobial peptides in the innate immunity system. These clip domains might be released during activation of the protease cascade to work as antimicrobial substances. Thus, the system shown in Fig. 1 may have dual actions: coagulation and the killing of invading microorganisms.

The clotting enzyme cleaves coagulogen of 175 amino acid residues at two sites, yielding a fragment referred to as peptide C (Thr19-Arg46), and the resulting coagulin, which consists of the NH_2-terminal A-chain (Ala1-Arg18) and the COOH-terminal B-chain (Gly47-Phe175), connected by two disulfide bridges, forms an insoluble gel by self-polymerization *(15,16)*. Crystal structural analysis of coagulogen has revealed an elongated molecule (approximate dimensions $60 \times 30 \times 20$ Å) with a topologic similarity to nerve growth factor *(11)*. The three-dimensional structure of coagulogen suggests a possible polymerization mechanism in which release of the helical peptide C would expose a hydrophobic cove on the "head," which interacts with the hydrophobic edge or "tail" of a second molecule, resulting in the formation of coagulin gel. We have

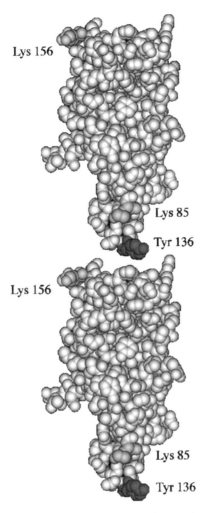

Fig. 2. A molecular model of the coagulin-coagulin interaction. Based on X-ray structural analysis, exposure of a hydrophobic cove on the head in response to the release of peptide C has been postulated *(11)*. A coagulin monomer lacking peptide C may polymerize through a head-to-tail interaction.

recently obtained evidence that the polymerization of coagulin proceeds through an interaction between the hydrophobic cove on the head and the hydrophobic tail *(17)*. The two lysine residues at positions 85 and 156, oppositely located at the head and tail regions of the elongated molecule, are chemically crosslinked intermolecularly (Fig. 2). An octapeptide containing Tyr136, which occupies the tail end of coagulin, inhibits the polymerization, and replacement of Tyr136 of the peptide with Ala results in a loss of inhibitory activity. The polymerization of coagulin possibly proceeds through an interaction between the newly exposed hydrophobic cove on the head and the wedge-shaped hydrophobic tail.

Several synthetic peptides corresponding to the NH$_2$-terminal regions of the fibrin α- and β-chains prevent the polymerization of fibrin monomers, and a peptide of Gly-Pro-

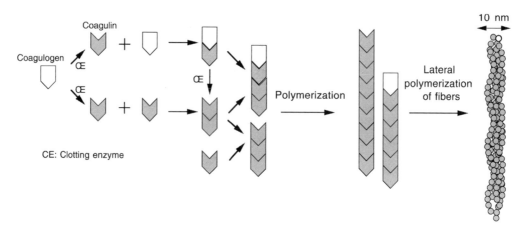

Fig. 3. A hypothetical scheme of coagulin polymerization.

Arg-Pro binds to fibrinogen *(18–20)* and to fragment D with $K_a = 0.5 \times 10^5 \ M^{-1}$ *(21,22)*. Coagulogen interacts with the immobilized coagulin through the tail of coagulogen and the head of coagulin, with $K_a = 1.7 \times 10^5 \ M^{-1}$. Not only the coagulin monomer, but also coagulogen, could be incorporated into a coagulin fiber and then converted to coagulin by the clotting enzyme, leading to an extension of the fiber (Fig. 3). Relative to this finding, if serine proteases in the coagulation cascade are scavenged in vivo by the horseshoe crab serine protease inhibitors *(23–25)*, coagulogen could regulate extension of the fiber to bind to the terminus. Coagulin fibers have a tendency to aggregate laterally to form a thicker fiber with a diameter of approx 10 nm, probably through other hydrophobic patches on the coagulogen surface *(11)*. The resulting thick fibers may form a reticulate, catching microorganisms invading from outside *(26)*. The binding site(s) for such a side-to-side interaction remains to be determined.

In the mammalian coagulation system, a plasma transglutaminase covalently crosslinks fibrin to convert a stable crosslinked fibrin with itself or with other proteins, which is essential for normal hemostasis and wound healing *(27)*. In horseshoe crab hemolymph, however, a transglutaminase is present in the cytosol of hemocytes, but not in the plasma *(28,29)*. Furthermore, coagulogen and coagulin themselves are not substrates for the hemocyte transglutaminase; the proteins of 8.6 and 80 kDa present in hemocytes serve as substrates for the transglutaminase *(5,28)*. These proteins may participate in forming the reticulate structure of the coagulin gel.

The activation of *Drosophila* Toll is also critical to the production of antibacterial and antifungal peptides as a response to microbial infection *(30,31)*. Although the molecular mechanism for the activation of Toll by spätzle is not currently known, many membrane receptors are known to be activated through ligand-induced dimerization or oligomerization *(32)*. Based on consideration of the polymerization process of coagulin, it seems possible that the ligand spätzle may also induce dimerization or oligomerization of *Drosophila* Toll, leading to activation of intercellular signaling *(33)*. Ideally, the polymerization mechanism demonstrated here in coagulin will contribute to the body of knowledge concerning proteolysis-induced associations of proteins in various biologic phenomena.

3. A LINK BETWEEN HEMOLYMPH COAGULATION AND PROPHENOLOXIDASE ACTIVATION

In insects and crustaceans, the prophenoloxidase activation system is an important part of the host defense, where it functions to detect and kill invading pathogens as well as to synthesize melanin for wound healing and encapsulation of pathogens *(34,35)*. Phenoloxidase, a copper-containing enzyme, is widely distributed not only in the animal kingdom but also in plants and fungi and is responsible for initiating the biosynthesis of melanin *(36)*. Under physiologic conditions, arthropod prophenoloxidases require proteolytic cleavage for activation by a specific protease: the freshwater crayfish prophenoloxidase with a molecular mass of 76 kDa is converted into a 62-kDa active form by the prophenoloxidase-activating enzyme *(37)*. The tarantula *Eurypelma californicum* hemocyanin expresses phenoloxidase activity after limited proteolysis with trypsin or chymotrypsin *(38)*, and it has recently been shown that the coagulation cascade of the horseshoe crab is linked to prophenoloxidase activation, with the oxygen carrier hemocyanin functioning as a substitute for prophenoloxidase *(39)*.

The clotting enzyme or factor $\overline{B}$ functionally transforms hemocyanin to phenoloxidase, and the conversion reaches a plateau at 1:1 stoichiometry without proteolytic cleavage. The active site-masked clotting enzyme also has the same effect, suggesting that complex formation of the clotting enzyme with hemocyanin is critical for the conversion. Interestingly, the zymogen of the clotting enzyme (proclotting enzyme) also induces the phenoloxidase activity. A common structural feature of the clotting enzyme and factor $\overline{B}$ is the presence of the NH_2-terminal clip domain, consisting of three disulfide bridges *(12,13)*, as mentioned previously. Homologous clip domains are also present in the NH_2-terminal regions of insect prophenoloxidase-activating enzymes *(40–42)*, but not in those of factor $\overline{C}$ and factor $\overline{G}$. Therefore, the clip domains of the clotting enzyme and factor $\overline{B}$ may mediate the interaction of these proteases with hemocyanin to turn on the switch for functional conversion. Arthropod prophenoloxidases are nonenzymatically activated by treatment with detergents, lipids, or organic solvents *(43)*. Hemocyanins from the crab *Carcinus maenas* and the lobster *Homarus americanus* express significant phenoloxidase activity in the presence of perchlorate *(44)*. Sodium dodecyl sulfate and phosphatidyl ethanolamine also induce the phenoloxidase activity of the horseshoe crab hemocyanin, and the specific activity for-methylcatechol is equal to that activated by the clotting enzyme *(39)*.

Arthropod hemocyanins display significant structural similarities to crustacean and insect prophenoloxidases, suggesting that the origin of arthropod hemocyanins is in ancient prophenoloxidase-like proteins *(45)*. The crystal structure of the American horseshoe crab *L. polyphemus* hemocyanin (subunit II) suggests the importance of Phe49 in allosteric cooperativity and the regulation of oxygen binding *(46,47)*. Furthermore, the crystal structure of catechol oxidase of the sweet potato *Ipomoea batatas* complexed with an inhibitor phenylthiourea indicates that the catalytic center could superimpose the oxygen-binding center of *L. polyphemus* hemocyanin *(48,49)*. The phenyl ring of Phe49 of *L. polyphemus* hemocyanin aligns perfectly with the aromatic ring of the phenylthiourea in the catechol oxidase-inhibitor complex. The shielding of Phe49 in *L. polyphemus* hemocyanin possibly inhibits the binding of phenolic substrates. In the case of octopus hemocyanin, the phenylalanine is substituted with a less bulky isoleucine, and the related phenoloxidase activity has been observed at pH 6.0 *(50)*.

Decker and Rimke *(38)* have hypothesized that the activation of tarantula hemo-cyanin creates a large entrance for phenolic substrates to the active site by removing the NH_2-terminal peptide containing Phe49 through limited proteolysis: Phe49 acts as a placeholder for the phenolic substrates while acting as an oxygen carrier to suppress the second function as a phenoloxidase. The Japanese horseshoe crab *T. tridentatus* hemocyanin also contains the conserved phenylalanine Phe48 *(51)*. Therefore, in response to specific binding of the clotting enzyme or factor $\overline{\text{B}}$, *T. tridentatus* hemo-cyanin can induce a conformational change or partial unfolding of the protein structure to pull Phe48 from the active site, creating an entrance for phenolic substrates.

The horseshoe crab coagulation cascade appears to be a highly rational and sophisti-cated system by which the host defense can simultaneously trigger both blood coagula-tion and prophenoloxidase activation. In insects and crustaceans, an ancestral protease cascade corresponding to the bifunctional cascade found in horseshoe crabs may have evolved into an exclusive system of prophenoloxidase activation.

4. NON-SELF-RECOGNIZING LECTINS

The innate immune system of the horseshoe crab recognizes invading pathogens through a combinatorial method using lectins with different specificities against carbo-hydrates exposed on pathogens *(52)*. Five types of lectins of the horseshoe crab, named tachylectins, have been identified in circulating hemocytes and hemolymph plasma. These tachylectins may serve synergistically to accomplish an effective host defense against invading microbes and foreign substances.

Tachylectin-1 interacts with Gram-negative bacteria, probably through 2-keto-3-deoxy-octonate, one of the constituents of LPS *(53)*. Tachylectin-1 exhibits no hemagglutinating activity, but it agglutinates sheep erythrocytes coated with LPS. Tachylectin-1 also binds to polysaccharides such as agarose and dextran with broad specificity. Tachylectin-1 is a sin-gle-chain protein consisting of 221 amino acid residues with no *N*-linked sugar chain and contains three intrachain disulfide bonds and a free Cys residue. An outstanding structural feature of tachylectin-1 is that it consists of six tandem repeats. Tachylectin-1 exists as a monomer in solution, judging from data obtained by gel-filtration chromatography.

A homolog of tachylectin-1 with unknown function has been identified in the myx-omycete *Physarum polycephalum* and named tectonin *(54)*. Tachylectin-1 shows 33% sequence identity to tectonin. This myxomycete in its plasmodial form feeds on bacte-ria and organic detritus by phagocytosis. Tectonin is located on the plasmodial surface, can therefore recognize LPS of Gram-negative bacteria for phagocytosis, and could have an affinity for several saccharides for non-self recognition.

Tachylectin-2 has hemagglutinating activity against human A-type erythrocytes *(55)*. Tachylectin-2 binds specifically to GlcNAc with a K_d of 0.05 m*M*, and detailed sugar-binding analysis has indicated that the acetamide group at the C-2 position and a free OH group at the C-4 position of GlcNAc are required for recognition by tachylectin-2. Tachylectin-2 consists of 236 amino acid residues, and the most interest-ing feature of the sequence is the presence of five tandem repeats of 47 amino acids. Tachylectin-2 contains no cysteine and no *N*- and *O*-linked sugars, and it is present as a monomer in solution, as judged from ultracentrifugal analysis.

Tachylectin-3 exhibits hemagglutinating activity specifically against human A-type ery-throcytes *(56)*. The hemagglutinating activity is equivalent to that of tachylectin-2, but it is not inhibited by D-GlcNAc or D-GalNAc. Interestingly, the hemagglutinating activity is completely inhibited by a synthetic pentasaccharide of a blood group A antigen and is more strongly inhibited by S-type LPS from several Gram-negative bacteria at concentration ranges of 5–10 ng/mL, but not by the corresponding R-type LPS. These results indicate a high specificity of tachylectin-3 against the O-antigens, and one of the most effective S-type LPS is from *Escherichia coli* 0111:B4 LPS. Tachylectin-3 contains 123 amino acid residues consisting of two repeating sequences and is present as a dimer in solution.

Tachylectin-4 containing 232 residues is an oligomeric glycoprotein of 470 kDa *(57)*. It has more potent hemagglutinating activity against human A-type erythrocytes than tachylectin-2 and tachylectin-3. Although L-fucose and *N*-acetylneuraminic acid at 100 mM completely inhibit the hemagglutinating activity of tachylectin-4, the activity is more strongly inhibited by bacterial S-type LPS than by R-type LPS, which is lacking an *O*-antigen. The most effective S-type LPS is from *E. coli* 0111:B4. The minimum concentration required for inhibiting agglutination against human A-type erythrocytes is 160-fold lower than those necessary for S-type LPS from *Salmonella minnesota*. Therefore, colitose (3-deoxy-L-fucose), a unique sugar present in the *O*-antigen of *E. coli* 0111:B4 with structural similarity to L-fucose, is the most probable candidate for a specific ligand of tachylectin-4.

Tachylectins-5A and -5B identified in hemolymph plasma show the strongest bacterial agglutinating activity among the five types of tachylectins, and they exhibit broad specificity against *N*-acetyl group-containing substances *(58)*. They agglutinate all types of human erythrocytes, indicating that the primary recognition substance is not a blood group antigen. Their hemagglutinating activities are inhibited by 5 mM EDTA, although this inhibition can be overcome by adding an excess amount of $CaCl_2$. Both lectins specifically recognize acetyl group-containing substances, including noncarbohydrates; the acetyl group is required and is sufficient for recognition. They also strongly agglutinate both Gram-negative and Gram-positive bacteria.

Hemolymph of horseshoe crabs contains another class of hemagglutinins that is structurally related to C-reactive protein (CRP) *(59)*. CRP was first recognized in human plasma as a nonimmunoglobulin capable of precipitating with C-polysaccharides derived from the cell wall of *Streptococcus pneunomiae (60)*. Limulin, a sialic acid- and phosphorylethanolamine-binding hemagglutinin in the hemolymph plasma of *L. polyphemus,* is a hemolytic CRP *(61)*. Three types of CRPs in the plasma of *T. tridentatus* have been purified based on different affinities against fetuin agarose and phosphorylethanolamine agarose. These CRPs are named *T. tridentatus* CRP-1 (tCRP-1), tCRP-2, and tCRP-3, each of which consists of several isoproteins *(62)*.

tCRP-2 and tCRP-3, but not tCRP-1, agglutinate mammalian erythrocytes. tCRP-1 is the most abundant CRP and exhibits the highest affinity to the phosphorylethanolamine-protein conjugate, but it lacks both sialic acid binding and hemolytic activity. tCRP-2 binds to both fetuin-agarose and phosphorylethanolamine-agarose and exhibits Ca^{2+}-dependent hemolytic and sialic acid binding activity. Furthermore, tCRP-2 exhibits a higher affinity to colominic acid, a bacterial polysialic acid. By contrast, tCRP-3 shows stronger hemolytic, sialic acid binding and hemagglutinating activities than tCRP-2. However, tCRP-3 has no affinity to phosphorylethanolamine agarose and colominic acid. tCRP-3, therefore, is a novel hemolytic CRP lacking a common characteristic of CRPs, phosphorylethanolamine-agarose binding affinity.

Twenty-two clones of tCRPs with different deduced amino acid sequences have been obtained *(62)*. These tCRP clones possess high molecular diversity and fall into three

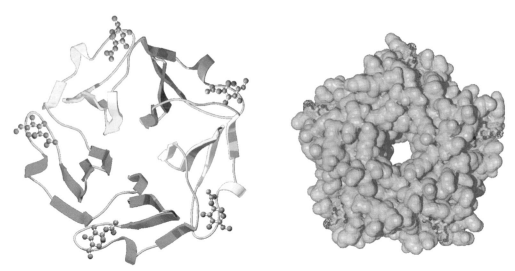

Fig. 4. A stereo ribbon plot (left) and a space-filling model (right) of tachylectin-2 complexed with GlcNAc as a ball-and-stick model.

related groups, consistent with classifications based on their biologic activities. Only tCRP-3 contains a unique hydrophobic nonapeptide sequence that appears in the transmembrane domain of an MHC class I heavy chain of rainbow trout, suggesting the importance of the hydrophobic patch to the hemolytic activity of tCRP-3. The structural and functional diversities of tCRPs provide a good model for the study of properties of innate immunity in invertebrates, which survive without the benefit of acquired immunity.

In the following sections we review recent functional and structural studies of tachylectin-2 and tachylectin-5, and we discuss a molecular mechanism in non-self-recognition.

4.1. Tachylectin-2

The X-ray structure of tachylectin-2 in a complex with GlcNAc has been solved at 2.0 Å resolution (Fig. 4) *(63)*. Tachylectin-2 is a fivefold β-propeller structure, and the single chain of tachylectin-2 is organized into five β-sheets arranged in consecutive order with fivefold symmetry around a central tunnel. Tachylectin-2 contains five equivalent binding sites with virtually identical occupancy and geometry in the crystal. The GlcNAc points its acetamide group to the bottom of the binding pocket, and the C6-OH group points outside into the solvent.

Tachylectin-2 shows virtually no change in main- or side-chain conformation on the binding of GlcNAc. The deviation (root mean square) between the free tachylectin-2 and the complex with the ligands is only 0.18 Å, suggesting no cooperativity in the ligand binding. The central tunnel is not a ligand binding site but is instead filled with water molecules. The water molecules are arranged in a pentagonal dodecahedron, a structural element that is also found in clathrate hydrates. However, the water cage in tachylectin-2 is empty, and no guest species has been observed in the cage. This water cage is not affected by the crystal packing of tachylectin-2 and is expected also to exist in solution, possibly contributing to stabilization of the protein fold.

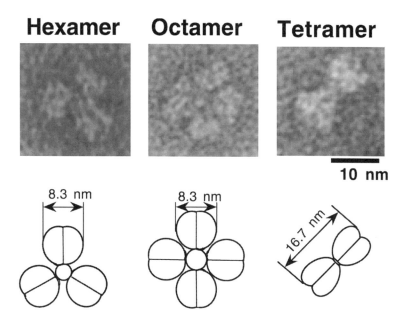

Fig. 5. Electron micrographs of negatively stained tachylectin-5A and tachylectin-5B. Tachylectin-5A forms a hexameric or octameric structure, and tachylectin-5B forms a tetrameric structure.

The nature of the binding pocket explains the strict specificity of tachylectin-2 for GlcNAc. The exoskeleton of the horseshoe crab contains a ubiquitous polysaccharide of β-1,4-linked GlcNAc, chitin. However, tachylectin-2 shows no significant binding affinity to chitin, primarily because there is no free 4-OH group in the β-1,4-linked GlcNAc units, except for the nonreducing end. The mechanism of self/nonself distinction is reinforced by a distance of two individual binding sites of 25 and 40 Å, respectively, which seems to prevent multiple binding to distant terminal GlcNAc units of chitin. Therefore, the high valency of five binding sites of the single molecule suggests the recognition of GlcNAc units on pathogens with a fairly high ligand density. Multiple binding of the five binding sites to repetitive structures on pathogens will generate very tight interactions.

4.2. Tachylectin-5

Tachylectin-5A is biosynthesized in the heart and intestine, and tachylectin-5B is synthesized only in hemocytes *(58)*. The overall sequence identity between tachylectin-5A of 269 residues and tachylectin-5B of 289 residues is 45%. Tachylectins-5A and -5B have significant sequence similarity with the COOH-terminal domains of fibrinogen β- and γ-chains and their related proteins such as ficolins, tenacins, and angiopoietins. Among the proteins, mammalian ficolins show striking sequence identity of up to 51%. Ficolins are composed of an NH_2-terminal cysteine-rich segment followed by a collagen-like region and a COOH-terminal fibrinogen-like globular domain *(64–66)*. Interestingly, a collagenous domain found in ficolins is missing in the corresponding regions of tachylectins-5A and -5B.

Based on electron microscopy, tachylectin-5A forms a three- or four-bladed propeller structure, and tachylectin-5B forms a two-bladed propeller structure (Fig. 5). If a ligand-binding site(s) is located in each blade, tachylectin-5A and -5B could have more avidity against ligands, with a high density on pathogens. Their polyvalent bindings of acetyl groups must be a key factor in binding to invading microorganisms. The horseshoe crab is equipped with a unique functional homolog of vertebrate fibrinogen, coagulogen, as the target protein of the clotting cascade. However, crystal analysis has indicated that coagulogen is a structural homolog of nerve growth factor *(11)*. The horseshoe crab has fibrinogen-related molecules in hemolymph plasma, but they function as non-self-recognizing lectins. An ancestor of fibrinogen-like proteins may have functioned as a non-self-recognizing protein. In fact, the human fibrinogen γ-chain contains a C-type lectin domain in the COOH-terminal portion.

5. ANTIMICROBIAL PEPTIDES

Arthropod antimicrobial peptides are very important for host defense related to the killing of invading microbes. Antimicrobial peptides purified from *T. tridentatus* hemocytes, including tachyplesin, big defensin, tachycitin, and tachystatins have an affinity to chitin, but none to other polysaccharides such as cellulose, mannan, xylan, and laminarin *(5,67)*. The antimicrobial and chitin binding activities of these peptides are summarized in Tables 1 and 2. Chitin is a component of the cell wall of fungi and is considered to be a target substance recognized by the innate immune system.

Tachyplesin, which consists of 17 residues, significantly inhibits the growth of Gram-negative and Gram-positive bacteria and fungi *(68,69)*. It forms a rigid hairpin loop constrained by two disulfide bridges and adopts the conformation of an antiparallel β-sheet connected to a β-turn *(70)*. In the planar conformation of tachyplesin, the five hydrophobic side chains are localized at one face, and the six cationic side chains are distributed on another face. The amphiphilic structure of tachyplesin is presumed to be closely associated with its bactericidal activity.

Big defensin, which consists of 79 residues, is distinct from the mammalian defensins in molecular size of 29–34 residues in common *(71)*. Big defensin is proteolytically divided into two domains by trypsin. The COOH-terminal domain shows sequence similarity with mammalian neutrophil-derived defensins. The disulfide motif in this domain is identical to that of β-defensin from bovine neutrophils. A noteworthy characteristic of big defensin is that there is a functional difference between the two domains. Big defensin has antimicrobial activity against both Gram-negative and Gram-positive bacteria. Interestingly, the NH$_2$-terminal hydrophobic domain is more effective than the COOH-terminal defensin domain against Gram-positive bacteria. In contrast, the COOH-terminal domain displays more potent activity than the NH$_2$-terminal domain against Gram-negative bacteria, suggesting a kind of chimera molecule. Big defensin may prove to represent a new class of the defensin family possessing two functional domains with different antimicrobial activities.

Tachystatins A, B, and C, which consist of 41–44 residues, exhibit a broad spectrum of antimicrobial activity against Gram-negative and Gram-positive bacteria and fungi *(72)*. Of these tachystatins, tachystatin C is most effective. Tachystatin A is homologous to tachystatin B. Tachystatin C contains the same disulfide motif as that found in tachystatin A, but it shows low sequence similarity to tachystatin A. Tachystatin A shows sequence similarity to ω-agatoxin-IVA of funnel web spider venom, a potent blocker of voltage-dependent calcium channels *(72)*. However, tachystatin A exhibits no blocking activity of

Table 1
Antimicrobial Activity of the Horseshoe Crab Chitin-Binding Peptides[a]

	Escherichia coli	Staphylococcus aureus	Candida albicans	Pichia pastoris
Tachyplesin	<2.5	0.3	0.2	0.1
Big defensin	2.5	<2.5	20.0	42.0
Tachystatin A	25.0	4.2	3.0	0.5
Tachystatin B	NI[b]	7.4	3.0	0.1
Tachystatin C	1.2	0.8	0.9	0.3
Tachycitin	33.0	56.0	52.0	41.0
Tachycitin	<33.0	<56.0	52.0	41.0

[a] Data are 50% growth-inhibitory concentration (IC_{50}), in µg/mL.
[b] No inhibition at 100 µg/mL.

Table 2
Chitin Binding Activities of the Horseshoe
Crab Antimicrobial Peptides

	Concentration required for 50% binding (µM)
Tachyplesin	6.6
Big defensin	25.4
Tachystatin A	8.4
Tachystatin B	4.3
Tachystatin C	5.2
Tachycitin	19.5

the P-type calcium channel in rat Purkinje cells. Tachystatins cause morphologic chages against a budding yeast, and tachystatin C has strong cell lysis activity. Furthermore, tachystatin C, but not tachystatins A and B, exhibits hemolytic activity. Tachystatin C shows sequence similarity to several insecticidal neurotoxins of spider venoms *(72)*. As horseshoe crabs are close relatives of spiders, tachystatins and spider neurotoxins may have evolved from a common ancestral peptide, with adaptive functions.

Tachycitin consists of 73 residues containing five disulfide bonds, but with no *N*-linked sugar *(67)*. The antimicrobial activity of tachycitin is not strong by itself, but it synergistically enhances the antimicrobial activity of big defensin: the 50% growth-inhibitory concentration (IC_{50}) value of big defensin against Gram-positive bacteria is decreased to 1/50 in the presence of a small amount of tachycitin. Tachylectins 5A and 5B also enhance the antimicrobial activity of big defensin against Gram-positive bacteria *(58)*. Interestingly, Tachylectins 5A and 5B do not enchance antimicrobial activity against Gram-negative bacteria. Recently, the solution structure of tachycitin has been determined by nuclear magnetic resonance (NMR) spectroscopy, which has provided the first three-dimensional structural information on invertebrate chitin binding protein *(73)*.

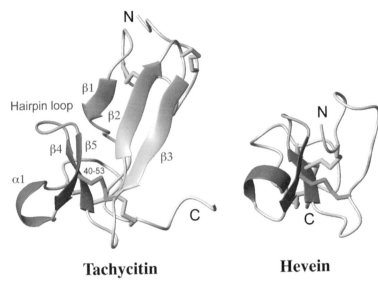

Tachycitin   **Hevein**

Fig. 6. A structural comparison of tachycitin and hevein.

5.1. Chitin Binding Structural Motif of Tachycitin

The structure of tachycitin is largely divided into NH_2-terminal and COOH-terminal domains. In the COOH-terminal domain, tachycitin forms a hairpin loop of a two-stranded β-sheet, which superimposes the structure of the chitin binding site of hevein without sequence similarity (Fig. 6). Hevein is an antifungal peptide from the rubber tree *Hevea brasiliensis (74)*. In hevein, the aromatic side chains of Trp21 and Trp23 in the loop directly interact with chitin-derived oligosaccharides through a hydrophobic interaction *(75,76)*. The side chains of Tyr49 and Val52 in tachycitin are perfectly superimposed on those of the two tryptophans in hevein (Fig. 7). Tachyplesin also contains a similar hairpin loop of a two-stranded β-sheet *(70)*. Therefore, in tachyplesin and tachycitin, the hydrophobic residues clustered on the one face of their β-hairpin loops probably function as chitin-binding sites.

Shen and Jacobs-Lorena *(77)* have hypothesized that chitin binding proteins in invertebrates and plants are correlated by a rare evolutional process, convergent evolution. Structural conservation of the chitin binding motif between the horseshoe crab and plants is faithful experimental evidence regarding this hypothesis. Chitin is a component of the cell wall of fungi and also a major structural component of arthropod exoskeletons. Therefore, the antimicrobial substances released from hemocytes probably recognize chitin exposed at the site of a lesion. They appear to serve not only as antibacterial molecules against invading microbes but also in wound healing, which may stimulate and accelerate chitin biosynthesis at the sites of injury.

5.2. Anti-LPS Factor

Horseshoe crab hemocytes contain a different type of antimicrobial proteins called anti-LPS factor. Anti-LPS factor, which consists of 102 residues, inhibits LPS-mediated hemolymph coagulation and shows antibacterial action against Gram-negative

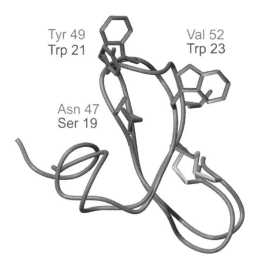

Fig. 7. The chitin binding site of hevein (Cys12-Ser32) superimposed onto the putative chitin binding site of tachycitin (Cys40-Gly60).

bacteria *(78–80)*. Anti-LPS factor is stored in L-granules, together with several clotting factors and protease inhibitors. Anti-LPS factor shows sequence similarity to the α-lactoalbumin/lysozyme family *(79)*. The crystal structure of anti-LPS factor is composed of a single domain consisting of three β-helices packed against a four-stranded β-sheet to form a wedge-shaped molecule with a striking charge distribution and amphiphilicity *(81)*. The binding site for LPS probably involves the extended amphiphilic loop, which represents an LPS binding motif shared by two mammalian proteins, LPS binding protein *(82)* and bactericidal/permeability-increasing protein *(83,84)*.

REFERENCES

1. Srimal S, Miyata T, Kawabata S, Miyata T, Iwanaga S. The complete amino acid sequence of coagulogen isolated from Southeast Asian horseshoe crab, *Carcinoscorpius rotundicauda*. J Biochem (Tokyo) 1985;98:305–318.
2. Hoffmann JA, Kafatos FC, Janeway CA, Ezekowitz RAB. Phylogenetic perspectives in innate immunity. Science 1999;284:1313–1318.
3. Toh Y, Mizutani A, Tokunaga F, Muta T, Iwanaga S. Morphology of the granular hemocytes of the Japanese horseshoe crab *Tachypleus tridentatus* and immunocytochemical localization of clotting factors and antimicrobial substances. Cell Tissue Res 1991;266:137–147.
4. Kawabata S, Muta T, Iwanaga S. Clotting cascade and defense molecules found in hemolymph of horseshoe crab. In: Söderhäll K, Iwanaga S, Vasta GR (eds.). New Directions in Invertebrate Immunology. Fairhaven, NJ: SOS Publications. 1996, pp. 255–283.
5. Iwanaga S, Kawabata S, Muta T. New types of clotting factors and defense molecules found in horseshoe crab hemolymph: their structures and functions. J Biochem (Tokyo) 1998;123:1–15.
6. Levin J, Bang FB. The role of endotoxin in the extracellular coagulation of *Limulus* blood. Bull Johns Hopkins Hosp 1964;115:265–274.
7. Levin J, Bang FB. Clottable protein in *Limulus:* its localization and kinetics of its coagulation by endotoxin. Thromb Diath Haemorrh 1968;19:186–197.
8. Belvin MP, Anderson KV. A conserved signaling pathway—the *Drosphila* toll-dorsal pathway. Annu Rev Cell Dev Biol 1996;12:393–416.

9. LeMosy EK, Hong CC, Hashimoto C. Signal transduction by a protease cascade. Trends Cell Biol 1999;9:102–107.

10. Smith CL, DeLotto R. A common domain within the proenzyme regions of the *Drosophila* snake and easter proteins and *Tachypleus* proclotting enzyme defines a new subfamily of serine proteases. Protein Sci 1992;1:1225–1226.

11. Bergner A, Oganessyan V, Muta T, et al. Crystal structure of a coagulogen, the clotting protein from horseshoe crab: a structural homologue of nerve growth factor. EMBO J 1996;15:6789–6797.

12. Muta T, Hashimoto R, Miyata T, et al. Proclotting enzyme from horseshoe crab hemocytes. cDNA cloning, disulfide locations, and subcellular localization. J Biol Chem 1990;265:22426–22433.

13. Muta T, Oda T, Iwanaga S. Horseshoe crab coagulation factor B. A unique serine protease zymogen activated by cleavage of an Ile-Ile bond. J Biol Chem 1993;268:21384–21388.

14. Jiang H, Kanost MR. The clip-domain family of serine proteases in arthropods. Insect Biochem Mol Biol 2000;30:95–105.

15. Nakamura S, Takagi T, Iwanaga S, Niwa M, Takahashi K. A clottable protein (coagulogen) of horseshoe crab hemocytes. Structural change of its polypeptide chain during gel formation. J Biochem (Tokyo) 1976;80:649–652.

16. Takagi T, Hokama Y, Miyata T, Morita T, Iwanaga S. Amino acid sequence of Japanese horseshoe crab *(Tachypleus tridentatus)* coagulogen B chain: completion of the coagulogen sequence. J Biochem (Tokyo) 1984;95:1445–1457.

17. Kawasaki H, Nose T, Muta T, et al. Head-to-tail polymerization of coagulin, a clottable protein of the horseshoe crab. J Biol Chem 2000;275:35297–35301.

18. Yee VC, Pratt KP, Cote HC, et al. Crystal structure of a 30 kDa C-terminal fragment from the gamma chain of human fibrinogen. Structure (Lond) 1997;5:125–138.

19. Pratt KP, Cote HC, Chung DW, Stenkamp RE, Davie EW. The primary fibrin polymerization pocket: three-dimensional structure of a 30-kDa C-terminal gamma chain fragment complexed with the peptide Gly-Pro-Arg-Pro. Proc Natl Acad Sci USA 1997;94:7176–7181.

20. Doolittle RF, Spraggon G, Everse SJ. Three-dimensional structural studies on fragments of fibrinogen and fibrin. Curr Opin Struct Biol 1998;8:792–798.

21. Laudano AP, Doolittle RF. Synthetic peptide derivatives that bind to fibrinogen and prevent the polymerization of fibrin monomers. Proc Natl Acad Sci USA 1978;75:3085–3089.

22. Laudano AP, Cottrell BA, Doolittle RF. Synthetic peptides modeled on fibrin polymerization sites. Ann NY Acad Sci 1983;408:315–329.

23. Miura Y, Kawabata S, Iwanaga S. A *Limulus* intracellular coagulation inhibitor with characteristics of the serpin superfamily. Purification, characterization, and cDNA cloning. J Biol Chem 1994;269:542–547.

24. Miura Y, Kawabata S, Wakamiya Y, Nakamura T, Iwanaga S. A *Limulus* intracellular coagulation inhibitor type 2. Purification, characterization, cDNA cloning, and tissue localization. J Biol Chem 1995;270:558–565.

25. Agarwala KL, Kawabata S, Miura Y, Kuroki Y, Iwanaga S. *Limulus* intracellular coagulation inhibitor type 3. Purification, characterization, cDNA cloning, and tissue localization. J Biol Chem 1996;271:23768–23774.

26. Liu T-Y, Minetti CAS, Fortes-Dias CL, et al. C-reactive protein, limunectin, liopopolysaccharide-binding protein, and coagulin. Ann NY Acad Sci 1994;712:146–154.

27. Lorand L, Credo RB, Janus, TJ. Factor XIII (fibrin-stabilizing factor). Methods Enzymol 1981;80:333–341.

28. Tokunaga F, Yamada M, Miyata T, et al. *Limulus* hemocyte transglutaminase. Its purification and characterization, and identification of the intracellular substrates. J Biol Chem 1993;268:252–261.

29. Tokunaga F, Muta T, Iwanaga S, et al. *Limulus* hemocyte transglutaminase. cDNA cloning, amino acid sequence, and tissue localization. J Biol Chem 1993;268:262–268.

30. Imler J-L, Hoffmann JA. signaling mechanisms in the antimicrobial host defense of *Drosophila*. Curr Opin Microbial 2000;3:16–22.

31. Anderson KV. Toll signaling pathways in the innate immune response. Curr Opin Immunol 2000;12:13–19.

32. Lemmon MA, Schlessinger J. Regulation of signal transduction and signal diversity by receptor oligomerization. Trends Biochem Sci 1994;19:459–463.

33. Mizuguchi K, Parker JS, Blundell TL, Gay NJ. Getting knotted: a model for the structure and activation of Spatzle. Trends Biochem Sci 1998;23:239–242.

34. Söderhäll K, Cerenius L. Role of the prophenoloxidase-activating system in invertebrate immunity. Curr Opin Immunol 1998;10:23–28.

35. Ashida M, Brey PT. Recent advances in research on the insect prophenoloxidase cascade. In; Brey PT, Hultmark D (eds.). Molecular Mechanism of Immune Responses in Insects. London: Chapman & Hall, 1998, pp. 135–172.

36. Solomon EI, Sundaram UM, Machonkin TE. Multicopper oxidases and oxygenases. Chem Rev 1996;96:2563–2605.

37. Aspan A, Huang TS, Cerenius L, Söderhäll K. cDNA cloning of prophenoloxidase from the freshwater crayfish *Pacifastacus leniusculus* and its activation. Proc Natl Acad Sci USA 1995;92:939–943.

38. Decker H, Rimke T. Tarantula hemocyanin shows phenoloxidase activity. J Biol Chem 1998;273:25889–25892.

39. Nagai T, Kawabata S. A link between blood coagulation and prophenol oxidase activation in arthropod host defense. J Biol Chem 2000;275:29264–29267.

40. Lee SY, Cho MY, Hyun JH, et al. Molecular cloning of cDNA for pro-phenol-oxidase-activating factor I, a serine protease is induced by lipopolysaccharide or 1,3-beta-glucan in coleopteran insect, *Holotrichia diomphalia* larvae. Eur J Biochem 1998;257:615–621.

41. Jiang HB, Wang Y, Kanost MR. Four serine proteinases expressed in *Manduca sexta* hemocytes. Insect Mol Biol 1999;8:39–53.

42. Satoh D, Horii A, Ochiai M, Ashida M. Prophenoloxidase-activating enzyme of the silkworm, *Bombyx mori*. Purification, characterization, and cDNA cloning. J Biol Chem 1999;274:7441–7453.

43. Ashida M, Yamazaki H. Biochemistry of the phenoloxidase system in insect: with special reference to its activation. In: Ohnishi E, Ishizaki H (eds.). Molting and Metamorphosis. Tokyo, Berlin: Japan Science Society Press/Springer-Verlag, 1990, pp. 239–265.

44. Zlateva T, Di Muro P, Salvato B, Beltramini M. The *o*-diphenol oxidase activity of arthropod hemocyanin. FEBS Lett 1996;384:251–254.

45. Burmester T, Scheller K. Common origin of arthropod tyrosinase, arthropod hemocyanin, insect hexamerin, and dipteran arylphorin receptor. J Mol Evol 1996;42:713–728.

46. Hazes B, Magnus KA, Bonaventura C, et al. Crystal structure of deoxygenated *Limulus polyphemus* subunit II hemocyanin at 2.18 Å resolution: clues for a mechanism for allosteric regulation. Protein Sci 1993;2:597–619.

47. Magnus KA, Hazes B, Ton-That H, et al. Crystallographic analysis of oxygenated and deoxygenated states of arthropod hemocyanin shows unusual differences. Proteins 1994;19:302–309.

48. Klabunde T, Eicken C, Sacchettini JC, Krebs B. Crystal structure of a plant catechol oxidase containing a dicopper center. Nat Struct Biol 1998;5:1084–1090.

49. Eicken C, Krebs B, Sacchettini JC. Catechol oxidase—structure and activity. Curr Opin Struct Biol 1999;9:677–683.

50. Salvato B, Santamaria M, Beltramini M, Alzuet G, Casella L. The enzymatic properties of *Octopus vulgaris* hemocyanin: *o*-diphenol oxidase activity. Biochemistry 1998;37:14065–14077.

51. Linzen B, Soeter NM, Riggs AF, et al. The structure of arthropod hemocyanins. Science 1985;229:519–524.

52. Kawabata S, Iwanaga S. Role of lectins in the innate immunity of horseshoe crab. Dev Comp Immunol 1999;23:391–400.

53. Saito T, Kawabata S, Hirata M, Iwanaga S. A novel type of *Limulus* lectin-L6. Purification, primary structure, and antibacterial activity. J Biol Chem 1995;270:14493–14499

54. Huh CG, Aldrich J, Mottahedeh J, et al. Cloning and characterization of *Physarum polycephalum* tectonins. Homologues of *Limulus* lectin L-6. J Biol Chem 1998;273:6565–6574.

55. Okino N, Kawabata S, Saito T, et al. Purification, characterization, and cDNA cloning of a 27-kDa lectin (L10) from horseshoe crab hemocytes. J Biol Chem 1995;270:31008–31015.

56. Inamori K, Saito T, Iwaki D, et al. A newly identified horseshoe crab lectin with specificity for blood group A antigen recognizes specific O-antigens of bacterial lipopolysaccharides. J Biol Chem 1999;274:3272–3278.

57. Saito T, Hatada M, Iwanaga S, Kawabata S. A newly identified horseshoe crab lectin with binding specificity to O-antigen of bacterial lipopolysaccharides. J Biol Chem 1997;272:30703–30708.

58. Gokudan S, Muta T, Tsuda R, et al. Horseshoe crab acetyl group-recognizing lectins involved in innate immunity are structurally related to fibrinogen. Proc Natl Acad Sci USA. 1999;96:10086–10091.

59. Nguyen NY, Suzuki A, Boykins RA, Liu TY. The amino acid sequence of *Limulus* C-reactive protein. Evidence of polymorphism. J Biol Chem 1986;261: 10456–10465.

60. Tillett WS, Francis TJ. Serological reactions in pneumonia with a nonprotein somatic fraction of pneumococcus. J Exp Med 1930;52:561–571.

61. Armstrong PB, Swarnakar S, Srimal S, et al. A cytolytic function for a sialic acid-binding lectin that is a member of the pentraxin family of proteins. J Biol Chem 1996;271:14717–14721.

62. Iwaki D, Osaki T, Mizunoe Y, et al. Functional and structural diversities of C-reactive proteins present in horseshoe crab hemolymph plasma. Eur J Biochem 1999;264:314–326.

63. Beisel HG, Kawabata S, Iwanaga S, Huber R, Bode W. Tachylectin-2: crystal structure of a specific GlcNAc/GalNAc-binding lectin involved in the innate immunity host defense of the Japanese horseshoe crab *Tachypleus tridentatus*. EMBO J 1999;18:2313–2322.

64. Ohashi T, Erickson HP. Two oligomeric forms of plasma ficolin have differential lectin activity. J Biol Chem 1997;272:14220–14226.

65. Hansen S, Holmskov U. Structural aspects of collectins and receptors for collectins. Immunobiology 1998;199:165–189.

66. Lu J, Le Y. Ficolins and the fibrinogen-like domain. Immunobiology 1998;199:190–199.

67. Kawabata S, Nagayama R, Hirata M, et al. Tachycitin, a small granular component in horseshoe crab hemocytes, is an antimicrobial protein with chitin-binding activity. J Biochem (Tokyo) 1996;120:1253–1260.

68. Nakamura T, Furunaka H, Miyata T, et al. Tachyplesin, a class of antimicrobial peptide from the hemocytes of the horseshoe crab *(Tachypleus tridentatus)*. Isolation and chemical structure. J Biol Chem 1988;263:16709–16713.

69. Iwanaga S, Muta T, Shigenaga T, et al. Structure-function relationships of tachyplesins and their analogues. Ciba Found Symp 1994;186:160–175.

70. Kawano K, Yoneya T, Miyata T, et al. Antimicrobial peptide, tachyplesin I, isolated from hemocytes of the horseshoe crab *(Tachypleus tridentatus)*. NMR determination of the beta-sheet structure. J Biol Chem 1990;265:15365–15367.

71. Saito T, Kawabata S, Shigenaga T, et al. A novel big defensin identified in horseshoe crab hemocytes: isolation, amino acid sequence, and antibacterial activity. J Biochem (Tokyo) 1995;117:1131–1137.

72. Osaki T, Omotezako M, Nagayama R, et al. Horseshoe crab hemocyte-derived antimicrobial polypeptides, tachystatins, with sequence similarity to spider neurotoxins. J Biol Chem 1999;274:26172–26178.

73. Suetake T, Tsuda S, Kawabata S, et al. Chitin-binding proteins in invertebrates and plants comprise a common chitin-binding structural motif. J Biol Chem 2000;275:17929–17932.

74. Broekaert W, Lee HI, Kush A, Chua NH, Raikhel N. Wound-induced accumulation of mRNA containing a hevein sequence in laticifers of rubber tree *(Hevea brasiliensis)*. Proc Natl Acad Sci USA 1990;87:7633–7637.
75. Asensio JL, Canada FJ, Bruix M, Rodriguez-Romero A, Jimenez-Barbero J. The interaction of hevein with N-acetylglucosamine-containing oligosaccharides. Solution structure of hevein complexed to chitobiose. Eur J Biochem 1995;230:621–633.
76. Asensio JL, Canada FJ, Bruix M, et al. NMR investigations of protein-carbohydrate interactions—refined three-dimensional structure of the complex between hevein and methyl beta-chitobioside. Glycobiology 1998;8:569–577.
77. Shen Z, Jacobs-Lorena M. Evolution of chitin-binding proteins in invertebrates. J Mol Evol 1999;48:341–347.
78. Morita T, Ohtsubo S, Nakamura T, et al. Isolation and biological activities of *Limulus* anticoagulant (anti-LPS factor) which interacts with lipopolysaccharide (LPS). J Biochem (Tokyo) 1985;97:1611–1620.
79. Aketagawa J, Miyata T, Ohtsubo S, et al. Primary structure of *Limulus* anticoagulant anti-lipopolysaccharide factor. J Biol Chem 1986;261:7357–7365.
80. Muta T, Miyata T, Tokunaga F, Nakamura T, Iwanaga S. Primary structure of anti-lipopolysaccharide factor from American horseshoe crab, *Limulus polyphemus*. J Biochem (Tokyo) 1987;101:1321–1330.
81. Hoess A, Watson S, Siber GR, Liddington R. Crystal structure of an endotoxin-neutralizing protein from the horseshoe crab, *Limulus* anti-LPS factor, at 1.5 Å resolution. EMBO J 1993;12:3351–3356.
82. Schumann RR, Leong SR, Flaggs GW, et al. Structure and function of lipopolysaccharide binding protein. Science 1990;249:1429–1431.
83. Marra MN, Wilde CG, Griffith JE, Snable JL, Scott RW. Bactericidal/permeability-increasing protein has endotoxin-neutralizing activity. J Immunol 1990;144:662–666.
84. Marra MN, Wilde CG, Collins MS, et al. The role of bactericidal/permeability-increasing protein as a natural inhibitor of bacterial endotoxin. J Immunol 1992;148:532–537.

7

Pattern Recognition Receptors in *Drosophila*

Mika Rämet, Alan Pearson, Kati Baksa, and Asha Harikrishnan

1. INTRODUCTION

The foundation of the innate immune system is the recognition of infectious non-self. Janeway *(1,2)* has proposed that this recognition is mediated by the binding of host pattern recognition proteins to pathogen-associated molecular patterns (PAMPs). PAMPs were originally defined as structures found on the surfaces of microorganisms but not present on normal host cells. More recently, this definition has been broadened to include intracellular components of microorganisms, such as CpG DNA *(3)*. There are several different classes of pattern recognition proteins including secreted, membrane-bound, and integral membrane proteins, and some pattern recognition molecules can exist in more than one of these forms. Recognition of PAMPs by pattern recognition proteins has several consequences, including the activation of induced cellular and humoral immune responses, such as the induction of antimicrobial genes in *Drosophila,* and the activation of T-cells in mammals. Pattern recognition proteins also participate in the effector mechanisms of the immune system, such as the complement (mammals) and prophenoloxidase (insect) cascades, as well as phagocytosis of microorganisms.

In this chapter we discuss what is known about the pattern recognition proteins of *Drosophila melanogaster.* We focus first on the secreted and membrane-bound pattern recognition molecules including the thioester-containing proteins, the Gram-negative binding proteins, and the peptidoglycan recognition proteins. Then we discuss what is known about the transmembrane pattern recognition molecules, focusing on the *Drosophila* scavenger receptors and hemomucin. We do not discuss the *Drosophila* Toll-like receptors, as these are discussed elsewhere in this book (*see,* Chaps. 5, 9, and 10). In addition, although in mammalian systems the Toll receptors may be pattern recognition receptors, this does not seem to be the case in *Drosophila.*

2. SECRETED AND MEMBRANE-BOUND PATTERN RECOGNITION RECEPTORS

2.1. ThioEster-Containing Proteins

The complement system plays a major role in vertebrate innate immunity. It can be activated through three distinct mechanisms, the classical, lectin and alternative pathways *(4),* which all converge at the C3 component. Proteolytic cleavage of C3 results in

From: *Infectious Disease: Innate Immunity*
Edited by: R. A. B. Ezekowitz and J. A. Hoffmann © Humana Press Inc., Totowa, NJ

an activated product that covalently attaches via a thioester bond to the surface of the pathogen, leading to phagocytosis or lysis of the pathogen. In the last few years, the identification in the sea urchin and horseshoe crab of proteins with structural similarities to the vertebrate C3 proteins has led to the concept that a complement system similar to that in vertebrates functions in the host defense of invertebrates. Another class of proteins that is similar to the vertebrate α_2-macroglobulins has also been recently identified in invertebrates. α_2-Macroglobulins are related to C3 proteins and are evolutionarily ancient protease inhibitors from which C3 is proposed to have arisen by gene duplication *(5)*. Interestingly, the *Limulus* (horseshoe crab) α_2-macroglobulin has been proposed to function as a protease inhibitor against proteases released by damaged tissue as a result of infection by pathogenic microorganisms *(6)*. It has been suggested that the early opsonic system may have relied simply on direct binding of α_2-macroglobulin to the protease-producing organism *(5)*. These findings have prompted a search for C3/α_2-macroglobulin-like proteins that may function in a primitive complement system in *Drosophila* and other insects.

Recently Lagueux et al. *(7)* have reported that *Drosophila* expresses at least four distinct proteins that exhibit overall sequence similarity to the proteins of the vertebrate complement C3/α_2-macroglobulin superfamily. These proteins contain the highly conserved thioester motifs and have been named thioester-containing proteins (TEPs 1–4). The protein sequences deduced from these genes show that TEPs 1–4 contain a highly conserved region of 30 amino acid residues harboring a canonical thioester motif, GCGEQ. They also have putative signal peptides, suggesting that these proteins are secreted. A unique feature of the TEPs is the highly conserved 126-amino acid stretch containing six cysteines in the C-terminal region of the protein. In contrast, the vertebrate proteins of the C3/α_2-macroglobulin family have a higher total number of cysteines but lack the C-terminal cysteine signature of the TEPs.

All four *Tep* genes show a low level of expression at the larval, pupal, and adult stages of development. The *Tep2* gene has five different splice isoforms, and the others have a single transcript each. Interestingly, *Tep1, Tep2,* and *Tep4* have been shown to be transcriptionally upregulated in larvae or adults upon immune challenge by bacteria. More detailed studies on *Tep1* show that it is strongly expressed in the fat body and to a lesser extent in the blood cells of immune-challenged larvae *(7)*. The fat body is known to express antimicrobial peptides strongly upon immune challenge, and two pathways, *Toll* and *imd,* have been shown to regulate the induction of these peptides. However, neither of these pathways appears to play a major role in mediating *Tep1* regulation. Instead, the *JAK* pathway, which was previously shown to play an important role in hemocyte development and in regulating the immune response in *Drosophila (8),* appears to regulate the expression of *Tep1*. A strong constitutive expression of *Tep1* is observed in *hop^Tuml* larvae, which carry a gain-of-function mutation in the *hop* gene. Conversely, in loss-of function *hop^M38* mutant larvae, there is reduced induction of *Tep1* by septic injury compared with wild type. These results suggest that JAK kinase may play a direct role in regulating *Tep1* function in *Drosophila* immunity.

More recently, Levashina et al. *(9)* have reported the identification of a novel TEP (*aTEP-1*) in the mosquito *Anopheles gambiae*. The translated sequence of *aTEP-1* has the canonical thioester motif (GCGEQ) and shows significant similarity both to mammalian complement factor C3 and to the related α_2-macroglobulin proteins. In contrast to the *Drosophila* TEPs, which are expressed mainly in the fat body, aTEP-1 is hemocyte-specific. These authors have provided the first functional evidence for an insect thioester-containing protein that behaves like complement to promote phagocytosis. They have shown that aTEP-1 is proteolytically cleaved in the hemolymph upon aseptic injury or bacterial challenge *(9)*. The cleaved product has been shown to bind *Escherichia coli* and *Staphylococcus aureus,* and this binding appears to depend on the presence of a functional thioester bond. Moreover, depletion of *aTEP1* in RNAi experiments using a hemocyte-like mosquito cell line suggests that *aTEP1* promotes phagocytosis of Gram-negative bacteria but not of Gram-positive bacteria.

These studies strengthen the view that the C3 complement system is not exclusive to vertebrate innate immunity and point to a common ancestral protein that functions in innate immunity of vertebrates and insects. The differences in the number and position of cysteines between the *Drosophila* TEPs and the vertebrate C3 proteins may support the view that TEPs either evolved independently or separated early from the common ancestor of C3/α_2-macroglobulins. Future studies on the mutant phenotypes of the various *Drosophila* TEPs as well as the regulation of their function by other genes will give us a clearer picture of the exact role that these proteins play in *Drosophila* innate immunity.

3. GRAM-NEGATIVE BACTERIA BINDING PROTEINS

Gram-Negative bacteria-binding protein (GNBP) was first isolated from the hemolymph of immunochallenged silkworm *(Bombyx mori)* larvae as a 50-kDa protein that bound specifically to the Gram-negative bacteria *Enterobacter cloacea* but only minimally to the Gram-positive bacteria *Bacillus licheniformis (10)*. In agreement with the notion that GNBP is a secreted protein, the cDNA encodes a protein with a putative N-terminal signal sequence. In addition, the C-terminal sequence may act as a glycosyl phosphatidyl inositol-4-phosphate (PIP) attachment site, suggesting that there may also be a membrane-bound form. The protein sequence also predicts two potential N-glycosylation sites in the N-terminal part of the protein. About one-third of the silk worm GNBP sequence shows considerable homology to bacterial gluconases and to the α-chain of the *Tachypleus tridentatus* serine protease (1,3)-B-D-glucan-sensitive coagulation factor G (identity 37%, similarity 68%). This gluconase homology region is probably responsible for the recognition/binding to bacterial cell walls. However, no gluconase activity was detected. The authors also found 21% homology and 46% overall similarity to human CD14.

Although low levels of constitutive GNBP expression are detected in the fat body and epidermis in naive silkworm larvae, transcription of GNBP is strongly induced in the fat body, and to a lesser degree in the cuticular epidermal cells surrounding the site of injury 6 hours after procuticular abrasion with bacteria *(10)*. Sterile injury alone could also slightly induce the GNBP RNA expression.

Recently, three *Drosophila* DGNBPs were cloned based on homology to the *Bombyx mori* GNBP *(11)*. DGNBP-1 was isolated from the mbn-2 cell library and has been molecularly characterized. DGNBP-2 and -3 were found by a homology search to DGNBP-1, with which they share 30 and 26% identity, respectively. All DGNBPs have a β-1,3-gluconase-like domain and are likely to lack gluconase activity since the critical amino acids necessary for enzyme activity are not conserved. DGNBP-1 mRNA is expressed throughout all developmental stages, whereas DGNBP-2 mRNA expression begins at the late embryonic stage and continues until later stages of development. DGNBP-3 mRNA is mainly expressed in larval and pupal stages. Induction studies for DGNBP-1 in adult flies and in cultured S2 and mbn-2 cells showed downregulation during the early phases (3–6 hours) of bacterial infection.

DGNBPs have a C-terminal hydrophobic tail containing a putative glycosylphos-phatidyl inositol (GPI) anchor attachment site that suggests an existence of a membrane-bound form. Indeed, the same authors *(11)* have found several lines of evidence that DGNBP-1 has both soluble and membrane-bound forms. First, a polyclonal antibody generated against DGNBP-1 bound to the surface of S2 cells. Second, in tissue culture experiments, overexpression of a mutant DGNBP-1 lacking the last 10 amino acids of the wild-type protein did not result in DGNBP-1 in the membrane fraction, whereas the full-length protein was present. Third, DGNBP-1-overexpressing cells treated with phosphatidylinositol-phospholipase C (PI-PLC) released DGNBP-1 from membrane to culture medium, demonstrating that DGNBP-1 is a GPI-anchored membrane protein. Finally, a small amount of soluble DGNBP-1 is always present in medium of the wild-type DGNBP-1-expressing cells *(11)*.

In addition to intact bacteria, DGNBPs have been shown to bind β-1,3-glucan and LPS. This is in contrast to the silk worm GNBP that binds β-1,3-glucan only poorly. DGNBP-1 fails to bind β-1-4-glucan and chitin. DGNBP-1 appears to be involved in the induction of the antimicrobial peptide genes attacin, cecropin, and drosomycin, as indicated by experiments showing that DGNBP-1-overexpressing cells are more responsive to LPS and β-1,3-glucan for the induction of these peptides. Furthermore, induction of antibacterial peptides can be significantly inhibited in S2 cells by pretreatment with DGNBP-1 antiserum *(11)*.

GNBP has also been cloned from mosquitoes *(Anopheles gambiae)* based on homology to the *Bombyx mori* protein *(12)*. Interestingly, mosquito GNPB seems to recognize both Gram-positive and Gram-negative bacteria when overexpressed in cultured cells *(12)*. *Anopheles* GNBP is induced by *Plasmodium* infection *(13)*, although it is possible that part of the induction can be accounted for by the resident bacteria of the gut, which get into the gut cells passively along with the *Plasmodium*.

These studies have identified an interesting protein family with homology to glu-conases. It would be beneficial to identify the binding specificity more precisely in all three organisms and to confirm the Gram-negative bacteria binding specificity, by comparing the binding of these proteins with additional Gram-negative and Gram-positive organisms. The possible functional homology between CD14 and of GNBPs is of potential future interest.

4. PEPTIDOGLYCAN RECOGNITION PROTEINS

Peptidoglycan, a major cell wall component of most bacteria, can induce both antimicrobial gene synthesis and activation of the hemolymph prophenoloxidase melanization cascade in insects. Using the silkworm *Bombyx mori,* Ashida and colleagues *(14)* were the first to purify a soluble hemolymph peptidoglycan binding protein capable of activating this cascade. Their subsequent cloning of the silkworm peptidoglycan recognition protein (PGRP) gene demonstrated that PGRPs are conserved from insects to mammals *(15,16)*. Those PGRPs tested have been shown to recognize peptidoglycan preferentially relative to chitin, α-glucan, or LPS *(14,15,17)*.

Recently, Hultmark and colleagues *(18)* have identified a 12-member family of PGRP genes in *Drosophila,* which they grouped into two classes. The seven short PGRP genes (PGRP-S) have short transcripts and 5′ UTRs and encode putative secreted proteins, much like the *Bombyx* PGRP. The five long PGRP genes (PGRP-L) have long transcripts and 5′ UTRs. Three of the PGRP-L genes encode putative transmembrane receptors, whereas the other two appear to lack signal sequences or transmembrane-like domains, suggesting that they may encode cytoplasmic PGRP molecules. In addition, most of the PGRP-L genes have multiple transcripts, some of which encode different putative protein isoforms.

The previously characterized insect PGRP genes were found to be expressed in hemocytes, the fat body, and the epidermis, and their expression was upregulated in response to bacterial challenge *(15,16)*. In *Drosophila,* expression of the different PGRP genes varies widely according to developmental stage, tissue specificity, and response to bacterial challenge. Most of the genes are expressed in many or all developmental stages, except for PGRP-SB2, which appears to be expressed exclusively in prepupae. At least four of the PGRP-S genes are strongly induced in response to bacterial challenge, whereas of the PGRP-L genes, only PGRP-LB is induced. The tissue expression pattern for these genes is quite complex, but in general, the short genes and the inducible genes are most highly expressed in the fat body but not in hemocytes. Two exceptions are PGRP-SA and PGRP-SD, which are constitutively expressed in hemocytes. In addition, PGRP-SA is strongly induced in the epidermis, whereas the PGRP-SC genes are constitutively expressed at high levels in the gut, both tissues that are known to be immune competent in *Drosophila.* In contrast to most of the short genes, the three PGRP-L genes containing transmembrane domains are expressed most strongly in hemocytes and the hemocyte-like mbn-2 cell line. It remains to be seen whether there are tissue-or infection-specific expression patterns for various PGRP-L isoforms.

PGRP-SA and PGRP-SC1B have been tested and shown to bind insoluble peptidoglycan and can thus be classified as pattern recognition proteins with peptidoglycan binding capabilities. However, it is possible that the many different PGRP proteins may have different specificities for microbial ligands. This, together with spatial and temporal differences in PGRP expression, could contribute to robustness in the *Drosophila* immune system. It is likely that, as in the silkworm, at least some of the soluble *Drosophila* PGRP proteins will participate in peptidoglycan-induced activation of the prophenoloxidase cascade. In addition, some soluble PGRPs might activate antibacterial gene induction pathways or act as opsonins to promote phagocytosis of bacteria by macrophages. It will be interesting to know whether any of the transmembrane PGRP-L proteins are able to recognize bacteria, as this would provide additional means beyond *Drosophila* class C scavenger receptor (dSR-CI) for the phagocytic uptake of pathogens. Furthermore, the PGRP-L genes are excellent candidates for the currently unknown receptor(s), which activates the major antibacterial gene pathway in *Drosophila,* the IMD pathway (*see* Chap.9).

Many of the *Drosophila* PGRP genes are no more closely related to each other than they are to mammalian PGRP genes, suggesting that much of the divergence in the

PGRP gene family occurred prior to the protostome/deuterostome split over 500 million years ago. This suggests that additional mammalian PGRP genes remain to be found. Indeed, Hultmark and colleagues *(18)* report the first sequences for a long-type mammalian PGRP that is more closely related to PGRP-LB than it is to the already known short-type mammalian PGRP. It will be exciting to see in the coming years how the functions of this ancient family of pattern recognition proteins have evolved as different lineages have been exposed to different microbial challenges during evolution.

5. TRANSMEMBRANE PATTERN RECOGNITION RECEPTORS

5.1. Drosophila *Class C Scavenger Receptors*

Scavenger receptor (SR) is a functional definition. Each molecule with an ability to bind chemically modified low-density lipoprotein (LDL) is classified as SR, regardless of the structure of the protein. Today, several structurally distinct SR classes are characterized *(19)*. Each class of SR is able to recognize common and unique ligands. For example, the mammalian class A scavenger receptors (SR-As) recognize polyanionic compounds like dextran sulfate, fucoidan, and polyinosinic acid (PolyI) and apoptotic cells in addition to oxidized and acetylated LDL *(20–22)*. The emphasis in SR-related research has been on their proposed role in the pathogenesis of atherosclerosis. However, it has been a longstanding observation that mammalian class A SRs recognize bacterial components [lipopolysaccharides (LPS) and lipoteichoic acid (LTA) in particular] and also both Gram-positive and Gram-negative bacteria *(20–22)*. Furthermore, studies on SR-AI/II-deficient mice indicate that class A SRs protect from *Listeria monocytogenes (24)* and *Staphylococcus aureus (25)* infections.

Drosophila embryonic macrophages and cultured Scheider S2 cells exhibit SR activity *(25),* and subsequently dSR-CI was identified using expression cloning *(26)*. Interestingly, dSR-CI has very similar ligand specificity to mammalian class A SRs (i.e., it recognizes both Gram-positive and Gram-negative bacteria, LTA, polyl, dextran sulfate, and acetylated LDL but not dextran, polycytidylic acid, LDL, or high-density lipoprotein) but bears no structural homology to SR-As *(26,27)*. dSR-CI is a type I integral membrane protein with hemocyte/macrophage-specific expression throughout development. It consists of two complement control protein (CCP) domains, MAM domains, a 48-amino acid somatomedin-like domain, and a 129-residue serine/threonine-rich region *(26)*. dSR-CI is the first member of a small family of proteins in *Drosophila.*

Currently three additional members have been described (shown schematically in Fig.1). dSR-CIII is also a type I integral membrane protein, whereas dSR-CIII and dSR-CIV are predicted to encode secreted proteins. dSR-CII appeared to be expressed only in the embryo, from 2 to 8 hours after egg laying, with no apparent hemocyte expression. dSR-CIII is expressed exclusively during the larval and pupal stages of development. No expression data are currently available for dSR-CI. At present, no data are available on the function of the other dSR-C family members besides dSR-CI.

Recently, dSR-CI was shown to be sufficient to bind both Gram-negative and Gram-positive *bacteria* when expressed in CHO or COS cells. Double-stranded RNA interference-based specific gene silencing of dSR-CI caused an approx 25% decrease in binding/phagocytosis of both *E. coli* and *S. aureus* in an in vitro *Drosophila* cell culture

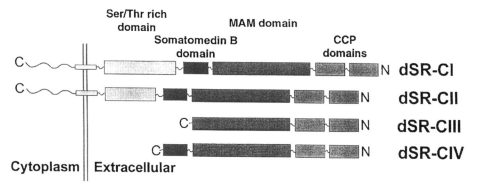

Fig. 1. Schematic representation of class C scavenger receptors (SR-Cs) indicating different domains. MAM, a domain find in *M*eprin, *A*5 antigen and RPTP *M*u. CCP, complement control protein domain.

assay (Rämet et al., unpublished data). Furthermore, extensive polymorphisms have been observed in wild populations of *Drosophila melanogaster and Drosophila simulans* (T. Schlenke and D. Begun, personal communication). This is consistent with dSR-CI playing a role in pattern recognition in host defense, because high-frequency polymorphism would be expected to confer some individual variation in the capacity to recognize pathogens. Although it remains to be determined what role dSR-CI has in phagocytosis in vivo, these results support the view that scavenger receptor bacterial recognition is conserved from insects to humans and may represent the most primitive form of microbial recognition. This suggests that SRs may mediate innate immunity-linked, evolutionarily conserved function.

6. HEMOMUCIN

Mucins are secreted and transmembrane glycoproteins that are heavily O-glycosylated. Membrane-bound mucins are known to have a role in cellular adherence and protection, whereas secreted mucins form a mucus layer that protects the epithelium. Mucins appear to have a role in vertebrate immunity. For example, they are involved in the attachment of leukocytes during an inflammatory response. At least nine different mucins have been described in humans.

Drosophila hemomucin was initially purified biochemically by affinity chromatography using the lectin A *hemagglutinin* from the snail *Helix pomatia* as a ligand *(28)*. Purification resulted in two proteins with molecular masses of 100 and 220 kDa. Based on several identical peptide sequences, these two proteins appear to be encoded by the same gene. The *Drosophila* hemomucin consists of four domains: an amino-terminal hydrophobic domain, a central domain with homology to the plant enzyme strictosidine synthase, a mucin domain, and a carboxyl-terminal domain. The *hemomucin* gene is expressed throughout development. In adults, high expression has been observed in hemocytes, in specific regions in the gut, and in the ovary *(28)*. Hemomucin is speculated to be involved in induction of antimicrobial peptides, but at the moment no direct evidence is available. Similarly, no data exist on whether hemomucin is involved in binding and phagocytosis of specific microbes by *Drosophila* hemocytes.

7. CONCLUSIONS

The last several years have seen the first significant progress toward a molecular understanding of pattern recognition in *Drosophila*. Some of the important pattern recognition molecules have now been identified, and screens in several labs for immunity-related genes may soon identify others. The completion of the *Drosophila* genome project and the development of the RNAi technique may also speed up the discovery of new pattern recognition proteins. It is now important to learn about the molecular consequences of pattern recognition by these proteins. For example, how do secreted recognition proteins activate the prophenoloxidase cascade? How do transmembrane receptors couple to the phagocytic machinery? How do pattern recognition receptors activate the antimicrobial gene response? Although the evolutionary lines leading to *Drosophila* and humans diverged 600 million years ago, the basic mechanisms of innate immunity, such as phagocytosis and the induction of antimicrobial activity, have been well conserved. Thus, although *Drosophila* pattern recognition molecules may differ in detail from those of humans, a better knowledge of these molecules and the mechanisms by which they work should contribute to our understanding of the human immune system.

NOTE IN PROOF

Several recent papers have now established a definitive role for PGRP-SA in the initiative of the *Drosophila* immune response to Gram positive bacteria along the Toll pathway *(29)* and for PGRP-LC in the recognition of Gram negative bacteria and the initiation of the *Drosophila* immune responses to Gram negative bacteria along the IMD pathway *(30–32)*.

REFERENCES

1. Janeway CA Jr. Approaching the asymptote? Evolution and revolution in immunology. Cold Spring Harbor Symp Quant Biol 1989;54:1–13.
2. Medzhitov R, Janeway CA Jr. Innate immunity: the virtues of a nonclonal system of recognition. Cell 1997;91:295–298.
3. Krieg AM. The role of CpG motifs in innate immunity. Curr Opin Immunol 2000;12:35–43.
4. Volanakis JE. Overview of the complement system. In: Volanakis JE, Frank MM (eds.). The Human Complement System in Health and Disease. New York: Marcel Dekker, 1998, pp:9–32.
5. Dodds AW, Law SK. The phylogeny and evolution of the thioester bond-containing proteins C3, C4 and alpha 2-macroglobulin. Immunol Rev 1998;166:15–26.
6. Armstrong PB, Melchior R, Swarnakar S, Quigley JP. α2-macroglobulin does not function as a C3 homologue in the plasma hemolytic system of the American horseshoe crab, *Limulus*. Mol Immunol 1998;35:47–53.
7. Lagueux M, Perrodou E, Levashina EA, Capovilla M, Hoffmann JA. Constitutive expression of a complement-like protein in Toll and JAK gain-of-function mutants of *Drosophila*. Proc Natl Acad Sci USA 2000;97:11427–11432.
8. Dearolf CR. JAKs and STATs in invertebrate model organisms. Cell Mol Life Sci 1999;55:1578–1584.
9. Levashina EA, Moita LF, Blandin S, et al. Conserved role of a complement-like protein in phagocytosis revealed by dsRNA knockout in cultured cells of the mosquito, *Anopheles gambiae*. Cell 2001;104:709–718.
10. Lee WJ, Lee JD, Kravchenko VV, Ulevitch RJ, Brey PT. Purification and molecular cloning of an inducible gram-negative bacteria-binding protein from the silkworm, *Bombyx mori*. Proc Natl Acad Sci USA 1996;93:7888–7893.

11. Kim YS, Ryu JH, Han SJ, et al. Gram-negative bacteria-binding protein, a pattern recognition receptor for lipopolysaccharide and beta-1,3-glucan that mediates the signaling for the induction of innate immune genes in *Drosophila melanogaster* cells. J Biol Chem 2000;275:32721–32727.

12. Dimopoulos G, Richman A, Muller HM, Kafatos FC. Molecular immune responses of the mosquito *Anopheles gambiae* to bacteria and malaria parasites. Proc Natl Acad Sci USA 1997;94:11508–11513.

13. Richman AM, Dimopoulos G, Seeley D, Kafatos FC. Plasmodium activates the innate immune response of *Anopheles gambiae* mosquitoes. EMBO J 1997;16:6114–6119.

14. Yoshida H, Kinoshita K, Ashida M. Purification of a peptidoglycan recognition protein from hemolymph of the silkworm, *Bombyx mori.* J Biol Chem 1996;271:13854–13860.

15. Ochiai M, Ashida M. A pattern recognition protein for peptidoglycan. Cloning the cDNA and the gene of the silkworm, *Bombyx mori.* J Biol Chem 1999;274:11854–11858.

16. Kang D, Liu G, Lundstrom A, Gelius E, Steiner H.A peptidoglycan recognition protein in innate immunity conserved from insects to humans. Proc Natl Acad Sci USA 1998;95:10078–10082.

17. Liu C, Gelius E, Liu G, Steiner H, Dziarski R. Mammalian peptidoglycan recognition protein binds peptidoglycan with high affinity, is expressed in neutrophils, and inhibits bacterial growth. J Biol Chem 2000;275:24490–24499.

18. Werner T, Liu G, Kang D, et al. A family of peptidoglycan recognition proteins in the fruit fly *Drosophila melanogaster.* Proc Natl Acad Sci USA 2000;97:13772–13777.

19. Gough PJ, Gordon S. The role of scavenger receptors in the innate immune system. Microbes Infect 2000;2:305–311.

20. Hampton RY, Golenbock DT, Penman M, Krieger M, Raetz CR. Recognition and plasma clearance of endotoxin by scavenger receptors. Nature 1991;352:342–344.

21. Ashkenas J, Penman M, Vasile E, Acton S, Freeman M, Krieger M. Structures and high and low affinity ligand binding properties of murine type I and type II macrophage scavenger receptors. J Lipid Res 1993;34:983–1000.

22. Dunne DW, Resnick D, Greenberg J, Krieger M, Joiner KA. The type 1 macrophage scavenger receptor binds to gram-positive bacteria and recognizes lipoteichoic acid. Proc Natl Acad Sci USA 1994;91:1863–1867.

23. Suzuki H, Kurihara Y, Takeya M, et al. A role for macrophage scavenger receptors in atherosclerosis and susceptibility to infection. Nature 1997;386:292–296.

24. Thomas C, Li Y, Kodoma T, et al. Protection from lethal Gram-positive infection by macrophage scavenger receptor-dependent phagocytosis. J Exp Med 2000;191:147–155.

25. Abrams JM, Lux A, Steller H, Krieger M. Macrophages in *Drosophila* embryos and L2 cells exhibit scavenger receptor-mediated endocytosis. Proc Natl Acad Sci USA 1992;89:10375–10379.

26. Pearson A, Lux A, Krieger M. Expression cloning of dSR-CI, a class C macrophage-specific scavenger receptor from *Drosophila melanogaster.* Proc Natl Acad Sci USA 1995;92:4056–4060.

27. Ramet M, Pearson A, Manfruelli P, et al. *Drosophila* scavenger receptor C1 is a pattern recognition receptor for bacteria. Immunity 2001;15:1027–1038.

28. Theopold U, Samakovlis C, Erdjument-Bromage et al. *Helix pomatia* lectin, an inducer of *Drosophila* immune response, binds to hemomucin, a novel surface mucin. J Biol Chem 1996;271:12708–12715.

29. Michel T, Reichhart JM, Hoffmann JA, Royet J. *Drosophila* Toll is activated by Gram-positive bacteria through a circulating peptidoglycan recognition protein. Nature 2001;414:756–759.

30. Ramet M, Manfruelli P, Pearson A, Mathey-Prevot B, Ezekowitz RA. Functional genomic analysis of phagocytosis and identification of a *Drosophila* receptor for *E. coli.* Nature 2002;416:644–648.

31. Gottar M, Gobert V, Michel T, et al. The *Drosophila* immune response against Gram-negative bacteria is mediated by a peptidoglycan recognition protein. Nature 2002;416:640–644.

32. Choe KM, Werner T, Stoven S, Hultmark D, Anderson KV. Requirement for a peptidoglycan recognition protein (PGRP) in Relish activation and antibacterial immune responses in *Drosophila.* Science 2002;296:359–362.

8

Humoral and Cellular Responses in *Drosophila* Innate Immunity

Julien Royet, Marie Meister, and Dominique Ferrandon

1. INTRODUCTION

The immune system of invertebrates has been the object of intense scrutiny ever since Elie Metchnikoff first discovered phagocytosis in starfish embryos in 1884 *(1)*. Not surprisingly, the cellular arm of the insect innate immune response was the first to be investigated at the turn of the 20th century. Glaser and Paillot, followed later on by Metalnikow, uncovered the existence of a humoral arm of the insect host defense *(2–5)*. However, the nature of the antimicrobial activity found in the hemolymph of immunized insects was not determined until the early 1980s, when Hans Boman's pioneering work led to the purification in the moth *Hyalophora cecropia* of small cationic peptides that were called cecropins *(6)*. Hundreds of peptides with antimicrobial activities were subsequently identified and characterized from insects of most orders (reviewed in ref. *7)*. Understanding the mechanisms responsible for their production is a major goal of recent research in innate immunity. For the last 10 years, *Drosophila* has been one major model system successfully used to dissect the molecular cascades controlling innate immunity in invertebrates. We describe here the current knowledge of the humoral and cellular arms of *Drosophila* immunity and highlight the similarities and disparities with the mammalian immune system.

2. HUMORAL IMMUNITY

A septic injury triggers a series of reactions that take place in the hemolymph. These include the activation of several protease cascades that lead to various defense phenomena such as melanization, coagulation, opsonization, or the synthesis of antimicrobial peptides. In this section, we limit ourselves to a description of the systemic antimicrobial response that is the hallmark of the humoral response in *Drosophila,* with concentrations of antimicrobial peptides in the hemolymph reaching overall values as high as 0.3 mM 24 hours after a septic injury (P. Bulet, personal communication). We discuss melanization in the section on cellular immunity, since the key enzyme of this cascade is secreted by a specific cell type found circulating in the hemolymph.

From: *Infectious Disease: Innate Immunity*
Edited by: R. A. B. Ezekowitz and J. A. Hoffmann © Humana Press Inc., Totowa, NJ

2.1. Drosophila *Antimicrobial Peptides*

In *Drosophila,* seven different families of antimicrobial peptides have been characterized molecularly or biochemically (*see* Chap. 5). These peptides are synthesized by the fat body, a tissue functionally equivalent to the liver of vertebrates. In contrast to mammalian antimicrobial peptides, *Drosophila* peptides induced during the immune response are active against a more restricted range of microorganisms. According to their main microbial targets, they can be divided into three groups: antifungal peptides, which include Drosomycin and Metchnikowin, peptides active against Gram-negative bacteria such as Diptericin, Attacins, Cecropins, and Drosocin, and peptides active against Gram-positive bacteria such as Defensin. Interestingly, it seems that the type of antimicrobial peptides produced by *Drosophila* is adapted, to some degree, to the nature of the invading microorganism *(8)*. For example, fungi and Gram-positive bacteria are better elicitors of *Drosomycin* expression than Gram-negative bacteria. In contrast, infection by Gram-negative bacteria induces preferentially the expression of the *Diptericin, Attacin, Cecropin,* and *Drosocin* genes. The specificity of the humoral host defense is well illustrated by the response occurring when flies are coated with spores of the entomopathogenous fungus *Beauveria bassiana.* Under these conditions, which mimic a natural infection, the antifungal, but not the antibacterial, peptide genes are induced *(8)*. The existence of distinct antimicrobial responses to various microorganisms suggests that the expression of the antimicrobial peptides is regulated via several pathways. The unraveling of these regulatory pathways is described below.

2.2. *Antimicrobial Peptide Gene Trancription Is Regulated by Rel Proteins*

Analysis of the promoters of antimicrobial peptide genes revealed the existence of relatively well conserved sequences that are reminiscent of κB binding sites for the vertebrate NF-κB factor, reviewed in Engström *(9)*. In the case of *Cecropin* and *Diptericin,* these sites were shown to be necessary and sufficient for one of the most important properties of the *Drosophila* immune response, its inducibility *(10–12)*. In vertebrates, κB sites are recognized by dimers of molecules of the Rel family of transcription factors such as NF-κB. This transcription factor plays a central role in the response to stress, most notably in inflammation *(13–15)*. NF-κB is already present in the cytoplasm but is prevented from moving to the nucleus by I-κB. Structurally, Rel family members are characterized by the presence of an N-terminal Rel DNA binding domain that also contains elements necessary for binding the ankyrin repeats of I-κB. When upstream signaling pathways are activated, a receptor-adaptor complex is formed and activates through phosphorylation an I-κB kinase (IKK) complex that targets I-κB for degradation by the proteasome. Consequently, NF-κB is free to move to the nucleus, where it regulates its target genes. Thus, the cardinal principle of NF-κB regulation resides in the control of the subcellular localization of this transcription factor. The major advantage of this system is that it allows for a response occurring within minutes of the stimulus since all components are already present in the responding cell. This property may be central to the evolutionary success of this signal transduction pathway that is used in different processes in the animal kingdom.

The first known member of the *Drosophila* Rel protein family, Dorsal, was isolated because of its role in the establishment of the embryonic dorsoventral polarity

(16). Further genetic screens led to the molecular characterization of multiple genes, which all belong to the same signaling pathway, named after one of the components, the transmembrane receptor Toll *(17,18)*. Activation of the Toll receptor by its putative ligand Spätzle in the ventral cells of the embryo triggers an intracellular transduction cascade that ultimately frees Dorsal from Cactus and allows its nuclear translocation. Interestingly, cactus is an ankyrin motif containing protein of the I-κB family. Loss of function mutants for *spätzle, Toll,* or *dorsal* generate embryos lacking ventral structures (dorsalized phenotype). In contrast, *cactus* mutants display a ventralized phenotype.

The *Toll* signaling pathway was, at that time, the only molecular cascade known to activate target genes through a Rel transcription factor. The effect of *Toll* pathway mutants was thus tested on *Drosophila* antimicrobial peptide inducibility *(19)*. Mutants of the *Toll* pathway were shown to be unable to express *Drosomycin* after fungal infection. Further experiments indicated that the *Toll* pathway components are necessary not only for the production of antimicrobial peptides in response to fungi, but also to Gram-positive bacteria. Interestingly, induction of the antibacterial peptide Diptericin by Gram-negative bacteria was unaffected in such mutants. In addition, flies carrying mutations in genes of the *Toll* pathway are highly susceptible to infection by Gram-positive bacteria or fungi but are as resistant as wild-type flies to infection by Gram-negative bacteria *(19–22)*. Thus, genes initially isolated for their developmental role proved to be key members of the pathway that controls the response to fungi and Gram-positive bacteria in *Drosophila*.

However, very surprisingly, flies lacking functional Dorsal protein are able to mount a normal immune response to bacterial and fungal infections *(19,23)*. Several laboratories thus investigated the putative role of two other *Drosophila* Rel proteins, Dorsal-related immune factor (DIF) and Relish in immunity *(24,25)*. When *Dif* mutant flies are challenged with fungal spores or Gram-positive bacteria, both the inducibility of *Drosomycin* and survival are strongly reduced compared with wild-type flies *(21,22)*. In addition, *cactus-Dif* double mutants present the *Dif* phenotype, suggesting that DIF is retained in the cytoplasm by Cactus. These results indicate that the DIF-Cactus complex is the downstream effector of the *Toll* pathway in adult host defense, whereas a dorsal-Cactus complex is used during embryonic development *(21,26,27)*.

The phenotype of *relish* mutants mirrors that of *Dif* mutants *(28)*. Although the response to Gram-positive bacteria and fungi is unaffected in *relish* mutants, the inducibility of the antibacterial peptide genes *Diptericin* or *Attacin* by Gram-negative bacteria is totally abolished. Flies carrying a *relish* mutation are highly susceptible to infection by Gram-negative bacteria but are as resistant as wild-type flies to Gram-positive bacterial and fungal infections. These phenotypes are reminiscent of that of the previously characterized *immune deficiency (imd)* mutation. The *imd* mutant was found serendipitously while investigating the potential role of a gene involved in melanization reactions *(29)*. It is historically the founding member of the Gram-negative antibacterial pathway.

In conclusion, the analysis of existing mutations allowed the delineation of at least two pathways, the *Toll* pathway, controlling the immunity against Gram-positive bacteria and fungi, and the *imd* pathway, regulating the host response to Gram-negative bacteria. Both pathways are variations on the theme of NF-κB regulation with receptors

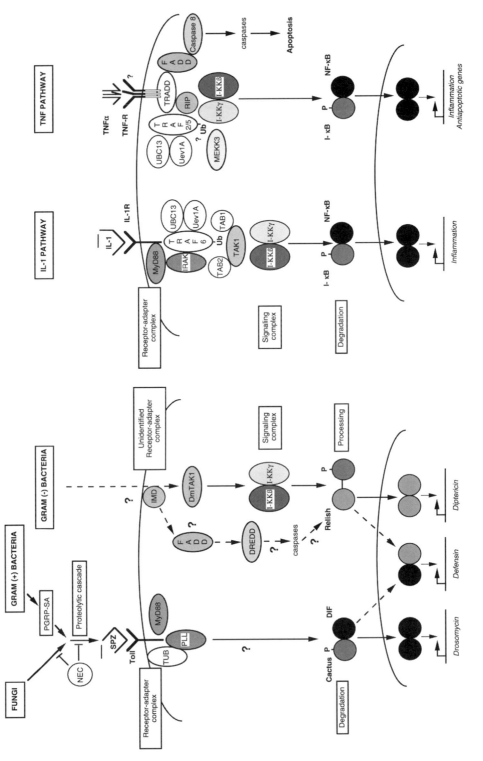

Fig. 1. Signal transduction pathways in innate immunity. The drawings present in a simplified form our knowledge of the signal transduction pathways used in the control of the *Drosophila* systemic antimicrobial response **(left)** and two of the numerous pathways of NF-κB activation found in mammals **(right)**. Genes belonging to the same family in the two phyla are shown with the same shade. Whereas the *Toll* and *imd* pathways are distinct in the fat body cell, in mammals both the IL-1 and the TNF pathways converge on the activation of the transcription factor NF-κB, a complex formed by the heterodimerization of two Rel subunits, *e.g.,* p50 and p65. In *Drosophila,* DIF and Relish may heterodimerize to control the transcription of some antimicrobial genes such as *Defensin, Cecropin,* and *Attacin,* since their expression is altered in either *Toll* or *imd* pathway mutants. The induction of apoptosis as shown in this scheme has actually been described in fibroblasts. In lymphocytes, RIP may also intervene in this apoptotic pathway *(73)*. *Abbreviations:* NEC, necrotic; SPZ, spätzle; MyD88, myeloid differentiation factor 88; TUB, Tube; PLL, Pelle; DIF, Dorsal-related immunity factor; IMD, immune deficiency; TAK1, transforming growth factor-β-activated kinase 1; I-KK, I-κB kinase; DmIKKβ, IRD5; DmIKKγ, Kenny; IL-1, interleukin-1; IL1-R, IL-1 receptor; IRAK, IL-1 receptor-associated kinase; TNF, tumor necrosis factor; TRADD, TNF receptor-associated death domain protein; TRAF6, TNF receptor-associated factor 6; MEKK3, mitogen-activated protein kinase/ERK kinase kinase 3; TAB2, TAK1 binding protein 2; UBC13, ubiquitin-conjugating enzyme 13; Uev1A, ubiquitin-conjugating E2 enzyme variant A; Ub, polyubiquitin chain crosslinked through Lys-63 of ubiquitin. TUB, PLL, MyD88, IMD, RIP, TRADD, and FADD proteins contain a death domain. MEKK3 and TAK1 are both MAPkinase kinase kinases.

triggering an intracellular transduction pathway that ultimately controls the nuclear uptake of *Drosophila* Rel family members (Fig. 1).

2.3. Control of Relish and DIF Nuclear Uptake

In contrast to Dorsal and DIF, Relish is a bipartite protein that contains both an N-terminal Rel DNA binding domain and six ankyrin repeats in its C-terminal half that supposedly maintain the protein in the cytoplasm. A similar arrangement is found in the vertebrate NF-κB precursors p105 and p100, which are processed by the proteasome to generate respectively the NF-κB subunits p50 and p52. Following activation of the *imd* pathway, Relish is rapidly cleaved, thus releasing two fragments *(30)*. The C-terminal domain that contains the ankyrin repeats remains in the cytoplasm, whereas the N-terminal Rel domain moves to the nucleus. The protease that cleaves Relish has not yet been formally identified. The Death-related ced-3/Nedd2-like (DREDD) caspase appears to play a key role in the process since Relish is no longer cleaved in the mutant *(30)* and since antibacterial peptides are no longer induced in *dredd* mutant flies *(31,32)*. However, biochemical and genetic data suggest that this apical caspase does not cleave Relish directly *(15,33)*. A possibility is that it triggers an executioner caspase that would cleave the protein since Relish processing is sensitive to caspase inhibitors *(15)*.

In mammals, p100 is partially processed in B-cells by the proteasome in a ubiquitin-dependent mechanism to yield the Rel protein p52. The available evidence points to a direct role of IKKα, which phosphorylates p100 in vitro, a post-translational modification that is likely to lead to its ubiquitination in vivo (*see* ref. *34* and references therein). In *Drosophila,* biochemical experiments have demonstrated that a complex composed of the IKKβ and IKKγ fly homologs is able to phosphorylate Relish and thus may target it for proteolytic cleavage *(35)*. Furthermore, the phenotypes of mutants affecting the two components of the *Drosophila* IKK signaling complex, *ird5* for IKKβ and *kenny* for IKKγ, are as severe as that of *relish (36,37)*. Gel retardation experiments performed with a *Diptericin* κB probe allowed the identification of a complex bound to that promoter fragment only in extracts from immune-challenged flies *(11)*. In *kenny* and in *relish* mutant extracts, the complex that binds to one of the *Diptericin* κB promoter fragments can no longer be observed. These experiments suggest that DmIKKγ is required for the processing/activation of relish *(36)*.

Even though the processing of mammalian p100 induced by IKKα may at first appear to have been conserved during evolution, namely, it is homologous to the proteolytic cleavage of Relish initiated by the *Drosophila* IKK signaling complex, one should point out that (1) Relish family members in the invertebrates and NF-κB precursors p105 and p100 in vertebrates originated after the separation between protostomes and deuterostomes *(25,38)*; (2) the *Drosophila* IKK kinase IRD5 appears to form an evolutionary subfamily of IKK kinases on its own *(15)*; and (3) p100 processing is proteasome-dependent, whereas Relish cleavage is not *(30,34)*. Thus, these two processes of transcription factor maturation may represent an example of convergent evolution at the molecular level.

In mammals, the IKK signaling complex phosphorylates I-κB on specific residues and thus targets it for proteasome-mediated degradation. Cactus is also phosphorylated in response to Toll signaling (*see* ref. *39* and references therein). However, the only known IKK signaling complex in *Drosophila,* even though it can phosphorylate Cactus *in vitro*, is not required physiologically in the *Toll* pathway since the response to Grampositive bacteria and fungi is normal in *kenny* and *ird5* mutants flies *(35–37,40)*. IK2, the only other kinase that presents some similarity to a mammalian IKK, has not been investigated so far. In addition, no gene obviously similar to *kenny* could be found in the fly genome. Thus, the nature of the Cactus kinase remains a mystery, during both early embryogenesis and the innate immune response. A second, functionally redundant kinase might replace DmIKKβ/IRD5 in phosphorylating cactus in *ird5* mutants *(37)*.

2.4. Upstream of the Signaling Complex in the imd Pathway

In mammals, the biochemical events that trigger the activation of the IKK signaling complex through phosphorylation of IKKβ have been deciphered (reviewed in ref. *15*). IKK is phosphorylated directly by the mitogen-activated protein (MAP) kinase transforming growth factor-activated kinase 1 (TAK1) *(41,42)*. TAK1, when bound to the TAK1 binding protein 1 (TAB 1) and TAB 2 proteins, is activated by an adapter protein called tumor necrosis factor receptor-activated factor 6 (TRAF6) in the interleukin-1 (IL-1) response pathway, only when TRAF6 has undergone a specific signal-dependent LYS63 polyubiquitination *(41,42)*. This reaction is catalyzed by the ubiquitin-conjugating enzyme (UBC) -13 and ubiquitin-conjugating E2 enzyme variant A (UEV1A). TRAF contains a RING finger, a domain thought to act in an ubiquitin ligase complex. In *Drosophila*, mutants have been isolated in the homolog of TAK1 *(43)*. The phenotype of the mutants as well as genetic epistatic analysis places it unambiguously in the *imd* pathway. Thus, DmTAK1 is a prime candidate for a fly IKK kinase. The analysis of the genome fails to reveal any obvious homolog of TAB1 and TAB2. However, there are some indications that the fly UBC13 and Uev1A may play a role in the control of *Diptericin* inducibility, at least in cell culture *(15)*. This result, however, awaits the identification of mutations in the cognate genes.

The most upstream component of the *imd* pathway identified so far is *imd* itself. It encodes a protein that contains a C-terminal death domain most similar to that of the receptor-interacting protein (RIP) of vertebrates *(33)*. RIP plays a crucial role in the activation of NF-κB by the tumor necrosis factor-α receptor (TNF-αR) and is part of the TNF-α receptor complex *(44)*. However, unlike its mammalian counterpart, IMD does not contain a kinase domain, which has been shown to be dispensable for TNF-α signaling. Overexpression of *imd* leads to the constitutive expression of antibacterial peptide genes in the absence of immune challenge, and this effect is blocked by mutations in the *dredd* or *kenny* genes *(33)*. Furthermore, *DmTAK1* has been shown genetically not to be upstream of *imd* and, by reference to the mammalian findings of direct activation of IKKβ by TAK1, the simplest hypothesis is that it acts downstream of *imd*. It should be noted that a direct interaction between RIP and IKKγ has been reported in the mammalian system in the context of the TNF-α receptor signaling complex *(45)*.

2.5. Upstream of the DIF-Cactus Complex in the Toll Pathway

Genetic epistasis experiments in the embryo placed the Pelle kinase and tube adaptor proteins between the Toll receptor and the NF-κB/I-κB complex *(18)*. Pelle and Tube form a heterodimer through interactions between their death domains *(46)*. *tube* was genetically shown to act upstream of *pelle,* a gene homologous to the mammalian IL-1 receptor-associated kinase (IRAK) gene *(47,48)*. Tube and Pelle are recruited to the membrane following Toll activation *(49)*. It is thus likely that Tube plays the role of an adapter between Toll and Pelle in the antifungal response pathway, a role held by the Myeloid Differentiation factor 88 (MyD88) protein in the mammalian IL-1 response pathway. A *Drosophila* MyD88 homolog is present in the genome and appears to be a component of the *Toll* pathway in the antifungal response *(50,51)*. The signaling events occurring downstream of the Tube-Pelle interaction are not understood.

2.6. Activation of the Toll Pathway

In embryonic dorsoventral patterning, Toll is activated by Spätzle, a secreted protein of the cystine-knot family of growth factors, which requires a processing step by proteolytic cleavage to become an active ligand. Spätzle proteolytic maturation in the extraembryonic fluid depends on the previous activation of a number of serine proteases including Easter and Snake *(52,53)*. Although mutations in *easter* and *snake* have dramatic effects on dorsoventral embryonic axis specification, they do not affect the *Toll*-dependent response to bacteria, indicating that a different cascade(s) is likely to be involved in the activation of Toll during the *Drosophila* immune response *(19)*. Indeed, mutations in the *necrotic (nec)* gene, which encodes a serine protease inhibitor, led to a *spätzle*-and *Toll*-dependent constitutive expression of *Drosomycin* but did not affect dorsoventral patterning *(54)*. The nature of the protease(s) involved in the activation of Spätzle during the immune response is not known.

These results indicate that the pathogen recognition step triggering the *Toll* pathway is an upstream event that may occur either in the fly hemolymph or locally in epithelia or blood cells. This situation contrasts with that of mammalian Toll-like receptors (TLRs) which are also involved in regulating innate immunity (reviewed in ref. *55*). TLR4 was shown to play a key role in the response to endotoxin, whereas TLR2 is required to mediate NF-κB activation following a bacterial Gram-positive challenge *(56,57)*. TLR3, TLR5, and TLR9 respectively mediate the response to viral double-stranded RNA, bacterial flagellin, and nonmethylated CpG bacterial DNA *(58–60)*. Several TLRs have been shown to be closely associated with microbial components such as lipopolysaccharide (LPS) of Gram-negative bacteria (TLR4) and may therefore be *bona fide* pattern recognition receptors (PRRs) *(61–64)*. PRRs were predicted by C. Janeway in a seminal paper published a decade ago *(65)*. They were postulated to have been selected during evolution for their ability to recognize relatively invariant patterns carried by microorganisms, for instance, LPS, double-stranded RNA, flagellin, ... These receptors inform the host of the presence of an infection and both activate and orient the adaptive arm of the immune system in higher vertebrates *(66)*.

If *Drosophila* Toll does not act as a PRR for Gram-positive bacteria or fungi, what then is the link between the detection of microorganisms and the maturation of Spätzle? Completion of the *Drosophila* sequence has led to the identification of numerous putative PRRs *(67)*. For example, the fly genome contains at least 12 predicted peptidoglycan recognition proteins (PGRPs), some of which are able to bind peptidoglycan, a major constituent of the Gram-positive bacterial cell wall *(68)*. We have recently generated a null mutation in one of the *Drosophila* PGRP genes *(20)*. Flies carrying a mutation in the *PGRP-SA* gene are highly susceptible to infection by Gram-positive bacteria but resist normally to natural infection with *Beauveria bassiana*. Interestingly, *Drosomycin* is induced by fungi but not by Gram-positive bacteria in this mutant background. These results provide the first *in vivo* functional evidence for a role of PRR in invertebrate immunity. They also point to the existence of distinct recognition systems for fungi and Gram-positive bacteria to activate the Toll pathway.

2.7. Activation of the imd Pathway

As opposed to the *Toll* pathway, the fat body cell receptor that triggers the *imd* pathway has not yet been identified. Bearing in mind the function of mammalian TLRs, it was tempting to propose that another member of the *Drosophila* Toll family could be this long-sought receptor. This family is composed of 10 members, *Toll1, 18-wheeler,* and *Toll3* to *Toll9*. It was reported that *Attacin* inducibility is reduced in *18-wheeler* mutant larvae, suggesting that 18-wheeler could be the *imd* pathway receptor *(69)*. However, adult *18-wheeler* mutants obtained using a new genetic combination are as resistant as wild-type flies to bacterial and fungal infections *(69a)*. It is likely that the effect described in the literature is nonspecific and caused by a maturation defect of the mutant larval fat body. Furthermore, chimeras allowing the formation of constitutively active receptors failed to reveal a role in the control of antibacterial gene expression for any of the *Drosophila* Tolls *(70)*.

What could then be the receptor(s)? A related question is that of the ligand(s) of this putative receptor(s). Does the detection of microorganisms take place directly on fat body cells through PRRs or is there, as in the *Toll* pathway, a cytokine-like signaling event? A protein that binds to Gram-negative bacteria (GNBP) was purified from extracts of the silkworm *Bombyx mori (71)*. In *Drosophila*, three members of the GNBP family have been described, and it was shown that one of them at least is a glycosyl phosphatidyl inositol (GPI)-anchored protein *(72)*. Since these proteins are secreted or anchored to the membrane, they have no way to transmit a signal directly through the membrane and are therefore at best co-receptors of Gram-negative bacteria, a condition reminiscent of the vertebrate LPS binding protein CD14. The identity of the receptor itself might be inferred from the identity of the adapter proteins that have been discovered so far, namely, IMD, a protein containing a death domain homologous to that of RIP, and DREDD, an initiator caspase. TNF-α signaling plays a role in mammalian inflammatory response through the RIP-dependent activation of NF-κB and is also involved in triggering apoptosis in lymphocytes *(73)*. RIP is however, not required in the IL-1 and endotoxin pathways.

Interestingly, overexpression of *imd* in flies induces apoptosis and the constitutive expression of antibacterial peptides in a *kenny* and *dredd*-dependent manner *(33)*. Both *imd* and *dredd* mutant pupae are more resistant than the wild type to ultraviolet irradiation, a treatment known to induce apoptosis. These experiments suggest that the *imd* pathway may be involved in triggering apoptosis in response to ultraviolet radiation. Finally, DREDD presents sequence similarity to mammalian caspases 8 and 10 and has been reported to bind to Fas-associated protein with death domain (FADD) *(74,75)*. Interestingly, TNF-α triggers apoptosis through FADD and caspase 8 in mammalian cells (Fig. 1). These phenotypes raise the possibility that *imd* may be involved in a TNF-α-like signaling pathway and that a TNF-α-like receptor could be upstream of the pathway.

In conclusion, the *Toll* and the *imd* pathways present striking similarities to vertebrate IL-1 and TNF-α pathways, respectively. However, for the time being none of them appears to be truly homologous to one single activation pathway. It is more likely that (like the multiple mammalian NF-κB activation pathways) they represent evolutionary invertebrate variations on a theme that was present in the last common ancestors of protostomes and deuterostomes.

3. CELLULAR IMMUNITY

Insect blood cells or hemocytes play an important role in host defense; however, the molecular mechanisms that underlie these aspects have hardly been investigated. Blood cell types in the various insect orders seem at first glance to be highly heterogeneous, but one can distinguish, in all species investigated, at least two conserved types *(76,77)*. A first cell type is responsible for phagocytosis. Such cells, called plasmatocytes in *Drosophila,* share morphologic and functional similarities with the mammalian monocyte/macrophage lineage. The second cell type, morphologically more variable among insect species, is characterized by the presence in the cytoplasm of abundant granules. Granule-packed blood cells were extensively analyzed in a related arthropod species, the horseshoe crab. Among a number of defense-related molecules, horseshoe crab granules contain high amounts of anti-microbial peptides (reviewed in ref. *78)*. These "granulocytes" are thus remotely reminiscent of mammalian neutrophils; they are, however, absent in higher Dipterans, namely, in *Drosophila.*

Drosophila hemocytes are responsible for phagocytosis. This involves the disposal of microorganisms, but also of apoptotic cells during embryogenesis and metamorphosis. In addition, hemocytes play several other roles that are predominantly related to defense reactions: humoral melanization, encapsulation, and production of opsonins,

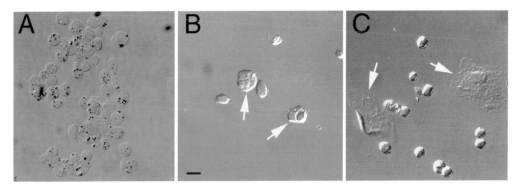

Fig. 2. Phase photomicrographs of *Drosophila* hemocytes. (**A**) Phagocytosis of India ink particles by plasmatocytes. (**B**) Two crystal cells (arrows) with conspicuous crystalline inclusions. (**C**) Two lamellocytes (arrows) and plasmatocytes. Scale bar = 10 μm.

signaling molecules, and antimicrobial peptides. These various aspects are reviewed below after a short description of blood cell types in this model (Fig. 2).

3.1. Blood Cells in Drosophila

In *Drosophila* larvae, three cell types (or hemocytes) are found in the circulation *(79,80)*. Most of them are plasmatocytes with a strong phagocytic capacity, and less than 5% are crystal cells. The latter contain large non-membrane-bound crystals within their cytoplasm; they are responsible for immune-related humoral melanization. The third cell population consists of a low percentage of small, undifferentiated prohemocytes.

An additional cell type, seldom present in healthy larvae, can differentiate under specific immune circumstances. The lamellocyte is a large flattened cell with few conspicuous cytoplasmic organelles and is specifically devoted to encapsulation *(79)*. Encapsulation is activated when an invader is too large to be phagocytosed by plasmatocytes. In association with melanization, it ensures the killing of the invader, which in the wild is frequently a parasitoid wasp egg (see below).

3.2. Hemocyte Functions

To establish the functional relevance of hemocytes during immune defense in *Drosophila*, two independent studies have used specific means to suppress their activity. Braun and coworkers *(81)* analyzed the survival of mutant larvae following bacteria injection. The mutants were *domino* larvae in which hemocytes fail to proliferate, *imd* larvae that do not produce antibacterial peptides, and *Black cell (Bc)*, larvae with no humoral melanization *(82)*. Larvae devoid of hemocytes, like *imd* or *Bc*, survived as efficiently as wild-type larvae under the challenge. However, if the absence of hemocytes was combined with absence of antibacterial peptides (*domino imd* double mutants) or absence of melanization (*domino Bc* double mutants), larvae became highly susceptible to bacterial infection. In keeping with these results, when the phagocytic function of adult hemocytes was saturated by injection of polystyrene beads into the abdomen, the susceptibility of *imd* pathway mutants to *E. coli* was significantly increased *(32)*. These experiments demonstrate that blood cells play an important role in *Drosophila* host defense, as they synergize with other immune effectors to provide full efficiency to the system.

3.3. Phagocytosis

Phagocytosis occurs in several steps, the first of which involves the binding of molecules carried by the target to specific receptors on blood cells. This triggers a signaling pathway leading to engulfment of phagocytosed material in phagosomes. It is eventually destroyed by lysosomal enzymes, reactive oxygen species, and nitric oxide. The main steps in phagocytosis are specific recognition, signal transduction, actin remodeling, and microtubule-dependent vesicle trafficking.

The primary step involves the existence of nonself receptors, which are discussed in Chapter 7. However, receptors for pathogens may not recognize the pathogen directly, but molecules that have been deposited by the host onto the microorganism, a process known as opsonization. Opsonins have occasionally been reported in insects, and recently four genes encoding proteins that have significant similarities with the thiolester-containing proteins of the complement C3/α_2-macroglobulin superfamily were found in the *Drosophila* genome *(83)*. The *Anopheles* homolog was shown to serve as a complement-like opsonin and to promote phagocytosis of Gram-negative bacteria *(84)*. Downstream of the recognition process, the engulfment mechanisms have so far not been investigated in *Drosophila,* but insights should be gained in the near future, as genetic screening is currently under way in several laboratories to identify phagocytosis mutants.

3.4. Encapsulation

Capsule formation occurs in *Drosophila* larvae in two circumstances: around eggs laid by endoparasitoid wasp species, or around melanotic tumors *(85,86)*. Both processes include surrounding of the invader/tumor by hemocytes (mainly lamellocytes) accompanied by blackening and hardening of the developing capsule through melanization.

When a parasitoid wasp lays an egg in a young nonpermissive larva, the egg is neutralized by the following sequence of events. It is initially recognized as nonself by plasmatocytes that are responsible for immune surveillance. They rapidly attach to the chorion of the wasp egg *(87)*. A few hours later, lamellocytes appear in the circulation as they massively differentiate in the hematopoietic organ *(88)*. They wrap around the invader as a multilayered capsule, cells eventually flatten, and all the surrounding layers undergo progressive blackening. The association of wrapping and melanization ensures efficient killing of the parasite, possibly by the local production of cytotoxic free radicals, quinones, or semiquinones, or by asphyxiation *(89,90)*.

Melanotic tumors or "pseudotumors" are often encountered in mutant fly stocks. They are not true tumors but rather noninvasive "autoimmune" reactions. It has been proposed that they correspond to the reaction of hemocytes against effete tissue fragments or that they result from dysregulated attack of blood cells against normal self *(91)*.

Encapsulation has been compared with granuloma formation in vertebrates; however, the molecular mechanisms that lead from recognition of the invader/effete self to capsule formation in *Drosophila* are not yet understood.

3.5. Melanization

Defense-related melanization produces black pigment as a result of the activation of a biochemical pathway that converts tyrosine to melanin (reviewed in refs. *92* and *93*). The key enzyme in the process is a phenoloxidase (PO) that catalyzes the oxidation of phenols to quinones, which then polymerize nonenzymatically to form melanin. Insect

POs are normally present in the circulation as zymogens, called prophenoloxidases (proPOs). It was shown in lepidopteran species that proPOs are activated by a serine protease cascade that is triggered by initial recognition of nonself molecular patterns such as β-1,3-glucans, peptidoglycan, LPS, or effete self. The identity of the components of this cascade are so far unknown; thus, an overlap with cascades upstream of the *Toll* or *imd* pathways cannot be excluded. Activated PO shows a tendency to associate and to form aggregates, which allows a tight control of the localization of melanization within the organism. This is essential, as a number of intermediate compounds formed during melanin synthesis are cytotoxic. Blood cells play a preponderant role in melanization. *Drosophila* proPOs are expressed specifically in crystal cells (M. Meister unpublished data), which, once activated, readily disrupt and deliver their content into the hemolymph, where the enzymes can function *(79)*.

Melanin that rapidly accumulates at wound sites in insects has been proposed to participate to the sealing of the wound, thus preceding the more elaborate wound healing process that takes several days *(94)*. In *Drosophila,* several mutations are known to affect melanization. Among them, two provoke a total suppression of humoral melanization: *lozenge (lz)* and *Bc (82,95)*. Strong *lz* mutations compromise the differentiation of crystal cells, whereas *Bc* results in death and blackening of differentiating crystal cells. Both *lz* and *Bc* mutants share the same phenotype of an absence of black spot formation at wound sites. They also fail to seal the wound and exhibit low survival to benign injury (T. Lebestky, personal communication) *(96)*. This indicates either that melanization ensures coagulation in *Drosophila* or that crystal cells are key players in a process parallel to melanization that leads to coagulation. In the horseshoe crab, the coagulation cascade has been totally elucidated and clearly triggers clotting via effectors that are not those of melanization, although both reactions may share components (reviewed in ref. *78*). Interestingly, some components of the melanization protease cascade are closely related to the proteases that activate Spätzle during *Drosophila* development. Furthermore, coagulogen, the target of the clotting cascade in *Limulus,* has a C-terminal half that belongs structurally to the cystine knot domain family, like Spätzle (*see* ref. *78* and references therein). It will thus be challenging to understand how melanization and coagulation are activated in *Drosophila,* to determine how closely they are related, and to identify the proteolytic cascades that are involved in these processes.

3.6. Communication with Other Immune-Competent Tissues

Last but not least, *Drosophila* hemocytes were clearly shown to produce signals that carry information to other tissues. In the case of wasp parasitization, the plasmatocytes are the primary cells that recognize the intruder and form a layer around its chorion. Hours later, lamellocytes are produced at a distance within the hematopoietic organ. It is therefore likely that the activated plasmatocytes send a differentiation signal to the latter.

An interesting set of experiments performed by B. Lemaitre and collaborators *(97)* suggests that under specific conditions the activation of the humoral immune response may also rely on communications between hemocytes and fat body cells. They used a natural infection system with the phytopathogenic bacteria *Erwinia carotovora.* Such an infection specifically induces and *imd* pathway-dependent antimicrobial peptide production in the fat body *(43,97)*. However, in *domino* or *l(3)hem* mutant larvae, which are characterized by a severely reduced hemocyte pool, this production was not significantly upregulated by such as an immune challenge. This finding demonstrates that hemocytes are required to activate antibacterial gene expression in the fat body after *E. carotovora* infection. The molecular identity of the signal is not known.

4. CONCLUSIONS

The field of *Drosophila* immunity has experienced exciting developments over the last few years. The most unexpected result was the discovery of significant similarities with the mammalian innate immune system. The intracellular signaling pathways that control the induction of *Drosophila* antimicrobial peptides share important similarities with those of the inflammatory response in mammals. In particular, the demonstration that Toll is a key player in host defense has had a major impact on our understanding of innate immunity. In spite of clear similarities, the molecular mechanisms that control activation of the Toll receptor, and more generally the recognition of microbial infections may differ significantly between insects and mammals. An understanding of upstream events that lead to the activation of the *imd* pathway is lacking at present. Finally, our knowledge of hematopoiesis, melanization, and coagulation remains largely descriptive in *Drosophila*. Finding the molecules involved in those processes will be one of the challenges of the coming years.

ACKNOWLEDGMENTS

We thank Jules Hoffmann and Jean-Marc Reichhart for critical reading of the manuscript. Work in the laboratory of the authors is supported by CNRS, NIH grant 1PO1 AI44220-02 to A. Ezekowitz and J. Hoffmann, the French Ministère de l'Education Nationale, de la Recherche et de la Technologie, EntoMed, Exelixis Inc., la Fondation pour la Recherche Médicale, and l'Association de la Recherche contre le Cancer.

REFERENCES

1. Metchnikoff E. Untersuchung über die intracellular Verdauung bei Wirbellosen Tieren. Arbeiten aus dem zoologischen Institut der universität zu Wien 1884;2:241.
2. Glaser RW. On the existence of immunity principles in insects. Psyche 1918;25:39–46.
3. Paillot A. Immunité naturelle chez les insectes. CR Acad Sci Paris 1919;169:202–204.
4. Paillot A. Contribution à l'étude de l'immunité humorale chez les insectes. CR Acad Sci Paris 1921;172:546–548.
5. Metalnikov S. Infection Microbienne et L'immunité chez la Mite des Abeilles *Galleria mellonella*. Paris: Masson, 1927.
6. Steiner H, Hultmark D, Engström A, Bennich H, Boman HG. Sequence and specificity of two antibacterial proteins involved in insect immunity. Nature 1981;292:246–248.
7. Bulet P, Hetru C, Dimarcq JL, Hoffmann D. Antimicrobial peptides in insects; structure and function. Dev Comp Immunol 1999;23:329–344.
8. Lemaitre B, Reichhart JM, Hoffmann JA. Drosophila host defense: differential display of antimicrobial peptide genes after infection by various classes of microorganisms. Proc Natl Acad Sci USA 1997;94:14614–14619.
9. Engström Y. Induction and regulation of antimicrobial peptides in *Drosophila*. Dev Comp Immunol 1999;23:345–358.
10. Engström Y, Kadalayil L, Sun S-C, et al. KappaB-like motifs regulate the induction of immune genes in *Drosophila*. J Mol Biol 1993;232:327–333.

11. Kappler C, Meister M, Lagueux M, et al. Insect immunity. Two 17-bp repeats nesting a kappaB-related sequence confer inducibility to the diptericin gene and bind a polypeptide in bacteria-challenged *Drosophila.* EMBO J 1993;12:1561–1568.
12. Meister M, Braun A, Kappler C, Reichhart J-M, Hoffmann JA. Insect immunity. A transgenic analysis in *Drosophila* defines several functional domains in the diptericin promoter. EMBO J 1994;13:5958–5966.
13. Karin M, Ben-Neriah Y. Phosphorylation meets ubiquitination: the control of NF-kappaB activity. Annu Rev Immunol 2000;18:621–663.
14. Pahl H. Activators and target genes of Rel/NF-κB transcription factors. Oncogene 1999;18:6853–6866.
15. Silverman N, Maniatis T. NF-kappaB signaling pathways in mammalian and insect innate immunity. Genes Dev 2001;15:2321–2342.
16. Nusslein-Volhard C, Lohs-Schardin M, Sander K, Cremer C. A dorso-ventral shift of embryonic primordia in a new maternal-effect mutant of *Drosophila.* Nature 1980;283:474–476.
17. St Johnston D, Nüsslein-Volhard C. The origin of pattern and polarity in the *Drosophila* embryo. Cell 1992;68:201–219.
18. Belvin MP, Anderson KV. A conserved signaling pathway: the *Drosophila* Toll-dorsal pathway. Annu Rev Cell Dev Biol 1996;12:393–416.
19. Lemaitre B, Nicolas E, Michaut L, Reichhart JM, Hoffmann JA. The dorsoventral regulatory gene cassette *spätzle/Toll/cactus* controls the potent antifungal response in *Drosophila* adults. Cell 1996;86:973–983.
20. Michel T, Reichhart J, Hoffmann JA, Royet J. *Drosophila* Toll is activated by Gram-positive bacteria through a circulating peptidoglycan recognition protein. Nature 2001;414:756–759.
21. Rutschmann S, Jung AC, Hetru C, et al. The Rel protein DIF mediates the antifungal, but not the antibacterial, response in *Drosophila.* Immunity 2000;12:569–580.
22. Rutschmann S, Kilinc A, Ferrandon D. The *Toll* pathway is required for resistance to Gram-positive bacterial infections in *Drosophila.* J Immunol 2002;168:1542–1546.
23. Lemaitre B, Meister M, Govind S, et al. Functional analysis and regulation of nuclear import of *dorsal* during the immune response in *Drosophila.* EMBO J 1995;14:536–545.
24. Ip YT, Reach M, Engstrom Y, et al. Dif, a dorsal-related gene that mediates an immune-response in *Drosophila.* Cell 1993;75:753–763.
25. Dushay MS, Asling B, Hultmark D. Origins of immunity: *Relish,* a compound Rel-like gene in the antibacterial defense of *Drosophila.* Proc Natl Acad Sci USA 1996;93:10343–10347.
26. Meng X, Khanuja BS, Ip YT. Toll receptor-mediated *Drosophila* immune response requires Dif, an NF-kappaB factor. Genes Dev 1999;13:792–797.
27. Manfruelli P, Reichhart JM, Steward R, Hoffmann JA, Lemaitre B. A mosaic analysis in *Drosophila* fat body cells of the control of antimicrobial peptide genes by the Rel proteins Dorsal and DIF. EMBO J 1999;18:3380–3391.
28. Hedengren M, Asling B, Dushay MS, et al. *Relish,* a central factor in the control of humoral but not cellular immunity in *Drosophila.* Mol Cell 1999;4:1–20.
29. Lemaitre B, Kromer-Metzger E, Michaut L, et al. A recessive mutation, *immune deficiency (imd),* defines two distinct control pathways in the *Drosophila* host defence. Proc Natl Acad Sci USA 1995;92:9465–9469.
30. Stöven S, Ando I, Kadalayil L, Engström Y, Hultmark D. Activation of the *Drosophila* NF-kappaB factor Relish by rapid endoproteolytic cleavage. EMBO Rep 2000;1:347–352.
31. Leulier F, Rodriguez A, Khush RS, Abrams JM, Lemaitre B. The *Drosophila* caspase Dredd is required to resist Gram-negative bacterial infections. EMBO Rep 2000;1:353–358.
32. Elrod-Erickson M, Mishra S, Schneider D. Interactions between the cellular and humoral immune responses in *Drosophila.* Curr Biol 2000;10:781–784.

33. Georgel P, Naitza S, Kappler C, et al. *Drosophila* immune deficiency (IMD) is a death domain protein that activates antibacterial defense and can promote apoptosis. Dev Cell 2001;1:503–514.
34. Senftleben U, Cao Y, Xiao G, et al. Activation by IKKalpha of a second, evolutionary conserved, NF-kappa B signaling pathway. Science 2001;293:1495–1499.
35. Silverman N, Zhou R, Stoven S, et al. A *Drosophila* IkappaB kinase complex required for Relish cleavage and antibacterial immunity. Genes Dev 2000;14:2461–2471.
36. Rutschmann S, Jung AC, Rui Z, et al. Role of *Drosophila* IKKγ in a Toll-independent antibacterial immune response. Nat Immunol 2000;1:342–347.
37. Lu Y, Wu LP, Anderson KV. The antibacterial arm of the *Drosophila* innate immune response requires an IkappaB kinase. Genes Dev 2001;15:104–110.
38. Huguet C, Crepieux P, Laudet V. Rel/NF-kappa B transcription factors and I kappa B inhibitors: evolution from a unique common ancestor. Oncogene 1997;15:2965–2974.
39. Fernandez NQ, Grosshans J, Goltz JS, Stein D. Separable and redundant regulatory determinants in Cactus mediate its dorsal group dependent degradation. Development 2001;128:2963–2974.
40. Kim YS, Han SJ, Ryu JH, et al. Lipopolysaccharide-activated kinase, an essential component for the induction of the antimicrobial peptide genes in *Drosophila melanogaster* cells. J Biol Chem 2000;275:2071–2079.
41. Wang C, Deng L, Hong M, et al. TAK1 is a ubiquitin-dependent kinase of MKK and IKK. Nature 2001;412:346–351.
42. Deng L, Wang C, Spencer E, et al. Activation of the IkappaB kinase complex by TRAF6 requires a dimeric ubiquitin-conjugating enzyme complex and a unique polyubiquitin chain. Cell 2000;103:351–361.
43. Vidal S, Khush RS, Leulier F, et al. Mutations in the *Drosophila dTAK1* gene reveal a conserved function for MAPKKKs in the control of rel/NF-κB dependent innate immune responses. Genes Dev 2001;15:1900–1912.
44. Kelliher MA, Grimm S, Ishida Y, et al. The death domain kinase RIP mediates the TNF-induced NF-kappaB signal. Immunity 1998;8:297–303.
45. Zhang SQ, Kovalenko A, Cantarella G, Wallach D. Recruitment of the IKK signalosome to the p55 TNF receptor: RIP and A20 bind to NEMO (IKKgamma) upon receptor stimulation. Immunity 2000;12:301–311.
46. Xiao T, Towb P, Wasserman SA, Sprang SR. Three-dimensional structure of a complex between the death domains of Pelle and Tube. Cell 1999;99:545–555.
47. Galindo RL, Edwards DN, Gillespie SK, Wasserman SA. Interaction of the pelle kinase with the membrane-associated protein tube is required for transduction of the dorsoventral signal in *Drosophila* embryos. Development 1995;121:2209–2218.
48. Grosshans, J, Bergmann A, Haffter P, Nüsslein-Volhard C. Activation of the kinase Pelle by Tube in the dorsoventral signal transduction pathway of *Drosophila* embryo. Nature 1994;372:563–566.
49. Towb P, Galindo RL, Wasserman SA. Recruitment of Tube and Pelle to signaling sites at the surface of the *Drosophila* embryo. Development 1998;125:2443–2450.
50. Horng T, Medzhitov R. *Drosophila* MyD88 is an adapter in the Toll signaling pathway. Proc Natl Acad Sci USA 2001;98:12654–12658.
51. Tauszig-Delamasure S, Bilak H, Capovilla M, Hoffmann JA, Imler JL. *Drosophila* MyD88 is required for the response to fungal and Gram-positive bacterial infections. Nat Immunol 2002;3:91–97.
52. LeMosy EK, Tan YQ, Hashimoto C. Activation of a protease cascade involved in patterning the *Drosophila* embryo. Proc Natl Acad Sci USA 2001;98:5055–5060.
53. Dissing M, Giordano H, DeLotto R. Autoproteolysis and feedback in a protease cascade directing *Drosophila* dorsal-ventral cell fate. EMBO J 2001;20:2387–2393.

54. Levashina EA, Langley E, Green C, et al. Constiutive activation of Toll-mediated antifungal defense in serpin-deficient *Drosophila.* Science 1999;285:1917–1919.

55. Imler J, Hoffmann JA. Toll receptors in innate immunity. Trends Cell Biol 2001;11:304–311.

56. Poltorak A, He X, Smirnova I, et al. Defective LPS signaling in C3H/HeJ and C57BL/10ScCr mice: mutations in Tlr4 gene. Science 1998;282:2085–2088.

57. Takeuchi O, Hoshino K, Kawai T, et al. Differential roles of TLR2 and TLR4 in recognition of gram-negative and gram-positive bacterial cell wall components. Immunity 1999;11:443–451.

58. Hayashi F, Smith KD, Ozinsky A, et al. The innate immune response to bacterial flagellin is mediated by Toll-like receptor 5. Nature 2001;410:1099–1103.

59. Hemmi H, Takeuchi O, Kawai T, et al. A Toll-like receptor recognizes bacterial DNA. Nature 2000;408:740–745.

60. Alexopoulou L, Holt AC, Medzhitov R, Flavell RA. Recognition of double-stranded RNA and activation of NF-kappaB by Toll-like receptor 3. Nature 2001;413:732–738.

61. da Silva Correia J, Soldau K, Christen U, Tobias PS, Ulevitch RJ. Lipopolysaccharide is in close proximity to each of the proteins in its membrane receptor complex: transfer from CD14 to TLR4 and MD-2. J Biol Chem 2001;276:21129–21135.

62. Lien E, Means TK, Heine H, et al. Toll-like receptor 4 imparts ligand-specific recognition of bacterial lipopolysaccharide. J Clin Invest 2000;105:497–504.

63. Poltorak A, Ricciardi-Castagnoli P, Citterio S, Beutler B. Physical contact between lipoplysaccharide and Toll-like receptor 4 revealed by genetic complementation. Proc Natl Acad Sci USA 2000;97:2163–2167.

64. Viriyakosol S, Tobias PS, Kitchens RL, Kirkland TN. MD-2 binds to bacterial lipopolysaccharide. J Biol Chem 2001;276:38044–38051.

65. Janeway CA. Approaching the asymptote: evolution and revolution in immunology. Cold Spring Harbor Symp Quant Biol 1989;54:1–13.

66. Schnare M, Barton GM, Holt AC, et al. Toll-like receptors control activation of adaptive immune responses. Nat Immunol 2001;2:947–950.

67. Rubin GM, Yandell MD, Wortman JR, et al. Comparative genomics of the eukaryotes. Science 2000;287:2204–2215.

68. Werner T, Liu G, Kang D, et al. A family of peptidoglycan recognition proteins in the fruit fly *Drosophila melanogaster.* Proc Natl Acad Sci USA 2000;97:13772–7.

69. Williams M, Rodriguez A, Kimbrell D, Eldon E. The 18-wheeler mutation reveals complex antibacterial gene regulation in *Drosophila* host defense. EMBO J 1997;15:6120–6130.

69a. Ligoxygakis P, Bulet P, Reichhart JM. Critical evaluation of the role of the Toll-like receptor 18-Wheeler in the host defense of *Drosophila.* EMBO Rep 2002;3:666–673.

70. Tauszig S, Jouanguy E, Hoffmann JA, Imler JL. Toll-related receptors and the control of antimicrobial peptide expression in *Drosophila.* Proc Natl Acad Sci USA 2000;97:10520–10525.

71. Lee WJ, Lee JD, Kravchenko VV, Ulevitch RJ, Brey PT. Purification and molecular cloning of an inducible gram-negative bacteria-binding protein from the silkworm, *Bombyx mori.* Proc Natl Acad Sci USA 1996;93:7888–7893.

72. Kim YS, Ryu JH, Han SJ, et al. Gram-negative bacteria-binding protein, a pattern recognition receptor for lipopolysaccharide and beta-1,3-glucan that mediates the signaling for the induction of innate immune genes in *Drosophila melanogaster* cells. J Biol Chem 2000;275:32721–32727.

73. Pimentel-Muinos FX, Seed B. Regulated commitment of TNF receptor signaling: a molecular switch for death or activation. Immunity 1999;11:783–793.

74. Chen P, Rodriguez A, Erskine R, Thach T, Abrams JM. Dredd, a novel effector of the apoptosis activators reaper, grim, and hid in *Drosophila.* Dev Biol 1998;201:202–216.

75. Hu S, Yang X. dFADD, a novel death domain-containing adapter protein for the *Drosophila* caspase DREDD. J Biol Chem 2000;275:30761–30764.

76. Zachary D, Hoffmann JA. The haemocytes of *Calliphora erythrocephala* (Meig.) (Diptera). Z Zellforsch Mikrosk Anat 1973;141:55–73.

77. Akai H, Sato S. Surface and internal ultrastructure of hemocytes of some insects. In: Gupta AP (ed.). Insect Hemocytes: Development, Forms, Functions and Techniques. Cambridge: Cambridge University Press, 1979, pp. 129–154.

78. Iwanaga S, Kawabata S. Evolution and phylogeny of defense molecules associated with innate immunity in horseshoe crab. Front Biosci 1998;3:D973–D984.

79. Rizki TM, Rizki RM. The cellular defense system of *Drosophila melanogaster.* In: King RC, Akai H (eds.). Insect Ultrastructure, vol 2. New York: Plenum, 1984, pp. 579–604.

80. Shrestha R, Gateff E. Ultrastructure and cytochemistry of the cell types in the larval hematopoietic organs and hemolymph of *Drosophila melanogaster.* Dev Growth Differ 1982;24:65–82.

81. Braun A, Hoffmann JA, Meister M. Analysis of the *Drosophila* host defense in domino mutant larvae, which are devoid of hemocytes. Proc Natl Acad Sci USA 1998;95:14337–14342.

82. Rizki TM, Rizki RM, Grell EH. A mutant affecting the crystal cells in *Drosophila melanogaster.* Wilhelm Rouxs Arch 1980;188:91–99.

83. Lagueux M, Perrodou E, Levashina EA, Capovilla M, Hoffmann JA. Constitutive expression of a complement-like protein in toll and JAK gain-of-function mutants of *Drosophila.* Proc Natl Acad Sci USA 2000;97:11427–11432.

84. Levashina EA, Moita LF, Blandin S, et al. Conserved role of a complement-like protein in phagocytosis revealed by dsRNA knockout in cultured cells of the mosquito, *Anopheles gambiae.* Cell 2001;104:709–718.

85. Carton Y, Nappi AJ. The *Drosophila* immune reaction and the parasitoid capacity to evade it: genetic and coevolutionary aspects. Acta Oecol 1991;12:89–104.

86. Sparrow JC. Melanotic tumours. In: Ashburner M, Wright TRF (eds.). The Genetics and Biology of *Drosophila,* vol 2B. New-York: Academic, 1978, pp. 277–313.

87. Russo J, Dupas S, Frey F, Carton Y, Brehelin M. Insect immunity: early events in the encapsulation process of parasitoid *(Leptopilina boulardi)* eggs in resistant and susceptible strains of *Drosophila.* Parasitology 1996;112:135–142.

88. Lanot R, Zachary D, Holder F, Meister M. Postembryonic hematopoiesis in *Drosophila.* Dev Biol 2001;230:243–257.

89. Nappi AJ, Ottaviani E. Cytotoxicity and cytotoxic molecules in invertebrates. Bioessays 2000;22:469–480.

90. Nappi AJ, Vass E. Melanogenesis and the generation of cytotoxic molecules during insect cellular immune reactions. Pigment Cell Res 1993;6:117–126.

91. Watson KL, Johnson TK, Denell RE. Lethal(1) aberrant immune response mutations leading to melanotic tumor formation in *Drosophila melanogaster.* Dev Genet 1991;12:173–187.

92. Ashida M, Brey P. Recent advances in research on the insect prophenoloxidase cascade. In: Brey PT, Hultmark D (eds.). Molecular Mechanisms of Immune Response in Insects. London: Chapman & Hall, 1997:135–172.

93. Soderhall K, Cerenius L. Role of the prophenoloxidase-activating system in invertebrate immunity. Curr Opin Immunol 1998;10:23–28.

94. Lai-Fook J. The repair of wounds in the integument of insects. J. Insect Physiol 1966;12:195–226.

95. Rizki TM, Rizki RM, Bellotti RA. Genetics of a *Drosophila* phenoloxidase. Mol Gen Genet 1985;201:7–13.

96. Ramet M, Lanot R, Zachary D, Manfruelli P. JNK signaling pathway is required for efficient wound healing in *Drosophila.* Dev Biol 2001;241:145–156.

97. Basset A, Khush RS, Braun A, et al. The phytopathogenic bacteria *Erwinia carotovora* infects *Drosophila* and activates an immune response. Proc Natl Acad Sci USA 2000;97:3376–3381.

9

Thioester-Containing Proteins of Protostomes

Elena A. Levashina, Stéphanie Blandin, Luis F. Moita, Marie Lagueux, and Fotis C. Kafatos

1. INTRODUCTION

The family of thioester-containing proteins (TEPs) appeared early in evolution: members of this family have been found in such diverse organisms as nematodes, insects, molluscs, fish, birds, and mammals *(1)*. They are characterized by homologous sequence features, including a unique intrachain β-cysteinyl-γ-glutamyl thioester, and a propensity for multiple conformationally sensitive binding interactions *(2)*. The presence of the highly reactive thioester bond renders the molecules unstable at elevated temperature and results in their autocatalytic fragmentation at the thioester site *(3,4)*. Moreover, when exposed, the thioester bond is readily hydrolyzed by water. To avoid precocious inactivation, the thioester in the native protein is protected by a shielded environment *(5,6)*. Proteolytic cleavage exposes a previously hidden thioester bond, which mediates covalent attachment through transacylation *(7)*. The reactivity associated with the thioester is one of the defining features of this protein family. Another important feature is the propensity for diverse conformationally sensitive interactions with other molecules. This includes covalent attachment to activating self and nonself surfaces (complement factors), covalent or noncovalent crosslinking to the attacking proteases [α2-macroglobulins (α2Ms)], interactions with receptors (complement factors and α2Ms), and binding of cleavage-generated products to corresponding receptors (anaphylatoxins of complement factors). In addition, α2Ms bind cytokines and growth factors and regulate their clearance and activity *(8,9)*.

Thioester-containing proteins are characterized by distinct structural forms. In this chapter we propose to use the following nomenclature. Complement factors C3, C4, and C5 are synthesized as single precursor molecules that are intracellularly processed into two- (C3 and C5) or three-*chain* (C4) molecules upon maturation. α2Ms exist in a monomeric form (single-chain molecule), in a dimeric form, composed of identical *subunits,* and in a tetrameric form, composed of four *subunits.* Heat denaturation causes fragmentation of thioester-containing proteins, resulting in autocatalytic *fragments,* whereas proteolytic activation generates *cleavage products.*

The diverse biochemical activities of the TEPs suggest that they are involved in multiple biologic functions. Indeed, in addition to the well-studied role of the complement

From: *Infectious Disease: Innate Immunity*
Edited by: R. A. B. Ezekowitz and J. A. Hoffmann © Humana Press Inc., Totowa, NJ

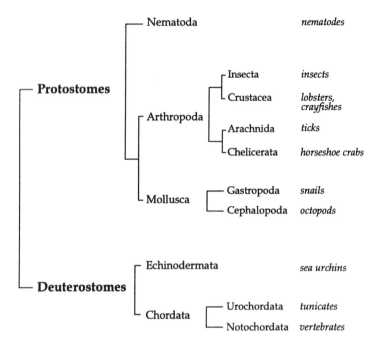

Fig. 1. Phylogenetic relationships between animal species discussed in this chapter.

factors in immune responses, it has been shown recently that *C3* is expressed in the regenerating limb blastema cells of urodeles *(10)*, suggesting that it plays a role in regenerative processes. Moreover, studies on *C5* knockdown mice have demonstrated the importance of C5a in liver regeneration *(11)*. Another report suggests that C3 is involved in fertilization, as it is associated with the extracellular matrix of eggs of an amphibian, *Bufo arenarum (12)*.

Considerable evidence implicates α_2Ms as important players in several biologic processes, yet the actual mechanisms underlying their influence are mostly unsolved. Decreased concentrations of human α_2M occur in states associated with proteolytic problems, for example, pancreatitis *(13)*. On the other hand, α_2Ms associate with a wide range of cytokines and growth factors and regulate their activity and distribution. Generation of mice deficient in either or both mouse α_2M and murinoglobulin-1 (MUG1), the single-chain protease inhibitor of the α_2M type, did not provide new insights into the protein function, as the knockdown mice are phenotypically normal under standard conditions *(14,15)*. In experimental conditions, the α_2M knockdown mice were more sensitive to a diet-induced model of pancreatitis than wild-type mice, and this sensibility correlated with both antiprotease and cytokine-binding activities of α_2M. Other important biologic functions of α_2Ms may not have been revealed by these studies.

A thorough understanding of any biologic system requires detailed knowledge of its origin, evolution, and diversity. It is becoming increasingly clear that both complement factors and α_2Ms derive from a common ancestor, prototypes of which can be found in invertebrates going back to Nematodes. Several recent reviews describe primitive complement-like system in tunicates *(16,17)* and sea urchins *(18,19)*. Here we summarize current knowledge of the TEPs of protostome invertebrates, with a specific emphasis on the potential of insect models to dissect the primitive functions of this protein family.

2. THIOESTER-CONTAINING PROTEINS OF PROTOSTOME INVERTEBRATES

A spectacular advance in the biochemical methods of protein purification and characterization occurred in the early eighties. One of the challenges of that time was to identify proteins responsible for diverse biochemical activities, e.g., proteases and protease inhibitors, by purification of active protein fractions. Following the original discovery of α_2M antiprotease activity in mammals *(20,21)*, this type of analysis was extended to invertebrate species *(22)*. All the TEPs of the protostome invertebrates, except for insects, have been purified from protein fractions selected for their α_2M-like antiprotease activity (*see* Fig. 1 for phylogenetic relationships between studied species). Most of these α_2Ms are dimers of two identical subunits; however, tetramers are not a unique feature of vertebrate α_2Ms, since such molecules are present in two species of gastropod molluscs (Table 1). Interestingly, protease-inhibitory activities of protostomal α_2Ms vary in their requirements for a functional thioester bond: most of the α_2Ms from Arthropoda are sensitive to methylamine treatment, whereas in molluscs, methylamine does not interfere with the protease-inhibitory activities. To date, complete sequence information is available only for the *Limulus* α_2M, and the absence of molecular data hampers phylogenetic analysis of TEPs in invertebrates.

2.1. α_2-Macroglobulins in Chelicerata

A TEP of an invertebrate was first detected in the hemolymph of the American horseshoe crab, *Limulus polyphemus,* by Quigley and Armstrong *(23)* in 1983. Up to now it is the best biochemically characterized α_2M in protostomes. This protein is synthesized by hemocytes and secreted into the hemolymph at a concentration of 50 nM *(24)*, whereas a minor portion is stored in the large granules of hemocytes, as demonstrated for the sister horseshoe crab species, *Tachypleus tridentatus (25)*. Immune or physical stimulation causes blood cell degranulation and α_2M secretion *(26)*. Like other TEPs, *Limulus* α_2M is a glycosylated protein with complex oligosaccharide chains *(25)*. Its molecular mass is 185 kDa *(27)*, and it circulates in the hemolymph mostly as a dimer of two disulphide-linked identical subunits *(28,29)*. However, the existence of a minor tetrameric form that dissociates into dimers upon activation has been reported *(30)*.

Comparison of the entire mature protein sequence of *Limulus* α_2M with human α_2M and C3 shows 31 and 23% similarities, respectively *(31)*. Interestingly, phylogenetic analysis clusters this protein with the clade of α_2M from vertebrates, indicating that the protein has retained the main features of this class of pan-protease inhibitors (Fig. 2). The sequence of *Limulus* α_2M displays a highly conserved thioester motif *(25)*, which is functional, as shown by the sensitivity of the native protein to autolytic fragmentation during heat denaturation: mild thermal treatment yielded fragments of 125 and 55 kDa *(32)*. Treatment with methylamine, a small nucleophilic molecule that is used to inactivate thioester, rendered the protein resistant to heat denaturation. The interpreta-

Table 1
Structure, Biochemical Activities, and Biologic Functions of Thioester-Containing Proteins in Protostomal Invertebrates[a]

Phylum	Subphylum	Class	Species	Name	Stoichiometry and size (kDa)
Arthropoda	Chelicerata	Merostoma	*Limulus*	L α_2M	2×185 *(28)*
			Tachypleus		ND
		Arachnida	*Ornithodoros*	TAM	$2 \times (92 + 92)$ *(58)*
	Mandibulata	Crustacea	*Homarus*	Lobster α_2M	2×180 *(62)*
			Pacifistacus	P α_2M	2×190 *(63)*
			Astacus	*Astacus* α_2M	2×185 *(64)*
		Insecta	*Drosophila*	Tep1	ND
				Tep2	ND
				Tep3	ND
				Tep4	ND
				Tep6	ND
			Anopheles	aTEP-I *(31)*	165 *(31)*
Mollusca		Cephalopoda	*Octopus*	Octopus α_2M	2×180 *(67)*
		Gastropoda	*Biomphalaria*	Snail α_2M	4×200 *(69)*
			Helix	Hp α_2M	4×195 *(70)*

ND, not determined; NA, nonapplicable; +TE, the specified function of the protein requires the thioester bond; α_2M, α_2-macroglobulin; TAM, tick α_2M. Numbers in parentheses indicate literature references.

tion that the thioester bond is involved in fragmentation was strengthened by the ability of *Limulus* α_2M to incorporate tritium-labeled glycerol *(28)*. Surprisingly, this incorporation was 10-fold higher than for human α_2M but was comparable to the glycerol incorporation seen with human C3. These results were interpreted as indicating that the *Limulus* α_2M and human C3 have similar binding preferences. However, this conclusion is premature and requires direct comparison of binding efficiencies to both labeled glycerol and glycine. Preferential binding to [^{3}H]glycerol is characteristic for human C3, whereas human α_2M is more efficient in incorporating [^{3}H]glycine *(33)*. This difference depends on a residue located at a site approx 100 amino acids downstream of the thioester site *(34)*. If this residue is a histidine, preferential binding to carboxyl groups is observed, whereas if it is an asparagine or an aspartic acid (as in many α_2Ms, including *Limulus* α_2M) formation of the amide bonds is favored.

The efficient binding to glycerol and the presence of methylamine-sensitive hemolytic activity in the hemolymph of *Limulus* led to the suggestion that *Limulus* α_2M might have dual properties, combining protease inhibitory and C3-like lytic activities *(28)*. The story became more complicated when the inhibitory effect of methylamine treatment on the cytolytic activity was shown to be dependent on the experimental procedure *(35)*. Later reports established that α_2M does not directly activate the hemolysis but modulates it through binding to another component of hemolymph, limulin *(36)*. Limulin, a member of the pentraxin protein family, is necessary and sufficient to induce lysis of sheep red blood cells by an unknown mechanism

Thioester			Function			
Sequence	Functionality	Catalytic residue	Protease inhibitor	Opsonization	Protein binding	Expression patterns
+ (25)	+ (32)	N (25)	+ TE (27)	ND	Limulin (39)	
					Coagulin (54)	Hemocytes (26)
ND	ND	ND	ND	ND	ND	Hemocytes (25)
+ (58)	+ (58)	ND	+ (58)	ND	ND	ND
+ (62)	+ (62)	ND	+ TE (62)	ND	ND	ND
+ (65)	+ (63)	ND	+ TE (63)	ND	ND	Hemocytes (66)
ND	+ (64)	ND	+ TE (64)	ND	ND	ND
+ (72)	ND	H (72)	ND	ND	ND	Fat body,
						hemocytes (72)
+	ND	D	ND	ND	ND	ND
+	ND	E	ND	ND	ND	ND
+	ND	Y	ND	ND	ND	ND
–	NA	NA	ND	ND	ND	ND
+ (31)	+ (31)	H (31)	ND	+TE (31)	ND	Hemocytes (31)
+ (67)	+ (67)	ND	+ (67)	ND	ND	ND
ND	+ (68)	ND	+ (68)	ND	ND	ND
+ (70)	+ (70)	ND	+ (70)	ND	ND	ND

that depends on sialic acid binding *(37,38)*. Native, unreacted α_2M has no effect on the hemolytic activity, but the thioester-reacted forms of *Limulus* α_2M bind limulin and thus indirectly prevent hemolysis *(39)*. Although the role of such modulatory mechanisms in immunity is not clear, vertebrate α_2Ms reportedly bind cytokines and growth factors and modulate their activity *(9)*. Thus, binding of *Limulus* α_2M to a pentraxin may represent another ancient property of these proteins as modulators of biologically reactive molecules.

Historically, protease inhibitory activity was detected in the horseshoe crab hemolymph before α_2M was purified and characterized *(22,23)*. This activity was sensitive to mild acidification and to methylamine treatment and inhibited a wide range of proteolytic enzymes from mammals and bacteria, including trypsin, chymotrypsin, plasmin, elastase, subtilisin, and thermolysin. The inhibited proteases retained the ability to cleave small molecular weight substrates. All these properties are specific to the α_2M family and, consequently, the detected activity was attributed to the presence of an α_2M in the hemolymph. This has been confirmed by purification of the protein *(27,32)* and cloning of the corresponding gene *(25)*.

Inhibition is initiated when the protease cleaves α_2M at a defined domain, the bait region. This domain contains multiple cleavage sites for a wide variety of proteases. It is the most variable part in thioester-containing molecules, even from phylogenetically close species, suggesting the possibility of evolutionary pressure *(40)*. Reaction of *Limulus* α_2M with trypsin generates cleavage products of 100 and 85 kDa, correspond-

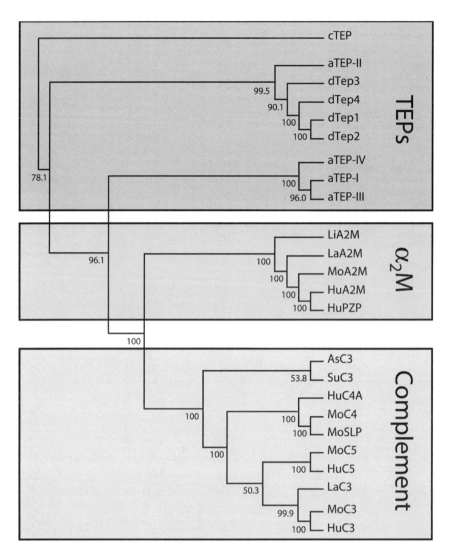

Fig. 2. Phylogenetic tree of thioester-containing proteins (TEPs). The tree is constructed using the neighbor-joining method based on alignment of the sequences using CLUSTAL_X. Numerals on the branches are bootstrap percentages to support the given partitioning. Clades of complement factors (Complement), α_2,-macroglobulins (α_2M), and insect/nematode TEPs (TEPs) are boxed.

ing to cleavage in the bait region, as well as three additional products with molecular masses greater than the native polypeptide *(41)*. Inactive proteases are not bound by *Limulus* α_2M, indicating that it has to be proteolytically activated before it can bind and exert its inhibitory activity *(42)*. The proteolytic activation of α_2M leads to its dramatic conformational change, causing the entrapment of the attacking protease *(21)*. Entrapment may or may not involve covalent binding through the amide bond formed between the activated thioester and amino groups of lysyl residues in the protease *(40)*. α_2M of *Limulus* entraps proteases mainly using the noncovalent mechanism. Interestingly, the "trapping" process is sensitive to methylamine; unlike the earlier cleavage of

α_2M in the bait region, the functional thioester crosslinks two α_2M subunits rather than the attacking protease. An isopeptide bond is formed between Lys254 of one α_2M subunit and the Glu residue of the thioester site in the second subunit *(43)*. It is believed that intersubunit crosslinking stabilizes the altered conformational structure of the reacted α_2M *(44)*. Only 1% of the attacking protease binds covalently to the *Limulus* α_2M *(28,41)*. It is important to note that both trypsin and methylamine treatment result in extensive compaction of the molecule, as evidenced by electron microscopy *(28,29)*. Such compaction results in a change of electrophoretic mobility of α_2Ms, a transition referred to as the slow to fast transformation *(45)*.

Proteolytic activation and protease entrapment exposes a receptor binding domain of α_2M *(46)*. This leads to receptor-mediated endocytosis of the α_2M-protease complexes from the circulation and their degradation in secondary lysosomes *(40)*. Clearance of *Limulus* α_2M from the hemolymph was evidenced by injecting the fluorescein-labeled proteins into the heart lumen and measuring fluorescence in the plasma and in the hemocytes *(42)*. Trypsin and α_2M-trypsin complexes were rapidly cleared from the hemolymph, in contrast to unreacted α_2M and the oxygen carrier hemocyanin, which remained in the circulation *(42)*. Blood cells bound the fluorescein isothiocyanate-labeled trypsin-reacted α_2M, demonstrating their involvement in α_2M clearance.

A wealth of biochemical data suggests that α_2M may play an important role in proteolytic homeostasis of *Limulus*. Interestingly, this pan-protease inhibitor does not inhibit the key serine proteases, which activate the coagulation cascade of the hemolymph in both *Limulus (47)* and the closely related species, *Tachypleus tridentatus (25)*. The coagulation cascade in the Japanese horseshoe crab has been well characterized at the molecular level *(48)*. Constituents of microbial cell walls, such as lipopolysaccharides and β-1,3-glucans, activate a cascade involving four serine proteases that are normally kept in check by endogenous serpins *(49–51)*. The proteolytic reaction culminates in the cleavage of soluble coagulogen into insoluble coagulin and the formation of a fibrillar extracellular clot *(52,53)*. Surprisingly, *Limulus* α_2M was found associated with the coagulin clot in a Ca^{2+}-dependent fashion *(54)*. The biologic role of these specific associations is not clear, but accumulation of the inhibitor may suppress degradation of the clot by microbial proteases *(54)*. In addition, the coagulation cascade triggers the activation of another immune reaction—the prophenol oxidase cascade *(55)*. Two clip-domain serine proteases of the coagulation cascade and an antimicrobial peptide, tachyplesin, convert hemocyanin to phenol oxidase, thus localizing the phenol oxidase activity to the site of infection *(56,57)*. Therefore the coagulation system in the horseshoe crab appears to be quite a sophisticated system. Invading microorganisms are locally trapped into a gelatinous clot, where their escape is prevented through inhibition of microbial proteases by high concentrations of α_2M; antimicrobial peptides (big defensin, tachyplesins, anti-LPS factor) then break microbial walls; and, finally, the *champ de bataille* is isolated from the healthy surroundings by a melanotic barrier.

Horseshoe crabs represent a convenient model for the biochemical analysis of these proteins, because large volumes of plasma and other biologic materials are readily available for analysis. However, a deeper understanding of biologic function requires the analysis of specific mutant phenotypes, which is not readily applicable to these live fossils.

2.2. α₂-Macroglobulins in Arachnida

A recent report identified α_2M as one of the major hemolymph glycoproteins in the soft tick, *Ornithodoros moubata (58)*. Although the complete protein sequence is unknown, partial sequencing confirmed that this protein is a new member of the family of TEPs; hence it was named TAM for tick α_2-macroglobulin. The structure of TAM is of particular interest, as it represents the first two-chain invertebrate α_2M in which two chains are held together by disulphide bridges. Such posttranslational processing of a precursor protein is a specific feature of the complement proteins C3, C4, and C5 *(59)*. However, a C3-like two-chain structure also exists in vertebrate α_2Ms from the plaice *Pleuronectes platessa (60)* and the carp *Cyprinus caprio (61)*. The native 400-kDa TAM is a dimer of two two-chain subunits. In contrast to *Limulus* α_2M, the TAM subunits are associated by bonds that are sensitive to sodium dodecyl sulfate polyacrylamide gel electrophoresis even in nonreducing conditions *(58)*, indicating that they are not disulphide or other covalent bridges. Purified TAM inhibits trypsin and thermolysin, and this activity is sensitive to methylamine treatment. The TAM-reacted trypsin is protected by steric interference against high molecular weight protease inhibitors, such as soybean trypsin inhibitor (SPI); it is still able to cleave low molecular weight substrates in the presence of the inhibitor. Further studies are needed to confirm the presence and functionality of the thioester bond in TAM and to clarify the mechanism of protease entrapment.

2.3. α₂-Macroglobulins in Crustacea

Although α_2M activity has been reported in several crustacean species *(44)*, the proteins have been purified only from the hemolymph of the American lobster *Homarus americanus (62)* and the crayfishes *Pacifastacus leniusculus (63)* and *Astacus astacus (64)*. The full-length protein sequences are not available for these proteins, the N-terminal amino acid sequences are strikingly similar *(64)*. In contrast, the similarity to the N-terminal sequence of the *Limulus* α_2M is less pronounced. All three proteins are dimers of two identical disulphide-linked subunits. Purified protein extracts inhibit trypsin proteolytic activity toward high molecular weight substrates but do not affect proteolysis of small molecular weight substrates. This inhibitory activity is sensitive to methylamine treatment. Consistently, the presence and functionality of the thioester bond was established by partial sequencing of the thioester-containing region in *Pacifastacus (65)* and *Homarus (62)*. Heat denaturation results in autolytic fragmentation of α_2Ms in all three species. It is unknown whether these proteins bind covalently to proteases or form intersubunit disulphide bridges like *Limulus* α_2M. The defense and recognition reactions of arthropods are to a great extent carried out by the blood cells (hemocytes). In *Pacifastacus,* α_2M is almost exclusively present in the hemocytes *(66)* and is continuously secreted into the plasma reaching the concentration of about 0.2 mg/ml *(65)*. Although a possible function of α_2M in regulating crayfish prophenol oxidase and/or clotting systems has been proposed *(65)*, the role of these proteins in Crustacea remains to be established.

2.4. α₂-Macroglobulins in Mollusca

The first α_2M protein identified in molluscs was purified from the hemolymph of a cephalopod, *Octopus vulgaris (67)*. The native glycoprotein forms a 360-kDa disulphide-bonded homodimer and inhibits three catalytic classes of proteases, serine-, met-allo-, and cysteine proteases *(67)*. Like other α_2Ms, the inhibitor does not interact with the active site of the proteases, but sterically shields it so that only protease inhibitors of molecular weight lower than 7 kDa are able to react with the encaged trypsin. Inter-estingly, proteolytic activation of octopus α_2M does not alter the apparent Stockes radius and, consequently, it is based on a type of conformational change different from that in α_2M from *Limulus,* or on an entirely different mechanism. In addition, the pro-tease entrapment does not require covalent binding *(67)*. The functionality of the con-served thioester site was not addressed in this study, and thus the possibility that octopus α_2M does not have a reactive thioester bond remains open.

All the invertebrate thioester-containing molecules discussed above form predomi-nantly homodimers, and only a minor fraction of *Limulus* α_2M was shown to exist as a tetramer prior to proteolytic activation *(30)*. The first tetrameric α_2M in invertebrates was purified from the hemolymph of the tropical planorbid snail, *Biomphalaria glabrata (68,69)*. The snail α_2M is similar to human α_2M in that the denatured mole-cule is composed of two subunits that form a disulphide-bonded dimer, whereas the native molecule consists of four subunits, each with a molecular mass of around 200 kDa *(69)*. Proteolytic activation of the snail inhibitor produces two cleavage products of 100–105 kDa, indicating that the bait region is located near the middle of the sub-unit. The snail α_2M is a glycosylated protein that displays wide-range protease-inhibit-ing activity. It exhibits the characteristic methylamine-sensitive autocatalytic fragmentation of TEPs. As in the octopus, methylamine treatment does not induce dra-matic conformational change and results in only a slight decrease in the protease inhibitory activity *(69)*. After complexing with trypsin, the native molecule undergoes a slow to fast transition, indicating that the snail α_2M uses a trapping mechanism simi-lar to that of octopus α_2M, in which protease is encaged by conformational changes caused by cleavage of the bait region. The protease entrapment is independent of thioester activation and does not require covalent binding to the protease nor covalent crosslinking of the subunits.

Recently an α_2M has been purified from the hemolymph of another gastropod mol-lusc, *Helix pomatia (70)*. The structure and inhibitory activities of the molecule are closely related to the above-discussed snail α_2M in that the native form consists of four subunits and shows protease inhibitory activity that is independent of the functional thioester bond. Thus the tetrameric forms of α_2M evolved quite early in evolution, and deeper characterization of these molecules could provide insight into the selective pres-sures that shaped their evolution.

3. THIOESTER-CONTAINING PROTEINS IN DIPTERAN INSECTS

Insects are able to mount a rapid and efficient response when confronting various microorganisms. This response is reminiscent of innate immune defenses of verte-brates and, because insects lack an adaptive immune response, it represents a valu-able model to study the "ante-antibody" immunity *(71)*. Characterization of immune responses in the fruitfly *Drosophila melanogaster* spearheads the research in the field owing to the exceptional experimental possibilities offered by this insect, including a myriad of molecular and genetic tools and the availability of the com-plete genome sequence.

Until recently, the major human malaria vector, the mosquito *Anopheles gambiae,* had few advantages, but in recent years this species has become an attractive insect model to study innate immunity. The recent completion of the *A. gambiae* genome sequencing project provides the first model of a parasitic disease in which full genome sequence information is available for all three constituents: *Plasmodium falciparum* (the causative agent of human malaria), *Homo sapiens* (the host), and *A. gambiae* (the vector). The interest of this model is highlighted by the fact that the protozoan parasite has to evade two related but distinct immune systems, those of the vertebrate host and those of the mosquito. Unraveling the mechanisms that underlie mosquito-parasite interactions, which is itself of substantial interest, may provide a simplified model for understanding some aspects of host-parasite interactions.

All the TEPs discussed above were purified as active protein fractions that exhibited protease inhibitory activity. In insects, the TEPs were identified by molecular cloning *in silico (D. melanogaster),* or by homology cloning *(A. gambiae)* that was guided by the evolutionary conservation of the thioester region.

3.1. Thioester-Containing Proteins in Drosophila melanogaster

A BLAST search of the Berkeley *Drosophila* Genome Sequencing Project Database with the amino acid sequence of the α-chain of human complement factor C3 produced six hits. All of them showed significant sequence similarities and were named Teps for *t*hioester-containing *p*roteins. Four genes of six contain a conserved thioester motif, whereas *Tep5* and *Tep6* display a modified sequence *(72,73;* M.L., unpublished data). One gene, *Tep5,* is present only in genomic sequences and is not discussed here. Full-length sequences are now available for *Tep1, Tep2, Tep3,* and *Tep4 (72)* and were used in phylogenetic analysis (see below). Three specific protein features are characteristic of four *Drosophila* Teps: (1) a highly conserved region of 30 amino acid residues harboring a canonical thioester motif GCGEQ; (2) a distinctive cysteine signature encompassing 126 residues in the C-terminal part of the molecule; and (3) a highly variable central region of about 60 residues in length. Interestingly, in *Tep2* this variable region is encoded by five distinct exons, which produce distinct transcripts as a result of alternative splicing *(72).* Should *Tep2* code for a protease inhibitor, alternative splicing of the bait region may extend the number of inhibited proteases. It may also represent a novel mechanism for recognition of noxious structural patterns in the absence of the large repertoire of receptors of the adaptive immune response in vertebrates.

Interestingly, so far alternative splicing had not been reported in TEPs. Such a mechanism is often employed by insects to produce closely related proteins with distinct properties without dramatically enlarging the size of the genome. The best characterized example is a serine protease inhibitor (serpin) from a tobacco hornworm, *Manduca sexta,* in which alternative splicing generates 12 serpin isoforms, each of which has a distinct protease inhibitory activity *(74).* The distribution of the *Tep2* splice isoforms is unknown, but it will be of great interest to learn the temporal and tissue-specific patterns of particular isoforms. All *Teps* are located on the left arm of the second chromosome. Interestingly, *Tep2* and *-3* form a discrete cluster in which genes are oriented head to head and are separated by 1.5 kb of putative regulatory sequences (M. L., unpublished data). This clustering may result from a recent duplication-inversion event. Surprisingly, according to phylogenetic analysis of sequences, all inducible Tep proteins 1, 2, and 4 (see below) cluster together, whereas the constitutively expressed Tep3 is somewhat divergent in sequence (Fig. 2).

TEPs are often acute-phase reactants *(40,75)*. In *Drosophila,* the expression of *Tep1, -2,* and, *-4* is strongly upregulated by bacterial challenge in larvae. During the adult stage, immune challenge markedly induces *Tep2* and *-4,* whereas the expression of *Tep1* is minor. To date, the expression pattern of *Tep1* in larvae is best characterized. This gene is mainly transcribed in the fat body after immune challenge, but it is also expressed in hemocytes in naive and challenged larvae. No expression of *Tep1* is detected in the *Drosophila l(2)mbn* and S2 Schneider cell lines.

The induction of immune responses in *Drosophila* is controlled by two distinct signaling pathways: the Toll pathway is primarily responsible for expression of the antifungal peptide gene *Drosomycin,* and the Imd pathway controls expression of most antibacterial peptide genes *(76,77)*. Somewhat surprisingly, the inducible expression of *Tep1* is not controlled by either of these pathways *(72)*. An indirect effect of the Toll pathway on *dTep1* expression is observed in *Toll* gain-of-function mutants and might be associated with the characteristic aggregation of blood cells into masses that tend to become melanized, a process referred to as melanotic tumor formation, in these mutants *(78)*. It has been suggested that Toll-induced melanotic tumor formation is mediated by the JAK kinase Hopscotch *(79)*. Remarkably, *Hopscotch* gain-of-function mutants constitutively express high levels of *Tep1*. Moreover, in *Hopscotch* loss-of-function mutants, the inducible expression of the gene dramatically levels off, suggesting a direct regulation of *Tep1* expression by the JAK pathway. Consistently, constitutive expression of the gene in *Toll* gain-of-function mutants is abolished in the *Hopscotch* loss-of-function background. It will be of interest to determine whether Toll-induced melanotic tumor formation is also abolished in the *Toll* gain-of-function/*Hopscotch* loss-of-function double mutants. If so, Tep1 may be involved in the aggregation of blood cells and the localized induction of melanization. Analysis of loss-of-function *Tep* mutants will provide crucial information on the role of this protein family in fly immunity and perhaps uncover new functions.

3.2. Thioester-Containing Proteins in Anopheles gambiae

A gene encoding a TEP, *aTEP-I,* has been cloned and characterized in detail in *A. gambiae (31)*. Recent evidence suggests the presence of at least three more members of the family: aTEP-II (E.A.L., L.F.M., and S.B., unpublished data), aTEP-III *(80)*, and aTEP-IV (IMCR-14) *(81)*. Expression of all these molecules is transcriptionally upregulated by bacterial challenge and by the *Plasmodium berghei* infectious blood meal *(81;* E.A.L., unpublished data).

aTEP-I is a typical representative of TEPs in the mosquito *A. gambiae*. The amino acid sequence deduced from a cDNA clone codes for a protein of 150 kDa. It contains a signal peptide-like hydrophobic N-terminal segment characteristic of secreted proteins. The sequence contains the canonical thioester motif, which is followed 100 amino acids downstream by a catalytic histidine residue. The most C-terminal part displays a cysteine signature, which is characteristic of the *Drosophila* Teps (see above). The protein is glycosylated and secreted into the hemolymph by mosquito hemocytes. In the hemolymph, the glycosylated aTEP-I is present as a full-length form of approx 165 kDa and as a smaller fragment of 80 kDa *(31),* indicating a constant low level of proteolytic cleavage of the protein. Interestingly, the same type of cleavage can be induced by both wounding and bacterial challenge. It is unknown whether cleavage occurs during activation or subsequent inactivation of the molecule.

Biochemical analysis and protein purification in the mosquito are hampered by the small size of the animal and the nanoliter quantities of its hemolymph. To overcome these limitations, functional studies on aTEP-I were performed using a mosquito cell line established by H.-M. Mueller *(82,83)*. Mosquito cells in vitro secrete aTEP-I into the conditioned medium, where it can be readily detected by affinity-purified rabbit polyclonal antibodies that recognize the full-length and the C-terminal fragment of the molecule *(31)*. All evidence obtained so far suggests that aTEP-I is secreted as a single-chain molecule, but only purification of the native protein will provide an ultimate proof.

The functionality of the thioester bond in aTEP-I is supported by experiments on denaturation-dependent autocatalytic fragmentation. Heat treatment of the conditioned medium leads to the appearance of a new C-terminal fragment of 50 kDa, resulting from fragmentation of the molecule at the thioester site. Methylamine treatment completely prevents this autocatalytic fragmentation *(31)*.

Cultured mosquito cells show phagocytic activity against latex beads and bacteria *(84)*. Interestingly, this activity can be enhanced by pretreating Gram-negative *Escherichia coli* with the conditioned cell medium, before exposing the bacteria to the cells *(31)*. Double-stranded RNA knockdown of aTEP-I and methylamine treatment of the conditioned medium both decrease the efficiency of bacteria uptake by 50%. These experiments revealed for the first time that a thioester protein of a protostome has an ancient complement-like function of opsonising Gram-negative bacteria for phagocytosis *(31)*. In the same experiments, the efficiency of phagocytosis of Gram-positive bacteria was shown to be very low and independent of opsonization by aTEP-I. Interestingly, aTEP-I opsonizes both Gram-positive and Gram-negative bacteria, binding to them in a thioester-dependent manner *(31)*. Therefore, the low uptake of Gram-positive bacteria by the mosquito cells is not caused by inefficient opsonization by aTEP-I.

A similar phenomenon has been described for the opsonization and phagocytosis of group A streptococci by polymorphonuclear leukocytes (PMNs) *(85)*. Streptococcal strains bearing M-surface antigens were totally resistant to phagocytosis by PMNs, whereas the M$^-$ strains were susceptible in a C3-dependent fashion. Both bacterial strains were opsonized by C3b activated by the alternative pathway. It was proposed that in the M$^+$ strains, the rigid α-helical M-protein blocks or physically hinders the receptor binding site of attached C3b, making it inaccessible for interaction with the leukocyte receptors *(85)*. It will be interesting to compare the phagocytic activity of the mosquito cells in culture with that of native hemocytes. This will allow us to discriminate between two broader explanations: (1) cultured cells may lack a component of the Gram-positive bacteria phagocytic receptor complex; or (2) the structure of the Gram-positive bacteria cell wall does not allow the opsonin to interact with the phagocytic receptors. In either case, the mosquito cell culture system provides a convenient model to address these questions.

Three additional genes encoding TEPs have been identified in *A. gambiae* thus far. In the phylogenetic tree, aTEP-I, aTEP-III, and aTEP-IV form a conspicuous cluster, suggesting that this cluster may result from a recent duplication event (Fig. 2). Future studies on the structure and function of all four aTEPs will provide valuable information pertinent to the broader question of functional evolution of this protein family. It is already clear that the TEPs represent a multimember family in both the fruitfly and the mosquito, probably reflecting the evolutionary importance of this family in the biology of insects. It is unknown as yet whether each aTEP has distinct functions, or whether these primitive molecules share common functions, possibly performing both protease inhibition and opsonization.

Of special interest is the role of aTEPs in the interactions between *Plasmodium* and the mosquito. The malaria parasite performs only part of its life cycle in the mammalian host, where it reaches and invades hepatocytes, then enters the circulation, and multiplies in the red blood cells. The remaining development of the parasite, including its sexual cycle, obligatorily occurs in the mosquito. During its complex passage through both the vertebrate host and the invertebrate vector, it now appears that the parasite repeatedly faces attacks from complement-like systems that represent more than 400 million years of evolutionary diversification. Interestingly, mosquito stages of parasite development in vitro are less resistant to complement than vertebrate blood-stage parasites *(86,87)*, indicating that some stage-specific factors may protect *Plasmodium* from the complement system in vivo. Dissection of the interactions between aTEPs and the parasite may provide new insights into the mechanisms of complement-parasite interactions.

5. CONCLUSIONS AND PERSPECTIVES

The mid-1980s evidenced an explosion of studies on the TEPs, especially on α_2Ms. In particular, several invertebrate species were analyzed for α_2M-like protease inhibitory activities, followed by purification and biochemical characterization of the relevant molecules. Animal size and the volume of hemolymph were important in selection of species for biochemical analysis. Big invertebrate species like the horseshoe crabs, crayfishes, octopuses, lobsters, and others discussed above were instrumental in demonstrating the presence of α_2M in protostomes and in revealing the amazing diversity of α_2M structural forms. Only dimeric α_2Ms were initially identified in invertebrates, leading to the belief that tetrameric forms are restricted to higher vertebrates. Recently tetrameric α_2Ms were characterized in two species of gastropod molluscs, and it is likely that insect TEPs are monomeric. Thus, monomeric, dimeric, and tetrameric TEPs might be widespread among animals. The protease inhibitory activity of tetrameric molecules appears to be less sensitive to methylamine than that of dimeric or putative monomeric molecules, in both invertebrate and vertebrate α_2Ms. The mechanism of protease entrapment in invertebrates has been characterized only for *Limulus* and represents a rather peculiar example, whereby the thioester forms a covalent bond with the opposite subunit of α_2M and not with the attacking protease.

Interestingly, not all thioester-containing molecules in invertebrates actually contain the thioester motif, e.g., *Drosophila* Tep6 lacks it. In vertebrates, complement factor C5 and ovostatin also lack this important protein signature, which would suggest that the thioester motif has been lost repeatedly during animal evolution. The overall picture suggests that the TEPs in the animal phyla undergo dramatic selective pressures that result in a set of polypeptides specific for each species. The nature of these selective pressures is unknown and can only be imagined when the functions of the proteins are more fully characterized.

Table 1 summarizes our present knowledge of the structure, biochemical activities, and biologic functions of TEP in protostomal invertebrates. Obviously, this field of research is only at an early stage of development, and "not determined" dominates the table. The recent discovery of TEPs proteins in *Drosophila* will certainly play a key role in understanding the function(s) of this protein family. The immune-inducible expression of *Tep1, 2,* and, *-4* suggests that *Drosophila* Teps may play a role in immune responses in the fruitfly. Mutant analysis may confirm this but may also reveal unexpected new functions. The mosquito represents a complementary model for functional analysis of this protein family. Cultured mosquito cells have provided a first quantitative phagocytic test and can potentially serve to dissect the molecules involved in regulation of phagocytosis. Another advantage of cell culture is the unlimited quantity of material available for biochemical studies; it will prove invaluable for purification of aTEPs and subsequent structure-functional analysis of the proteins. Most importantly, the mosquito represents an elegant model for studying the role of TEPs during the response to parasitic infections. The malaria parasite faces the complement system and α_2Ms in the vertebrate host, as well as aTEPs in the mosquito, and is still able to complete its life cycle. Understanding the mechanisms of parasite evasion from the mosquito TEPs may extend our knowledge of parasite resistance to the mammalian complement system and to α_2M, with potential implications for the treatment of human disease.

Current data suggest that the TEPs in protostomes are mostly represented by α_2Ms (Table 1). However, this idea should be treated with caution, as most of the invertebrate proteins were purified as extracts that displayed α_2M-like protease inhibitory activity. Insect TEPs are the first example of a genomics-based approach for unbiased study of these proteins. Future systematic investigations on the invertebrate TEPs are very likely to break up the accepted view of a rigid separation of this family into complement factors and α_2M. This will open new perspectives for understanding the fascinating diverse and (probably) multifunctional TEP family.

ACKNOWLEDGMENTS

The authors thank Prof. Jules A. Hoffmann for critical reading of the manucript. Work in our laboratories has received support from the National Institutes of Health, grant 1PO1 AI44220, and from the European Commission Human Potential—Research Training Networks Programme, grant HPRN-CT-2000-00080.

REFERENCES

1. Nonaka M. Origin and evolution of the complement system. In: Du Pasquier L, Litman GW (eds.). Origin and Evolution of the Vertebrate Immune System, vol 248. New York: Springer-Verlag, 2000, pp. 37–50.
2. Chu CT, Pizzo SV. Alpha 2-macroglobulin, complement, and biologic defense: antigens, growth factors, microbial proteases, and receptor ligation. Lab Invest 1994;71:792–812.
3. Harpel PC, Hayes MB, Hugli TE. Heat-induced fragmentation of human alpha 2-macroglobulin. J Biol Chem 1979;254:8669–8678.

4. Howard JB. Methylamine reaction and denaturation-dependent fragmentation of complement component 3. Comparison with alpha2-macroglobulin. J Biol Chem 1980;255:7082–7084.

5. Salvesen GS, Sayers CA, Barrett AJ. Further characterization of the covalent linking reaction of alpha 2-macroglobulin. Biochem J 1981;195:453–461.

6. Sim RB, Sim E. Autolytic fragmentation of complement components C3 and C4 under denaturing conditions, a property shared with alpha 2-macroglobulin. Biochem J 1981;193:129–141.

7. Law SK, Dodds AW. The internal thioester and the covalent binding properties of the complement proteins C3 and C4. Protein Sci 1997;6:263–274.

8. Lysiak JJ, Hussaini IM, Webb DJ, et al. Alpha 2-macroglobulin functions as a cytokine carrier to induce nitric oxide synthesis and cause nitric oxide-dependent cytotoxicity in the RAW 264.7 macrophage cell line. J Biol Chem 1995;270:21919–21927.

9. Webb DJ, Wen J, Lysiak JJ, et al. Murine alpha-macroglobulins demonstrate divergent activities as neutralizers of transforming growth factor-beta and as inducers of nitric oxide synthesis. A possible mechanism for the endotoxin insensitivity of the alpha2-macroglobulin gene knock-out mouse. J Biol Chem 1996;271:24982–24988.

10. Del Rio-Tsonis K, Tsonis PA, Zarkadis IK, Tsagas AG, Lambris JD. Expression of the third component of complement, C3, in regenerating limb blastema cells of urodeles. J Immunol 1998;161:6819–6824.

11. Mastellos D, Papadimitriou JC, Franchini S, Tsonis PA, Lambris JD. A novel role of complement: mice deficient in the fifth component of complement (C5) exhibit impaired liver regeneration. J Immunol 2001;166:2479–2486.

12. Llanos RJ, Whitacre CM, Miceli DC. Potential involvement of C(3) complement factor in amphibian fertilization. Comp Biochem Physiol A Mol Integr Physiol 2000;127:29–38.

13. McMahon MJ, Bowen M, Mayer AD, Cooper EH. Relation of alpha 2-macroglobulin and other antiproteases to the clinical features of acute pancreatitis. Am J Surg 1984;147:164–170.

14. Umans L, Serneels L, Overbergh L, et al. Targeted inactivation of the mouse alpha 2-macroglobulin gene. J Biol Chem 1995;270:19778–19785.

15. Umans L, Serneels L, Overbergh L, Stas L, Van Leuven F. Alpha2-macroglobulin- and murinoglobulin-1-deficient mice. A mouse model for acute pancreatitis. Am J Pathol 1999;155:983–993.

16. Nonaka M. Origin and evolution of the complement system. Curr Top Microbiol Immunol 2000;248:37–50.

17. Nonaka M. Evolution of the complement system. Curr Opin Immunol 2001;13:69–73.

18. Smith LC, Azumi K, Nonaka M. Complement systems in invertebrates. The ancient alternative and lectin pathways. Immunopharmacology 1999;42:107–120.

19. Smith LC, Clow LA, Terwilliger DP. The ancestral complement system in sea urchins. Immunol Rev 2001;180:16–34.

20. Starkey PM, Barrett AJ. Inhibition by alpha-macroglobulin and other serum proteins. Biochem J 1973;131:823–831.

21. Barrett AJ, Starkey PM. The interaction of alpha 2-macroglobulin with proteinases. Characteristics and specificity of the reaction, and a hypothesis concerning its molecular mechanism. Biochem J 1973;133:709–724.

22. Starkey PM, Barrett AJ. Evolution of alpha 2-macroglobulin. The demonstration in a variety of vertebrate species of a protein resembling human alpha 2-macroglobulin. Biochem J 1982;205:91–95.

23. Quigley JP, Armstrong PB. An endopeptidase inhibitor, similar to mammalian alpha 2-macroglobulin, detected in the hemolymph of an invertebrate, *Limulus polyphemus.* J Biol Chem 1983;258:7903–7906.

24. Swarnakar S, Melchior R, Quigley JP. Regulation of the plasma cytolytic pathway of *Limulus polyphemus* α_2-macroglobulin. Biol Bull 1995;189:226–227.

25. Iwaki D, Kawabata S, Miura Y, et al. Molecular cloning of *Limulus* alpha 2-macroglobulin. Eur J Biochem 1996;242:822–831.

26. Armstrong PB, Quigley JP. The *Limulus* blood cell secretes α_2-macroglobulin when activated. Biol Bull 1990;178:137–143.

27. Quigley JP, Armstrong PB. A homologue of alpha 2-macroglobulin purified from the hemolymph of the horseshoe crab *Limulus polyphemus*. J Biol Chem 1985;260:12715–12719.

28. Enghild JJ, Thogersen IB, Salvesen G, et al. Alpha-macroglobulin from *Limulus polyphemus* exhibits proteinase inhibitory activity and participates in a hemolytic system. Biochemistry 1990;29:10070–10080.

29. Armstrong PB, Mangel WF, Wall JS, et al. Structure of alpha 2-macroglobulin from the arthropod *Limulus polyphemus*. J Biol Chem 1991;266:2526–2530.

30. Bowen ME, Armstrong PB, Quigley JP, Gettins PG. Comparison of *Limulus* alpha-macroglobulin with human alpha2-macroglobulin: thiol ester characterization, subunit organization, and conformational change. Arch Biochem Biophys 1997;337:191–201.

31. Levashina EA, Moita LF, Blandin S, et al. Conserved role of a complement-like protein in phagocytosis revealed by dsRNA knockout in cultured cells of the mosquito, *Anopheles gambiae*. Cell 2001;104:709–718.

32. Armstrong PB, Quigley JP. *Limulus* alpha 2-macroglobulin. First evidence in an invertebrate for a protein containing an internal thiol ester bond. Biochem J 1987;248:703–707.

33. Dodds AW, Law SK. Structural basis of the binding specificity of the thioester-containing proteins, C4, C3 and alpha-2-macroglobulin. Complement 1988;5:89–97.

34. Sepp A, Dodds AW, Anderson MJ, et al. Covalent binding properties of the human complement protein C4 and hydrolysis rate of the internal thioester upon activation. Protein Sci 1993;2:706–716.

35. Armstrong PB, Armstrong MT, Quigley JP. Involvement of alpha2-macroglobulin and C-reactive protein in a complement-like hemolytic system in the arthropod *Limulus polyphemus*. Mol Immunol 1993;30:929–934.

36. Armstrong PB, Melchior R, Swarnakar S, Quigley JP. Alpha2-macroglobulin does not function as a C3 homologue in the plasma hemolytic system of the American horseshoe crab, *Limulus*. Mol Immunol 1998;35:47–53.

37. Armstrong PB, Misquith S, Srimal S, Melchior R, Quigley JP. Identification of limulin as a major cytolytic protein in the plasma of the American horseshoe crab, *Limulus polyphemus*. Biol Bull 1994;187:227–228.

38. Armstrong PB, Swarnakar S, Srimal S, et al. A cytolytic function for a sialic acid-binding lectin that is a member of the pentraxin family of proteins. J Biol Chem 1996;271:14717–14721.

39. Swarnakar S, Asokan R, Quigley JP, Armstrong PB. Binding of alpha2-macroglobulin and limulin: regulation of the plasma haemolytic system of the American horseshoe crab, *Limulus*. Biochem J 2000;347:679–685.

40. Sottrup-Jensen L. Alpha-macroglobulins: structure, shape, and mechanism of proteinase complex formation. J Biol Chem 1989;264:11539–11542.

41. Quigley JP, Ikai A, Arakawa H, Osada T, Armstrong PB. Reaction of proteinases with alpha 2-macroglobulin from the American horseshoe crab, *Limulus*. J Biol Chem 1991;266:19426–19431.

42. Melchior R, Quigley JP, Armstrong PB. Alpha 2-macroglobulin-mediated clearance of proteases from the plasma of the American horseshoe crab, *Limulus polyphemus*. J Biol Chem 1995;270:13496–13502.

43. Dolmer K, Husted LB, Armstrong PB, Sottrup-Jensen L. Localisation of the major reactive lysine residue involved in the self-crosslinking of proteinase-activated *Limulus* alpha 2-macroglobulin. FEBS Lett 1996;393:37–40.

44. Armstrong PB, Quigley JP. Alpha2-macroglobulin: an evolutionarily conserved arm of the innate immune system. Dev Comp Immunol 1999;23:375–390.

45. Barrett AJ, Brown MA, Sayers CA. The electrophoretically 'slow' and 'fast' forms of the alpha2-macroglobulin molecule. Biochem J 1979;181:401–418.

46. Van Leuven F, Marynen P, Sottrup-Jensen L, Cassiman JJ, Van den Berghe H. The receptor-binding domain of human α_2-macroglobulin. Isolation after limited proteolysis with a bacterial proteinase. J Biol Chem 1986;261:11369–11373.

47. Armstrong PB, Levin J, Quigley JP. Role of endogenous protease inhibitors in the regulation of the blood clotting system of the horseshoe crab, *Limulus polyphemus.* Thromb Haemost 1984;52:117–120.

48. Iwanaga S, Kawabata S, Muta T. New types of clotting factors and defense molecules found in horseshoe crab hemolymph: their structures and functions. J Biochem (Tokyo) 1998;123:1–15.

49. Miura Y, Kawabata S, Iwanaga S. A *Limulus* intracellular coagulation inhibitor with characteristics of the serpin superfamily: purification, characterization and cDNA cloning. J Biol Chem 1994;269:542–547.

50. Miura Y, Kawabata S, Wakamiya Y, Nakamura T, Iwanaga S. A *Limulus* intracellular coagulation inhibitor type 2. Purification, characterization, cDNA cloning, and tissue localization. J Biol Chem 1995;270:558–565.

51. Agarwala KL, Kawabata S, Miura Y, Kuroki Y, Iwanaga S. *Limulus* intracellular coagulation inhibitor type 3. Purification, characterization, cDNA cloning, and tissue localization. J Biol Chem 1996;271:23768–23774.

52. Iwanaga S, Morita T, Miyata T, et al. The *Limulus* Coagulation System Is Sensitive to Bacterial Endotoxins. Heidelberg: Verlag Chemie, 1983, pp. 365–382.

53. Muta T, Seki N, Takaki Y, et al. Horseshoe crab factor G: a new heterodimeric serine protease zymogen sensitive to $(1 \rightarrow 3)$-beta-D-glucan. Adv Exp Med Biol 1996;389:79–85.

54. Asokan R, Armstrong MT, Armstrong PB. Association of alpha2-macroglobulin with the coagulin clot in the American horseshoe crab, *Limulus polyphemus:* a potential role in stabilization from proteolysis. Biol Bull 2000;199:190–192.

55. Ashida M. The prophenoloxidase cascade in insect immunity. Res Immunol 1990;141:908–910.

56. Nagai T, Kawabata S. A link between blood coagulation and prophenol oxidase activation in arthropod host defense. J Biol Chem 2000;275:29264–29267.

57. Nagai T, Osaki T, Kawabata S. Functional conversion of hemocyanin to phenoloxidase by horseshoe crab antimicrobial peptides. J Biol Chem 2001;276:27166–27170.

58. Kopacek P, Weise C, Saravanan T, Vitova K, Grubhoffer L. Characterization of an alpha-macroglobulin-like glycoprotein isolated from the plasma of the soft tick *Ornithodoros moubata.* Eur J Biochem 2000;267:465–475.

59. Dodds AW, Law SK. The phylogeny and evolution of the thioester bond-containing proteins C3, C4 and alpha 2-macroglobulin. Immunol Rev 1998;166:15–26.

60. Starkey PM, Barrett AJ. Evolution of alpha 2-macroglobulin. The structure of a protein homologous with human alpha 2-macroglobulin from plaice (*Pleuronectes platessa* L.) plasma. Biochem J 1982;205:105–115.

61. Mutsuro J, Nakao M, Fujiki K, Yano T. Multiple forms of alpha2-macroglobulin from a bony fish, the common carp *(Cyprinus carpio):* striking sequence diversity in functional sites. Immunogenetics 2000;51:847–855.

62. Spycher SE, Arya S, Isenman DE, Painter RH. A functional, thioester-containing alpha 2-macroglobulin homologue isolated from the hemolymph of the American lobster *(Homarus americanus).* J Biol Chem 1987;262:14606–14611.

63. Hergenhahn HG, Hall M, Soderhall K. Purification and characterization of an alpha 2-macroglobulin-like proteinase inhibitor from plasma of the crayfish *Pacifastacus leniusculus.* Biochem J 1988;255:801–806.

64. Stocker W, Breit S, Sottrup-Jensen L, Zwilling R. Alpha2-macroglobulin from hemolymph of the freshwater crayfish *Astacus astacus.* Comp Biochem Physiol B 1991;98:501–509.

65. Hall M, Soderhall K, Sottrup-Jensen L. Amino acid sequence around the thiolester of alpha 2-macroglobulin from plasma of the crayfish, *Pacifastacus leniusculus.* FEBS Lett 1989;254:111–114.

66. Liang Z, Lindblad P, Beauvais A, et al. Crayfish alpha-macroglobulin and 76-kDa protein: their biosynthesis and subcellular localization of the 76-kDa protein. J Insect Physiol 1992;38:987–995.

67. Thogersen IB, Salvesen G, Brucato FH, Pizzo SV, Enghild JJ. Purification and characterization of an alpha-macroglobulin proteinase inhibitor from the mollusc *Octopus vulgaris.* Biochem J 1992;285:521–527.

68. Bender RC, Fryer SE, Bayne CJ. Proteinase inhibitory activity in the plasma of a mollusc: evidence for the presence of alpha-macroglobulin in *Biomphalaria glabrata.* Comp Biochem Physiol B 1992;102:821–824.

69. Bender RC, Bayne CJ. Purification and characterization of a tetrameric alpha-macroglobulin proteinase inhibitor from the gastropod mollusc *Biomphalaria glabrata.* Biochem J 1996;316:893–900.

70. Yigzaw Y, Gielens C, Preaux G. Isolation and characterization of an alpha-macroglobulin from the gastropod mollusc *Helix pomatia* with tetrameric structure and preserved activity after methylamine treatment. Biochim Biophys Acta 2001;1545:104–113.

71. Hoffmann JA, Kafatos FC, Janeway CA, Ezekowitz RA. Phylogenetic perspectives in innate immunity. Science 1999;284:1313–1318.

72. Lagueux M, Perrodou E, Levashina EA, Capovilla M, Hoffmann JA. Constitutive expression of a complement-like protein in *Toll* and *JAK* gain-of-function mutants of *Drosophila.* Proc Natl Acad Sci USA 2000;97:11427–11432.

73. Crowley TE, Hoey T, Liu JK, et al. A new factor related to TATA-binding protein has highly restricted expression patterns in *Drosophila.* Nature 1993;361:557–561.

74. Jiang H, Kanost MR. Characterization and functional analysis of 12 naturally occurring reactive site variants of serpin-1 from *Manduca sexta.* J Biol Chem 1997;272:1082–1087.

75. Volanakis JE. Transcriptional regulation of complement genes. Annu Rev Immunol 1995;13:277–305.

76. Anderson KV. Toll signaling pathways in the innate immune response. Curr Opin Immunol 2000;12:13–19.

77. Imler JL, Hoffmann JA. Signaling mechanisms in the antimicrobial host defense of *Drosophila.* Curr Opin Microbiol 2000;3:16–22.

78. Qiu P, Pan PC, Govind S. A role for the *Drosophila* Toll/Cactus pathway in larval hematopoiesis. Development 1998;125:1909–1920.

79. Mathey-Prevot B, Perrimon N. Mammalian and *Drosophila* blood: JAK of all trades? Cell 1998;92:697–700.

80. Dimopoulos G, Casavant TL, Chang S, et al. *Anopheles gambiae* pilot gene discovery project: identification of mosquito innate immunity genes from expressed sequence tags generated from immune-competent cell lines. Proc Natl Acad Sci USA 2000;97:6619–6624.

81. Oduol F, Xu J, Niare O, Natarajan R, Vernick KD. Genes identified by an expression screen of the vector mosquito *Anopheles gambiae* display differential molecular immune response to malaria parasites and bacteria. Proc Natl Acad Sci USA 2000;97:11397–11402.

82. Müller HM, Dimopoulos G, Blass C, Kafatos FC. A hemocyte-like cell line established from the malaria vector *Anopheles gambiae* expresses six prophenoloxidase genes. J Biol Chem 1999;274:11727–11735.

83. Catteruccia F, Nolan T, Blass C, et al. Toward *Anopheles* transformation: *Minos* element activity in anopheline cells and embryos. Proc Natl Acad Sci USA 2000;97:2157–2162.

84. Dimopoulos G, Müller HM, Kafatos FC. How does *Anopheles gambiae* kill malaria parasites? Parassitologia 1999;41:169–175.
85. Weis JJ, Law SK, Levine RP, Cleary PP. Resistance to phagocytosis by group A streptococci: failure of deposited complement opsonins to interact with cellular receptors. J Immunol 1985;134:500–505.
86. Touray MG, Warburg A, Laughinghouse A, Krettli AU, Miller LH. Developmentally regulated infectivity of malaria sporozoites for mosquito salivary glands and the vertebrate host. J Exp Med 1992;175:1607–1612.
87. Margos G, Navarette S, Butcher G, et al. Interaction between host complement and mosquito-midgut-stage *Plasmodium berghei*. Infect Immun 2001;69:5064–5071.

Section III

Mammalian Host Defenses:
Pattern Recognition Receptors

Section Editor: Siamon Gordon

Selected topics reviewed in this section provide a natural link between related molecules, pathways, and functions in invertebrate host defenses (Section II) and the induction of acquired immunity (Section IV). The topics chosen, Toll-like receptors (TLR), lipopolysaccharide binding protein (LBP) and CD14, macrophage mannose receptor (MMR), complement control proteins (CCP), and lung collectins, illustrate the variety of molecular and cellular mechanisms and consequences of host recognition of an increasingly diverse range of ligands. Whilst the original concept of pattern recognition retains considerable merit for heuristic purposes, it is clear that these molecules interact selectively not only with a range of exogenous molecules displayed by pathogens or harmless 'foreign' organisms, but also with endogenous modified self-components, consistent with a broader role in tissue homeostasis, as part of host defenses.

An overview of this section provides several interesting features, briefly noted here and explained in detail in each individual chapter. We find examples of protein interactions with proteins, lipids, saccharides, and even nucleic acids, on cell surfaces and in solution. Structural features are described in detail, perhaps best illustrated in the case of short consensus repeats (SCR) of complement control proteins, which are able to accommodate substantial sequence variability and therefore interact with a multiplicity of ligands. Multidomain receptors are also able to bind diverse ligand structures, and thus perform multiple functions, resulting in an expanded repertoire.

Lipopolysaccharide has been a powerful stimulus to both cells and research in this area, but the range of microbial structures that serve as ligands has expanded considerably to include constituents of bacteria, fungi, viruses, and parasites, microorganisms which exploit (or evade) cellular receptors for their own purposes, even while subject to host defenses and immune recognition. The emphasis is on complexity (whole

From: *Infectious Disease: Innate Immunity*
Edited by: R. A. B. Ezekowitz and J. A. Hoffmann © Humana Press Inc., Totowa, NJ

organisms rather than individual components), and interactions within the living host (which may express or lack a key molecule, as a result of genetic manipulation). Viral homologs such as vaccinia-derived proteins are useful in the study of complement control and may even provide inhibitors to regulate complement activation. However, a range of modified and stress-induced host proteins are also now shown to be ligands, in addition to apoptotic cells and denatured molecules destined for clearance.

The range of cells which utilize innate recognition receptors is also expanding—apart from macrophages, dendritic and natural killer cells, epithelia, such as type II alveolar cells are also able to participate in innate defenses. Each cell type may express its own profile of receptors, depending on its local microenvironment, such as the lung. Recognition can be opsonic, e.g., via surfactant proteins or LBP, or it can be direct, and induce adhesion, uptake, and destruction of target organisms, as well as lead to cell migration, secretion, and adaptive immunity. The deciphering of the signal is a complex process involving interactions of multiple proteins at the plasma membrane, and in both cytosol and nucleus. For example, CD14 may be surrounded by associated surface proteins, relaying signals through TLRs and their partners.

Some of the genetic and *in vivo* functional studies have yielded surprises, others revealed a complexity beyond the findings of simpler *in vitro* models. Thus surfactant protein A is critical for host defense against infection *in vivo*, whereas surfactant protein D also plays a role in surfactant homeostasis and protection against oxidant injury in the lung. CD14 knockout animals show variable susceptibility to infection, perhaps reflecting the importance of genetic background, including polymorphisms, and the complexity of infectious processes within the host.

Overall, the outcome of recognition can be host protective or give rise to toxicity, shock, or allergy. As our knowledge grows, it should bring improved understanding of health, disease, and possibilities for intervention.

Siamon Gordon

10

Toll-Like Receptors

Tsuneyasu Kaisho and Shizuo Akira

1. INTRODUCTION

Mammalian host defense is categorized into innate and adaptive immunity. Adaptive immunity is mediated by B- and T-lymphocytes, which carry antigen-specific receptors that can bind antigen with high affinity owing to somatic gene recombination. In infection, adaptive immunity is advantageous because of high-affinity recognition and memory responses but is disadvantageous because the response is gradual. Innate immunity is mediated by macrophages and dendritic cells (DCs), generically known as antigen-presenting cells (APCs). Innate immunity is a rapid response, thereby playing major roles, especially in the early phase of infection. For decades, it was considered that the way macrophages recognize pathogens is nonspecific, based on the fact that they do not carry rearranged receptors. However, accumulating evidence suggests that innate immunity can discriminate pathogens as nonself from self through a group of transmembrane proteins called the Toll-like receptor (TLR) family (1,2). In this chapter, we describe the current knowledge of this receptor family.

2. DISCOVERY OF MAMMALIAN TOLL-LIKE RECEPTORS

Insects do not possess any lymphocytes and therefore do not have adaptive immunity. Nevertheless, insects can cope with invasion of microorganisms efficiently by producing antimicrobial peptides. Synthesis of the peptides is triggered by differential activation of distinct Toll family receptors. For example, Toll signaling can lead to production of an antifungal peptide, drosomycin (3). Another Toll family member, 18W, can transduce the signal for synthesis of antibacterial peptides such as attacin (4). Toll family members show common molecular structures, characterized by their extracellular regions with leucine-rich repeat (LRR) and intracytoplasmic regions, called Toll/interleukin-1 receptor (IL-1R) homology (TIR) domains. The intracytoplasmic regions were so designated based on their similarity to those of mammalian IL-1R family members. The IL-1R family was initially thought to be a mammalian counterpart of the *Drosophila* Toll family because their intracytoplasmic regions are similar. However, Janeway's group identified the first mammalian Toll homolog whose extracellular and intracytoplasmic portions are structurally similar to Toll (5). At present 10 members (TLR1–10) have been shown to belong to the mammalian TLR family (6–10).

From: *Infectious Disease: Innate Immunity*
Edited by: R. A. B. Ezekowitz and J. A. Hoffmann © Humana Press Inc., Totowa, NJ

Table 1
TLR Family Members and Their Ligands

TLR	Origin of ligand	Ligand
TLR2	Gram-positive bacteria	Lipoproteins
		Peptidoglycan (TLR2/6 or TLR2/X)[a]
		Lipoteichoic acids
		Lipopeptides (TLR2/X)
	Mycoplasma	Lipoproteins
	Mycobacteria	Lipopeptides (including MALP-2,
	Spirochetes	TLR2/6)
	Mycobacteria	Lipoarabinomannan
	Porphyromonas	LPS
	Spirochetes (*Leptospira*)	
	Yeast	Zymosan (TLR2/6)
	Trypanosoma cruzi	GPI anchors
	Neisseria meningitidis	Soluble factor (TLR1/2)
TRL3[b]	Virus	Double-stranded RNA
TLR4	Gram-negative bacteria	LPS
	Gram-positive bacteria	Lipoteichoic acids
	Plant	Taxol
	RS virus	Fusion protein
	Host	HSP60
		Fibronectin EDA domain, fibrinogen
TLR5	Bacteria with flagella	Flagellin
TRL7[c]	Chemical compound	Imidazoquinolines
TLR9	Bacteria	Unmethylated CpG DNA
TLR1, -8, -10	Unknown	

Abbreviations: EDA, extra domain A; GPI, glycosylphosphatidyl inositol; HSP60, heat shock protein 60; LPS, lipopolysaccharide; MALP-2, macrophage-activating lipoprotein-2; TLR, Toll-like receptor.

[a] TLR2 recognizes some PAMPs by heterodimerizing with TLR1, TLR6, or unknown TLR (TLRX).

[b,c] Recently, TRL3 and TRL7 have been shown to recognize double-stranded RNA *(61)* and antiviral chemical compounds, imidazoquinolines *(62)*, respectively.

3. PATHOGEN SENSING BY TLRS

TLRs mainly function as sensors for pathogens. So far a number of TLR ligands have been identified (Table 1), and most of them can be classified as pathogen-associated molecular patterns (PAMPs) *(11)*. Some ligands are non-PAMPs, but, as described below, not only PAMPs but also non-PAMPs should play critical roles through TLRs in host immune and inflammatory responses.

3.1. TLR4 as the Signal Transducer for LPS

Lipopolysaccharide (LPS) is the most well-known PAMP. LPS is a major component of the outer membrane of Gram-negative bacteria and contains a hydrophilic polysaccharide and a hydrophobic lipid A, which is a biologically active component. LPS can stimulate APCs to produce proinflammatory cytokines and can upregulate surface

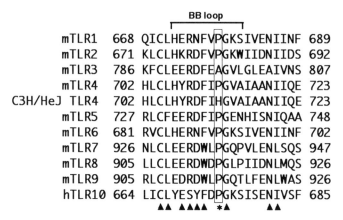

Fig. 1. Sequence alignment of the regions surrounding the BB loop of the TIR domain. The BB loop is located between the second β-strand and the second α-helix and creates a protrusion on the surface of the structure *(60)*. In C3H/HeJ mice, the 712th amino acid, proline, of TLR4 is replaced with histidine (boxed and indicated by asterisk). Residues conserved in at least seven TLRs are indicated by arrowheads. The amino acid sequence of mouse TLR10 is not available.

expression of costimulatory molecules such as CD40. Excess amounts of LPS can also cause endotoxin shock with high mortality.

LPS binds to LPS binding protein (LBP) in the serum and is then transferred to target cells. Most target cells carry another LPS binding molecule, CD14, on the cell surface. CD14 is critical in retaining LPS, but CD14 alone cannot transduce signals because it is a glycosylphosphatidyl inositol (GPI)-anchoring molecule. Genetic studies revealed that TLR4 is responsible for LPS signaling. A mutant mouse strain, C3H/HeJ, is known for its hyporesponsiveness to LPS *(12)*. The intracytoplasmic region of C3H/HeJ-derived TLR4 has a point mutation, which is a replacement of well-conserved proline with histidine (Fig. 1) *(13,14)*. In fact, this mutation could abrogate the function of TLR2 and TLR4 *(15,16)*. Another mutant strain, C57BL/10ScCr, also possesses chromosomal deletion in the TLR4 gene locus *(13,14)*. Furthermore, gene targeting of TLR4 also results in unresponsiveness to LPS *(16)*. These findings demonstrate that TLR4 is a critical signal tranducer for LPS (Table 1).

3.2. TLR2 Senses a Variety of Lipoproteins

Similar to Gram-negative bacteria, Gram-positive bacteria can provoke not only immune responses but also shock status. However, Gram-positive bacteria do not possess LPS in the cell wall. Instead, they carry a thick layer of peptideglycan (PGN), which is an alternating β(1,4)-linked *N*-acetylmuramyl and *N*-acetylglucosaminyl glycan crosslinked with tetrapeptides and can induce macrophages to produce inflammatory cytokines. Analysis with TLR2-deficient mice revealed that PGN acts as a PAMP through TLR2 *(17)*. Furthermore, another microorganism, *Mycoplasma,* although it lacks cell walls, carries lipoproteins and lipopeptides in the cytoplasmic membrane, and these components can stimulate macrophages to provoke inflammatory responses. One of the macrophage-activating lipopeptides from *Mycoplasma fermentans,* MALP-2, was found to utilize TLR2 as the receptor *(18)*. Furthermore, TLR2 can recognize a variety of lipopeptides or lipoproteins, mycobacterial lipoarabinomannan, yeast extracts, and GPI-anchoring proteins from *Treponema pallidum* (Table 1) *(2)*.

Initial studies suggest that TLR2 is involved in LPS signaling, because overexpression of TLR2 can confer LPS responsiveness on the cell lines. However, TLR2-, but not TLR4-, deficient mice retained the responses to LPS. The discrepancy can be ascribed to the high sensitivity of TLR2-overexpressing cell lines and TLR2 agonistic activity of contaminants in commercial LPS preparations *(19)*. However, LPS from *Porphyromonas gingivalis (20)* or *Leptospira (21)* was shown to act through TLR2. *P. gingivalis* is a Gram-negative anaerobic bacterium that is considered to play major roles in the pathogenesis of periodontal diseases. This LPS is structurally different from enterobacterial LPS in that it contains branched fatty acids with 15–17 carbon chains and lacks a phosphoryl group at position 4′ of the nonreducing glucosamine *(22)*. The difference can account for the inability of polymyxin B to inhibit the effects of *P. gingivalis* LPS. Meanwhile, *Leptospira* belongs to the Spirochaetales order and is different from Gram-positive and -negative bacteria. *Leptospira* LPS can be regarded as an atypical LPS in its several biochemical characteristics *(21)*. Thus, although LPS from these microorganisms can act through TLR2, they are structurally different from the typical LPS from *E. coli* or *Salmonella*. Therefore it is generally accepted that TLR4, rather than TLR2, is responsible for inflammatory responses provoked by LPS from most of the Gram-negative bacteria.

3.3. TLR5 Recognizes Flagellin

Most bacilli, including *Salmonella,* harbor common protein structures termed flagella, which project from the bacterial cell surface and are involved in motility. Flagellin, a monomeric subunit of flagella, can show a proinflammatory activity such as induction of IL-8 or inducible nitric oxide (NO) synthase in intestinal epithelial cells *(23,24)*. Several lines of evidence suggest that TLR5 can sense flagellin *(25)*. First, TLR5 expression conferred responding ability to flagellin on flagellin-unresponsive cell lines. In addition, *Salmonella typhimurium* lacking the flagellin gene cannot activate TLR5-expressing cell lines. Furthermore, flagellin expression rendered nonflagellated *E. coli* capable of activating TLR5. Analysis of TLR5-deficient mice should also be performed to confirm the conclusions.

Salmonella translocates flagellin across intestinal epithelia, possibly through a type III secretion apparatus, and can elicit inflammatory responses with flagellin *(26)*. Flagellin can act through the basolateral, but not apical, surface, probably because of the basolateral expression of TLR5 *(27)*. Thus, interestingly, the host prevents a nonpathogenic microorganism in the lumen from causing inflammation through polarized expression of TLR5, whereas pathogens manage to provoke inflammatory cascades through flagellin translocation.

3.4. TLR9 Recognizes Bacterial DNA

A *Mycobacterium bovis* strain, bacillus Calmette-Guèrin (BCG), has been well known as one of the effective adjuvants for inducing cell-mediated immunity. In the mid-1980s, Tokunaga et al. *(28)* found that BCG-derived DNA contributed to immunostimulatory activity of BCG. They have also shown that the DNA inhibited the growth of tumors, enhanced natural killer cell activity, and induced interferons (IFNs) from lymphocytes *(28)*. By utilizing synthetic oligonucleotides, the unmethylated cytidine-phosphate-guanosine (CpG) motif was found to be responsible for the activity. Furthermore, the motif could activate B-cells *(29)*. This motif is rare and is mostly methylated in vertebrate DNAs, which lack the immunostimulatory activity. Therefore, DNA containing this unmethylated CpG motif can also be regarded as a PAMP. All effects of CpG DNA were abolished in TLR9-deficient mice, indicating that TLR9 is a critical signal transducer for CpG DNA *(9)*.

Another group identified DNA-dependent protein kinase (DNA-PK) as the receptor for CpG DNA *(30)*. DNA-PK is a member of the phosphatidylinositol-3-kinase (PI3K)-like family and is involved in repair of DNA double-stranded breaks *(31)*. DNA-PK deficiency results in impairment of adaptive immunity *(31)*. Thus the idea is intriguing that a single enzyme is critical for both innate and adaptive immunity. However, the relationship between the TLR9 signaling pathway and DNA-PK activation remains unclear.

3.5. TLR4 Recognizes not Only PAMPs but Also a Variety of Products Including Host Proteins

TLR4 recognizes a variety of ligands other than lipids. For example, TLR4 can recognize a diterpene, taxol, which is a plant-derived product *(32)*. Moreover, TLR4 can sense a protein from respiratory syncytial virus (RSV) *(33)*. TLR4-deficient mice cannot eradicate RSV efficiently, suggesting that TLR4 is also critical in viral infection. Interestingly, vaccinia virus carries two protein products with similar amino acid structures to TIR domains, through which IL-1 and TLR4 signaling can be inhibited *(34)*. It can be assumed that the virus incorporates those proteins into the genome for its survival, strengthening the importance of TLR4 in viral infection.

Furthermore, it is also noteworthy that TLR4 can recognize host-derived products. During inflammation or tissue injury, extracellular matrix components such as fibronectin or collagen are degraded by proteases. These degraded products then trigger the inflammatory cascades. One of these products, a fragment of fibronectin, can stimulate TLR4 *(35)*. Furthermore, during inflammation, plasma fibrinogen is extravasated owing to endothelial cell retraction, and local deposition of fibrin or fibrinogen increases. Fibrinogen can stimulate chemokine production from macrophages in a TLR4-dependent manner *(36)*. Thus, TLR4 senses several proteins generated during the inflammatory process.

TLR4 is also involved in sensing another host-derived molecule, heat shock protein 60 (HSP60) *(37,38)*. A set of endogeneous molecules including HSP60 and calreticulin, which have potent immunostimulatory activity, are released upon necrotic, but not apoptotic, cell death *(39)*. This finding fits well with danger theory, which says that the immune system does not distinguish self from nonself but can detect danger signals released by damaged cells *(40)*. Therefore, interaction of TLRs and HSPs can be the molecular basis of the danger theory. CD91, which does not belong to TLR family, has been identified as a receptor for HSPs *(41)*. It is likely that HSPs endocytosed by CD91 activate TLRs to induce immune activation. However, further studies are necessary to clarify how HSPs activate cells through CD91 and TLRs.

4. RECOGNITION MECHANISM THROUGH TLRS

Ligands for TLR2 or TLR4 are quite heterogeneous in terms of their origins and molecular structures. How can such a variety of molecules be recognized by limited numbers of TLRs? Cytokines bind to their receptors with high affinity. Indeed, some cytokine receptors have been molecularly cloned or characterized through this high-affinity interaction. In contrast, none of the ligands have been identified on the basis of their binding activity to their TLRs. Therefore, we can surmise that TLRs recognize their ligands with low affinity. However, some molecules exist that can assist TLR recognition. For example, CD14, which is localized near TLR4 on the cell surface, retains and presents LPS to TLR4, thereby facilitating their interaction. In addition, TLR-associated molecules can also contribute to the interaction. A secreted molecule, MD-2, can confer LPS responsiveness on TLR4 by associating with TLR4 *(42)*. MD-2 can also directly bind to LPS independently of CD14 and LBP *(42,43)*. Furthermore, Triantafilou et al. *(44)* have shown that functional LPS receptor complexes contain HSPs and a chemokine receptor. These molecules coordinately function to facilitate the recognizing ability of TLR4.

Heterodimerization can also contribute to the diversification of the molecular repertoire recognized by TLRs *(45)*. Although expression of TLR4 alone can confer LPS responsiveness, expression of TLR2 is not sufficient for restoring responsiveness to zymosan, Gram-positive bacteria, or PGN. However, coexpression of TLR2 with TLR6 can confer the ability to respond to these stimuli. Furthermore, the responses were inhibited by dominant negative forms of either TLR2 (TLR2 DN) or TLR6 (TLR6 DN). Both TLR2 and TLR6 are recruited to macrophage phagosomes and physically interact with each other, demonstrating that TLR2 and TLR6 cooperatively interact to achieve their microbial recognition *(45)*. Notably, responses to bacterial lipopeptides (BLPs) can be inhibited by TLR2 DN, but not by TLR6 DN, suggesting that TLR2 can heterodimerize with other TLRs for BLP recognition. In vivo analysis using TLR2- or TLR6-deficient mice also supported this idea *(46)*. That is, responses to both BLP and MALP-2 were abolished in TLR2-deficient macrophages, whereas only the response to MALP-2 was abolished in TLR6-deficient macrophages. BLP is triacylated at the N-terminal cysteine residue, whereas MALP-2 is diacylated at the corresponding residue. Therefore, TLR2 discriminates this subtle molecular difference by heterodimerizing with distinct TLRs: TLR2/TLRX for BLP and TLR2/TLR6 for MALP-2. TLR1 is a possible candidate for TLRX, because TLR1 is genealogically close to TLR6 and can functionally heterodimerize with TLR2 for recognizing soluble factors from *Neisseria meningitidis (47)*.

5. TLR SIGNALING PATHWAY

5.1. Phylogenetic Conservation of the Pathway

After recognizing the ligands, TLRs activate signal transduction pathways leading to expression of cytokines. Because both TLR and IL-1R families possess TIR domains in their intracytoplasmic regions, they can activate similar signaling cascades (Fig. 2). All TLR and IL-1R family members associate with a cytoplasmic adapter molecule, MyD88, and sequentially activate a serine-threonine kinase, IL-1R-associated kinase (IRAK). Then I-κB kinase (IKK) complexes are activated through a scaffold protein, tumor necrosis factor receptor-associated factor 6 (TRAF6). I-κB phosphorylation induced by the IKK complex induces I-κB degradation, and nuclear factor κB (NF-κB) is liberated to enter the nucleus. In addition to NF-κB, other transcription factors such

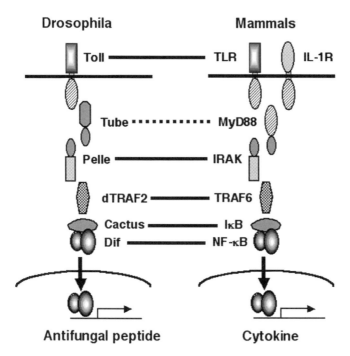

Fig. 2. Phylogenetic conservation of *Drosophila* Toll and mammalian interleukin-1 receptor/Toll-like receptor (IL-1R/TLR) signaling pathways. Both pathways stimulate similar sets of signaling components. Molecules with similar structures are indicated by thick solid lines. MyD88 carries both the TIR domain and the death domain (DD), whereas Tube carries only DD. Therefore, similarity between Tube and MyD88 is lower than other components. IRAK, IL-IR-associated kinase; TRAF, tumor necrosis factor receptor-activated protein.

as mitogen-activated protein kinases (MAPKs) are also activated. *Drosophila* Toll can also stimulate similar signaling components (Fig. 2) *(48)*. Thus, the Toll and TLR families utilize phylogenetically conserved signaling pathways.

5.2. Critical Roles of MyD88 in TLR Signaling

MyD88-deficient cells lack activation of NF-κB and MAPKs in response to IL-1 or IL-18 *(49)*. Furthermore, all biologic responses to these cytokines were completely abolished in MyD88-deficient mice, suggesting that MyD88 is an essential adapter for IL-1R family signaling pathways.

In addition, NF-κB activation was abrogated in MyD88-deficient cells stimulated with TLR2 ligand, indicating that MyD88 plays critical roles in TLR2 signaling *(18)*. However, LPS can induce activation of NF-κB and MAPKs, albeit with delayed kinetics, in MyD88-deficient cells *(50)*, indicating that a MyD88-independent pathway exists in TLR4 signaling. In response to LPS, MyD88-deficient mice lack any responses including cytokine or NO production from macrophages and B-cell blastogenesis, and they manifest no sign of endotoxin shock *(50)*. Therefore, the biologic significance of the MyD88-independent pathway was initially, unclear.

This question was clarified through analysis with DCs. MyD88-deficient DCs, both in vitro and in vivo, showed some characteristics of maturation, i.e., enhanced expression of their costimulatory molecules including CD40 and CD86 in response to LPS *(51,52)*. Costimulatory molecules are involved in DC-T-cell interaction, and therefore these biologic responses are quite important in linking innate and adaptive immunity *(2)*. Meanwhile, cytokine production in response to LPS was completely abolished in MyD88-deficient DCs, consistent with the results from macrophages *(50)*. The results clearly demonstrate that cytokine production induced by TLR and IL-1R families is totally dependent on MyD88 and that TLR4 can induce DC maturation in a MyD88-independent manner.

5.3. Molecular Basis for the MyD88-Independent Pathway

At present, the molecular mechanism underlying the MyD88-independent pathway is not clear. C3H/HeJ-derived bone marrow DCs showed impairment of both cytokine and costimulatory molecule induction in response to LPS *(51)*. This indicates that the conserved proline residue in TLR4 is critical for both MyD88-dependent and -independent pathways and that both pathways originate from the intracytoplasmic region of TLR4. IRAK appears to be an integral component of the MyD88-dependent pathway, as IRAK activation is abolished in MyD88-deficient DCs. Furthermore, in response to LPS, TRAF6-deficient embryonic fibroblasts exhibited impaired, but still detectable levels of NF-κB activation with delayed kinetics *(53)*. Taken together, these results suggest that the MyD88-independent pathway bifurcates at the intracytoplasmic region of TLR4 but converges again at or just downstream of TRAF6 (Fig. 3).

Subtractive hybridization analysis revealed that several IFN-inducible genes, including a CXC chemokine, IFN-inducible protein-10 (IP-10) and an IFN-regulated gene-1 (IRG-1), were induced in MyD88-deficient macrophages in response to LPS *(53)*. IP-10 gene induction requires IFN regulatory factor-3 (IRF-3) *(54)*, and nuclear translocation of IRF-3 in response to LPS is observed in MyD88-deficient cells *(53)*. Therefore, it is likely that IRF-3 activation contributes to the MyD88-independent pathway. Furthermore, in response to LPS, MyD88-deficient liver macrophages, i.e., Kuppfer cells, can secrete the active form of IL-18 in a caspase 1-dependent manner *(55)*. At present, it is unclear how IRF-3 or caspase 1 is activated downstream of TLR4.

Another adapter protein, called TIR domain-containing adapter protein (TIRAP) or MyD88-adapter-like protein (MAL), was shown to be associated with TLR4 and to be involved in the MyD88-independent pathway *(56,57)*. TIRAP/MAL can also associate with and activate double-stranded RNA (dsRNA)-activated protein kinase PKR *(56)*, which was now found to be another molecular component in the MyD88-independent pathway.

5.4. DIVERSITY OF THE TLR FAMILY SIGNALING

It is quite interesting how TLR signaling is different among the family members. For example, TLR9 signaling induces similar effects to TLR4 signaling, i.e., cytokine induction and costimulatory molecule upregulation. However, in contrast to TLR4, all the effects induced by TLR9 signaling are dependent on MyD88 (Fig. 3) *(51)*. The results indicate that TLR4 and TLR9 can activate distinct signaling mechanisms, leading to similar biologic effects. The fact that TIRAP/MAL can associate with TLR4, but not with TLR9, can account for the inability for TLR9 signaling to activate the MyD88-independent pathway *(56)*. However, it remains an intriguing puzzle why cos-

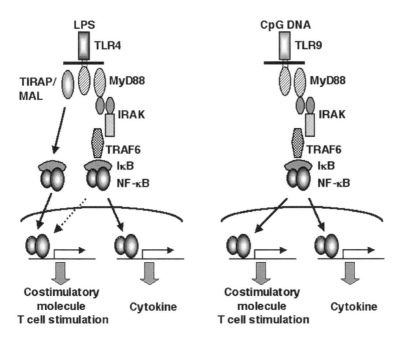

Fig. 3. TLR4 and TLR9 signaling pathways. TLR4 can activate two pathways emanating from the intracytoplasmic region of TLR4. One is the MyD88-dependent pathway, which is essential for cytokine production. The other is mediated through another adapter protein, Toll/interleukin-1 receptor domain-containing adaptor protein/macrophage activating protein (TIRAP/MAL), and can lead to upregulation of costimulatory molecules in the absence of MyD88. TLR9 signaling cannot activate the TIRAP/MAL-mediated pathway, but it can still lead to both cytokine production and upregulation of costimulatory molecules in an MyD88-dependent manner. LPS, lipopolysaccharide. For other abbreviations, see fig. 1 legend.

timulatory molecule expression is differentially regulated between TLR4 and TLR9 signaling.

As described above, TLR2 signaling requires heterodimerization with either TLR1 or TLR6. In contrast, homodimerization of TLR4 is sufficient for transducing the signal. This is another piece of evidence indicating that TIR domains among TLR family members are not equivalent. TLR2 signaling can induce activation of the Rho GTPases Rac1 and PI3K and recruitment of them to the intracytoplasmic domain of TLR2 *(58)*. Then protein kinase Akt is activated and sequentially stimulates the transactivating ability of nuclear p65. This signaling requires phosphorylation of two tyrosine residues of TLR2. However, one of two residues, located in a YXXM motif that potentially contributes to TLR2 association with PI3K, is present in TLR1, TLR2, and TLR6 but absent in TLR3, TLR4, and TLR5. This might further indicate that TLR2 signaling is distinct from other TLR signaling.

Concerning diversity of TLR signaling, TLR3 should also be mentioned. TLR3 is the only TLR family member that possesses an alanine residue instead of a conserved proline residue in the intracytoplasmic region (Fig. 1). This amino acid replacement is observed in both human and mouse TLR3. In addition to identifying the TLR3 ligand, it should also be important to clarify the signaling mechanism through TLR3.

6. CONCLUSIONS

TLR family signaling can induce a variety of adjuvant effects on various cells or tissues including macrophages, DCs, and epithelial cells. However, ligands for all TLRs have not yet been clarified. TLR ligands identified so far mainly activate DCs to produce inflammatory cytokines such as IL-12, thereby conferring the ability to support Th1 cell differentiation on DCs. DCs can be functionally divided into two subsets that are involved in instructing T-cells to differentiate into Th1 or Th2 cells. Considering the diversity of the TLR signaling pathways, it is an interesting possibility that some pathogen-derived products can induce DCs to support T_H2 cell differentiation through certain TLRs.

Most of the TLRs are ubiquitously expressed, but certain cell populations show differential expression of TLR family members. For example, TLR2 and TLR4 are expressed on monocyte-derived DCs, whereas TLR9 is expressed on plasmacytoid DCs *(59)*. Furthermore, it is possible that TLR expression is upregulated in certain inflammatory or autoimmune diseases such as Crohn's disease. Thus, it would be important to investigate the expression of TLRs not only among various cell populations but also in some pathologic conditions. Knowledge of ligands, signaling pathways, and expression patterns of TLRs should help to clarify the pathogenesis not only of infectious diseases but also of various kinds of inflammation and should facilitate the development of effective vaccination protocols.

ACKNOWLEDGMENTS

We thank our lab members and Dr. Chihiro Sasakawa for useful discussions and suggestions. This work was supported by grants from the Ministry of Education, Culture, Sports, Science, and Technology in Japan and from the Japan Science and Technology Corporation.

REFERENCES

1. Aderem A, Ulevitch RJ. Toll-like receptors in the induction of the innate immune response. Nature 2000;406:782–787.
2. Akira S, Takeda K, Kaisho T. Toll-like receptors: critical proteins linking innate and acquired immunity. Nat Immunol 2001;2:675–680.
3. Lemaitre B, Nicolas E, Michaut L, Reichhart JM, Hoffmann JA. The dorsoventral regulatory gene cassette spatzle/Toll/cactus controls the potent antifungal response in *Drosophila* adults. Cell 1996;86:973–983.
4. Williams MJ, Rodriguez A, Kimbrell DA, Eldon ED. The 18-wheeler mutation reveals complex antibacterial gene regulation in *Drosophila* host defense. EMBO J 1997;16:6120–6130.
5. Medzhitov R, Preston-Hurlburt P, Janeway CA Jr. A human homologue of the *Drosophila* Toll protein signals activation of adaptive immunity. Nature 1997;388:394–397.
6. Rock FL, Hardiman G, Timans JC, Kastelein RA, Bazan JF. A family of human receptors structurally related to *Drosophila* Toll. Proc Natl Acad Sci USA 1998;95:588–593.
7. Takeuchi O, Kawai T, Sanjo H, et al. TLR6: A novel member of an expanding toll-like receptor family. Gene 1999;231:59–65.
8. Du X, Poltorak A, Wei Y, Beutler B. Three novel mammalian toll like receptors: gene structure, expression, and evolution. Eur Cytokine Netw 2000;11:362–371.
9. Hemmi H, Takeuchi O, Kawai T, et al. A Toll-like receptor recognizes bacterial DNA. Nature 2000;408:740–745.

10. Chuang T, Ulevitch RJ. Identification of hTLR10: a novel human Toll-like receptor preferentially expressed in immune cells. Biochim Biophys Acta 2001;1518:157–161.
11. Medzhitov R, Janeway CA Jr. Innate immunity: the virtues of a nonclonal system of recognition. Cell 1997;91:295–298.
12. Sultzer BM. Genetic control of leucocyte responses to endotoxin. Nature 1968;219:1253–1254.
13. Poltorak A, He X, Smirnova I, et al. Defective LPS signaling in C3H/HeJ and C57BL/10ScCr mice: mutations in Tlr4 gene. Science 1998;282:2085–2088.
14. Qureshi ST, Lariviere L, Leveque G, et al. Endotoxin-tolerant mice have mutations in Toll-like receptor 4 (Tlr4). J Exp Med 1999;189:615–625.
15. Underhill DM, Ozinsky A, Smith KD, Aderem A. Toll-like receptor-2 mediates mycobacteria-induced proinflammatory signaling in macrophages. Proc Natl Acad Sci USA 1999;96:14459–14463.
16. Hoshino K, Takeuchi O, Kawai T, et al. Cutting edge: Toll-like receptor 4 (TLR4)-deficient mice are hyporesponsive to lipopolysaccharide: evidence for TLR4 as the Lps gene product. J Immunol 1999;162:3749–3752.
17. Takeuchi O, Hoshino K, Kawai T, et al. Differential roles of TLR2 and TLR4 in recognition of gram-negative and gram-positive bacterial cell wall components. Immunity 1999;11:443–451.
18. Takeuchi O, Kaufmann A, Grote K, et al. Cutting edge: preferentially the R-stereoisomer of the mycoplasmal lipopeptide macrophage-activating lipopeptide-2 activates immune cells through a toll-like receptor 2-and MyD88 dependent signaling pathway. J Immunol 2000;164:554–557.
19. Hirschfeld M, Ma Y, Weis JH, Vogel SN, Weis JJ. Cutting edge: repurification of lipopolysaccharide eliminates signaling through both human and murine toll-like receptor 2. J Immunol 2000;165:618–622.
20. Hirschfeld M, Weis JJ, Toshchakov V, et al. Signaling by toll-like receptor 2 and 4 agonists results in differential gene expression in murine macrophages. Infect Immun 2001;69:1477–1482.
21. Werts C, Tapping RI, Mathison JC, et al. Leptospiral lipopolysaccharide activates cells through a TLR2-dependent mechanism. Nat Immunol 2001;2:346–352.
22. Tanamoto K, Azumi S, Haishima Y, Kumada H, Umemoto T. The lipid A moiety of *Porphyromonas gingivalis* lipopolysaccharide specifically mediates the activation of C3H/HeJ mice. J Immunol 1997;158:4430–4436.
23. Steiner TS, Nataro JP, Poteet-Smith CE, Smith JA, Guerrant RL. Enteroaggregative *Escherichia coli* expresses a novel flagellin that causes IL-8 release from intestinal epithelial cells. J Clin Invest 2000;105:1769–1777.
24. Eaves-Pyles T, Murthy K, Liaudet L, et al. Flagellin, a novel mediator of *Salmonella*-induced epithelial activation and systemic inflammation: IκBα degradation, induction of nitric oxide synthase, induction of proinflammatory mediators, and cardiovascular dysfunction. J Immunol 2001;166:1248–1260.
25. Hayashi F, Smith KD, Ozinsky A, et al. The innate immune response to bacterial flagellin is mediated by Toll-like receptor-5. Nature 2001;410:1099–1103.
26. Gewirtz AT, Simon J, Schmitt CK, et al. *Salmonella typhimurium* translocates flagellin across intestinal epithelia, inducing a proinflammatory response. J Clin Invest 2001;107:99–109.
27. Gewirtz AT, Navas TA, Lyons S, Godowski PJ, Madara JL. Cutting edge: bacterial flagellin activates basolaterally expressed TLR5 to induce epithelial proinflammatory gene expression. J Immunol 2001;167:1882–1885.
28. Tokunaga T, Yamamoto H, Shimada S, et al. Antitumor activity of deoxyribonucleic acid fraction from *Mycobacterium bovis* BCG. I. Isolation, physicochemical characterization, and antitumor activity. J Natl Cancer Inst 1984;72:955–962.
29. Krieg AM, Yi AK, Matson S, et al. CpG motifs in bacterial DNA trigger direct B cell activation. Nature 1995;374:546–549.

30. Chu W, Gong X, Li Z, et al. DNA-PKcs is required for activation of innate immunity by immunostimulatory DNA. Cell 2000;103:909–918.
31. Smith GC, Jackson SP. The DNA-dependent protein kinase. Genes Dev 1999;13:916–934.
32. Kawasaki K, Akashi S, Shimazu R, et al. Mouse toll-like receptor 4.MD-2 complex mediates lipopolysaccharide-mimetic signal transduction by Taxol. J Biol Chem 2000;275:2251–2254.
33. Kurt-Jones EA, Popova L, Kwinn L, et al. Pattern recognition receptors TLR4 and CD14 mediate response to respiratory syncytial virus. Nat Immunol 2000;1:398–401.
34. Bowie A, Kiss-Toth E, Symons JA, et al. A46R and A52R from vaccinia virus are antagonists of host IL-1 and toll-like receptor signaling. Proc Natl Acad Sci USA 2000;97:10162–10167.
35. Okamura Y, Watari M, Jerud ES, et al. The EDA domain of fibronectin activates toll-like receptor 4. J Biol Chem 2001;276:10229–10233.
36. Smiley ST, King JA, Hancock WW. Fibrinogen stimulates macrophage chemokine secretion through Toll-like receptor 4. J Immunol 2001;167:2887–2894.
37. Ohashi K, Burkart V, Flohe S, Kolb H. Cutting edge: heat shock protein 60 is a putative endogenous ligand of the toll-like receptor-4 complex. J Immunol 2000;164:558–561.
38. Vabulas RM, Ahmad-Nejad P, da Costa C, et al. Endocytosed hsp60s use toll-like receptor 2 (tlr2) and tlr4 to activate the toll/interleukin-1 receptor signaling pathway in innate immune cells. J Biol Chem 2001;276:31332–31339.
39. Basu S, Binder RJ, Suto R, Anderson KM, Srivastava PK. Necrotic but not apoptotic cell death releases heat shock proteins, which deliver a partial maturation signal to dendritic cells and activate the NF-κB pathway. Int Immunol 2000;12:1539–1546.
40. Matzinger P. Tolerance, danger, and the extended family. Annu Rev Immunol 1994;12:991–1045.
41. Basu S, Binder RJ, Ramalingam T, Srivastava PK. CD91 is a common receptor for heat shock proteins gp96, hsp90, hsp70, and calreticulin. Immunity 2001;14:303–313.
42. Shimazu R, Akashi S, Ogata H, et al. MD-2, a molecule that confers lipopolysaccharide responsiveness on Toll-like receptor 4. J Exp Med 1999;189:1777–1782.
43. Viroyakosol S, Tobias PS, Kitchens RL, Kirkland TN. MD-2 binds to bacterial lipopolysaccharide. J Biol Chem, 2002;276:38044–38051.
44. Triantafilou K, Triantafilou M, Dedrick RL. A CD14-independent LPS receptor cluster. Nat Immunol 2001;2:338–345.
45. Ozinsky A, Underhill DM, Fontenot JD, et al. The repertoire for pattern recognition of pathogens by the innate immune system is defined by cooperation between toll-like receptors. Proc Natl Acad Sci USA 2000;97:13766–13771.
46. Takeuchi O, Kawai T, Muhlradt PF, et al. Discrimination of bacterial lipoproteins by Toll-like receptor 6. Int Immunol 2001;13:933–940.
47. Wyllie DH, Kiss-Toth E, Visintin A, et al. Evidence for an accessory protein function for Toll-like receptor 1 in anti-bacterial responses. J Immunol 2000;165:7125–7132.
48. Imler JL, Hoffmann JA. Toll receptors in innate immunity. Trends Cell Biol 2001;11:304–311.
49. Adachi O, Kawai T, Takeda K, et al. Targeted disruption of the MyD88 gene results in loss of IL-1-and IL-18-mediated function. Immunity 1998;9:143–150.
50. Kawai T, Adachi O, Ogawa T, Takeda K, Akira S. Unresponsiveness of MyD88-deficient mice to endotoxin. Immunity 1999;11:115–122.
51. Kaisho T, Takeuchi O, Kawai T, Hoshino K, Akira S. Endotoxin induced maturation of MyD88-deficient dendritic cells. J Immunol 2001;166:5688–5694.
52. Kaisho T, Akira S. Dendritic-cell function in Toll-like receptor-and MyD88-knockout mice. Trends Immunol 2001;22:78–83.
53. Kawai T, Takeuchi O, Fujita T, et al. Lipopolysaccharide stimulates the MyD88-independent pathway and results in activation of IRF-3 and the expression of a subset of LPS-inducible genes. J Immunol 2001;167:5887–5894.

54. Nakaya T, Sato M, Hata N, et al. Gene induction pathways mediated by distinct IRFs during viral infection. Biochem Biophys Res Commun 2001;283:1150–1156.

55. Seki E, Tsutsui H, Nakano H, et al. Lipopolysaccharide-induced IL-18 secretion from murine Kupffer cells independently of myeloid differentiation factor 88 that is critically involved in induction of production of IL-12 and IL-1beta. J Immunol 2001;166:2651–2657.

56. Horng T, Barton GM, Medzhitov R. TIRAP: an adapter molecule in the Toll signaling pathway. Nat Immunol 2001;2:835–841.

57. Fitzegerald KA, Palsson-McDermott EM, Bowie AG, et al. Mal (MyD88-adapter-like) is required for Toll-like receptor-4 signal transduction. Nature 2001;413:78–83.

58. Arbibe L, Mira JP, Teusch N, et al. Toll-like receptor 2-mediated NF-κB activation requires a Rac1-dependent pathway. Nat Immunol 2000;1:533–540.

59. Bauer S, Kirschning CJ, Hacker H, et al. Human TLR9 confers responsiveness to bacterial DNA via species-specific CpG motif recognition. Proc Natl Acad Sci USA 2001;98:9237–9242.

60. Xu Y, Tao X, Shen B, et al. Structural basis for signal transduction by the Toll/interleukin-1 receptor domains. Nature 2000;408:111–115.

61. Alexopoulou L, Holt AC, Medzhitov R, Flavell RA. Recognition of double-stranded RNA and activation of NF-κB by Toll-like receptor 3. Nature 2001;413:732–738.

62. Hemmi H, Kaisho T, Takeuchi O, et al. Small antiviral compounds activate immune cells via TLR7 MyD88-dependent signaling pathway. Nat Immunol 2002;3:196–200.

11

The Macrophage Mannose Receptor and Innate Immunity

Thiruvamoor P. Ramkumar, Djilali Hammache, and Philip D. Stahl

1. INTRODUCTION

Multilectin receptors, as the name implies, have multiple lectin domains present within a single peptide backbone. There are four known members in this class of molecules, the best studied of which is the macrophage mannose receptor (MR). This chapter discusses the structure and function of the multilectin receptors as represented by the macrophage MR and its proposed role in the innate immune response (for recent review articles on the mannose receptor, *see* refs. *1–3*).

Pathogenic organisms including bacteria, yeast, viruses, and parasitic protozoa display an array of carbohydrate structures on their surfaces. These carbohydrate structures are ideal molecular patterns that can be used to recognize the pathogens *(4)*. The class of molecules that recognize these carbohydrates structures is called lectins, which include collectins, multilectins and selectins among them. All lectins have a structurally homologous domain called the carbohydrate recognition domain (CRD). The interaction between a unique CRD and its corresponding oligosaccharide ligand is generally weak and requires the recognition of multiple oligosaccharides or multiple sites on an oligosaccharide to provide high-affinity interaction *(5)*. Formation of lectin multimers is also a frequently observed strategy to overcome the weak affinity. Lectins are also capable of recognizing sugars with various spatial arrangements, i.e., sugars coupled via different glycosidic linkages, as is common in branched oligosaccharides. Certain types of receptors, like the MR, appear to recognize only terminal sugars, and its binding seems to be unaffected by the pentultimate and other underlying sugar residues *(6)*. Microbial oligo-and polysaccharide structures are often different from those of mammalian origin, possibly reflecting the differences in their synthetic pathways and biological requirements. Among the potential targets that are recognized by CRDs are mannans, glucans, lipophosphoglycans, and glycoinositol-phospholipids with mannose, glucose, fucose or *N*-acetylglucosamine as terminal hexoses (Table 1).

In higher organisms, protection from invading pathogens is handled by two distinct yet closely coordinated defense mechanisms—the innate and the adaptive immune

From: *Infectious Disease: Innate Immunity*
Edited by: R. A. B. Ezekowitz and J. A. Hoffmann © Humana Press Inc., Totowa, NJ

Table 1
Pathogenic and Host-Derived ᴊigands for Mannose Receptor

Ligand	Reference
Bacterial	
Mycobacterium tuberculosis (lipoarabinomannan)	*71*
Klebsiella pneumoniae (capsular polysaccharide)	*72*
Pseudomonas aeruginosa	*73*
Escherichia coli	*74*
Listeria monocytogenes	Alvarez-Domingez and Stahl, unpublished observations
Fungal	
Candida albicans (mannan)	*75*
Saccharomyces cerevisiae (zymosan)	*23*
Pneumocystis carinii (gpA)	*76*
Viral	
HIV (gp 120)	*77*
Influenzavirus	*78*
Protozoan	
Leishmania donovani	*79*
Trypanosoma cruzi	*80*
Host derived	
Type I procollagen propeptide	*81*
Lysosomal hydrolases	*18*
Neutrophil myeloperoxidase	*82*
Tissue plasminogen activator	*83*
Thyrotropin and lutropin	*84*
Sialoadhesin and CD45 glycoform	*28*
Thyroglobulin	*46*

responses. The better studied of the two, the adaptive immune response, is mediated by clonally selected lymphocytes that can mount a specific response against virtually any pathogen that the host might encounter via an endless repertoire of antibodies with random specificities. However, the adaptive immune response suffers from an inherent time lag resulting from the selection and propagation of specific lymphocyte populations, before an effective systemic response can be mounted. Hence the requirement for a quiescent but rapidly triggered response that will act as the first line of host defense, a function that is served by the innate immune response.

In contrast to the adaptive response, the evolutionarily older innate immune response is activated by the recognition of pathogenic ligands by germline-encoded receptors. Almost all multicellular organisms have a remarkably conserved innate immune system and at times rely on it exclusively. Charles Janeway in 1992 *(7)* hypothesized that innate immunity is based on sensors and receptors that have been selected through evolution to recognize highly conserved and widely distributed features of common pathogens. The requirement of distinguishing self from nonself molecules places an additional level of specificity on these receptors. The invariant features on microbial pathogens are commonly referred to as pathogen-associated molecular patterns (PAMPs), and the molecules that recognize them are termed pattern recognition receptors (PRR). These PRRs have a broad ligand specificity that can recognize pathogens but may fail to discriminate between them. They are expressed by a particular subset of cells, such as macrophages, dendritic cells, and natural killer cells. They are probably also found in the epithelium and endothelium of the skin, lung, and gastrointestinal tract, since these are the sites that are immediately exposed to the environment. Upon binding to a ligand expressed on the surface of an invading microorganism, the PRRs can mediate their phagocytic uptake and/or generate intracellular signals leading to host cell activation. These signals may also play a role in activating the appropriate adaptive immune response, which details the nature of the antigens and the appropriate type of response to be induced (e.g., Th1-versus Th2-regulated effector mechanisms).

2. MR AS A MACROPHAGE MARKER

Macrophages play an important role in innate and acquired immunity, as well as in the maintenance of tissue homeostasis. These cells are found throughout the body, with varying characteristics depending on the local environment in which they differentiate. Because of the heterogeneous nature of tissue macrophages, phenotypic markers have been used extensively to characterize macrophage subpopulations and to study their differentiation and development. The heterogenous phenotype of the macrophage undoubtedly reflects distinct functional roles tailored to their tissue specificity. The expression pattern of MR is a characteristic marker of macrophages, with inflammatory macrophages showing high levels and activated macrophages showing low levels of expression *(8)*. In addition, numerous macrophage-like cells are known to express MR, although its regulation in these cell types has not been examined. Among the cell types identified as MR-expressing are retinal pigment epithelium *(9)*, osteoclasts *(10)*, mesangial cells of the kidney *(11)*, microglia *(12)*, astrocytes *(13)*, hepatic endothelial cells *(14)* and dendritic cells *(15)*.

3. MR ACTIVITY IN VIVO: *CLEARANCE AND ANTIGEN DELIVERY*

Studies on the recognition and clearance of lysosomal hydrolases *in vivo* led to the discovery of a novel oligosaccharide-specific receptor expressed in mononuclear phagocytes, specifically Kupffer cells and hepatic endothelial cells. This clearance of lysosomal enzymes was observed to be sensitive to organophosphate exposure and competition by glycoproteins with terminal *N*-acetylglucosamine *(16)*. It was also noted that in vivo clearance of RNase B was dependent on terminal mannose residues *(17)*. Further experiments showed that clearance of GlcNAc-terminal glycoproteins could be effectively competed for by mannan, mannose, fucose, and glucose, indicating a single receptor with multiple terminal sugar specificities. This receptor, subsequently called mannose receptor, was initially characterized in alveolar macrophages with neoglycoproteins as ligands *(18)*. Later, a variety of macrophage preparations, including bone marrow-derived macrophages, monocyte-derived macrophages, peritoneal macrophages, and microglia were shown to exhibit MR activity. Studies have localized MR to the spleen and almost all tissues harboring macrophages *(19)*.

Analysis of spent media taken from macrophage cultures led to the identification of a soluble form of MR, which is fully active with respect to mannose binding. The soluble mannose receptor is produced by a proteolytic clip and is present in normal sera

(20). To examine possible functions of soluble MR, Gordon and colleagues used a chimeric fusion protein that consisted of the cysteine-rich (CR) domain fused to the Fc fragment of lgG. This construct was then used to probe tissues for possible ligands. The experiments that followed identified certain forms of sialoadhesin as a possible ligand and several populations of macrophages in spleen and lymph node as possible targets. The results suggest that the soluble receptor could transport antigen to a specific subset of cells as part of the immune response against specific targets *(21).*

4. MR STRUCTURE AND FUNCTION

Sequences from proteolytic cleavage products of isolated mannose receptor from human placenta were used to screen placental and macrophage cDNA libraries to obtain the complete coding sequence *(22,23).* The primary structure of the MR gene indicates that the receptor is encoded by 30 exons *(24).* Only one potential polymorphism has been identified in the human sequences, and this polymorphism does not alter the sequence of the encoded protein molecule. Fluorescence *in situ* hybridization experiments have confirmed that MR is encoded by a single gene and is located in the short arm of chromosome 10 (10p 13) *(25),* a region that is syntenic to the proximal end of the mouse chromosome 2, where the mouse homolog is located *(26).* The primary sequence of the mature form of MR has 1438 amino acids and indicates that the receptor is a type 1 transmembrane protein. Sequence and homology analysis allows us to divide the protein into five distinct domains: the N-terminus CR domain, a fibronectin type II-like repeat, the multiple carbohydrate recognition domains, the transmembrane region, and the C-terminus cytoplasmic tail.

The CR domain is made up of 140 amino acids in the N terminus, 6 of which are cysteines; it seems to have a distinct specificity for sulphated carbohydrates. This domain has been observed to play a role in the recognition of pituitary hormones like luteinizing hormone and thyroid-stimulating hormone *(27)* and is also involved in binding sialoadhesin *(28).* The MR population that is expressed in the hepatic endothelial cells and the Kupffer cells is thought to use this affinity to influence the circulatory half-life of the hormones. Biochemical studies on the specificity of the CR region for sulphated sugars have found that *N*-glycans and chondroitin terminating with 4-SO4-GalNAc, as well as sulphated blood group chains terminating with 3-SO4-Gal, are recognized ligands. The crystal structure of this domain has recently been obtained, and the sulphate groups of the ligands are shown to form extensive hydrogen bonds with the peptide backbone and the side-chain atoms of MR *(29).* The amino acid, Trp117 seems to play an important role in the stacking of the sugar ring required for optimal binding.

The fibronectin type ll repeat domain is adjacent to the CR domain, and no significant function has as yet been assigned to this region of MR. These repeats are also found in a few other proteins like gelatinases and the cation-independent mannose 6-phosphate receptor.

C-terminal to the fibronectin domain is a tandem repeat of eight lectin sites, more commonly called carbohydrate recognition domains (CRD). MR and the other members of the family are among the only known proteins to have more than one lectin domain on the same peptide backbone (with the possible exception of the CI mannose phosphate receptor). The lectins found in the mannose receptor are C-type lectins, with an absolute requirement for calcium to facilitate sugar recognition *(30)*. The CRDs, which form a hydrophobic pocket, are about 120 amino acids each in length and are marked by two conserved cysteine residues. The crystal structure of CRD-4 has recently been solved; it is similar to the C-type CRD from mannose binding protein *(31)*. Two sets of-helixes and β-sheets seem to characterize these structures.

MR has a transmembrane domain followed by a relatively short 45, amino acid C-terminal cytoplasmic tail, which has no homology to the tails of any other known receptor. A tyrosine residue similar to that present in low-density lipoprotein (LDL) receptor and known to be critical for the localization and internalization of some endocytic receptors in clathrin-coated pits, is also seen in MR *(32)*. Deletion of the cytoplasmic tail seems to abolish the ability of the receptor to internalize ligands and to phagocytose yeast particles *(33)*. Although there are a few potential phosphorylation sites, none has yet been shown to be a target site for a cellular kinase.

5. CELL BIOLOGY

Scatchard analysis of binding of labeled mannose bovine serum albumin (man-BSA) at 4°C in rat alveolar macrophages revealed the presence of about 10^5 binding sites per cell with a K_d of about 10 nM with man-BSA as ligand *(34)*. Uptake was saturable, with increasing ligand concentrations, and uptake *vs.* time was linear at high concentrations of the ligand. Ligand bound at 4°C was sensitive to both EDTA and trypsin, but at 37°C complete receptor/ligand internalization was found to occur within 5 minutes. Internalized MRs rapidly recycle back to the plasma membrane, and this mechanism is not affected by cycloheximide, an inhibitor of protein synthesis. The reversibility of the receptor binding to its ligand is pH-dependent, and dissociation requires a pH of less than 6 *(35)*. Timed endocytosis studies have shown that the receptor with the ligand enters the endosomal fraction in minutes and that individual MRs appear to recycle many times during their lifetime ($t_{1/2} > 30$ hours). In macrophages, internalized ligands reach the lysosomes within 20 minutes *(36)*. MR has been localized to clathrin-coated vesicles, and internalization via this mechanism appears to rely on the internalization motif in the cytoplasmic tail of the receptor. Recent work also indicates that other motifs in the cytoplasmic tail of the MR may play a role in receptor recycling during endocytosis *(32)*.

MR also mediates phagocytosis by what appears to be a zipper mechanism. Particles internalized via the MR make their way to the lysosomal compartment, although the rate appears to be much slower than with particles internalized via the lgG Fc receptor (Funato and Stahl, unpublished observations). Ezekowitz and colleagues showed that COS cells expressing full-length MR efficiently internalized particles and that the cytoplasmic tail of the MR was required for internalization *(33)*. Since phagocytosis and receptor-mediated endocytosis are essentially different processes requiring different cellular proteins and exhibiting sensitivity to different inhibitors, the question of how MR can carry out both processes poses intriguing possibilities (Fig. 1). Moreover, as discussed below, MR expression and function are both highly responsive to cytokine treatment, suggesting that, apart from other functions, phagocytosis by MR is dependent on the expression and/or activation of certain proteins.

Other than the ubiquitous exon splicing and polyadenylation, no unique posttranscriptional processing is known to occur on the MR transcript. It should be noted that

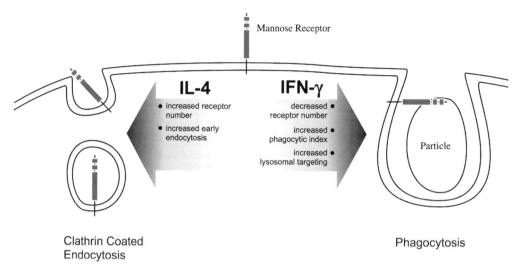

Fig. 1. Mannose receptor (MR) is both an endocytic and a phagocytic receptor. Treatment of macrophages with interleukin-4 (IL-4) elevates MR expression and enhances mannose glyco-conjugate uptake. Concomitant with elevated MR expression, the endocytic apparatus of macrophages is selectively expanded, reflecting elevated membrane traffic. Treatment of macrophages with interferon-γ (IFN-γ) results in a reduction in MR expression. Receptor-mediated endocytosis via the MR is correspondingly reduced. However, the efficiency of endocytosis via the MR (the phagocytic index) is enhanced. IFN-γ treatment, unlike IL-4 results in elevated particle sorting to the lysosomal compartment *(48)*.

there is evidence for alternative splicing of an MR-related molecule, Endo180, in fetal liver *(37)*. MR, being an integral membrane protein, is synthesized in the rough endoplasmic reticulum (ER) and is shuttled via the Golgi body to the plasma membrane. Pulse chase experiments with newly synthesized MR provide evidence for N- and O-linked oligosaccharide chain additions during maturation. An initial signal peptide cleavage step is also observed before ER docking. Sodium dodecyl sulfate polyacrylamide gel electrophoresis analysis of newly synthesized MR indicates that MR is initially synthesized as a 154-Kda. protein and is subsequently modified to a glycoprotein with an apparent mass of 165–180 Kda. The initially synthesized form of MR is inactive and unable to bind to ligands. An activation event, which may involve the formation of disulphide bonds, is required for MR to gain competency for ligand binding. Kinetic studies indicate that the half-life for acquiring normal physiologic activity following synthesis in the ER is about 40 minutes *(38)*.

6. BINDING PROPERTIES

MR was initially characterized by its ability to endocytose lysosomal enzymes and glycoproteins in a sugar-specific manner *(18,39)*. The terminal sugar moieties determine the affinity of MR for a glycosyl group. MR was also found to have a high affinity for L-fucose and then mannose, GlcNAc, glucose, and D-xylose, in that order *(40)*. It was also determined that galactose, L-arabinose, and D-fucose were unable to inhibit MR binding. Along with the terminal sugar itself, the glycosidic linkages seem to influence binding too. α1-6 mannan has a higher affinity for mannose receptor than α1-2 or α1-3 mannan *(41)*. Experiments comparing branched and linear oligosaccharides show a marked preference for branched glycosyl groups, while two terminal mannoses provided high-affinity binding *(42)*. A methyl modification of mannose increases affinity by five-fold, which suggests hydrophobic interactions as part of the mechanism of recognition. Experiments performed with partial MR constructs, containing various sections of the eight tandem CRDs, show that not all CRDs are similar in their affinities to sugars. An MR construct with the N-terminal CR and FN domains deleted was still able to endocytose *(43)*. A soluble construct containing only CRD4–8 retained mannose binding activity at levels similar to those of the endogenous receptor, whereas CRD1–3 were incapable of binding to a mannose-Sepharose column.

Further delineation of the CRDs showed that CRD4 alone was able to bind mannose-BSA in a calcium-dependent manner but with significantly reduced affinity. Additional experiments indicated that the central binding activity is mediated by CRD4 and CRD5, whereas CRD6–8 provide stability to the complex and enhance affinity. CRD1–3 seem to provide no detectable binding activity to the receptor *(44)*. The binding of sugar to CRD4 has been shown to be completely dependent on calcium *(45)*. It has been suggested that CRD4, mannose, and calcium form a ternary structure that stabilizes the interaction, similar to that observed with mannose binding protein A. Moreover, site-directed mutagenesis of the residue involved in binding calcium seems to obliterate sugar binding. Apart from the nature of ligand binding, an important question is the identity of natural ligands for the MR. Linehan et al. *(46)* have used a CRD4-7Fc chimera construct to identify MR ligands in various tissues. They found that many secretory cells were enriched in MR ligand, e.g., thyroglobulin, and that interstitial macrophages were always found in close proximity to such secretory cells, suggesting that MR may function in secretory product uptake.

7. REGULATION OF EXPRESSION

Cytokines have been shown to regulate the expression of MR in cultured macrophages. The interleukins IL-4 and IL-13 are strong stimulators of MR expression. Mouse peritoneal macrophages treated with IL-4 show a 10-fold increase in MR expression and a 15-fold increase in endocytosis, whereas IL-13 is slightly less effective *(8,47)*. Another Th2-derived cytokine, IL-10, seems to reduce the MR-mediated endocytosis in monocyte-derived macrophages. Strangely, the same molecule increases MR-mediated endocytosis and increases MR expression in dendritic cells *(48)*. The Th1 cytokine interferon-γ (IFN-γ) downregulates MR expression and endocytosis in both human and mouse macrophages *(49)*. Surprisingly, in spite of this downregulation in expression, IFN-γ seems to increase the phagocytic capacity of treated monocyte-derived macrophages *(50)*. During macrophage differentiation, addition of IgG2 increased MR expression in the early stages of the cultures but had no effect on MR expression when the cultures had terminally differentiated. This effect was found to be both isotype and subclass-specific *(51)*, hinting that this observation could be physiologically relevant as a mechanism by which IgG-secreting B-lymphocytes may control MR expression in macrophage populations. The active form of vitamin D has also been shown to promote differentiation of macrophages and to upregulate MR expression in the process *(52)*. Prostaglandin E is (PGE) another cellular factor that may drive macrophage differentiation; it has been found to up-regulate MR expression dramatically in mouse but not human cells (Pontow and Stahl, unpublished observations) *(53)*. PGE induced MR expression 2–3 days earlier than untreated controls, which could be physiologically relevant in the mouse bone marrow. The steroid dexamethasone has been shown to increase MR expression at the transcription level *(49)*.

Lipopolysaccharides (LPS) are one of the most potent inhibitors of MR activity, and in conjunction with phorbol myristate acetate (PMA) can reduce the available surface receptors by 70% *(54)*. Not surprisingly, MR-mediated endocytosis is also downregulated by exposure to infectious agents like *Leishmania donovani* and *Candida albicans* *(55,56)*. It is interesting to note that hydrogen peroxide treatment can cause a reduction of up to 80% in MR-mediated endocytosis within 30 minutes, and this effect has been linked to the inability of MR to recycle to the cell surface *(57)*. A probable explanation is the susceptibility of the MR-ligand dissociation to the presence of oxidative species.

MR is a phagocytic receptor responsible for the uptake of *Pneumocystis carinii* and a variety of other pathogen-bearing MR ligands *(58)*. Several papers have appeared suggesting that engagement of MR via the phagocytic route activates a signal transduction pathway leading to cytokine production *(59–62)*. It is not unique for a scavenger receptor to engage a signal transduction pathway. LDL receptors have been reported to activate a signal transduction pathway and the phospholipase A2 (PLA$_2$) receptor, a member of the MR family of receptors, clearly does activate transcriptional events following ligand binding *(63)*. Toll receptors, charter members of the innate immune system, clearly are signal-generating units. The fact that MR only transmits a signal when in the phagocytic mode is unique and suggests that MR is a multifunctional receptor.

8. MR FAMILY OF MULTILECTIN RECEPTORS

The MR family now consists of four members (Fig. 2). The PLA$_2$ receptor was first identified in 1995 and was subsequently cloned by two groups *(64,65)*. The PLA$_2$-receptor (R) is topologically very similar to the MR and shares about 30% identity in overall sequence. The only known ligand for PLA$_2$-R is PLA$_2$ (which surprisingly has no covalently bound sugar). A large group of secretory PLAs exist that have been placed in as many as 10 groups. Only a few of these have been identified as ligands for PLA$_2$-R. PLA$_2$ appears to bind to CRD5 on the PLA$_2$-R molecule. Importantly, interaction of PLA$_2$ with PLA$_2$-R leads to a signal transduction event that results in the production of arachidonic acid (unrelated to the enzymatic activity of the ligand). A targeted knockout of the PLA$_2$-R knockout has been reported, and the phenotype shows increased sensitivity to endotoxin *(66)*. Localization of PLA$_2$-R has not been determined with any degree of specificity. Although initially identified in muscle, it is known that many different cell types respond to added PLA$_2$, suggesting that the receptor is widely expressed *(67)*.

Endo 180, the third member of the MR family, was initially cloned by Lasky and colleagues in the mouse *(37)*. Subsequently, lssacke and coworkers *(68)*, based on earlier work with a specific monoclonal antibody (Endo 180), and Behrendt et al. *(69)*, using chemical crosslinking coupling to mass spectrometry, identified the human gene product. The latter group found the receptor to exist in a complex with urokinase plasminogen-activated receptor (uPAR) the receptor for plasminogen activator that is a glycosylphosphatidyl inositol (GPI)-linked membrane protein. Ligands for endo

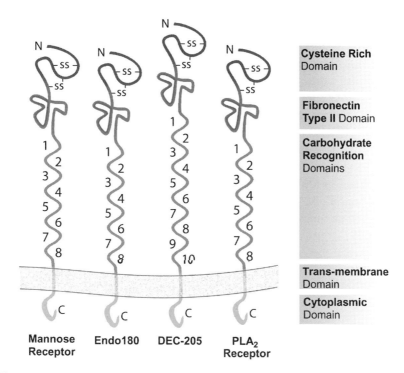

Fig. 2. The mannose receptor family of receptors. The mannose receptor is the prototype of a new family of proteins currently made up of four members. The family includes (1) the mannose receptor, (2) the receptor for secretory phospholipase A2 (PLA$_2$R), (3) DEC-205, which functions in the internalization of the antigens for processing and presentation in dendritic cells, and (4) Endo 180/uPARAP, the newest member, which is associated with the urokinase-type plasminogen activator receptor and recognizes *N*-acetylglucosamine moieties. The MR family of receptors are type 1 membrane proteins that are very similar in overall structural organization, with high homology at the amino acid level in certain regions. Sequence and homology studies have delineated distinct domains, and a consensus structure predicts the presence of an N-terminal cysteine-rich (CR) domain, a fibronectin type II (FNII)-like domain, a variable number of carbohydrate recognition domains (CRDs), a transmembrane region, and a short cytoplasmic tail. The latter possesses a tyrosine-based internalization motif.

180/uPAR associated protein (uPARAP) include *N*-acetylglucosamine-derivitized proteins. Endo180/uPAR is widely expressed in the endothelium, and some evidence exists for its expression in macrophages, trophoblasts, and chondrocytes.

DEC-205 is the fourth member of the MR family. Apart from having 10 CRDs, 2 more than the other members of the family, DEC-205 is topologically very similar to MR *(70)*. DEC205 appears to be exclusively expressed in dendritic cells and is thought to mediate the uptake of glycosylated antigens, although no ligand specific for any of the CRDs in DEC-205 has been identified.

9. FUTURE DIRECTIONS

The MR family of endocytosis receptors represents, it would appear, an important arm of the innate immune system. At the present time, there are four known members of the MR family, expressed by a variety of cell types. The primary function of the MR receptor family is to identify, bind, and internalize macromolecular ligands bearing determinants that mark them either as foreign or as intracellular proteins that have been misrouted to the extracellular compartment (e.g., lysosomal enzymes). The library of MR family ligands is quite small at the present time, but it could be substantial considering that among the four known receptors there are potentially as many as 42 recognition sites (34 CRDs, 4 FNII repeats, and 4 CR domains). It is also possible that individual receptors could form macromolecular aggregates or couple with other proteins in the plasma membrane, as has been reported for uPARAP/endo 180, to generate additional ligand-specific binding sites. Furthermore, it is conceivable that additional members of the family, as yet unidentified, exist in the higher eukaryote genome. Since MRs are part of an innate immune system, several functions may be attached to the MR family: clearing or scavenging proteins, glycoproteins, and complex glycoconjugates from the extracellular compartment; (2) phagocytosis of pathogens and other particulate matter; (3) activating or modulating gene expression of host defense factors; (4) providing cell-cell recognition during development; and (4) participating in adaptive immunity via endocytosis of antigens and the transport of antigens via soluble receptor to the spleen or lymph nodes.

REFERENCES

1. Stahl PD, Ezekowitz RA. The mannose receptor is a pattern recognition receptor involved in host defense. Curr Opin Immunol 1998;10:50–55.
2. Linehan SA, Martinez-Pomares L, Gordon S. Macrophage lectins in host defence. Microbes Infect 2000;2:279–288.
3. Taylor ME. Structure and function of the macrophage mannose receptor. Results Probl Cell Differ 2001;33:105–121.
4. Medzhitov R, Janeway CA Jr. Innate immunity: impact on the adaptive immune response. Curr Opin Immunol 1997;9:4–9.
5. Hille-Rehfeld A. Mannose 6-phosphate receptors in sorting and transport of lysosomal enzymes. Biochim Biophys Acta 1995;1241:177–194.
6. Stahl PD, Wileman TE, Diment S, Shepherd VL. Mannose-specific oligosaccharide recognition by mononuclear phagocytes. Biol Cell 1984;51:215–218.
7. Janeway CA Jr. The immune system evolved to discriminate infectious nonself from noninfectious self. Immunol Today 1992;13:11–16.
8. Doyle AG, Herbein G, Montaner LJ, et al. Interleukin-13 alters the activation state of murine macrophages in vitro: comparison with interleukin-4 and interferon-gamma. Eur J Immunol 1994;24;1441–1445.
9. McLaughlin BJ, Tarnowski BI, Shepherd VL. Identification of mannose 6-phosphate and mannose receptors in dystrophic and normal retinal pigment epithelium. Prog Clin Biol Res 1987;247:243–257.
10. Palokangas H, Mulari M, Vaananen HK. Endocytic pathway from the basal plasma membrane to the ruffled border membrane in bone-resorbing osteoclasts. J Cell Sci 1997;110:1767–1780.
11. Liu ZH, Striker GE, Stetler-Stevenson M, et al. TNF-alpha and IL-1 alpha induce mannose receptors and apoptosis in glomerular mesangial but not endothelial cells. Am J Physiol 1996;270:C1595–601.
12. Marzolo MP, von Bernhardi R, Inestrosa NC. Mannose receptor is present in a functional state in rat microglial cells. J Neurosci Res 1999;58:387–395.

13. Burudi EM, Riese S, Stahl PD, Regnier-Vigouroux A. Identification and functional characterization of the mannose receptor in astrocytes. Glia 1999;25:44–55.
14. Seydel W, Stang E, Roos N, Krause J. Endocytosis of the recombinant tissue plasminogen activator alteplase by hepatic endothelial cells. Arzneimittelforschung 1991;41:182–186.
15. Dong X, Storkus WJ, Salter RD. Binding and uptake of agalactosyl IgG by mannose receptor on macrophages and dendritic cells. J Immunol 1999;163:5427–5434.
16. Stahl P, Schlesinger PH, Rodman JS, Doebber T. Recognition of lysosomal glycosidases in vivo inhibitied by modified glycoproteins. Nature 1976;264:86–88.
17. Baynes JW, Wold F. Effect of glycosylation on the in vivo circulating half-life of ribonuclease. J Biol Chem 1976;251:6016–6024.
18. Stahl PD, Rodman JS, Miller MJ, Schlesinger PH. Evidence for receptor-mediated binding of glycoproteins, glycoconjugates, and lysosomal glycosidases by alveolar macrophages. Proc Natl Acad Sci USA 1978;75:1399–1403.
19. Linehan SA, Martinez-Pomares L, Stahl PD, Gordon S. Mannose receptor and its putative ligands in normal murine lymphoid and nonlymphoid organs: in situ expression of mannose receptor by selected macrophages, endothelial cells, perivascular microglia, and mesangial cells, but not dendritic cells. J Exp Med 1999;189:1961–1972.
20. Martinez-Pomares L, Mahoney JA, Kaposzta R, et al. A functional soluble form of the murine mannose receptor is produced by macrophages in vitro and is present in mouse serum. J Biol Chem 1998;273:23376–23380.
21. Martinez-Pomares L, Gordon S. Potential role of the mannose receptor in antigen transport. Immunol Lett 1999;65:9–13.
22. Taylor ME, Conary JT, Lennartz MR, Stahl PD, Drickamer K. Primary structure of the mannose receptor contains multiple motifs resembling carbohydrate-recognition domains. J Biol Chem 1990;265:12156–12162.
23. Ezekowitz RA, Sastry K, Bailly P, Warner A. Molecular characterization of the human macrophage mannose receptor: demonstration of multiple carbohydrate recognition-like domains and phagocytosis of yeasts in Cos-1 cells. J Exp Med 1990;172:1785–1794.
24. Kim SJ, Ruiz N, Bezouska K, Drickamer K. Organization of the gene encoding the human macrophage mannose receptor (MRC1). Genomics 1992;14:721–727.
25. Eichbaum Q, Clerc P, Bruns G, McKeon F, Ezekowitz RA. Assignment of the human macrophage mannose receptor gene (MRC1) to 10p13 by in situ hybridization and PCR-based somatic cell hybrid mapping. Genomics 1994;22:656–658.
26. Harris N, Peters LL, Eicher EM, et al. The exon-intron structure and chromosomal localization of the mouse macrophage mannose receptor gene Mrc1: identification of a Ricin-like domain at the N-terminus of the receptor. Biochem Biophys Res Commun 1994;198:682–692.
27. Roseman DS, Baenziger JU. Molecular basis of lutropin recognition by the mannose/GalNAc-4-SO4 receptor. Proc Natl Acad Sci USA 2000;97:9949–9954.
28. Martinez-Pomares L, Crocker PR, Da Silva R et al. Cell-specific glycoforms of sialoadhesin and CD45 are counter-receptors for the cysteine-rich domain of the mannose receptor. J Biol Chem 1999;274:35211–35218.
29. Liu Y, Misulovin Z, Bjorkman PJ. The molecular mechanism of sulfated carbohydrate recognition by the cysteine-rich domain of mannose receptor. J Mol Biol 2001; 305:481–490.
30. Lennartz MR, Wileman TE, Stahl PD. Isolation and characterization of a mannose-specific endocytosis receptor from rabbit alveolar macrophages. Biochem J 1987; 245:705–711.
31. Feinberg H, Park-Snyder S, Kolatkar AR, et al. Structure of a C-type carbohydrate recognition domain from the macrophage mannose receptor. J Biol Chem 2000; 275:21539–21548.
32. Schweizer A, Stahl PD, Rohrer J. A di-aromatic motif in the cytosolic tail of the mannose receptor mediates endosomal sorting. J Biol Chem 2000; 275:29694–29700.

33. Kruskal BA, Sastry K, Warner AB, Mathieu CE, Ezekowitz RA. Phagocytic chimeric receptors require both transmembrane and cytoplasmic domains from the mannose receptor. J Exp Med 1992; 176:1673–1680.

34. Stahl P, Schlesinger PH, Sigardson E, Rodman JS, Lee YC. Receptor-mediated pinocytosis of mannose glycoconjugates by macrophages: characterization and evidence for receptor recycling. Cell 1980; 19:207–215.

35. Tietze C, Schlesinger P, Stahl P. Mannose-specific endocytosis receptor of alveolar macrophages: demonstration of two functionally distinct intracellular pools of receptor and their roles in receptor recycling. J Cell Biol 1982; 92:417–424.

36. Wileman T, Boshans RL, Schlesinger P, Stahl P. Monesin inhibits recycling of macrophage mannose-glycoprotein receptors and ligand delivery to lysosomes. Biochem J 1984; 220:665–675.

37. Wu K, Yuan J, Lasky LA. Characterization of a novel member of the macrophage mannose receptor type C lectin family. J Biol Chem 1996; 271:21323–21330.

38. Pontow SE, Blum JS, Stahl PD. Delayed activation of the mannose receptor following synthesis. Requirement for exit from the endoplasmic reticulum. J Biol Chem 1996; 271:30736–30740.

39. Hubbard AL, Stukenbrok H. An electron microscope autoradiographic study of the carbohydrate recognition systems in rat liver. II. Intracellular fates of the 125l-ligands. J Cell Biol 1979; 83:65–81.

40. Shepherd VL, Lee YC, Schlesinger PH, Stahl PD. L-Fucose-terminated glycoconjugates are recognized by pinocytosis receptors on macrophages. Proc Natl Acad Sci USA 1981; 78:1019–1022.

41. Achord DT, Brot FE, Bell CE, Sly WS. Human beta-glucuronidase: in vivo clearance and in vitro uptake by a glycoprotein recognition system on reticuloendothelial cells. Cell 1978; 15:269–278.

42. Kery V, Krepinsky JJ, Warren CD, Capek P, Stahl PD. Ligand recognition by purified human mannose receptor. Arch Biochem Biophys 1992; 298:49–55.

43. Taylor ME, Drickamer K. Expression and purification of the cytoplasmic tail of an endocytic receptor by fusion to a carbohydrate-recognition domain. Protein Expr Purif 1992; 3:308–312.

44. Taylor ME, Drickamer K. Structural requirements for high affinity binding of complex ligands by the macrophage mannose receptor. J Biol Chem 1993; 268:399–404.

45. Mullin NP, Hall KT, Taylor ME. Characterization of ligand binding to a carbohydrate-recognition domain of the macrophage mannose receptor. J Biol Chem 1994; 269:28405–28413.

46. Linehan SA, Martinez-Pomares L, da Silva RP, Gordon S. Endogenous ligands of carbohydrate recognition domains of the mannose receptor in murine macrophages, endothelial cells and secretory cells; potential relevance to inflammation and immunity. Eur J Immunol 2001; 31:1857–1866.

47. Stein M, Keshave S, Harris N, Gordon S. Interleukin 4 potently enhances murine macrophage mannose receptor activity: a marker of alternative immunologic macrophage activation. J Exp Med 1992; 176:287–292.

48. Montaner LJ, da Silva RP, Sun J, et al. Type 1 and type 2 cytokine regulation of macrophage endocytosis: differential activation by IL-4/IL-13 as opposed to IFN-gamma or IL-10. J Immunol 1999; 162:4606–4613.

49. Mokoena T, Gordon S. Human macrophage activation. Modulation of mannosyl, fucosyl receptor activity in vitro by lymphokines, gamma and alpha interferons, and dexamethasone. J Clin Invest 1985; 75:624–631.

50. Marodi L, Johnston RB Jr. Enhancement of macrophage candidacidal activity by interferon-gamma. Immunodeficiency 1993; 4:181–185.

51. Schreiber S, Blum JS, Stenson WF, et al. Monomeric IgG2a promotes maturation of bone-marrow macrophages and expression of the mannose receptor. Proc Natl Acad Sci USA 1991; 88:1616–1620.

52. Clohisy DR, Bar-Shavit Z, Chappel JC, Teitelbaum SL. 1,25-Dihydroxyvitamin D3 modulates bone marrow macrophage precursor proliferation and differentiation. Up-regulation of the mannose receptor. J Biol Chem 1987; 262:15922–15929.

53. Schreiber S, Perkins SL, Teitelbaum SL, et al. Regulation of mouse bone marrow macrophage mannose receptor expression and activation by prostaglandin E and IFN-gamma. J Immunol 1993; 151:4973–4981.

54. Shepherd VL, Abdolrasulnia R, Garrett M, Cowan HB. Down-regulation of mannose receptor activity in macrophages after treatment with lipopolysaccharide and phorbol esters. J Immunol 1990; 145:1530–1536.

55. Basu N, Sett R, Das PK. Down-regulation of mannose receptors on macrophages after infection with *Leishmania donovani.* Biochem J 1991; 277:451–456.

56. Shepherd VL, Lane KB, Abdolrasulnia R. Ingestion of *Candida albicans* down-regulates mannose receptor expression on rat macrophages. Arch Biochem Biophys 1997; 344:350–356.

57. Bozeman PM, Hoidal JR, Shepherd VL. Oxidant-mediated inhibition of ligand uptake by the macrophage mannose receptor. J Biol Chem 1988; 263:1240–1247.

58. Ezekowitz RA, Williams DJ, Koziel H, et al. Uptake of *Pneumocystis carinii* mediated by the macrophage mannose receptor. Nature 1991; 351:155–158.

59. Yamamoto Y, Klein TW, Friedman H. Involvement of mannose receptor in cytokine interleukin-1beta (IL-1beta), IL-6, and granulocyte-macrophage colony-stimulating factor responses, but not in chemokine macrophage inflammatory protein 1beta (MIP-1beta), MIP-2, and KC responses, caused by attachment of *Candida albicans* to macrophages. Infect Immun 1997; 65:1077–1082.

60. Shibata Y, Metzger WJ, Myrvik QN. Chitin particle-induced cell-mediated immunity is inhibited by soluble mannan: mannose receptor-mediated phagocytosis initiates IL-12 production. J Immunol 1997; 159:2462–2467.

61. Nigou J, Zelle-Rieser C, Gilleron M, Thurnher M, Puzo G. Mannosylated lipoarabinomannans inhibit IL-12 production by human dendritic cells: evidence for a negative signal delivered through the mannose receptor. J Immunol 2001; 166:7477–7485.

62. Fonteh AN, Atsumi G, Porte T, Chilton FH. Secretory phospholipase A2 receptor-mediated activation of cytosolic phospholipase A2 in murine bone marrow-derived mast cells. J Immunol 2000; 165:2773–2782.

63. Triggiani M, Granata F, Oriente A, et al. Secretory phospholipases A2 induce beta-glucuronidase release and IL-6 production from human lung macrophages. J Immunol 2000; 164:4908–4915.

64. Arita H, Hanasaki K. Physiological aspects of a high affinity binding site for pancreatic-type phospholipase A2. J Lipid Mediat 1993; 6:217–222.

65. Lambeau G, Ancian P, Barhanin J, Lazdunski M. Cloning and expression of a membrane receptor for secretory phospholipases A2. J Biol Chem 1994; 269:1575–1578.

66. Hanasaki K, Yokota Y, Ishizaki J, Itoh T, Arita H. Resistance to endotoxic shock in phospholipase A2 receptor-deficient mice. J Biol Chem 1997; 272:32792–32797.

67. Hanasaki K, Arita H. Biological and pathological functions of phospholipase A(2) receptor. Arch Biochem Biophys 1999; 372:215–223.

68. Sheikh H, Yarwood H, Ashworth A, Isacke CM. Endo180, an endocytic recycling glycoprotein related to the macrophage mannose receptor is expressed on fibroblasts, endothelial cells and macrophages and functions as a lectin receptor. J Cell Sci 2000; 113:1021–1032.

69. Behrendt N, Jensen ON, Engelholm LH, et al. A urokinase receptor-associated protein with specific collagen binding properties. J Biol Chem 2000; 275:1993–2002.

70. Jiang W, Swiggard WJ, Heufler C, et al. The receptor DEC-205 expressed by dendritic cells and thymic epithelial cells is involved in antigen processing. Nature 1995; 375:151–155.

71. Kang BK, Schlesinger LS. Characterization of mannose receptor-dependent phagocytosis mediated by *Mycobacterium tuberculosis* lipoarabinomannan. Infect Immun 1998; 66:2769–2777.
72. Ofek I, Crouch E, Keisari Y. The role of C-type lectins in the innate immunity against pulmonary pathogens. Adv Exp Med Biol 2000; 479:27–36.
73. Speert DP, Wright SD, Silverstein SC, Mah B. Functional characterization of macrophage receptors for in vitro phagocytosis of unopsonized *Pseudomonas aeruginosa*. J Clin Invest 1998; 82:872–879.
74. Felipe I, Bochio EE, Martins NB, Pacheco C. Inhibition of macrophage phagocytosis of *Escherichia coli* by mannose and mannan. Braz J Med Biol Res 1991; 24:919–924.
75. Marodi L, Korchak HM, Johnston RB Jr. Mechanisms of host defense against *Candida* species. I. Phagocytosis by monocytes and monocyte-derived macrophages. J Immunol 1991; 146:2783–2789.
76. O'Riordan DM, Standing JE, Limper AH. *Pneumocystis carinii* glycoprotein A binds macrophage mannose receptors. Infect Immun 1995; 63:779–784.
77. Curtis BM, Scharnowske S, Watson AJ. Sequence and expression of a membrane-associated C-type lectin that exhibits CD4-independent binding of human immunodeficiency virus envelope glycoprotein gp120. Proc Natl Acad Sci USA 1992; 89:8356–8360.
79. Chakraborty P, Bhaduri AN, Das PK. Neoglycoproteins as carriers for receptor-mediated drug targeting in the treatment of experimental visceral leishmaniasis. J Protozool 1990; 37:358–364.
80. Soeiro M, Paiva MM, Barbosa HS, Meirelles Mde N, Araujo-Jorge TC. A cardiomyocyte mannose receptor system is involved in *Trypanosoma cruzi* invasion and is down-modulated after infection. Cell Struct Funct 1999; 24:139–149.
81. Smedsrod B, Melkko J Risteli L, Risteli J. Circulating C-terminal propeptide of type I procollagen is cleared mainly via the mannose receptor in liver endothelial cells. Biochem J 1990; 271:345–350.
82 Shepherd VL, Hoidal JR. Clearance of neutrophil-derived myeloperoxidase by the macrophage mannose receptor. Am J Respir Cell Mol Biol 1990; 2:335–340.
83 Smedsrod B, Einarsson M. Clearance of tissue plasminogen activator by mannose and galactose receptors in the liver. Thromb Haemost 1990; 63:60–66.
84 Fiete DJ, Beranek MC, Baenziger JU. A cysteine-rich domain of the "mannose" receptor mediates GalNAc-4-SO4 binding. Proc Natl Acad Sci USA 1998; 95:2089–2093.

12
Diverse Roles of Lung Collectins in Pulmonary Innate Immunity

Erika C. Crouch and Jeffrey A. Whitsett

1. INTRODUCTION

The lung is constantly challenged by a wide variety of infectious agents, organic antigens, and other potentially toxic substances. The relative infrequency of serious or life-threatening infections and lung injury among otherwise normal individuals demonstrates the efficiency of the lung's system of host defense and immune and inflammatory regulation. Consistent with the diversity of potential challenges, this defense system is complex and multilayered and includes anatomic and cellular components, as well as secreted molecules of the natural and acquired immune system. The airways and airspaces of the lung are lined by a biochemically and functionally heterogenous material that is ideally positioned to participate in the ongoing process of neutralization and clearance of inhaled microorganisms and the "detoxification" of other injurious substances. Two important components of this innate and natural defense system are surfactant protein A (SP-A) and surfactant protein D (SP-D) *(1–5)*.

The goal of this review is to examine the roles of SP-A and SP-D in pulmonary innate immunity. Particular emphasis is placed on integrating the in vitro biologic activities of these proteins, with alterations in the host response observed in the context of in vivo models of microbial or antigenic challenge, lung injury, and collectin deficiency. The roles of collectins in the general processes of microbial clearance and neutralization, as well as regulation of the inflammatory and oxidant response to microbial challenge, is examined.

In the initial sections we summarize what is currently known about collectin structure and biosynthesis. We also briefly review the in vitro interactions of these molecules with various classes of ligands, including microorganisms, and their interactions with ligands or receptors expressed on host cells. The remainder of the chapter attempts to integrate in vitro and in vivo findings within the context of selected model systems.

2. OVERVIEW

The lung collectins are now recognized as members of a growing family of collagenous C-type lectins that also includes serum mannose binding lectin (MBL; also

From: *Infectious Disease: Innate Immunity*
Edited by: R. A. B. Ezekowitz and J. A. Hoffmann © Humana Press Inc., Totowa, NJ

known as mannose binding protein). In ruminants there are at least two additional serum collectins (conglutinin and CL-43) *(1,4,6)* and a novel intracellular collectin, CL-L1 *(7)*. Significantly, all the secreted collectins demonstrate calcium-dependent lectin activity and show potential host-defense activities in vitro *(5)*.

2.1. Historical Perspective

SP-A was first identified as the major surfactant-associated protein. It is a component of airspace tubular myelin, is isolated from the lung in association with surfactant lipids, and can modify the surface-active properties of isolated surfactant. Although in vitro studies supported the concept that SP-A influenced the uptake and secretion of surfactant phospholipids by alveolar type II cells *(8)*, in vivo studies do not support a major role for SP-A in surfactant lipid homeostasis or function. A few early studies described interactions with microorganisms or phagocytic cells, but most papers published prior to the development of transgenic models of SP-A deficiency in the mid-1990s emphasized potential roles in surfactant function or homeostasis. However, interest in host defense functions rapidly grew with the realization that SP-A null mice showed no readily discernible respiratory impairment or surfactant abnormality *(9,10)* but had impaired responses to various microorganisms *(11–18)*.

By contrast, SP-D was first identified as an SP-A-like, collagenous glycoprotein (CP4) that is secreted as a soluble protein by isolated rat alveolar epithelial cells *(19,20)*. Although a fraction of lung SP-D is isolated in association with surfactant, early studies suggested no role in regulating surface activity in vitro, and roles in host defense were proposed based on the capacity to bind and aggregate Gram-negative bacteria *(21)*. Thus, most papers published prior to the development of transgenic models of SP-D deficiency in the late-1990s emphasized these potential host defense roles. General interest among lung biologists increased significantly with the discovery that SP-D null mice develop a marked alveolar lipoidosis *(22–24)* and emphysema *(25)*, suggesting roles in surfactant metabolism and inflammatory regulation, respectively. However, consistent with the abundant in vitro data, SP-D-deficient animals also show abnormal responses to microbial challenge attributable to the absence of SP-D *(13,26)*.

2.2. Sites of Collectin Expression and Accumulation

The lung collectins are synthesized and secreted into the pulmonary airspaces and airways by alveolar type II cells and subsets of bronchiolar epithelial cells *(1)*. In some species SP-A is also expressed in submucosal glands in the trachea, eustachian tube, and possibly a few other tissue sites *(27,28)*. By contrast, there is evidence that SP-D is widely expressed at many epithelial sites including the upper airways, tracheal-bronchial glands, and oropharynx *(29)*. Although both proteins are isolated from lung washings, they may not be microanatomically codistributed in vivo. Most of the SP-A is isolated from the lung in association with surfactant lipid and is a component of tubular myelin *(8)*, whereas a large fraction of the SP-D is recovered as a "soluble" protein *(1)*.

2.3. Evolutionary Relationships

Both proteins probably evolved through exon shuffling and gene duplication events involving primordial collagen cassettes and C-type lectin domains *(30)*. In this regard,

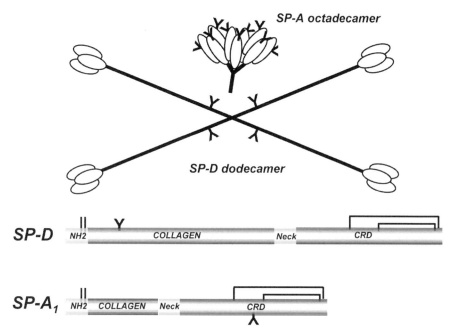

Fig. 1. Structure of lung collectins. Schematic diagrams of lung collectin monomers and molecules are shown. Each protein has an amino-terminal (NH_2-) crosslinking domain, a collagenous domain, a neck or linking domain, and a C-type lectin carbohydrate recognition domain (CRD). The sites of N-linked glycosylation (Y) in human SP-A and SP-D and the positions of intrachain disulfide crosslinks that stablize the CRD are indicated. SP-A is predominantly assembled as 18-chain molecules consisting of six homo- or heterotrimers. SP-D is preferentially assembled as 12-chain molecules consisting of four homotrimeric molecules. The two proteins show marked differences in the spatial distribution of trimeric CRDs. Accordingly, they have very different capacities to participate in bridging interactions between spatially separated ligands.

the genes for SP-A, SP-D, and MBL occupy a "collectin locus" on the long arm of human chromosome 10 *(31)*, and these genes are similarly clustered in the genome of at least some other species. SP-A is expressed in mammals, reptiles, amphibians, and birds, as well as by actinopterygiian fish and lungfish *(32)*. Interestingly, SP-A was also identified in the swimbladder of goldfish, consistent with roles independent of respiratory function. Humans and some other mammals have two SP-A genes. However, a single SP-D gene has been identified in mammals—from mouse to human—and in birds and amphibians *(33)*. Conglutinin and CL-43 are believed to have evolved from SP-D through gene duplication in ruminants *(4)*. The C-type lectin domain is of course much older in evolutionary terms; for example, at least 19 proteins with a similar C-type lectin domain are encoded in the genome of *Caenorhabditis elegans (34)*.

2.4. Collectin Structure

The minimum functional unit of each collectin is a trimer *(35)*, which confers high-affinity saccharide binding. Each trimeric subunit consists of a short, amino-terminal crosslinking domain; a triple helical collagenous domain; a trimeric coiled-coil linking or neck domain; and a mannose-subtype, C-type lectin carbohydrate recognition domain (CRD) *(6)* (Fig. 1). The amino-terminal association and crosslinking of trimeric subunits permits bridging interactions between spatially separated ligands.

All the known, secreted collectins fall into two structurally distinct families, one resembling SP-A and the other related to SP-D. SP-A and MBL ultrastructurally resemble C1q and are characterized by relatively short and interrupted collagen domains and the propensity to form bouquet-like octamers of trimeric subunits (18 chains). By contrast, SP-D and the evolutionarily related bovine serum lectins (conglutinin and CL-43) are characterized by relatively long and uninterrupted collagen domains. In the case of SP-D and conglutinin, the trimeric subunits preferentially associate as cruciform tetramers (12 chains). For both classes of proteins, smaller and larger orders of multimers can be observed, and the proportions of various multimeric forms can vary with the species and among individuals *(36,37)*.

In the case of primate SP-As, an additional complexity relates to the capacity of the molecules to assemble as heterotrimers of the two, genetically different, chain types *(38)* that are subject to differential regulation *(39,40)*. By contrast, MBL and all the known members of the SP-D family are assembled as homotrimers. The functional significance of these heteropolymers is unknown.

Although the lung collectins show comparable domain structures, there is significant divergence in primary sequence, within all domains of the molecule. The CRDs share the essential and most of the highly conserved elements of the C-type lectin fold but diverge in the intervening sequences, as well as within and surrounding the coordinated calcium that mediates saccharide binding *(6,35)*. The short collagen domain of SP-A shows little obvious homology with the collagen domain of SP-D, except for a hydrophilic region at the amino-terminal end of the collagen domain. Both neck domains encode an amphipathic α-helical structure that mediates trimerization; however, within these conformational restraints the overall homology is low. Sequence differences in the carboxy-terminal region of the neck domain could influence the binding activities of the CRD, directly or through alterations of the spatial distribution of the CRDs within a trimeric subunit.

There are also conspicuous differences in the distribution of attached carbohydrates that could influence function or interactions with microbial lectins. In particular, the collectins vary with respect to asparagine-linked glycosylation *(41)*. Although there are species variations in the number and sites of Asn-linked glycosylation, all known SP-Ds and SP-As contain at least one conserved complex oligosaccharide. The conserved sugar in SP-A is within the CRD, whereas the sugar in SP-D is usually confined to Asn70 within the collagen domain. As discussed below, the sialylated oligosaccharide associated with the SP-A CRD is required for interactions with certain microorganisms, particularly viruses. Thus far, no functional differences between wild-type rat SP-D and a mutant with a deleted consensus for Asn-linked glycosylation have been described. SP-D, conglutinin, CL-43, and MBL also contain hydroxylysine-linked glycosides within the collagen domain, but there is no hydroxylysine in SP-A. Lastly, a variant form of human SP-D has been shown to contain threonine-conjugated, O-linked carbohydrate within the amino-terminal domain *(42)*.

2.5. Production of Lung Collectins

SP-D is constitutively expressed by rat alveolar type II cells *(20)*, and a large fraction of human SP-A is similarly secreted in a constitutive fashion independent of surfactant lamellar bodies *(43)*. However, SP-A and SP-D have been localized to the same or overlapping populations of secretory granules in rat nonciliated bronchiolar cells *(44)*, suggesting that they are subject to regulated secretion at these sites.

Little is currently known about the regulation of lung collectin expression in vivo, at least in relation to their host defense functions. The expression of lung collectins is increased following a variety of types of lung injury *(1)*. For example, the production of both proteins is quite rapidly increased following intratracheal instillation of bacterial endotoxin [lipopolysaccharide (LPS)] in rats, leading to the suggestion that they are pulmonary "acute-phase proteins" *(45)*. Hyperoxia is also a potent stimulus in vivo *(46–48)*. However, the specific regulatory mechanisms have not been elucidated.

SP-A is increased following the exposure of human fetal lung explants to epidermal growth factor (EGF), cAMP, interferon-γ, interleukin-1β (IL-1β), and certain other mediators *(49–52)* and inhibited by glucocorticoid. Regulation of SP-A and SP-D gene expression is distinct *(53)*. Like surfactant proteins B and C, SP-A gene transcription requires the activity of the homeodomain-containing nuclear factor thyroid transcription factor-1 (TTF-1) *(54)*. In contrast, SP-D expression does not require TTF-1 and is expressed in numerous tissues. Cell culture studies of SP-D expression have been complicated by the rapid loss of epithelial expression following cell isolation and the limited utility of available suitable tumor cell lines. Modifications of the culture system used for freshly isolated rat type II cells have been developed that support more sustained expression. Notably, the production of both proteins is maintained or increased in the presence of keratinocyte growth factor, an important mediator of alveolar cell proliferation following lung injury *(55)*. The upstream regulatory sequences of SP-A and SP-D contain binding sites for transcription factors that may contribute to the regulation of the response to injury. For example, the SP-D gene contains a conserved AP-1 element *(56)*, as well as multiple sites for the binding of CCAAT-enhancer binding proteins, as observed in the genes of many hepatic acute-phase proteins.

3. BINDING INTERACTIONS IN VITRO

3.1. Collectin Ligands

The lung collectins bind to a variety of purified saccharides, as well as specific phospholipids and glycolipids. With a few exceptions, the carboxy-terminal domains mediate these binding activities. However, binding affinity and outcome of these neck+CRD-dependent interactions can be influenced by the state of multimerization of the trimeric subunits, as determined by the amino-terminal and collagen domains.

The saccharide preferences of both proteins in solid-phase binding assays are different but partially overlapping. SP-D preferentially binds maltose, inositol, and glucose, whereas SP-A prefers *N*-acetylmannosamine or mannose relative to glucose *(57–59)*. Both react relatively poorly with *N*-acetylglucosamine, the preferred ligand for conglutinin. Despite such differences in relative selectivity for carbohydrates, both proteins have similar CRD-dependent interactions with certain glycoproteins. For example, as discussed below, both proteins can bind to gp140, a heavily mannosylated glycoprotein associated with the cell wall of *Pneumocystis carinii.*

In other cases, SP-A and SP-D bind to the same glycoconjugates but through different mechanisms *(60).* One example is Gram-negative endotoxin (bacterial LPS). SP-D has CRD-dependent interactions with conserved core oligosaccharides of LPS that contain glucose residues or other potential saccharide ligands. By contrast, SP-A preferentially interacts with the acylated lipid A domain. Likewise, SP-A and SP-D interact via distinct molecular mechanisms with influenza A hemagglutinin (the sialic acid receptor that binds to the host cell). In this case, SP-D binds to Asn-linked oligomannose residues near the sialic acid binding site of the hemagglutinin, whereas the sialylated residues in the Asn-linked sugar of the CRD of SP-A are recognized by the viral hemagglutinin.

There is less apparent overlap of binding activities between SP-A and SP-D with respect to lipid ligands. SP-A preferentially binds to dipalmitoylphosphatidyl choline (DPPC), the most abundant phospholipid in lung surfactant, whereas SP-D binds to phosphatidylinositol (PI), a variably minor component of surfactant *(8).* In the case of glycolipids, it appears that both collectins primarily recognize the associated sugar, e.g., SP-D binds to glucosylceramide, but not galactosyl ceramide, whereas the opposite is true for SP-A *(61,62).*

Interactions of the collectins with phospholipids are more complex. For example, there is indirect evidence that SP-D interacts through CRD-dependent binding to the inositol headgroup of PI but also through other substituents of the phospholipid, possibly the acyl side chains *(63–65).* In addition, studies with chimeric collectins demonstrated distinct contributions of the C-terminal end of the CRD *(66).*

3.2. Interactions with Host Cells

As a group, the collectins interact with at least two classes of cellular receptors or binding molecules on host cells *(4,8,60).* However, the identity and signaling pathways mediating the effects of either collectin on various target cells remains poorly understood. These include glycoconjugates (such as glycolipids or glycoproteins reactive with the lectin domain) and membrane proteins that interact with other regions of the molecule. SP-A may interact with the calreticulin C1q receptor and C1qR$_p$, the phagocytic C1q receptor. However, there is no evidence that the ClqR$_p$ is a physiologic receptor for SP-A. SPR-210, a surface protein expressed by type II cells, alveolar macrophages, and lymphocytes, has been implicated in the SP-A-dependent inhibition of T-lymphocyte proliferation *(67)* and the uptake of mycobacteria by alveolar macrophages *(68,69).* At least two additional binding sites have been described on alveolar epithelial cells, but the mechanisms of interaction, their collectin specificity, and their specific functional roles (whether in signaling, recycling, or catabolism of SP-A) have not yet been elucidated.

Both SP-D and SP-A can also interact with soluble CD14, suggesting possible interactions with the membrane-associated form of the LPS receptor complex, mCD14 *(70).* The binding of SP-D involves interactions of the lectin domain with N-linked oligosaccharides on CD14, whereas SP-A interacts with the protein backbone. Both proteins also show calcium-dependent, but lectin-independent, interactions with the gp340 scavenger protein salivary agglutinin *(71–73).* Although gp340 has been identified on alveolar macrophages, it lacks a transmembrane domain, and there is currently no evidence that gp340 represents a cellular receptor for either protein.

As indicated above, the collectins may also interact with other cell surface glyco-conjugates, such as phospholipids or glycolipids. For example, SP-D binds to PI associated with the outer leaflet of the plasma membrane *(74)*.

Thus, there remains considerable uncertainty regarding the mechanism of lung collectin interactions with host cells. In some situations, collectin receptors are not necessary to modulate cellular function. For example, collectin-mediated aggregation of influenza A virus can alter the presentation of the virions to their sialylated cellular receptors on phagocytes and thereby alter the cell's response to the virus *(75)*.

4. ROLES IN MICROBIAL CLEARANCE AND NEUTRALIZATION

SP-A and SP-D interact with or modify the phagocyte response to a wide variety of microorganisms including many Gram-negative bacteria, certain Gram-positive pathogens, classical fungi, *P. carinii,* several respiratory viruses, and mycobacteria (Tables 1 and 2). Because the mechanisms and functional consequences of these interactions have been discussed in the recent literature *(5,60),* they will not be retabulated or critically reexamined. In brief, published studies have described a variety of different consequences of microbial binding (e.g., enhanced uptake with increased or decreased killing, decreased phagocytic uptake and killing, enhanced oxidant responses of the phagocyte to the bound organism, and varying degrees of microbial aggregation or agglutination with differing effects on uptake). Some of these activities are attributable to direct effects of the collectin on the phagocyte, whereas other effects involve prior recognition or opsonization of the organism by the collectin. There are also some apparent discrepancies in the literature that are probably attributable to other differences in experimental design including microbial strain differences, differences in microbial growth conditions, differences in the type or state of activation of the target cells, and differences in the state of multimerization or purity of the collectin preparation.

Unquestionably, an impressive array of microbial interactions and potential antimicrobial activities has been observed in vitro. However, the following discussion will focus on interactions that have found some confirmation in recent in vivo studies. To illustrate these interactions, we have selected the most extensively characterized examples relating to bacterial, fungal, and viral respiratory pathogens. We do not wish to imply that the examples are truly representative of the entire class of interactions. However, together they confirm innate immune functions and suggest possible mechanisms.

4.1. Model: Clearance of **Pseudomonas aeruginosa** and Other Bacterial Pathways

P. aeruginosa is a particularly important human pathogen and the most common cause of Gram-negative sepsis among hospitalized patients of all ages. In addition, certain mucoid strains of this organism are major causes of morbidity in the setting of cystic fibrosis. SP-A and SP-D bind to clinical isolates of *P. aeruginosa (21,76).* At least one of the ligands for SP-D is the LPS *(59,77).* Studies by Wright and coworkers have demonstrated that both proteins can enhance the binding, internalization, and killing of some mucoid and nonmucoid strains by alveolar macrophages *(78)* in vivo *(79).*

Table 1
"Antimicrobial" Activities of SP-A

Organism	Reference
Gram-negative bacteria	
Pseudomonas aeruginosa	*14*
Klebsiella pneumoniae (cap+ with Manα2/3M)	*129*
Escherichia coli (rough)	*130*
	103
Haemophilus influenzae, type A	*131*
	76
	13
Gram-positive bacteria	
Staphylococcus aureus	*132*
	133
	134
	135
Streptococcus pneumoniae	*134*
	76
	132
Group B streptococci	*16*
	13
	17
Fungi	
Aspergillus fumigatus	*80*
	136
	81
	82
Cryptococcus neoformans (cap–)	*137*
Pneumocystis carinii	*83*
	84
	86
Respiratory viruses	
Influenza A (IAV)	*138*
	139
Respiratory syncytial virus (RSV)	*15*
	100
	140
	98
Herpes simplex	*141*
	142
Cytomegalovirus	*143*
Other	
Mycobacterium tuberculosis	*144*
	145
Mycoplasma pneumoniae	*146*

Table 2
"Antimicrobial" Activities of SP-D

Organism	Reference
Gram-negative bacteria	
Pseudomonas aeruginosa	79
Klebsiella penumoniae (cap–)	147
	148
Escherichia coli	130
Haemophilus influenzae	13
Gram-positive bacteria	
Staphylococcus aureus	134
Streptococcus pneumoniae	134
Group B streptococci	13
Fungi	
Aspergillus fumigatus	80
	136
	81
	82
Cryptococcus neoformans (cap–)	137
Candida albicans	149
Pneumocystis carinii	85
	87
Respiratory viruses	
Influenza A (IAV)	150
	95
Respiratory syncytial virus (RSV)	99
	15
Other	
Mycobacterium tuberculosis	151

In vivo studies in which SP-A$^{-/-}$ mice were intratracheally treated with *P. aerugi-nosa* confirmed the important role of SP-A in innate immunity to this organism *(14)*. Clearance of *P. aeruginosa* from the lung in vivo was decreased in the SP-A$^{-/-}$ mice 6 and 24 hours after infection. The defects in clearance were associated with decreased macrophage uptake, increased leukocyte infiltration, and increased expression of inflammatory cytokines tumor necrosis factor-α (TNF-α), IL-6, and macrophage inflammatory protein-2 (MIP-2). Oxidant production by neutrophils was normal in the SP-A$^{-/-}$ mice following infection, supporting the concept that SP-A is primarily required for optimal alveolar macrophage function in vivo.

Similarly, SP-A$^{-/-}$ mice show increased susceptibility to bacterial infection by *Klebsiella pneumoniae, Escherichia coli, Haemophilus influenza,* and group B streptococcus (GBS) *(12,13,16,17)*. For example, in the GBS infection model, clearance of the organism was markedly impaired in the SP-A$^{-/-}$ mice and was associated with increased systemic spread from the lung. Opsonization, uptake, and killing of GBS by alveolar macrophages were impaired in the SP-A$^{-/-}$ mice, and oxidant production was markedly diminished following exposure to GBS. Repletion of native SP-A to the SP-A$^{-/-}$ mice at the time of infection completely restored bacterial clearance in the GBS model, enhancing oxidant production and decreasing lung inflammation. Thus, in vivo experiments with a number of pulmonary bacterial pathogens demonstrate a critical role of SP-A in innate antibacterial defense of the lung. Interestingly, SP-D$^{-/-}$ mice did not show decreased killing of *H. influenza,* GBS, *K. pneumonia,* or *P. aeruginosa,* perhaps reflecting the increased activation of alveolar macrophage functions typical of the SP-D$^{-/-}$ mice prior to infection *(13).* However, internalization of the organisms by alveolar macrophages was significantly decreased.

4.2. Model: Clearance of Aspergillus fumigatus

Human SP-A and SP-D show CRD-dependent binding to N-linked oligosaccharides of cell wall glycoproteins of *A. fumigatus (80,81).* In a recent study, circumstantial evidence was presented that SP-D may also interact with β(1–6)-glucans associated with the *aspergillus* cell wall. Pustulan, a β(1–6) glucose homopolymer, but not a β(1–3) homopolymer, was found to be a potent inhibitor of SP-D binding to *Aspergillus fumigatus* and *Saccharomyces cerevisiae.*

Madan and coworkers *(80)* observed CRD-dependent agglutination of the fungi, as well as enhanced killing of *Aspergillus* conidia by human neutrophils and macrophages in vitro in the presence of human SP-A and SP-D. The increased killing was associated with an enhanced respiratory burst response. By contrast, Allen and coworkers *(81)* found no evidence for the enhanced association of conidia by rat SP-A or SP-D with rat alveolar macrophages. Although rat SP-A did not bind, they confirmed CRD-dependent interactions of rat SP-D, as well as human SP-A and SP-D, with the conidia. Thus, there could be important species differences in these interactions. Interestingly, human surfactant lipids significantly inhibited the effects of SP-A, but not the effects of SP-D.

In an important recent study, Madan and coworkers *(82)* demonstrated that SP-D can play a protective role in the host defense against *A. fumigatus* in vivo. Using a murine model of fatal, invasive aspergillosis, they found that intranasal administration of human lung collectins, or recombinant, trimeric human SP-D neck+CRDs markedly enhanced survival (0% survival for untreated mice; 80% for mice treated with SP-D). Given the in vitro findings described above, it is notable that the SP-D preparations appeared significantly more potent than SP-A. Interestingly, the protective effects of either collectin were greater than those achieved with the antimycotic agent amphotericin B (20% survival).

4.3. Model: Clearance of Pneumocystis carinii

Pneumocystis carinii (PC) is an important opportunistic pathogen that leads to morbidity and mortality among individuals with various forms of acquired immunodeficiency and the very young. Infection is often characterized by massive accumulations of organisms within the airspace, often in association with characteristic foamy exudates that contain surfactant lipids and proteins. SP-A and SP-D show CRD-dependent binding to the "trophozoites" and cyst forms of PC *(83–85).* This in part involves CRD-dependent interactions with a heavily mannosylated, cell wall glycoprotein, gpA (gp140) *(85,86).* There is also evidence that SP-D binds to β-glucans, which are associated with the cell wall *(87).* The lung collectins increase the attachment of PC to rat alveolar macrophages *(83,88)*. However, there are discrepancies in the literature regarding the effects of binding of the collectin on internalization of PC. Some studies have observed no effect of human SP-A or rat SP-D on PC uptake by rat alveolar macrophages *(83,88)*, whereas another study found that human SP-A enhanced the binding and internalization of the organism by these cells *(89)*. However, yet another study found decreased binding and uptake of PC by human alveolar macrophages after addition of SP-A *(90)*.

There is evidence that PC infection is associated with alterations in the concentrations of SP-A and SP-D in the lung. For example, PC infection in the rat is associated with increased SP-A *(91)*. In addition, SP-A levels are increased in the lavage fluid from HIV+ patients with PC pneumonia compared with HIV+ controls *(92)*. In another study using the rat model, the levels of SP-D were markedly increased (> three-fold), whereas the levels of SP-A and the hydrophobic surfactant proteins were maintained or decreased, respectively *(93)*. In wild-type mice, SP-D concentrations were significantly increased during PC pneumonia *(94)*.

Although the levels of the collectins are influenced by PC infection and these proteins can alter the interactions of PC with alveolar macrophages, it has been unclear whether they serve a protective role or are, in fact, utilized by PC for attachment and infections. However, recent in vivo studies demonstrated the susceptibility of SP-A$^{-/-}$ mice to PC infection *(18)*. Increased PC cysts and foamy macrophage infiltration were observed in the SP-A$^{-/-}$ mice, whether the organism was acquired by cohabitation with infected mice or by direct intratracheal infection with cysts.

4.4. Model: Neutralization of Influenza A and Respiratory Syncytial Virus

4.4.1. Influenza A Virus

SP-D and SP-A interact with viral envelope proteins of the influenza A virus (IAV) *(95)*. SP-D binds to high-mannose oligosaccharides associated with the globular hemagglutinin (HA)$_1$ domain of the HA molecule. These interactions of SP-D with IAV are calcium-dependent and are inhibited by saccharide ligands. As indicated above, the activity of SP-A involves the binding of viral lectins to Asn-linked sugars on SP-A. Nevertheless, both inhibit the hemagglutination activity and infectivity of IAV in vitro. SP-D also inhibits the activity of the viral neuraminidase, an envelope protein that contributes to the dissemination of new viral particles from infected cells *(96)*.

Because the oligosaccharide on the HA$_1$ domain overlies the sialic acid binding pocket (i.e., the cell attachment site), the binding of SP-D to the HA, or the binding of the HA to SP-A, can similarly inhibit hemagglutinin activity and thereby decrease viral attachment to host cells. These differences in binding mechanism are consistent with the observation that SP-A inhibits the hemagglutinin activity and infectivity of certain "collectin-resistant" laboratory strains of IAV that do not bind to SP-D or the serum collectins because of the absence of oligosaccharide attachments on HA$_1$.

SP-D induces massive CRD-dependent agglutination of IAV particles. The size of the resulting aggregates is much larger than those observed for optimal concentrations SP-A or MBL. The degree of SP-D-dependent agglutination correlates with the multimerization state of the protein. Although highly multimerized preparations are significantly more potent than dodecamers, trimeric CRDs induce minimal agglutination. SP-D-mediated agglutination enhances the binding and internalization of virus by neutrophils through increased binding of the virus to sialic acid receptors on the neutrophil. Increased binding is accompanied by increased production of hydrogen peroxide and decreased "deactivation" of the neutrophil by IAV.

Additional evidence for a role of lung collectins in the host defense against IAV has come from in vivo studies using wild-type or collectin-deficient mice. Reading and coworkers *(96)* demonstrated a strong inverse correlation between the number of oligosaccharide attachments on the HA of specific IAV strains and the ability of SP-D to inhibit viral infectivity or enhance clearance in vivo. The coadministration of mannan as a competitor of C-type lectin activity increases the replication SP-D-sensitive strains of IAV in the lung. SP-D-sensitive IAV strains also replicate to higher titers in lungs of hyperglycemic diabetic mice compared with nondiabetic controls *(97)*, whereas the SP-D-insensitive PR-8 strain replicates to the same extent in diabetic and control animals. Viral replication was positively correlated with the level of blood glucose and decreased following insulin treatment. Significantly, glucose concentrations comparable to those encountered in the blood of diabetic mice inhibited the interaction of SP-D with IAV in vitro.

The in vitro findings, supporting the importance of both SP-A and SP-D in innate defense against IAV, are strongly supported by in vivo data derived from SP-A$^{-/-}$ and SP-D$^{-/-}$ mice *(97a,97b)*. Both lung collectin-deficient mice were highly susceptible to IAV infection in vivo. Viral load, inflammation, the expression of proinflammatory cytokines (including TNF-α, IL-1β, IL-6, and MIP-2) were increased in the lungs of SP-A$^{-/-}$ and SP-D$^{-/-}$ mice. Uptake of IAV by alveolar macrophages was markedly impaired in the SP-D$^{-/-}$ mice. In general, the effects were much more dramatic for SP-D than SP-A deficiency. In both SP-D$^{-/-}$ and SP-A$^{-/-}$ mice, repletion of native SP-A and SP-D at the time of infection diminished inflammatory responses during IAV infection. Thus, both SP-A and SP-D play important roles in innate defense during IAV infection of the lung, enhancing uptake and clearance of the virus and suppressing inflammatory responses in vivo. These studies also suggest that differences in the mechanisms by which SP-A and SP-D interact with pathogens and host defense cells could broaden the range of potential viral interactions in vivo.

4.4.2. Respiratory Syncytial Virus

Respiratory syncytial virus (RSV) is the most important cause of clinically significant viral respiratory tract infections among neonates and infants. Both SP-A and SP-D bind to RSV particles *(98,99)*. These interactions involve the lectin-dependent binding of the collectin to the viral G protein, a heavily glycosylated attachment protein. SP-A has also been shown to enhance the uptake of RSV by macrophages and epithelial cells, and it alters the cytokine response to internalized virus *(98,100)*.

Similar to findings with IAV infection, SP-A$^{-/-}$ and SP-D$^{-/-}$ mice were highly susceptible to pulmonary RSV infection in vivo *(15)* (LeVine et al., in preparation). Decreased viral clearance, increased expression of proinflammatory cytokines, and increased neutrophilic infiltrates were observed in both gene-targeted mice. Clearance of RSV was reversed by coadministration of SP-A to the SP-A$^{-/-}$ mice. Hickling and coworkers *(99)* have shown that SP-D and recombinant, trimeric SP-D neck+CRDs decrease infectivity and viral proliferation in cell monolayers and in vivo in BALB/C mice.

Pulmonary SP-D levels, but not the levels of serum mannose binding lectin, markedly increased after IAV infection *(96)* (LeVine et al., in preparation). However, the concentrations of SP-A and SP-D were decreased in bronchoalveolar lavage fluid from children with severe RSV bronchiolitis and pneumonia *(101)*.

5. REGULATION OF THE INFLAMMATORY RESPONSE TO MICROBIAL CHALLENGE

There is considerable evidence that the lectins modulate the host response to LPS and possibly to other biologically active molecules released by microorganisms. Both SP-A and SP-D bind to LPS, particularly rough forms that lack extended O-antigens *(21,102,103)*. However, in vitro studies suggest that the effects of collectin response of macrophages to LPS could involve several mechanisms. These can include direct effects on the cellular responsiveness to LPS *(104,105)*. For example, SP-A was found to decrease TNF-α activity in the conditioned medium of macrophages stimulated with smooth LPS, which binds poorly to SP-A *(106)*. In addition, SP-A inhibited TNF-α mRNA levels and secretion by U937 cells in response to smooth (but not rough) LPS *(107)*. This finding contrasts with the results obtained using the THP-1 macrophage cell line, which showed increased production of proinflammatory cytokines in response to purified SP-A or SP-A in combination with smooth LPS *(108)*.

The interactions of collectins with LPS could also result in altered or decreased presentation of LPS to host cell receptors, alterations in the cellular metabolism of LPS, or effects on the interactions of LPS binding proteins or receptors to LPS. For example, SP-D "scavenges" intratracheally instilled LPS in rats, and the resulting complexes are rapidly internalized into lysosomal compartments in alveolar macrophages *(109)*; human SP-A increases alveolar macrophage uptake and deacylation of tritiated *E. coli* LPS *(110)*. In addition, both SP-A and SP-D bind to soluble CD14 *(70)*, and SP-A can decrease the cellular response to smooth LPS, apparently through its interaction with CD14 *(107)*.

In vivo, SP-A-and SP-D-deficient mice are highly susceptible to LPS-induced pulmonary inflammation. Intratracheal administration of *Salmonella* endotoxin to SP-A$^{-/-}$ mice increased neutrophilic infiltration and inflammatory cytokine production, compared with wild-type mice *(105)*. Similarly, pulmonary inflammation was increased in the SP-D$^{-/-}$ mice treated with LPS *(111)*.

As indicated in the introductory section, the intratracheal administration of endotoxin in rats is associated with quite rapid changes in the production or concentrations of SP-A and SP-D *(45)*. In other studies, SP-A was increased or decreased following exposure to bacterial endotoxin *(112–114)*. The variability is probably related to differences among species, dose, and type of endotoxin. These potential interrelationships are schematized in Fig. 2.

6. MODULATION OF REACTIVE OXYGEN METABOLISM AND THE OXIDANT RESPONSE TO MICROBIAL CHALLENGE

A recent study suggested that SP-A and SP-D had direct inhibitory effects on lipid peroxidation, protecting lipoproteins, surfactant phospholipids, and macrophages from oxidation *(115)*. However, it is unclear whether the antioxidant activity copurified with the SP-A and SP-D. On the other hand, oxidants and certain free radicals have been

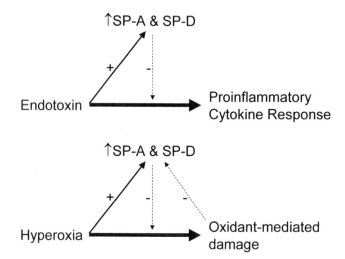

Fig. 2. Lung collectins and the response to endotoxin and hyperoxia. The diagrams illustrate potential interrelationships suggested by *in vitro* and *in vivo* studies for two of the selected models. Please see the corresponding text for details. SP, surfactant protein.

shown to modify SP-A and decrease certain CRD-dependent activities in vitro. For example, hydrogen peroxide treatment of SP-A leads to the disruption of inter-subunit disulfide bonds, with decreased multimer size and associated decreased in lectin activity *(116)*. In vitro, peroxynitrite caused nitration of SP-A without disruption of its oligomeric structure. The nitrated protein shows decreased lipid aggregation and is defective in enhancing the binding or uptake of *Pneumocystis* organisms to alveolar macrophages *(89,117)*.

At present, there is relatively little information relating to the effects of lung collectins on oxidant metabolism in vivo. However, alveolar macrophages from SP-D null mice show a marked elevation in hydrogen peroxide production *(25)*, as well as increased superoxide and hydrogen peroxide production in response to bacterial challenge *(13)*. It has been suggested that increased oxidants contribute to metalloproteinase activation, with resulting emphysema. Although SP-A-deficient mice show no abnormalities in basal oxidant metabolism, they show decreased oxidant responses to RSV and GBS challenge relative to controls *(13,15,16)*. There may also be some dependence on the specific microbial challenge or target cell. For example, SP-A-deficient and control mice challenged with *P. aeruginosa* show similar levels of superoxide production by neutrophils *(14)*.

In contrast to findings in SP-A–/– mice, basal oxidant production by alveolar macrophages from SP-D–/– mice was markedly increased. Likewise, oxidized lipid species accumulated in the lungs of SP-D–/– mice. Alveolar macrophages from SP-D–/– mice expressed high levels of the metalloproteinases MMP-2, MMP-9, and MMP-12, in part mediated by activation and nuclear translocation of NF-κB. Apocynin, an inhibitor of oxidant production, blocked both NF-κB activity and metalloproteinase expression in alveolar macrophages isolated from the SP-D–/– mice *(118)*. Therefore, SP-D appears to play a critical role in both regulation of oxidant production and alveolar macrophage activation, at least in part by regulation of the activity of NF-κB.

As indicated in the introductory section, there is considerable evidence that hyperoxia is associated with the increased expression of SP-A and SP-D by lung epithelial cells. Given the in vitro and in vivo findings, it may be particularly significant that the levels of SP-D are increased in a situation in which the risk of oxidative damage is increased. These potential interrelationships are summarized in Fig. 2 (bottom).

7. AT THE CROSSROADS OF INNATE AND ADAPTIVE IMMUNITY

7.1. Model: Regulation of the Immune Response to Aspergillus fumigatus

Allergic hypersensitivity to *A. fumigatus* is a well-recognized complication of asthma that may follow fungal colonization of mucus within the asthmatic airways with the release of complex fungal antigens. The resulting immune reactions can be manifest as eosinophilic pneumonia, mucus plugging of the airways, bronchocentric granulomatous inflammation with bronchiectasis, and obliterative changes in small airways. These reactions are believed to involve IgE-stimulated release of mediators from mast cells and eosinophils, as well as immune complex-mediated tissue injury.

As indicated above, SP-A and SP-D show CRD-dependent binding to major glycoprotein allergens associated with the cell walls of, and released by, *A. fumigatus (80)*. This binding can inhibit specific IgE binding to the allergens, as well as block histamine release from sensitized basophils. Madan and coworkers *(119)* also developed a murine model of *A. fumigatus* hypersensitivity that develops following intranasal instillation and intraperitoneal injection of fungal antigen for 4 weeks. These animals develop specific IgG and IgE antibodies, peripheral eosinophilia, pulmonary eosinophilic infiltrates, and elevated splenic IL-2 and Th2-type cytokines, including IL-4 and IL-5; they also exhibit decreased interferon-α. The administration of SP-A, SP-D, or recombinant trimeric SP-D neck+CRD decreases specific IgG and IgE levels, decreases peripheral and pulmonary eosinophilia, and decreases splenic IL-2, IL-4, and IL-5. Given the in vitro data, it is likely that these effects involve the CRD-dependent inhibition of binding of specific Ig to the fungal antigen. The lung collectins can also interact with the major dust mite allergen *(120)* and certain pollens *(121)*, suggesting more general roles of the collectins in modulating responses to complex organic antigens. SP-A can also decrease the production and release of IL-8 by eosinophils *(122)*.

These findings are of particular interest given that some patients with asthma and individuals with hypersensitivity to organic antigens show alterations in the level, structure, or activity of lung collectins. For example, increased levels of SP-A and SP-D were found in the lung washings of asthmatic patients *(123)*, possibly secondary to the epithelial inflammatory reaction. However, in an earlier study, levels of immunoreactive SP-A were reported to be decreased in asthmatic patients *(124)*.

SP-A and SP-D were found to decrease the allergen-induced proliferation of peripheral blood lymphocytes from healthy children and children with stable asthma *(125)*. However, lymphocytes isolated from children with unstable asthma showed a diminished inhibitory response. Interestingly, Hickling and coworkers *(36)* found an increased proportion of small oligomeric forms of SP-A in patients with pollen allergy compared with controls.

Given the potentially important role of IL-4 in the hypersensitivity response, it is interesting that transgenic mice overexpressing IL-4 in nonciliated bronchiolar cells show very marked increases in lung SP-D (approx 90-fold) *(126)*.

7.2. Other Potential Interactions with Acquired Immunity

Both SP-A and SP-D can also decrease IL-2-dependent T-lymphocyte proliferation *(127,128)*. In the case of SP-A, there is evidence that a region of collagen domain containing an RGD motif is required, suggesting possible integrin involvement *(67)*. Mutagenesis of the saccharide binding site did not effect inhibition. Although the effect was not blocked with competing C1q, antibodies to the 210-kDa SP-A receptor blocked the inhibitory activity.

In other studies, natural SP-A and SP-D and the neck+CRD of SP-D were similarly found to inhibit the proliferation of peripheral blood mononuclear cells *(125)*. However, the neck+CRD of SP-D was also inhibitory, and the effects of both collectins were inhibited with maltose, suggesting a lectin-dependent activity. These effects appeared to involve direct interactions with lymphocytes and were associated with decreased expression of CD11b.

At present, little is known about the *in vivo* significance of collectin-dependent alterations in lymphocyte proliferation. However, it may be significant that SP-D-deficient mice show an apparent expansion of peribronchial lymphoid tissue *(22,25)*. Given the numerous interactions of lung collectins and macrophages and the effects of these proteins on the internalization of certain organisms or complex organic antigens, it seems likely that they may modulate processes of antigen presentation involving dendritic cells or other pulmonary antigen-presenting cells. This exciting possibility awaits examination.

8. MODULATION OF SURFACTANT HOMEOSTASIS

One of the most surprising results from analysis of the SP-D$^{-/-}$ mice was the observed marked accumulation of surfactant lipids. Increased phospholipids, specifically saturated phosphatidylcholine (SatPC), were observed as early as 2 days following birth and persisted thereafter. Whereas phospholipid pools generally decreased in the mammalian lung postnatally, both alveolar and total lung phospholipid content remained remarkably elevated in the SP-D$^{-/-}$ mice. In contrast, the contents of other surfactant proteins (SP-A, SP-B, and SP-C) were relatively decreased in relationship to PC content, a finding in marked contrast to that in the alveolar proteinosis seen in animals deficient in granulocyte/macrophage colony-stimulating factor. Thus, SP-D deficiency results in selective impairment in the regulation of surfactant phospholipids. Clearance of surfactant phospholipids from the lungs of SP-D$^{-/-}$ mice was relatively normal. Likewise, uptake and catabolism of surfactant lipids by alveolar macrophages from the SP-D$^{-/-}$ mice were relatively unimpaired. Large intracellular and extracellular pool sizes of saturated phosphatidylcholine that accumulate in the lungs of SP-D$^{-/-}$ mice suggest that SP-D plays an important role in establishing intracellular pools of surfactant lipids, in turn influencing intracellular and extracellular surfactant homeostasis. Although the mechanisms regulating surfactant lipid homeostasis in the SP-D$^{-/-}$ mice are incompletely known, evidence to date supports the concept that SP-D plays a critical role in the regulation of surfactant metabolism in the type II epithelial cell. Thus, collectins may orchestrate a complex dialogue between synthetic and catabolic activities of both the epithelium and alveolar macrophages that determine the composition and functional capacities of materials forming the interface between the lung and the environment. Therefore the "host defense roles" of these proteins may be considerably broader than antimicrobial host defense.

9. CONCLUSIONS

A large and growing body of *in vitro* and *in vivo* data strongly support important roles of lung collectins in the defense against a variety of pulmonary pathogens, and more generally in the regulation of inflammatory and immune processes within the lung. Both proteins are constitutively secreted, and their production is rapidly increased in response to a variety of lung injuries and challenges. Furthermore, both proteins can recognize several pathogen-associated molecular patterns and facilitate cell-mediated clearance of the pathogen. In these respects SP-A and SP-D resemble other pattern recognition molecules. Although a number of observations suggest that these proteins may fulfill other specialized roles that involve specific host cell recognition in the absence of a pathogen or exogenous complex antigen, we speculate that these functions may also fall within the realm of innate defense. In this case, pattern recognition may extend to the recognition of potential patterns resulting from environmental modifications of host components (e.g., the oxidation of lipids).

ACKNOWLEDGMENTS

We acknowledge grant support from the National Institutes of Health [HL-61646 (to J.A.W.) and HL-29594 and HL-44015 (to E.C.C.),] and the excellent secretarial assistance of Janet North and Ann Maher.

REFERENCES

1. Crouch EC. Collectins and pulmonary host defense. Am J Respir Cell Mol Biol 1998;19:177–201.
2. Wright JR. Immunomodulatory functions of surfactant. Physiol Rev 1997;77:931–962.
3. Haagsman HP. Interactions of surfactant protein A with pathogens. Biochim Biophys Acta 1998;1408:264–277.
4. Holmskov UL. Collectins and collectin receptors in innate immunity. APMIS Suppl 2000;100:1–59.
5. Lawson PR, Reid KB. The roles of surfactant proteins A and D in innate immunity. Immunol Rev 2000;173:66–78.
6. Hakansson K, Reid KB. Collectin structure: a review. Protein Sci 2000;9:1607–1617.
7. Ohtani K, Suzuki Y, Eda S, et al. Molecular cloning of a novel human collectin from liver (CL-L1). J Biol Chem 1999;274:13681–13689.
8. Hawgood S, Poulain FR. The pulmonary collectins and surfactant metabolism. Annu Rev Physiol 2001;63:495–519.
9. Ikegami M, Korfhagen TR, Whitsett JA, et al. Characteristics of surfactant from SP-A-deficient mice. Am J Physiol (Lung Cell Mol Physiol) 1998;19:L247–L254.
10. Korfhagen TR, Bruno MD, Ross GF, et al. Altered surfactant function and structure in SP-A gene targeted mice. Proc Natl Acad Sci USA 1996;93:9594–9599.
11. Harrod KS, Trapnell BC, Otake K, Korfhagen TR, Whitsett JA. SP-A enhances viral clearance and inhibits inflammation after pulmonary adenoviral infection. Am J Physiol 1999;277:L580–L588.

12. Korfhagen T, Bruno MD, Whitsett JA, LeVine AM. Enhanced *K. pneumoniae* pulmonary infection in mice lacking SP-A. Am J Respir Crit Care Med 2000;161:A514.

13. LeVine AM, Whitsett JA, Gwozdz JA, et al. Distinct effects of surfactant protein A or D deficiency during bacterial infection on the lung. J Immunol 2000;165:3934–3940.

14. LeVine AM, Kurak KE, Bruno MD et al. Surfactant protein-A-deficient mice are susceptible to *Pseudomonas aeruginosa* infection. Am J Respir Cell Mol Biol 1998;19:700–708.

15. LeVine AM, Gwozdz J, Stark J, et al. Surfactant protein-A enhances respiratory syncytial virus clearance in vivo. J Clin Invest 1999;103:1015–1021.

16. LeVine AM, Kurak KE, Wright JR, et al. Surfactant protein-A binds group B streptococcus enhancing phagocytosis and clearance from lungs of surfactant protein-A-deficient mice. Am J Respir Cell Mol Biol 1999;20:279–286.

17. LeVine AM, Bruno MD, Huelsman KM, et al. Surfactant protein A-deficient mice are susceptible to group B streptococcal infection. J Immunol 1997;158:4336–4340.

18. Linke MJ, Harris CE, Korfhagen TR, et al. Immunosuppressed surfactant protein A-deficient mice have increased susceptibility to *Pneumocystis carinii* infection. J Infect Dis 2001;183:943–952.

19. Persson A, Chang D, Rust K, et al. Purification and biochemical characterization of CP4 (SP-D), a collagenous surfactant-associated protein. Biochemistry 1989;28:6361–6367.

20. Persson A, Rust K, Chang D, et al. CP4: a pneumocyte-derived collagenous surfactant-associated protein. Evidence for heterogeneity of collagenous surfactant proteins. Biochemistry 1988;27:8576–8584.

21. Kuan SF, Rust K, Crouch E. Interactions of surfactant protein D with bacterial lipopolysaccharides. Surfactant protein D is an *Escherichia coli*-binding protein in bronchoalveolar lavage. J Clin Invest 1992;90:97–106.

22. Botas C, Poulain F, Akiyama J, et al. Altered surfactant homeostasis and alveolar type II cell morphology in mice lacking surfactant protein D. Proc Natl Acad Sci USA 1998;95:11869–11874.

23. Korfhagen TR, Sheftelyevich V, Burhans MS, et al. Surfactant protein-D regulates surfactant phospholipid homeostasis in vivo. J Biol Chem 1998;273:28438–28443.

24. Ikegami M, Whitsett JA, Jobe AH, et al. Alterations in surfactant homeostasis resulting from SP-D deficiency. Am J Respir Crit Care Med 2000;161:A44.

25. Wert SE, Yoshida M, LeVine AM, et al. Increased metalloproteinase activity, oxidant production, and emphysema in surfactant protein D gene-inactivated mice. Proc Natl Acad Sci USA 2000;97:5972–5977.

26. LeVine AM, Gwozdz J, Fisher J, Whitsett J, Korfhagen T. Surfactant protein-D modulates lung inflammation with respiratory syncytial virus infection *in vivo*. Am J Respir Crit Care Med 2000;161:A515.

27. Khoor A, Gray ME, Hull WM, Whitsett JA, Stahlman MT. Developmental expression of SP-A and SP-A mRNA in the proximal and distal respiratory epithelium in the human fetus and newborn. J Histochem Cytochem 1993;41:1311–1319.

28. Khubchandani KR, Snyder JM. Surfactant protein A (SP-A): the alveolus and beyond. FASEB J 2001;15:59–69.

29. Madsen J, Kliem A, Tornoe I, et al. Localization of lung surfactant protein D (SP-D) on mucosal surfaces in human tissues. J Immunol 2000;164:5866–5870.

30. Drickamer K. Evolution of Ca^{2+} dependent animal lectins. In: Cohn WE, Moldave K (eds.). Progress in Nucleic Acid Research and Molecular Biology. New York: Academic, 1993, pp. 207–232.

31. Hoover RR, Floros J. Organization of the human SP-A and SP-D loci t 10q22-q23. Physical and radiation hybrid mapping reveal gene order and orientation. Am J Respir Cell Mol Biol 1998;18:353–362.

32. Sullivan LC, Daniels CB, Phillips ID, Orgeig S, Whitsett JA. Conservation of surfactant protein A: evidence for a single origin for vertebrate pulmonary surfactant. J Mol Evol 1998;46:131–138.

33. Lawson PR, Perkins VC, Holmskov U, Reid KB. Genomic organization of the mouse gene for lung surfactant protein D. Am J Respir Cell Mol Biol 1999;20:953–963.

34. Drickamer K, Dodd RB. C-Type lectin-like domains in *Caenorhabditis elegans:* predictions from the complete genome sequence. Glycobiology 1999;9:1357–1369.

35. Hakansson K, Lim NK, Hoppe HJ, Reid KB. Crystal structure of the trimeric alpha-helical coiled-coil and the three lectin domains of human lung surfactant protein D. Structure Fold Des 1999;7:255–264.

36. Hickling TP, Malhotra R, Sim RB. Human lung surfactant protein A exists in several different oligomeric states: oligomer size distribution varies between patient groups. Mol Med 1998;4:266–275.

37. Crouch E, Persson A, Chang D. Accumulation of surfactant protein D in human pulmonary alveolar proteinosis. Am J Pathol 1993;142:241–248.

38. Voss T, Melchers K, Scheirle G, Schafer KP. Structural comparison of recombinant pulmonary surfactant protein SP-A derived from two human coding sequences: implications for the chain composition of natural human SP-A. Am J Respir Cell Mol Biol 1991;4:88–94.

39. Karinch AM, Deiter G, Ballard PL, Floros J. Regulation of expression of human SP-A1 and SP-A2 genes in fetal lung explant culture. Biochim Biophys Acta 1998;1398:192–202.

40. McCormick SM, Mendelson CR. Human SP-A1 and SP-A2 genes are differentially regulated during development and by cAMP and glucocorticoids. Am J Physiol 1994;266:L367–L374.

41. Van Eijk M, Haagsman HP, Skinner T, et al. Porcine lung surfactant protein D: complementary DNA cloning, chromosomal localization, and tissue distribution. J Immunol 2000;164:1442–1450.

42. Mason RJ, Nielson LD, Kuroki Y, et al. A 50-kDa variant form of human surfactant protein D. Eur Respir J 1998;12:1147–1155.

43. Froh D, Gonzales LW, Ballard PL. Secretion of surfactant protein A and phosphatidylcholine from type II cells of human fetal lung. Am J Respir Cell Mol Biol 1993;8:556–561.

44. Voorhout WF, Veenendaal T, Kuroki Y, et al. Immunocytochemical localization of surfactant protein D (SP-D) in type II cells, Clara cells, and alveolar macrophages of rat lung. J Histochem Cytochem 1992;40:1589–1597.

45. McIntosh JC, Swyers AH, Fisher JH, Wright JR. Surfactant proteins A and D increase in response to intratracheal lipopolysaccharide. Am J Respir Cell Mol Biol 1996;15:509–519.

46. Nogee LM, Wispe JR, Clark JC, Whitsett JA. Increased synthesis and mRNA of surfactant protein A in oxygen-exposed rats. Am J Respir Cell Mol Biol 1989;1:119–125.

47. Aderibigbe AO, Thomas RF, Mercer RR, Auten RL. Brief exposure to 95% oxygen alters surfactant protein D and mRNA in adult rat alveolar and bronchiolar epithelium. Am J Respir Cell Mol Biol 1999;20:219–227.

48. Horowitz S, Watkins RH, Auten RL, Jr, Mercier CE, Cheng ER. Differential accumulation of surfactant protein A, B, and C mRNAs in two epithelial cell types of hyperoxic lung. Am J Respir Cell Mol Biol 1991;5:511–515.

49. Dhar V, Hallman M, Lappalainen U, Bry K. Interleukin-1 alpha upregulates the expression of surfactant protein-A in rabbit lung explants. Biol Neonate 1997;71:46–52.

50. Ballard PL, Liley HG, Gonzales LW, et al. Interferon-gamma and synthesis of surfactant components by cultured human fetal lung. Am J Respir Cell Mol Biol 1990;2:137–143.

51. Whitsett JA, Weaver TE, Lieberman MA, Clark JC, Daugherty C. Differential effects of epidermal growth factor and transforming growth factor-beta on synthesis of Mr = 35,000 surfactant-associated protein in fetal lung. J Biol Chem 1987;262:7908–7913.

52. Whitsett JA, Pilot T, Clark JC, Weaver TE. Induction of surfactant protein in fetal lung. Effects of cAMP and dexamethasone on SAP-35 RNA and synthesis. J Biol Chem 1987;262:5256–5261.

53. Dulkerian SJ, Gonzales LW, Ning Y, Ballard PL. Regulation of surfactant protein D in human fetal lung. Am J Respir Cell Mol Biol 1996;15:781–786.

54. Bohinski RJ, Di Lauro R, Whitsett JA. The lung-specific surfactant protein B gene promoter is a target for thyroid transcription factor 1 and hepatocyte nuclear factor 3, indicating common factors for organ-specific gene expression along the foregut axis. Mol Cell Biochem 1994;94:5671–5681.

55. Xu X, McCormick-Shannon K, Voelker DR, Mason RJ. KGF increases SP-A and SP-D mRNA levels and secretion in cultured rat alveolar type II cells. Am J Respir Cell Mol Biol 1998;18:168–178.

56. He Y, Crouch EC, Rust K, Spaite E, Brody SL. Proximal promoter of the surfactant protein D gene. Regulatory roles of AP-1, forkhead box, and GT box binding proteins. J Biol Chem 2000;275:31051–31060.

57. Haagsman HP, Hawgood S, Sargeant T, et al. The major lung surfactant protein, SP 28-36, is a calcium-dependent, carbohydrate-binding protein. J Biol Chem 1987;262:13877–13880.

58. Persson A, Chang D, Crouch E. Surfactant protein D is a divalent cation-dependent carbohydrate-binding protein. J Biol Chem 1990;265:5755–5760.

59. Lim BL, Wang JY, Holmskov U, Hoppe HJ, Reid KB. Expression of the carbohydrate recognition domain of lung surfactant protein D and demonstration of its binding to lipopolysaccharides of gram-negative bacteria. Biochem Biophys Res Commun 1994;202:1674–1680.

60. Crouch E, Wright JR. Surfactant proteins A and D and pulmonary host defense. Annu Rev Physiol 2001;63:521–554.

61. Momoeda K, Hirota K, Utsuki T, et al. Developmental changes of neutral glycophingolipids as receptors for pulmonary surfactant protein SP-A in alveolar epithelium of murine lung. J Biochem 1996;119:1189–1195.

62. Kuroki Y, Gasa S, Ogasawara Y, Makita A, Akino T. Binding of pulmonary surfactant protein A to galactosylceramide and asialo-GM2. Arch Biochem Biophys 1992;299:261–267.

63. Persson AV, Gibbons BJ, Shoemaker JD, Moxley MA, Longmore WJ. The major glycolipid recognized by SP-D in surfactant is phosphatidylinositol. Biochemistry 1992;31:12183–12189.

64. Ogasawara Y, Kuroki Y, Akino T. Pulmonary surfactant protein D specifically binds to phosphatidylinositol. J Biol Chem 1992;267:21244–21249.

65. Ogasawara Y, McCormack FX, Mason RJ, Voelker DR. Chimeras of surfactant proteins A and D identify the carbohydrate recognition domains as essential for phospholipid interaction. J Biol Chem 1994;269:29785–29792.

66. Saitoh M, Sano H, Chiba H, et al. Importance of the carboxy-terminal 25 amino acid residues of lung collectins in interactions with lipids and alveolar type II cells. Biochemistry 2000;39:1059–1066.

67. Borron P, McCormack FX, Elhalwagi BM, et al. Surfactant protein A inhibits T cell proliferation via its collagen-like tail and a 210-kDa receptor. Am J Psychol 1998;275:L679–L686.

68. Chroneos ZC, Abdolrasulnia R, Whitsett JA, Rice WR, Shepherd VL. Purification of a cell-surface receptor for surfactant protein A. J Biol Chem 1996;271:16375–16383.

69. Weikert LF, Lopez JP, Abdolrasulnia R, Chroneos ZC, Shepherd VL. Surfactant protein A enhances mycobacterial killing by rat macrophages through a nitric oxide-dependent pathway. Am J Physiol (Lung Cell Mol Physiol) 2000;279:L216–L223.

70. Sano H, Chiba H, Iwaki D, et al. Surfactant proteins A and D bind CD14 by different mechanisms. J Biol Chem 2000;275:22442–22451.

71. Prakobphol A, Xu F, Hoang VM, et al. Salivary agglutinin, which binds *Streptococcus mutans* and *Helicobacter pylori* is the lung scavenger receptor cysteine-rich protein gp-340 [in process citation]. J Biol Chem 2000;275:39860–39866.

72. Holmskov U, Mollenhauer J, Madsen J, et al. Cloning of gp-340, a putative opsonin receptor for lung surfactant protein D. Proc Natl Acad Sci USA 1999;96:10794–10799.

73. Tino MJ, Wright JR. Glycoprotein-340 binds surfactant protein-A (SP-A) and stimulates alveolar macrophage migration in an SP-A-independent manner. Am J Respir Cell Mol Biol 1999;20:759–768.

74. Dong Q, Wright JR. Binding of surfactant protein D (SP-D) to membrane glycolipids on alveolar macrophages. FASEB J 1998;12:A180.

75. Crouch E, Hartshorn K, Ofek I. Collectins and pulmonary innate immunity. Immunol Rev 2000;173:52–65.

76. Tino MJ, Wright JR. Surfactant protein A stimulates phagocytosis of specific pulmonary pathogens by alveolar macrophages. Am J Physiol 1996;270:L677–L688.

77. Kishore U, Wang JY, Hoppe HJ, Reid KBM. The alpha-helical neck region of human surfactant protein D is essential for the binding of the carbohydrate recognition domains to lipopolysacharides and phospholipids. Biochem J 1996;318:505–511.

78. Mariencheck WI, Savov J, Dong Q, Tino MJ, Wright JR. Surfactant protein A enhances alveolar macrophage phagocytosis of a live, mucoid strain of *P. aeruginosa*. Am J Physiol (Lung Cell Mol Physiol) 1999;277:L777–L786.

79. Restrepo C, Dong Q, Savov J, Mariencheck W, Wright JR. Surfactant protein D stimulates phagocytosis of *Pseudomonas aeruginosa* by alveolar macrophages. Am J Respir Cell Mol Biol 1998;21:576–585.

80. Madan T, Kishore U, Shah A, et al. Lung surfactant proteins A and D can inhibit specific IgE binding to the allergens of *Aspergillus fumigatus* and block allergen-induced histamine release from human basophils. Clin Exp Immunol 1997;110:241–249.

81. Allen MJ, Harbeck R, Smith B, Voelker DR, Mason RJ. Binding of rat and human surfactant proteins A and D to *Aspergillus fumigatus* conidia. Infect Immun 1999;67:4563–4569.

82. Madan T, Kishore U, Singh M, et al. Protective role of lung surfactant protein D in a murine model of invasive pulmonary aspergillosis. Infect Immun 2001;69:2728–2731.

83. Williams MD, Wright JR, March KL, Martin WJ. Human surfactant protein A enhances attachment of *pneumocystis carinii* to rat alveolar macrophages. Am J Respir Cell Mol Biol 1996;14:232–238.

84. Zimmerman PE, Voelker DR, McCormack FX, Paulsrud JR, Martin WJ2.120-kD surface glycoprotein of *Pneumocystis carinii* is a ligand for surfactant protein A. J Clin Invest 1992;89:143–149.

85. O'Riordan DM, Standing JE, Kwon KY, et al. Surfactant protein D interacts with *Pneumocystis carinii* and mediates organism adherence to alveolar macrophages. J Clin Invest 1995;95:2699–2710.

86. McCormack FX, Festa AL, Andrews RP, Linke M, Walzer PD. The carbohydrate recognition domain of surfactant protein A mediates binding to the major surface glycoprotein of *Pneumocystis carinii*. Biochemistry 1997;36:8092–8099.

87. Vuk-Pavlovic Z, Diaz-Montes T, Standing JE, Limper AH. Surfactant protein-D binds to cell wall β-glucans. Am J Respir Cell Mol Bio 1998;157:A236.

88. Limper AH, Crouch EC, O'Riordan DM, et al. Surfactant protein D modulates interaction of *Pneumocystis carinii* with alveolar macrophages. J Lab Clin Med 1995;126:416–422.

89. Zhu S, Kachel DL, Martin WJ, Matalon S. Nitrated SP-A does not enhance adherence of *Pneumocystis carinii* to alveolar macrophages. Am J Physiol 1998;275:L1031–L1039.

90. Koziel H, Phelps DS, Fishman JA, et al. Surfactant protein-A reduces binding and phagocytosis of *Pneumocystis carinii* by human alveolar macrophages in vitro. Am J Respir Cell Mol Biol 1998;18:834–843.

91. Phelps DS, Umstead TM, Rose RM, Fishman JA. Surfactant protein-A levels increase during *Pneumocystis carinii* pneumonia in the rat. Eur Respir J 1996;9:565–570.

92. Sternberg RI, Whitsett JA, Hull WM, Baughman RP. *Pneumocystis carinii* alters surfactant protein A concentrations in bronchoalveolar lavage fluid. J Lab Clin Med 1995;125:462–469.
93. Atochina EN, Beers MF, Scanlon ST, Preston AM, Beck JM. *P. carinii* induces selective alterations in component expression and biophysical activity of lung surfactant. Am J Physio Lung Cell Mol Physio 2000;278:L599–L609.
94. Paine R, Preston AM, Wilcoxen S, et al. Granulocyte- macrophage colony-stimulating factor in the innate immune response to *Pneumocystis carinii* pneumonia in mice. J Immunol 2000;164:2602–2609.
95. Hartshorn K, White MR, Voelker D, et al. Mechanism of binding of surfactant protein D to influenza A viruses: importance of binding to hemagglutinin to antiviral activity. Biochem J 2000;351:449–458.
96. Reading PC, Morey LS, Crouch EC, Anders EM. Collectin-mediated antiviral host defence of the lung: evidence from influenza virus infection of mice. J Virol 1997;71:8204–8212.
97. Reading PC, Allison J, Crouch EC, Anders EM. Increased susceptibility of diabetic mice to influenza virus infection: compromise of collectin-mediated host defence of the lung by glucose? J Viol 1999;72:6884–6887.
97a. LeVine AM, Whitsett JA, Hartshorn KL, et al. Surfactant protein D enhances clearance of influenza A virus from the lung in vivo. J Immunol 2001;167:5868.
97b. LeVine AMK, Hartshorn J, Elliott J, et al. Absence of SP-A modulates innate and adaptive defense responses to pulmonary influenza infection. Am J Physiol (Lung Cell Mol Physiol) 2002;282:L563–L572.
98. Hickling TP, Malhotra R, Bright H, et al. Lung surfactant protein A provides a route of entry for respiratory syncytical virus into host cells. Viral Immunol 2000;13:125–135.
99. Hickling TP, Bright H, Wing K, et al. A recombinant trimeric surfactant protein D carbohydrate recognition domain inhibits respiratory syncytial virus infection in vitro and in vivo. Eur J Immunol 1999;29:3478–3484.
100. Barr FE, Pedigo H, Johnson TR, Shepherd VL. Surfactant protein-A enhances uptake of respiratory syncytial virus by monocytes and U937 macrophages. Am J Respir Cell Mol Biol 2000;23:586–592.
101. Kerr MH, Paton JY. Surfactant protein levels in severe respiratory syncytial virus infection. Am J Respir Crit Care Med 1999;159:1115–1118.
102. Kalina M, Blau H, Riklis S, Kravtsov V. Interaction of surfactant protein A with bacterial lipopolysaccharide may affect some biological functions. Am J Physiol 1995;268:L144–51.
103. Van Iwaarden JF, Pikaar JC, Storm J, et al. Binding of surfactant protein A to the lipid A moiety of bacterial lipopolysaccharides. Biochem J 1994;303:407–411.
104. Stamme C, Wright JR. Surfactant protein A enhances interferon γ-induced nitric oxide but inhibits LPS-induced nitric oxide by alveolar macrophages. Am J Respir Crit Care Med 2000;161:A515.
105. Borron P, McIntosh JC, Korfhagen TR, et al. Surfactant-associated protein A inhibits LPS-induced cytokine and nitric oxide production in vivo. Am J Physiol (Lung Cell Mol Physiol) 2000;278:L840–L847.
106. McIntosh JC, Mervinblake S, Conner E, Wright JR. Surfactant protein A protects growing cells and reduces TNF-alpha activity from LPS-stumulated macrophages. Am J Physiol (Lung Cell Mol Physiol) 1996;15:L 310–L 319.
107. Sano H, Sohma H, Muta T, et al. Pulmonary surfactant protein A modulates the cellular response to smooth and rough lipopolysaccharides by interaction with CD14. J Immunol 1999;163:387–395.
108. Song M, Phelps DS. Interaction of surfactant protein A with lipopolysaccharide and regulation of inflammatory cytokines in the THP-1 monocytic cell line. Infect Immun 2000;68:6611–6617.

109. Van Rozendall BAWM, Van de Lest CHA, Van Eijk M, et al. Aerosolized endotoxin is immediately bound by pulmonary surfactant protein D in vivo. Biochim Biophys Acta Mol Basis Dis 1999;1454:261–269.

110. Stamme C, Wright JR. Surfactant protein A enhances the binding and deacylation of *E. coli* LPS by alveolar macrophages. Am J Physiol 1999;276:L540–L547.

111. Greene KE, Whitsett JA, Korfhagen TR, Fisher JH. SP-D expression regulates endotoxin mediated lung inflammation in vivo. Am J Respir Crit Care Med 2000;161:A515.

112. Mora R, Arold S, Marzan Y, Suki B, Ingenito EP. Determinants of surfactant function in acute lung injury and early recovery. Am J Physiol (Lung Cell Mol Physiol) 2000;279:L342–L349.

113. Viviano CJ, Bakewell WE, Dixon D, Dethloff LA, Hook GE. Altered regulation of surfactant phospholipid and protein A during acute pulmonary inflammation. Biochim Biophys Acta 1995;1259:235–244.

114. Sugahara K, Iyama K, Sano K, et al. Overexpression of surfactant protein SP-A, SP-B, and SP-C mRNA in rat lungs with lipopolysaccharide-induced injury. Lab Invest 1996;96:209–220.

115. Bridges JP, Davis HW, Damodarasamy M, et al. Pulmonary surfactant proteins A and D are potent endogenous inhibitors of lipid peroxidation and oxidative cellular injury. J Biol Chem 2000;275:38,848–38,855.

116. Stuart GR, Sim RB, Malhotra R. Characterization of radioiodinated lung surfactant protein A (SP-A) and the effects of oxidation on SP-A quarternary structure and activity. Exp Lung Res 1996;22:467–487.

117. Haddad IY, Crow JP, Hu P, et al. Concurrent generation of nitric oxide and superoxide damages surfactant protein A. Am J Physiol 1994;267:L242–L249.

118. Yoshida M, Korhagen TR, Whitsett JA. Surfactant protein D regulates NF-κB and matrix metalloproteinase production in alveolar macrophages via oxidant-sensitive pathways. J Immunol 2001;49:108–112.

119. Madan T, Kishore U, Singh M, et al. Surfactant proteins A and D protect mice against pulmonary hypersensitivity induced by *Aspergillus fumigatus* antigens and allergens. J Clin Invest 2001;107:467–475.

120. Wang JY, Kishore U, Lim BL, Strong P, Reid KBM. Interaction of human lung surfactant proteins A and D with mite *(Dermatophagoides pteronyssinus)* allergens. Clin Exp Immunol 1996;106:367–373.

121. Malhotra R, Haurum J, Thiel S, Jensenius JC, Sim RB. Pollen grains bind to lung alveolar type II cells (A549) via lung surfactant protein A (SP-A). Biosci Rep 1993;13:79–90.

122. Cheng G, Ueda T, Nakajima H, et al. Suppressive effects of SP-A on ionomycin-induced IL-8 production and release by eosinophils. Int Arch Allergy Immunol 1998;suppl1:59–62.

123. Cheng G, Ueda T, Numao T, et al. Increased levels of surfactant protein A and D in bronchoalveolar lavage fluids in patients with bronchial ashtma. Eur Respir J 2000;16:831–835.

124. van de Graaff EA, Jansen HM, Lutter R, et al. Surfactant protein A in bronchoalveolar lavage fluid. J Lab Clin Med 1992;120:252–263.

125. Wang JY, Shieh CC, You PF, Lei HY, Reid KB. Inhibitory effect of pulmonary surfactant proteins A and D on allergen-induced lymphocyte proliferation and histamine release in children with asthma. Am J Respir Crit Care Med 1998;158:510–518.

126. Ikegami M, Whitsett JA, Chroneos ZC, et al. IL-4 increases surfactant and regulates metabolism in vivo. Am J Physiol (Lung Cell Mol Physiol) 2000;278:L75–L80.

127. Borron P, Veldhuizen RAW, Lewis JE, et al. Surfactant associated protein-A inhibits human lymphocyte proliferation and IL-2 production. Am J Respir Cell Mol Biol 1996;15:115–121.

128. Borron PJ, Crouch EC, Lewis JF, et al. Recombinant rat surfactant-associated protein D inhibits human T lymphocyte proliferation and IL-2 production. J Immunol 1998;161:4599–4603.

129. Kabha K, Schmegner J, Keisari Y, et al. SP-A enhances phagocytosis of *Klebsiella* by interaction with capsular polysaccharides and alveolar macrophages. Am J Physiol (Lung Cell Mol Physiol) 1997;272:L344–L352.

130. Pikaar JC, van Golde LMG, van Strijp JAG, Van Iwaarden JF. Opsonic activities of surfactant proteins A and D in phagocytosis of gram-negative bacteria by alveolar macrophages. J Infect Dis 1995;172:481–489.

131. McNeely TB, Coonrod JD. Aggregation and opsonization of type A but not type B *Hemophilus influenzae* by surfactant protein A. Am J Respir Cell Mol Biol 1994;11:114–122.

132. McNeely TB, Coonrod JD. Comparison of the opsonic activity of human surfactant protein A for *Staphylococcus aureus* and *Streptococcus pneumoniae* with rabbit and human macrophages. J Infect Dis 1993;167:91–97.

133. Geertsma MF, Nibbering PH, Haagsman HP, Daha MR, van Furth R. Binding of surfactant protein A to C1q receptors mediates phagocytosis of *Staphylococcus aureus* by monocytes. Am J Physiol 1994;267:L578–L584.

134. Hartshorn KL, Crouch E, White MR, et al. Pulmonary surfactant proteins A and D enhance neutrophil uptake of bacteria. Am J Physiol 1998;274:L958–L969.

135. Manz-Keinke H, Plattner H, Schlepper-Schafer J. Lung surfactant protein A (SP-A) enhances serum-independent phagocytosis of bacteria by alveolar macrophages. Eur J Cell Biol 1992;57:95–100.

136. Madan T, Eggleton P, Kishore U, et al. Binding of pulmonary surfactant proteins A and D to *Aspergillus fumigatus* conidia enhances phagocytosis and killing by human neutrophils and alveolar macrophages. Infect Immun 1997;65:3171–3179.

137. Schelenz S, Malhotra R, Sim RB, Holmskov U, Bancroft GJ. Binding of host collectins to the pathogenic yeast *Cryptococcus neoformans:* human surfactant protein D acts as an agglutinin for acapsular yeast cells. Infect Immun 1995;63:3360–3366.

138. Benne CA, Kraaijeveld CA, van Strijp JA, et al. Interactions of surfactant protein A with influenza A viruses: binding and neutralization. J Infect Dis 1995;171:335–341.

139. Benne CA, Benaissa-Trouw B, van Strijp JA, Kraaijeveld CA, Van Iwaarden JF. Surfactant protein A, but not surfactant protein D, is an opsonin for influenza A virus phagocytosis by rat alveolar macrophages. Eur J Immunol 1997;27:886–890.

140. Ghildyal R, Hartley C, Varrasso A, et al. Surfactant protein a binds to the fusion glycoprotein of respiratory syncytial virus and neutralizes virion infectivity. J Infect Dis 1999;180:2009–2013.

141. van IJF, van SJA, Ebskamp MJ, et al. Surfactant protein A is opsonin in phagocytosis of herpes simplex virus type 1 by rat alveolar macrophages. Am J Physiol 1991;261:L204–9.

142. Van Iwaarden JF, van Strijp JA, Visser H, et al. Binding of surfactant protein A (SP-A) to herpes simplex virus type 1-infected cells is mediated by the carbohydrate moiety of SP-A. J Biol Chem 1992;267:25039–25043.

143. Weyer C, Sabat R, Wissel H, et al. Surfactant protein A binding to cytomegalovirus proteins enhances virus entry into rat lung cells. Am J Respir Cell Mol Biol 2000;23:71–78.

144. Downing JF, Pasula R, Wright JR, Twigg HL, Martin WJ. Surfactant protein A promotes attachment of *Mycobacterium tuberculosis* to alveolar macrophages during infection with human immunodeficiency virus. Proc Natl Acad Sci USA 1995;92:4848–4852.

145. Gaynor CD, McCormack FX, Voelker DR, McGowan SE, Schlesinger LS. Pulmonary surfactant protein A mediates enhanced phagocytosis of *Mycobacterium tuberculosis* by a direct interaction with human macrophages. J Immunol 1995;155:5343–5351.

146. Hickman-Davis JM, Lindsey JR, Zhu S, Matalon S. Surfactant protein A mediates mycoplasmacidal activity of alveolar macrophages. Am J Physiol (Lung Cell Mol Physiol) 1998;18:L270–L277.

147. Ofek I, Crouch E. Interactions of microbial glycoconjugates with collectins: implications for pulmonary host defense. In: Doyle RJ, (ed.). Glycomicrobiology. London: Plenum, 2000, pp. 517–537.

148. Ofek I, Kabha K, Keisari Y, et al. Recognition of *Klebsiella pneumoniae* by pulmonary C-type lectins. Nova Acta Leopold 1997;NF75:43–54.

149. van Rozendaal BA, van Spriel AB, van De Winkel JG, Haagsman HP. Role of pulmonary surfactant protein D in innate defense against *Candida albicans.* J Infect Dis 2000;182:917–922.

150. Hartshorn KL, Crouch EC, White MR, et al. Evidence for a protective role of pulmonary surfactant protein D (SP-D) against influenza A viruses. J Clin Invest 1994;94:311–319.

151. Ferguson JS, Voelker DR, McCormack FX, Schlesinger LS. Surfactant protein D binds to *Mycobacterium tuberculosis* bacilli and lipoarabinomannan via carbohydrate-lectin interactions resulting in reduced phagocytosis of the bacteria by macrophages. J Immunol 1999;163:312–321.

Structures of Complement Control Proteins

Thilo Stehle and Mykol Larvie

1. INTRODUCTION

Complement is an element of innate immunity consisting of a system of approx 30 interacting plasma proteins and cell surface receptors. This system can be activated by antibody clustering (the classical pathway), binding of mannose-binding lectin (MBL) to carbohydrates in bacterial cell walls (the MBL pathway), or cleavage of C3, a plasma complement protein, and deposition of one of its fragments, C3b, on cell surfaces (the alternative pathway). Initiation of any of these pathways leads to a serial cascade of proteolysis-mediated activation of proteins in the plasma (fluid phase) and on cell surfaces (solid phase). The three initiation pathways converge on a common pathway that results in the formation of the membrane attack complex (MAC), a multiprotein pore-forming structure capable of lysing cells. Since activation through any of these pathways can occur almost instantly and without the participation of cellular elements, the complement system is an essential first line of attack against microbial infection.

Tight regulation of this system is essential to prevent injury to host tissues. This is achieved in part by mechanisms that prevent the inappropriate activation of complement on autologous cells and tissues. One aspect of this protection is the cell surface expression of proteins that inhibit complement activity. A family of proteins known as the regulators of complement activation (RCA) plays a key role in this process by interacting with fragments of complement proteins C3 and/or C4. Members of this family are defined by the presence of short consensus repeat (SCR) domains, the ability to bind complement molecules C3b and C4b, and their clustering on chromosome 1 at the q3.2 locus (1,2). The RCA family includes the soluble plasma proteins C4 binding protein (C4bp) and factor H as well as the integral membrane proteins CD46 (membrane cofactor protein), CD55 (decay accelerating factor), CD35 (complement receptor type 1), and CD21 (complement receptor type 2). Table 1 lists some properties and functions of the RCA family members. A C9 binding protein known as the membrane attack complex inhibition factor is also able to inhibit complement activation but is not formally considered an RCA protein.

In addition to their function in complement regulation, many RCA family members are used as receptors by a surprisingly large and diverse number of pathogens. CD46 is

From: *Infectious Disease: Innate Immunity*
Edited by: R. A. B. Ezekowitz and J. A. Hoffmann © Humana Press Inc., Totowa, NJ

Table 1
The Regulators of Complement Activation

Molecule	Number of SCRs	Function
Soluble plasma proteins		
C4 binding protein (C4bp)	8 (α-chain) 3 (β-chain)	Accelerates decay of classical pathway C3 convertase; acts as a cofactor for factor I cleavage ofC3b and C4b
Factor H (fH)	20	Accelerates decay of alternative pathway C3 convertase; acts as a cofactor for factor I cleavage of C3b and C4b
Integral membrane proteins		
Membrane cofactor protein (MCP, CD46)	4	Acts as a cofactor for factor I cleavage of C3b and C4b
Complement receptor type 1 (CR1, CD35)	30	Accelerates dissociation of alternative and classical pathway C3 convertases; acts as a cofactor for factor I cleavage of C3b and C4b
Complement receptor type 2 (CR2, CD21)	15	Binds C3d attached to antigen; acts as a cofactor for factor I cleavage of C3b and C4b
Decay accelerating factor (DAF, CD55)	4	Accelerates dissociation of classical and alternative pathway C3 convertases

a receptor for measles virus *(3,4)*, group A *Streptococcus pyogenes (5)*, *Neisseria gonorrhoeae* and *Neisseria meningitidis (6)*, and human herpesvirus 6 *(7)*. CD55 has been identified as a receptor for enterovirus 70 *(8)*, some echoviruses *(9–11)*, and some coxsackieviruses *(12,13)*. CD21 is a receptor for Epstein-Barr virus *(14–16)*. The plasma proteins factor H and C4bp bind to *Streptococcus pyogenes (17,18)*, and factor H also binds to the surface protein OspE of *Borrelia burgdorferi (19)*. The interactions of RCA family proteins with complement proteins and pathogens probably use the same principles and share similar features. For example, the envelope glycoprotein gp350/220 of Epstein-Barr virus is thought to mimic features of the natural CD21 ligand C3d *(20)*.

The proteins in the RCA family have been reviewed extensively in the past *(1,2,21–24)*. In this review, we focus on recent advances in the structural and functional analysis of some members of the RCA family. We discuss the crystal structures of key portions of CD46 *(25)* and CD21 *(26)*, as well as the likely solution structure of full-length factor H *(27)*. In addition, we discuss the atomic structure of vaccinia virus complement control protein, a viral protein that mimics the regulators of complement activation *(28)*. Using these structures, we highlight key features of RCA family members and describe some of the challenges that lie ahead on our quest for a better understanding of complement regulation at the structural and functional level.

2. THE RCA FAMILY AND SHORT CONSENSUS REPEATS

The members of the RCA family contain short consensus repeats (SCRs), modules of about 60 amino acids with four invariant cysteines linked in a Cys1-Cys3, Cys2-Cys4 pattern *(2)*. A striking feature of these molecules is that they each have several SCR domains concatenated in an uninterrupted series. The number of SCRs found in RCA family members varies substantially: CD46 and CD55 contain 4 SCRs, CD21 contains 15 SCRs, factor H contains 20 SCRs, CD35 contains 30 SCRs, and the α- and β-chains of the C4 binding protein contain 8 and 3 SCRs, respectively. SCR domains are by no means limited to RCA family members; they are present in a wide variety of other cell surface receptors [such as the γ-aminobutyric acid (GABA) receptor, the interleukin-2 (IL-2) receptor, and E-, L- and P-selectins] and soluble proteins (such as $\beta2$-glycoprotein I, coagulation factor XIII, and haptoglobin). Moreover, a number of complement proteins (e.g., C1s, C6, and C7) or complement factors (e.g., C3/C5 convertase) contain SCR domains, as does the mannose binding lectin-associated serine protease (MASP) of the MBL pathway. In all these molecules, the SCR domains are arranged in a contiguous series with at least two SCRs. That SCR domains are not found singly in proteins suggests that a two-domain fragment is the smallest stable module of protein sequence comprising SCR motifs.

Structures of the SCR domain have been determined by nuclear magnetic resonance (NMR) *(29–34)* and by X-ray crystallography *(25,26,28,35–37)*. These studies have established details of the architecture of a single SCR domain and provide insights into their organization in extended concatamers. The SCR domain adopts a β-barrel fold that consists of a central four-stranded antiparallel β-sheet. This β-sheet packs against an N-terminal coil and is, in some cases, surrounded by several additional short β-strands at either end of the domain. SCR domains frequently contain N-linked glycosylation sites. Most often there is a single glycosylation site per repeat, but as many as three have been predicted. The SCR fold efficiently exposes most of the side chains to the solvent, giving these domains a high surface-to-volume ratio. Figure 1 is a comprehensive sequence alignment of all SCR domains of human RCA family members. The alignment shows that this motif is defined primarily by only five invariant residues: four cysteine residues forming two disulfide bridges, and one tryptophan in the small hydrophobic core of the domain. Apart from these conserved residues, there is striking sequence diversity between SCR domains. Figure 2A shows the structure of an SCR domain, using SCR1 of CD46 as an example. The five strictly conserved residues are shown. The four cysteines link the N and C termini of the domain to the domain body, which is probably crucial for the stability of the domain fold. The invariant tryptophan is buried in the small hydrophobic core of the domain, and its side chain forms a hydrogen bond with an amide at the N terminus, thereby anchoring the N-terminal coil to the domain. The tryptophan also packs against one of the disulfide bridges.

The large differences in sequence translate into a profound heterogeneity of SCR domains at the structural level. A comparison of all known structures of SCR domains *(25,26,28,32–37)* reveals striking differences among them (Fig. 2B). The domains can be superimposed onto each other with root-mean-square deviations of approx 1.8 Å for 25–59 C_α atoms, depending on the individual case. The only structural elements that superimpose well are the central β-strand (strand C, Fig. 2A) and a small part of the

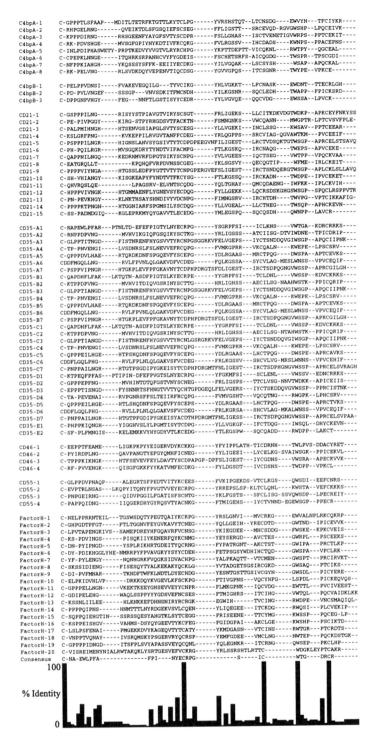

Fig. 1. Alignment of amino acid sequences of human RCA proteins. Below the alignment a bar plot of the sequence identity is shown in which the percentage of sequences containing the most common residue at each position is plotted. C4bpA, C4 binding protein chain A; C4bpB, C4 binding protein chain B.

A　　　　**B**

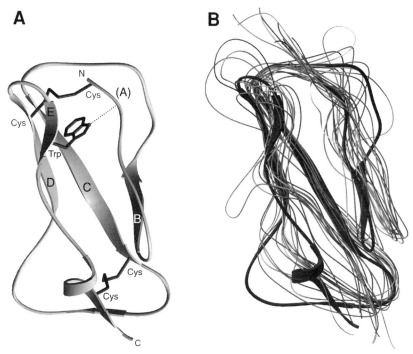

Fig. 2. Three-dimensional structure of the SCR domain. **(A)** Ribbon drawing of the first repeat of CD46. The core of the domain contains a small, central β-sheet (strands B, C, D, and E) connected by loops. Some SCR domains contain an additional short strand, labeled (A), at the top of the domain. The side chains of the five strictly conserved residues defining the domain (four cysteines and a tryptophan) are shown. The cysteines form two disulfide bridges that provide structural stability. The conserved tryptophan is buried in the small hydrophobic core of the domain, and its side chain forms a hydrogen bond with a main chain nitrogen at the N terminus (indicated with a dotted line). This particular domain also contains a short helix near its C terminus, which is absent in other domains. **(B)** Superposition of all structurally known SCR domains. The superposition includes SCR1 and SCR2 of CD46 *(25)*, SCR1 and SCR2 of CD21 *(26)*, SCR2 of the C1s complement protein *(37)*, SCR15 and SCR16 of factor H *(32)*, and the SCR1-SCR4 domains of the vaccinia virus complement control protein *(28)* and β-glyco-protein I *(36)*. SCR1 of CD46 is shown in black and thicker lines, including secondary structure elements. The other repeats are shown as thin gray ribbons. The superimposition was performed in program O *(82)* by maximizing the number of superimposed C_α atoms while maintaining a root-mean-square deviation of 2.0 Å or less. The numbers of C_α atoms used for this procedure range from 25 to 59 for each domain. Figure prepared with RIBBONS *(83)*.

surrounding β-sheet structure. The remaining regions and especially the surface loops differ substantially in structure.

2.1. CD46 (Membrane Cofactor Protein)

CD46, also known as membrane cofactor protein, is a type I integral membrane glycoprotein with a single transmembrane domain. The extracellular portion of the molecule contains four SCR domains and a 25-amino acid sequence that is relatively rich in serine, threonine, and proline residues (the STP region). The CD46 ectodomain is followed by a transmembrane region and a short cytoplasmic tail. Two alternate exons encode the cytoplasmic domain, and four alternate exons encode variations of the STP region. These can combine to form eight different versions of CD46, although it appears that four of these variants are most common *(2)*. There are three N-linked glycosylation sites, one each in SCR1, SCR2, and SCR4, and several O-linked glycosylation sites in the STP region.

CD46 is widely distributed. Its expression was first examined in hematopoietic tissues, where it was found on platelets, granulocytes, helper T-cells, cytotoxic T-cells, B-cells, natural killer cells, monocytes, neutrophils, monocytes, and cells of epithelial, endothelial, and fibroblast origin *(2,38,39)*. In fact, with the notable exception of erythrocytes, CD46 expression has been identified on every cell type examined *(40)*. A soluble form of CD46 has been identified in numerous secretions and is especially rich in semen and vaginal fluids *(41)*. Recombinant soluble forms of CD46 are able to inhibit complement activation *(42,43)*, and thus they have a potential use as complement-suppressing agents in tissue transplantation *(44)*. Recombinant forms of CD46 are also able to inhibit measles virus infections *(45)*.

CD46 inhibits complement activation by binding separately to C3b or C4b and stabilizing them for proteolytic inactivation by factor I, a plasma protein in the trypsin protease family *(46)*. Inactivation of C3b and C4b, in either the fluid or solid phase, inhibits continued complement activation and the progression of the pathway to MAC assembly. In the alternative pathway, for example, C3b that is generated from spontaneous hydrolysis (the so-called C3 tickover) might lead to a critical level of C3 convertase, thereby triggering a positive feedback cycle of further C3b production, if there were no constitutive mechanism to inactivate C3b. CD46 provides an intrinsic defense in that it protects cells on whose surface it is expressed. Its broad tissue distribution is accounted for by the necessity of guarding any cells that may be exposed to complement from its inappropriate activation.

A curious feature of CD46 is the use that multiple pathogenic microbes make of it as a receptor. The best known of these is the measles virus *(3,4)*, although this finding is currently the subject of skeptical review following the discovery of another receptor (SLAM/CDw150) that appears to account better for the pathogenesis of measles virus infection *(47,48)*. Group A *S. pyogenes (5)*, *N. gonorrhoeae*, *N. meningitidis (6)*, and human herpes virus 6 *(7)* have all been found to utilize CD46 as a specific cellular receptor. Some of these interactions have been mapped to specific regions of CD46. Binding to measles virus involves SCR1 and SCR2 of CD46 *(49–52)*, and *N. gonorrhoeae* recognizes the SCR3 domain and the STP region of CD46 *(53)*.

The structure of the measles virus binding SCR1-SCR2 portion of CD46 was determined using X-ray crystallography *(25)*. A ribbon drawing of the structure is shown in Fig. 3A. The polypeptide chain folds into two concatenated β-barrels, each containing two disulfide bonds and one N-linked glycan attached to the "top" of the domain. The two glycans cover a significant portion of the concave side of the molecule and approach each other owing to a pronounced bend of approx 60° between the two SCR domains. The analyzed crystals contain six independent copies of the CD46 fragment. These assume somewhat different conformations, and the interdomain angle varies by about 15° among the six molecules. Thus, some flexibility exists at the interface between SCR1 and SCR2. Up to seven carbohydrate residues are seen at each of the

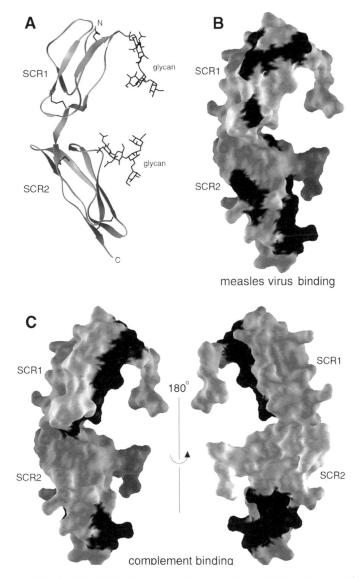

Fig. 3. Structure of the SCR1-SCR2 fragment of human CD46 *(25)* and interaction with ligands. **(A)** Ribbon drawing of the crystallized fragment. The polypeptide chain folds into two concatenated β-barrels, each containing two disulfide bonds and one N-linked glycan attached to the "top" of the domain. The two glycans cover a significant portion of the concave side of the molecule and approach each other owing to a pronounced bend of approx 60° from a linear conformation. The molecule has substantial mobility (about 15°) at the SCR1-SCR2 interface. **(B)** Interaction with measles virus. Surface representation of CD46 SCR1-SCR2, with residues implicated in measles virus binding shown in black. Residues Glu24, Arg25, Pro39, Ile45-Arg48, Tyr67, Asp70, and Phe85-Ile104 define an extended measles virus-binding surface that spans both domains. See ref. *25* for details. **(C)** Two views of the CD46 surface with areas predicted to be involved in C4b interaction and regulation highlighted in black. Three such areas (residues 47–61, 94–103, and 120–122) have been identified *(58)*. These residues cluster in two areas: underneath the glycan moiety of SCR1 and at the base of SCR2, next to and partially overlapping residues involved in measles virus binding. **A** was prepared with RIBBONS *(83)*, and **B** and **C** were produced with GRASP *(84)*.

two N-linked glycosylation sites, and the position of the glycans at the same side of the molecule suggests that they play a role both in maintaining the interdomain orientation of the fragment and in limiting flexibility.

The CD46 residues involved in measles virus binding define a large, glycan-free surface that extends from the top of the first to the bottom of the second repeat (Fig. 3B) *(25)*. The proposed virus binding surface is spread over a large area spanning two flexibly linked domains, in contrast to other known examples, in which virus-receptor interactions occur at a single, smaller site at the tip of an inflexible domain (reviewed in ref *54*). Although the glycan attached to SCR2 has been implicated in the interaction with measles virus *(55)*, it most likely does so indirectly by helping to maintain the conformation of the virus binding surface.

How does CD46 interact with complement proteins C3b and C4b? Although less is known about these interactions than about those of the protein with measles virus, some details are beginning to emerge. Earlier studies suggested that binding to complement involves SCR2, SCR3, and SCR4, which includes sites that are physically distinct from the measles virus binding surface defined by SCR1 and SCR2 *(50,56)*. The glycans at SCR2 and SCR4 of CD46 were found to be necessary for interaction with complement, whereas the glycan at SCR1 is not required *(57)*. More recent mutagenesis and peptide inhibition studies have now implicated all four SCR domains in complement binding *(58)*. These studies also indicates that the C3b and C4b binding sites are not identical. Three areas likely to be involved in C4b binding and regulation are located within SCR1-SCR2, and their location can now be examined using the structure of the SCR1-SCR2 fragment of CD46. Inspection of the structure shows that they cluster on one face of SCR1 and at the base of SCR2 (Fig. 3C). Of note, the site at the base of SCR2 is close to the predicted measles virus binding surface of CD46 shown in Fig. 3B, leading to speculation that measles virus and C4b use a similar site for docking to CD46 and therefore might share some structural homology *(58)*. However, the binding surfaces for measles virus and C4b on SCR2, although close to each other, appear to involve some non-overlapping regions (Fig. 3B and C). The sites are even more distinct in SCR1, where the predicted complement-regulatory site lies primarily underneath the glycan, whereas residues thought to be involved in measles virus binding are exposed and lie on the side opposite to the glycan.

Other predicted complement binding regions in domains SCR1-SCR4 of CD46 involve sequences that contain multiple prolines, especially so in SCR3 and SCR4 *(58)*. No structural information about CD46 domains SCR3 and SCR4 is available, and the role of these proline residues remains unclear. We note that a prominent loop in SCR1, which is predicted to be involved in measles virus binding, also contains two consecutive proline residues.

The association of CD46 with complement proteins C3b and C4b is among both the more relevant and the least understood of its known actions. Aside from the above-described advances, little is known about the specific nature of its interactions with C4b and C3b. The inappropriate activation of complement, which CD46 acts to inhibit, is a major cause of tissue injury in many disease states. It follows, then, that a better knowledge of CD46-mediated complement regulation may lead to useful interventions in sepsis and autoimmune diseases. Ultimately, such knowledge will have to await the structural analysis of the remaining SCR domains of CD46 and the complexes with its ligands.

2.2. CD21 *(Complement Receptor Type 2)*

Complement receptor type 2 (CD21) is a key interface between innate and adaptive immunity *(59)*. The molecule is primarily expressed on mature B-lymphocytes and follicular dendritic cells and serves as a receptor for complement component C3d *(15,60)*. C3d-bound antigens bind to CD21 via C3d and to the B-cell receptor via the antigen, thus amplifying B-lymphocyte activation. In addition, CD21 also serves as a ligand for Epstein-Barr virus *(14)* and the IgE receptor CD23 *(61,62)*. All three interactions require the presence of the first two of the 15 SCR domains of CD21, and the binding sites for Epstein-Barr virus and C3d overlap *(20,63)*. The recently determined crystal structure of a complex between C3d and the first two repeats of CD21, shown in Fig. 4, has demonstrated for the first time how protein-ligand interactions are mediated by SCR domains *(26)*. The complex consists of a V-shaped CD21 SCR1-SCR2 receptor fragment bound to a globular C3d ligand. Several unexpected findings are revealed by this structure:

1. The CD21 fragment exhibits a pronounced bend between SCR1 and SCR2, resulting in a V-like shape that is strikingly different from the more extended conformations seen in all other known structures of fragments with two or more SCR domains *(25,28,32–36)*. Although CD21 is so far the only example for a ligand-receptor complex in this family, it is unlikely that the V-like conformation is induced by ligand binding since the crystals contain a second, unliganded CD21 molecule in an essentially identical conformation. Thus the V-like arrangement of its two N-terminal domains appears to be an inherent property of CD21.
2. The structure of the CD21/C3d complex reveals that only one of the CD21 repeats, SCR2, directly contacts the C3d ligand. It was previously shown that both repeats are required for C3d binding *(64,65)*. Since the two domains are engaged in extensive side-by-side contacts, the most likely explanation for the requirement of both domains for C3d binding is that the presence of SCR1 stabilizes the three-dimensional structure of the two-domain fragment and therefore the C3d binding site on SCR2 *(26)*.
3. Finally, the crystals contain a dimer of CD21, although one of the monomers in this dimer is not liganded to a C3d molecule. Interactions within the CD21 dimer are generated by contacts between the SCR1 domains. Is this dimer physiologic? Although the molecule is monomeric in solution, it is conceivable that it forms a dimer under the presumably more constrained conditions at the cell surface.

How does CD21 recognize its ligand? The interaction between C3d and CD21 is to a large extend defined through hydrogen bonds involving main chain atoms. With the exception of one residue (Asn170), all hydrogen bonds to CD21 involve main chain atoms of C3d. Thus, specificity for the complex seems to be achieved through the overall complementarity of the interacting surfaces rather than through specific side chain interactions. The CD21/C3d interaction was found earlier to be substantially affected by salt concentrations, indicating that complex formation involves strong hydrogen bonds and perhaps salt bridges *(26)*. Ionic interactions in particular are affected by the ionic strength of the surrounding environment: high salt concentration weakens such interactions, whereas low salt concentration stabilizes them. The analysis of the CD21/C3d interface does not easily explain the dependence of the interaction on ionic

240   *Stehle and Larvie*

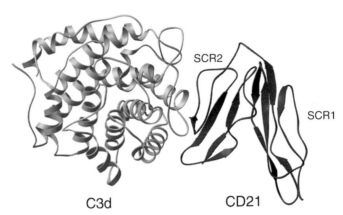

Fig. 4. Crystal structure of the complex between CD21 SCR1-SCR2 and complement protein C3d *(26)*. The two SCR domains of CD21 form a severely bent, V-shaped structure. The severe bend is unique among known SCR structures. It is most likely made possible by the long, eight-residue linker between SCR1 and SCR2. All other multidomain structures of SCR-containing repeats determined to date have shorter linkers of four residues and a more extended conformation. Figure prepared with RIBBONS *(83)*.

strength, since no salt bridges are seen in the complex. However, an unusual interaction involves Arg84 of CD21, which is located at the edge of a loop and is coordinated by an anion-hole formed by four carbonyl oxygens at the carboxy terminus of a helix in C3d. Thus the positively charged Arg84 side chain acts as a "capping residue" for the negatively charged helix dipole moment. It is conceivable that this interaction, which is comparable in strength to a strong hydrogen bond or a salt bridge, is affected by salt concentrations, thus explaining the earlier findings. The CD21/C3d complex was crystallized in the presence of zinc, and the interface contains two zinc ions. The zinc is probably a crystal artifact. It is not known whether other cations (which might be replaced by zinc in the structure) play a physiologic role in the C3d/CD21 interaction. It is possible that the presence of zinc distorts the view of the interactions between CD21 and C3d, since acidic residues coordinating the zinc ions in the complex might otherwise be free to form salt bridges with positively charged lysine or arginine residues.

The C3d/CD21 interaction illustrates the limitations of mutagenesis and antibody inhibition studies that have attempted to identify interacting residues in the absence of structural information. The interaction of CD21 with C3d has been the focus of numerous studies, and the crystal structure of C3d has been available for several years *(66)*. Residues at the CD21 SCR1-SCR2 interface were identified as possible ligands for C3d *(65)* through antibody inhibition studies; these residues do not contact C3d in the crystal structure, although they are in the vicinity of the site of interaction. Mutagenesis experiments identified two clusters of acidic C3d residues as important CD21-contacting regions *(67)*. Both clusters are not contacting CD21, and one of the clusters (Glu37/Glu39) is in fact located opposite to the surface that interacts with CD21. Finally, two CD21 residues (Ser16 and Tyr68) were identified as potential ligands for

C3d and the Epstein-Barr virus glycoprotein gp350/220, two proteins that are thought to have overlapping but distinct binding sites on CD21 *(20)*. The structure of the complex shows that neither residue contacts C3d.

2.3. Factor H

Factor H, a plasma protein, functions as a cofactor for the enzyme factor I in the breakdown of C3b and iC3b. The molecule contains 20 SCR domains, and it was the first member of the RCA family for which structural information was available. To date, structures of factor H SCR5,SCR16, and a fragment containing SCR15-SCR16 have been determined *(29–32)*. Although none of these structures contain known ligand binding sites, they have been very useful in helping to identify key features of the SCR fold, such as the two conserved disulfide bridges and the small hydrophobic core. A complement-regulatory site of factor H lies within the N-terminal four SCR domains, and two additional sites are believed to be involved in C3b binding [reviewed in ref. *(22)*]. Factor H is also a receptor for *S. pyogenes,* and SCR7 has been implicated in this interaction *(17,68)*.

Factor H is interesting partly because it is a soluble complement-regulatory protein, in contrast to the membrane-bound receptors CD46 and CD21. Thus its conformation is less restrained owing to the absence of a membrane anchor. Recent work by Aslam and Perkins *(27)* has shed some light on how we might envision the conformation of the long, 20-SCR factor H molecule in solution. When fully extended, the factor H chain would span a distance of about 750 Å. A structural analysis of such a long and presumably flexible molecule by NMR or protein crystallography is not feasible, and so Aslam and Perkins used low-angle X-ray and neutron scattering, analytical ultracentrifugation, and molecular simulation experiments to study the conformation of the factor H chain in solution. They found, surprisingly, that the 20 SCR domains are likely to assume a folded-back structure rather than adopting an elongated, linear conformation *(27)*. Of note, the factor H sequence has several especially long interdomain linkers around its midpoint. The longest of these is an eight-residue linker between SCR12 and SCR13 (Fig. 1), and such a long linker would allow for a V-shaped arrangement similar to that seen in the crystal structure of CD21 (Fig. 3). Domains SCR10-SCR11, SCR11-SCR12, SCR13-SCR14, and SCR18-SCR19 also have linkers of at least six amino acids, and thus flexibility and bending is likely to occur at these sites.

3. VIRAL COMPLEMENT CONTROL PROTEINS

Preventing the inappropriate activation of complement is of great importance. Molecules that regulate complement are central to achieving this goal, and any interference with these molecules can lead to serious harm. It is therefore not too surprising that viruses have evolved strategies to evade immunity mediated by antibodies and complement and to manipulate the inflammatory response mounted by a host. These strategies include the incorporation of host complement-regulatory proteins into the virion envelope and the expression of viral proteins that mimic complement regulators *(69,70)*. A well-known example for the latter strategy is the vaccinia virus complement control protein (VCP) *(71)*, which is synthesized by poxviruses. VCP can inhibit both the classical and alternative pathways of complement activation by binding to complement components C3b and C4b, as well as through its ability to accelerate the decay of the

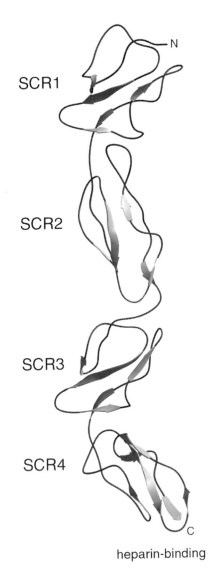

SCR1

SCR2

SCR3

SCR4

heparin-binding

Fig. 5. Structure of the vaccinia virus complement control protein (VCP) *(28)*. The crystallized protein contains all four SCR domains and assumes an extended structure. Figure prepared with RIBBONS *(83)*.

C3 convertase complex. By interfering with the host's complement system in this manner, the virus can escape neutralization through antibodies and can protect virion progeny from host complement attack. The VCP protein mimics the members of the RCA family; it contains four SCR domains that are closely related to the A chain of C4 binding protein (C4bpA). In fact, VCP so closely mimics the function of human C4bp that it has been shown to inhibit the classical pathway of complement activation with greater potency than C4bp *(72)*.

The recently determined crystal structure of VCP, shown in Fig. 5, has shed some light on how this protein interacts with complement *(28)*. Although VCP is not a member of the RCA family, it is useful to consider it in this review because it closely mimics the function of RCA family members and because it is so far the only "complete" atomic structure of a protein that contains SCR domains and regulates complement. The VCP molecule has an extended conformation, with all four domains stacked end to end (Fig. 5). Interdomain contacts are limited to interactions between consecutive SCR domains, which is similar to the way the two SCR domains are arranged in CD46 SCR1-SCR2 but different from the side-to-side packing seen in the CD21 SCR1-SCR2 structure. The VCP molecule shows little flexibility, since five independently determined structures of the molecule can be superimposed with minimal root-mean-square deviations *(28)*. This would suggest that crystal packing forces are not responsible for the observed conformation, which has led to the suggestion that VCP adopts this conformation in solution *(28)*. However, the orientation of SCR2 with respect to SCR3 in the crystals differs dramatically from that seen in the NMR structure of a VCP SCR2-SCR3 fragment *(34)*. One explanation for this discrepancy is that the SCR2-SCR3 linkage is flexible under some conditions. A small contact area and substantial flexibility between SCR2 and SCR3 were shown earlier to be important properties of VCP *(73)*. It is unlikely that the presence of SCR1 and SCR4, which are included in the crystallized protein but not in the NMR structure of VCP SCR2-SCR3, has any bearing on the flexibility between SCR2 and SCR3 since they do not engage in contacts with this region (Fig. 5). The available structural data thus offer conflicting views about the molecule's conformation in solution.

How does the VCP structure inform us about the interaction with the C3b and C4b complement proteins? Most of the available data implicate domains SCR1 and SCR2 in complement inhibition. An ionic interaction has been proposed, and a face formed by SCR1 and SCR2 does in fact contain numerous positively charged residues that are thought to interact with a negatively charged surface on the complement proteins *(28)*. Additional information about complement binding comes from similarities in sequence between CD46 and VCP. Many of the CD46 residues likely to be involved in complement binding *(58)* are conserved in VCP, suggesting that complement binding itself is at least partially conserved in CD46 and VCP. Most of the conserved residues are located in SCR2. A second binding site in the VCP SCR4 domain has been predicted as well *(28)*. This site lies next to a proposed heparin binding surface at the base of the molecule. Interaction with heparin is thought to be used by VCP as a means for cell surface association. Thus vaccinia virus seems to have arrived at an elegant solution for targeting a soluble protein to the membrane surface and making it functionally equivalent to membrane-associated complement regulators such as CD46; although the mechanism of surface adhesion is different in both cases.

4. EMERGING PRINCIPLES

The RCA family members are constructed from a large number of SCR domains, as many as 30 in the case of CD35. Thus the design of these molecules is highly modular. It is also apparent that gene duplication has played a significant role in the construction of several of these proteins. The CD21 chain, for example, appears to have been generated through the repeat of a basic unit of four consecutive SCRs, whereas the CD35 sequence seems to have a basic repeated unit of seven SCR domains. With almost 2500 amino acids, CD35 is the largest RCA family member. Its 30 SCR domains, when fully extended, would span a distance of more than 1000 Å. It seems intuitive that such a long molecule would need to have both some degree of conformational order and also some degree of flexibility. What, then, are the parameters that define conformation and flexibility? It is useful to compare the existing structures in order to identify principles of construction that would allow a better understanding of conformation and flexibility and perhaps also help with the prediction of homotypic and heterotypic interactions.

4.1. Conformation

The database of known structures of two or more concatenated SCR domains is still very small, and new structures continue to offer surprises. The following analysis is therefore constrained by the available data. Figure 6A shows a superposition of the 10 existing structures of two-domain fragments of SCR-containing proteins *(25,26,28,32,34,36)*. There is a surprisingly large variation in the orientation of one SCR relative to the next, and no preferred conformation seems to exist. In the crystal structure of the CD21 SCR1-SCR2/C3d complex, the two SCRs are folded back on each other so that they form a tight V shape (Fig. 4) *(26)*. In contrast, β-glycoprotein I has several linkages that are very nearly linear *(35,36)*. Several other structures have somewhat bent conformations *(25,28,32,35)*, but the degree and direction of the observed bends are quite variable. How variable are these bends, and what are the parameters that define them?

To address this question in a more rigorous manner, we calculated and plotted parameters of the interdomain orientations between the two SCR domains of all 10 available SCR pairs. Several methods have been employed for this purpose *(33,36)*, and our analysis is based on the calculation of the *tilt* and *twist* angles *(36)* (Fig. 6B). The tilt angle describes the deviation of a two-domain structure from a fully extended conformation, whereas the twist angle describes a rotation along the central axis of the domain in order to align the β-sheets of the two domains. Plotting the tilt and twist angles for each two-domain fragment, as shown in Fig. 6B, reveals that the parameters of 7 of 10 structures cluster in the upper left quadrant of the plot, with both tilt and twist values between 0° and 180°. Thus, although their precise conformations differ, the molecules in this region have generally similar interdomain angles.

The similar direction of the tilt of most molecules is obvious from Fig. 6A, which shows that the tilt is predominantly to the left. The only two structures tilting to the right are CD46 SCR1-SCR2 *(25)* and the crystal structure of VCP domains SCR2 and SCR3 *(28,34)*. The conformation of the latter is in question as it differs from the solution structure of VCP SCR2-SCR3 *(34)*. The conformation of CD46 SCR1-SCR2, on the other hand, is probably accurate, as it is nearly identical in two unrelated crystal forms with a total of 12 independent copies of this fragment *(25)* (T.S. and M.L., unpublished data). The unique tilt of the CD46 SCR1-SCR2 fragment may be related to the especially protruding DE-loop in SCR2, as hypothesized earlier *(25)*. In most structures, the N-terminal SCR domain bends over the DE-loop of the C-terminal domain, partially covering it (Fig. 6A). The DE-loop of CD46-SCR2 carries an insertion not present in most other domains (Fig. 1), which results in an extension of strands D and E in a more protruding loop conformation. Because of its protruding nature and rigidity, the DE-loop may force the SCR1 domain to tilt away from it in order to prevent steric clashes.

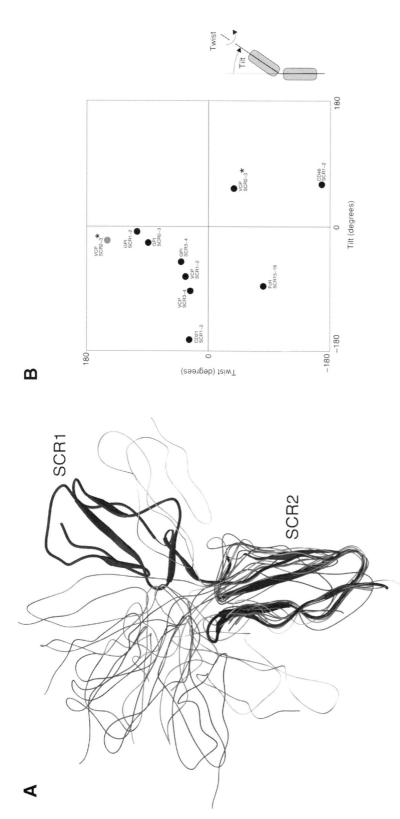

Fig. 6. Orientational differences in fragments with two consecutive SCR domains. (**A**) Superimposition of all available structures with two consecutive SCR domains. The superimposition is based on the C-terminal repeat of each two-domain fragment and was performed as described in the legend to Fig. 2. The CD46 SCR1-SCR2 structure (25) is shown in black and thicker lines, including β-strands. Other structures are shown as thin gray ribbons and include CD21 SCR1-SCR2 (26), factor H SCR15–SCR16 (32), VCP fragments SCR1-SCR2, SCR2-SCR3, and SCR3-SCR4 (28), and β₂-glycoprotein I fragments SCR1-SCR2, SCR2-SCR3, and SCR3-SCR4 (36). (**B**) Two-dimensional plot of the distribution of tilt and twist angles in each of the two-domain fragments shown in **A**. GPI, β₂-glycoprotein I; fH, factor H. Two sets of angles are shown for the VCP SCR2-SCR3 fragment (marked with an asterisk). One set corresponds to the conformation observed in the crystal structure of VCP SCR1-SCR4 (28) (gray dot), and the other corresponds to the conformation seen in an NMR structure of the VCP SCR2-SCR3 fragment (34) (black dot). A was prepared with RIBBONS (83).

245

Most of the observed tilt angles are less than 90°. The only molecule with a significantly more severe tilt is CD21 SCR1-SCR2. This extreme tilt is accommodated by the unusually long eight-residue linker between those two repeats. All other structures determined to date have four-residue linkers, and, based on the currently available data, it appears that a four-residue linker is incompatible with a tilt in excess of 90°.

The twist direction is also similar for most structures. Seven of the 10 molecules have twist angles between 0 and 180°, with most clustered in a narrower range between 0 and 90°. Thus, two consecutive domains seem to face in roughly similar directions. The molecules that deviate most sharply from this arrangement are CD46 SCR1-SCR2, the X-ray structure of VCP SCR2-SCR3, and factor H SCR15-SCR16. The interfaces of the latter two structures are likely to be flexible *(32,73)*, and the VCP SCR2-SCR3 interface has a dramatically different conformation in solution *(34)*.

4.2. Flexibility

The degree of flexibility between consecutive SCR domains is difficult to determine from the experimental data. In structures determined in solution by NMR, flexibility can sometimes be estimated directly from the primary data. Although crystal structures represent a more static picture of a molecule, information about flexibility can sometimes be obtained from the comparison of conformations of multiple copies of a molecule in the crystallographic asymmetric unit. The crystal structure of the SCR1-SCR2 fragment of CD46 shows that SCR2 can move about 15° with respect to SCR1 *(25)*, which arises from flexibility between the two repeats. The NMR structural analysis of the two-domain fragment of factor H has revealed even greater interdomain flexibility, with very few contacts between the two repeats *(32)*. On the other hand, the interdomain linkers between the four SCR modules of VCP appear to be surprisingly rigid, since all five independent molecules in the crystals assume almost identical conformations *(28)*. The CD21 SCR1-SCR2 fragment, which shows no evidence of flexibility, is unusual in that it is the only one that features side-by-side packing.

What structural features affect flexibility? The known structures suggest four such parameters: length of the interdomain linker, sequence of the interdomain linker, glycosylation, and structure of the loops at the interdomain interface.

1. The length of the interdomain linker, defined here as the residues between the C-terminal cysteine of one domain and the N-terminal cysteine of the second domain, is arguably the most important parameter affecting flexibility. These linkers vary from two to eight residues (Fig. 1). A shorter linker is expected to create a tighter interface between consecutive domains, whereas a longer linker allows for more movement. This is probably the reason for the observed flexibility of full-length factor H, which has several long linkers around its midpoint *(27)*. In CD21, an eight-residue linker allows for a folded-over orientation with extensive face-to-face contacts between two SCR domains, although there is no evidence for interdomain flexibility *(26)*.

2. The sequence of the linker plays a role as well—some of the more flexible linkers contain proline and/or glycine residues *(27,32)*. Prolines probably prevent the formation of hydrogen bonds and secondary structure elements (such as the β-strand conformation adopted by the linker in CD46 SCR1-SCR2), and the presence of glycines usually increases polypeptide flexibility.

3. Glycosylation is probably an important factor in determining relative domain orientations. The structures of glycosylated CD46 SCR1-SCR2 suggest that the glycans limit

the molecule's flexibility. Both carbohydrate moieties are located on the same side of the molecule and face toward each other, thus helping to maintain the molecule's conformation (Fig. 3).

4. The structures and lengths of surface loops are significant determinants of the orientations available to adjoining SCRs, but the database of structures is presently too small to define stereotypic mechanisms for these effects.

4.3. Interaction with Ligands

Proteins constructed from SCR domains are generally thought to require more than one repeat for interaction with ligands. For example, the first two repeats of CD46 are both necessary and sufficient for the interaction with measles virus *(49–52),* and all four CD46 repeats appear to be required for interaction with C3b and C4b *(58).* Experiments probing the binding areas of other RCA family members have produced similar results *(74–76).* It is important to realize, however, that these studies are usually based on site-directed mutagenesis experiments, antibody-inhibition assays, or peptide binding studies. It is not clear, therefore, whether the identified residues directly contact a particular ligand or whether they are merely required for the structural integrity of a domain or a multidomain fragment. It is clear that a mutation in one area of a protein can affect the structure of a region that is distant to it *(77).* Moreover, even a highly conservative mutation such as Met→ Leu can severely destabilize a protein and cause it to unfold partially, as seen in the case of a squash trypsin inhibitor *(78).*

To date, the only direct structural information about how SCR domains interact with a protein ligand comes from the crystallographic analysis of the CD21-C3d complex *(26).* Surprisingly, this structure revealed that C3d only contacts a single SCR domain (SCR2) of CD21, although repeats 1 and 2 had previously been implicated in the interaction with C3d *(65).* The linker between the two CD21 repeats, with eight amino acids, is unusually long (Fig. 1) and allows for a severely bent conformation that is essentially identical in the presence and absence of the C3d ligand *(26).* The extensive contacts between the two domains may explain why mutations in SCR1 (which does not contact C3d) might still affect C3d binding through indirect effects. It is unlikely that the CD21-C3d complex can serve as a model for other interactions since most of the interdomain linkers in the RCA family are shorter than eight residues, and the conformations of the molecules are likely to be more extended and have fewer interdomain contacts. The structure of one domain would therefore depend less on the structural integrity of the next, and mutations would be less likely to have long-range effects. Thus, interactions involving a larger surface spanning multiple domains, such as the measles virus binding surface of CD46 *(25),* are likely to occur in other RCA family members. The potential role of ions in mediating these interactions is poorly understood. A dependence on Ca^{2+} is an important property of the interaction between CD55 and CD97 *(76),* and the crystal structure of CD46 contains a calcium ion at the SCR1-SCR2 interface that probably helps to stabilize the conformation of this fragment *(25).* Zn^{2+} ions are involved in the interaction between CD21 and C3d *(26),* although these ions are present in the crystallization buffer in high concentration and it is not clear whether they replace physiologic divalent cations at the CD21/C3d interface or not.

4.4. Oligomerization

A problem with the structural analysis of small, soluble fragments of membrane protein receptors is that the results reveal little about the conformation of the entire molecule and the ligand binding surfaces as they appear on the cell surface. Moreover, the structures do not show the molecules in the context of the lipid and protein environment in which they function. The crystal structures of CD46 SCR1-SCR2 and CD21 SCR1-SCR2 have revealed the presence of distinct oligomers (a trimer in the case of CD46, a dimer in the case of CD21) in the crystals. In the case of CD46, an identical trimer was seen in two unrelated crystal forms *(25)*. As cell surface proteins, CD46 and CD21 are constrained within the outer leaflet of the cell membrane, where oligomers might form more easily than is possible in solution. In this regard, it is conceivable that the crystallographic environment more closely mimics the environment at the cell surface in that the higher effective protein concentration allows the stabilization of physiologically relevant oligomers. Of course, it is possible that the observed multimers are crystallographic artifacts. However, it is useful to recall the cases of human CD4 and human intercellular adhesion molecule-1. Both cell surface receptors were found to dimerize in the crystals, and these dimers are probably of physiologic relevance *(79–81)*.

5. CONCLUSIONS

The regulators of complement activation are proteins constructed from short consensus repeats (SCRs). Several properties of these repeats render them well suited for their function as modular protein-protein interaction components. Their small size and open conformation result in a large surface area that efficiently exposes the amino acid side chains to solvent. The SCR architecture can accommodate substantial sequence variety—there are relatively few conserved residues, and the extended conformation of the protein backbone imposes few constraints on side-chain orientation. The divergence in sequence and also in structure reflects the adaptation of SCR domains to specialized functions, such as the ability to bind complement proteins seen in members of the RCA family. This structural variability is also exploited by the numerous pathogens that use SCR-containing proteins as their cellular receptors. SCR domains, then, are essentially diversity scaffolds in which the variety of their surface properties is achieved through both sequence and conformational heterogeneity.

The available structures of SCR domains demonstrate both significant conformational heterogeneity at the domain level and a wide variation in the interdomain orientation of SCRs. Although the structure of an individual SCR domain can be reasonably inferred from known structures, their relative orientation and the overall conformation of a multi-SCR protein cannot yet be predicted with reasonable accuracy. Nevertheless, we show here that the conformations of two-domain SCR domain fragments are not random. Preferred orientations do exist, as many of the known structures cluster in a defined region of the available conformational space. In the absence of additional information, this knowledge can be used to form a working hypothesis for understanding a particular SCR-SCR conformation. In addition, some predictions can be made about the effect of the linker between SCRs on the conformation and flexibility of SCR concatamers. Most of the known structures have short, four-residue linkers and reasonably fixed conformations—probably a significant reason why they were amenable to structural analysis at all. Longer linkers (around six residues) allow for increased flexibility and can accommodate less extended conformations, as suggested by the analysis of full-length factor H *(27)*. Extremely long linkers (eight residues or longer) can permit a rigid, folded-back conformation, as seen in CD21 *(26)*.

Most SCR structures have been determined during the last 2 years. It can be expected that the database for these structures will swell dramatically in the future, and this will undoubtedly help to establish principles of structural organization of molecules containing concatenated SCR domains. A larger number of available structures, and structures of complexes, will also help to shed light on the mechanisms by which SCR domains mediate both homo- and heterotypic protein-protein interactions. A wealth of biochemical data has been accumulated that identifies residues or regions of RCA family members involved in interactions with ligands. Although the nature of these interactions is at present poorly understood, this is likely to change in the near future if the structural studies of these abundant and still enigmatic domains continue at their present pace.

ACKNOWLEDGMENTS

This work was supported by NIH grant R01-45716 to T.S. Additional support was provided by the Milton Foundation at Harvard Medical School (to T.S.).

REFERENCES

1. Hourcade D, Holers VM, Atkinson JP. The regulators of complement activation (RCA) gene cluster. Adv Immunol 1989;45:381–416.
2. Liszewski MK, Post TW, Atkinson JP. Membrane cofactor protein (MCP or CD46): newest member of the regulators of complement activation gene cluster. Annu Rev Biochem 1991;9:431–455.
3. Dörig RE, Marcil A, Chopra A, Richardson CD. The human CD46 molecule is a receptor for measles virus (Edmonston strain). Cell 1993;75:295–305.
4. Naniche D, Varior-Krishnan G, Cervoni F, et al. Human membrane cofactor protein (CD46) acts as a cellular receptor for measles virus. J Virol 1993;67:6025–6032.
5. Okada N, Liszewski MK, Atkinson JP, Caparon M. Membrane cofactor protein (CD46) is a keratinocyte receptor for the M protein of the group A *Streptococcus*. Proc Natl Acad Sci USA 1995;92:2489–2493.
6. Kallstrom H, Liszewski MK, Atkinson JP, Jonsson AB. Membrane cofactor protein (MCP or CD46) is a cellular pilus receptor for pathogenic *Neisseria*. Mol Microbiol 1997;25:639–647.
7. Santoro F, Kennedy PE, Locatelli G, et al. CD46 is a cellular receptor for human herpesvirus 6. Cell 1999;99:817–827.
8. Karnauchow TM, Dawe S, Lublin DM, Dimock K. Short consensus repeat domain 1 of decay-accelerating factor is required for enterovirus 70 binding. J Virol 1998;72:9380–9383.
9. Bergelson JM, Chan M, Solomon KR, et al. Decay- accelerating factor (CD55), a glycosylphosphatidyl-inositol-anchored complement regulatory protein, is a receptor for several echoviruses. Proc Natl Acad Sci USA 1994;91:6245–6249.
10. Ward T, Pipkin PA, Clarkson NA, et al. Decay-accelerating factor CD55 is identified as the receptor for echovirus-7 using CELICS, a rapid immuno-focal cloning method. EMBO J 1994;13:5070–5074.
11. Clarkson NA, Kaufman R, Lublin DM, et al. Characterization of the echovirus 7 receptor: domains of CD55 critical for virus binding. J Virol 1995;69:5497–5501.

12. Bergelson JM, Modlin JF, Wieland-Alter W, et al. Clinical coxsackievirus B isolates differ from laboratory strains in their interaction with two cell-surface receptors. J Infect Dis 1997;175:697–700.

13. Bergelson JM, Cunningham JA, Droguett G, et al. Isolation of a common receptor for coxsackie B viruses and adenoviruses 2 and 5. Science 1997;275:1320–1323.

14. Fingeroth JD, Weis JJ, Tedder TF, et al. Epstein-Barr virus receptor of human B lymphocytes is the C3d receptor CR2. Proc Natl Acad Sci USA 1984;81:4510–4514.

15. Weis JJ, Tedder TF, Fearon DT. Identification of a 145,000 Mr membrane protein as the C3d receptor (CR2) of human B lymphocytes. Proc Natl Acad Sci USA, 1984;81:881–885.

16. Nemerow GR, Wolfert R, McNaughton ME, Cooper NR. Identification and characterization of the Epstein-Barr virus receptor on human B lymphocytes and its relationship to the C3d complement receptor (CR2). J Virol 1985;55:347–351.

17. Sharma AK, Pangburn MK. Localization by site-directed mutagenesis of the site in human complement factor H that binds to *Streptococcus pyogenes* M protein. Infect Immun 1997;65:484–487.

18. Thern A, Stenberg L, Dahlback B, Lindahl G. Ig-binding surface proteins of *Streptococcus pyogenes* also bind human C4b-binding protein (C4BP), a regulatory component of the complement system. J Immunol 1995;154:375–386.

19. Hellwage J, Meri T, Heikkila T, et al. The complement regulator factor H binds to the surface protein. OspE of *Borrelia burgdorferi*. J Biol Chem 2001;276:8427–8435.

20. Martin DR, Marlowe RL, Ahearn JM. Determination of the role for CD21 during Epstein-Barr virus infection of B-lymphoblastoid cells. J Virol 1994;68:4716–4726.

21. Hourcade D, Liszewski MK, Krych-Goldberg M, Atkinson JP. Functional domains, structural variations and pathogen interactions of MCP, DAF and CRI. Immunopharmacology 2000;49:103–116.

22. Pangburn MK. Host recognition and target differentiation by factor H, a regulator of the alternative pathway of complement. Immunopharmacology 2000;49:149–157.

23. Kirkitadze MD, Barlow PN. Structure and flexibility of the multiple domain proteins that regulate complement activation. Immunol Rev 2001;180:146–161.

24. Kirschfink M. Targeting complement in therapy. Immunol Rev 2001;180:177–189.

25. Casasnovas JM, Larvie M, Stehle T. Crystal structure of two CD46 domains reveals an extended measles virus-binding surface. EMBO J 1999;18:2911–2922.

26. Szakonyi G, Guthridge JM, et al. Structure of complement receptor 2 in complex with its C3d ligand. Science 2001;292:1725–1728.

27. Aslam M, Perkins SJ. Folded-back solution structure of monomeric factor H of human complement by synchrotron X-ray and neutron scattering. Analytical ultracentrifugation and constrained molecular modelling. J Mol Biol 2001;309:1117–1138.

28. Murthy KHM, Smith SA, Ganesh VK, et al. Crystal structure of a complement control protein that regulates both pathways of complement activation and binds heparan sulfate proteoglycans. Cell 2001;104:301–311.

29. Norman DG, Barlow PN, Baron M, et al. Three-dimensional structure of a complement control protein module in solution. J Mol Biol 1991;219:717–725.

30. Barlow PN, Baron M, Norman DG, et al. Secondary structure of a complement control protein module by two-dimensional ^{1}H NMR. Biochemistry 1991;30:997–1004.

31. Barlow PN, Norman DG, Steinkasserer A, et al. Solution structure of the fifth repeat of factor H: a second example of the complement control protein module. Biochemistry 1992;31:3626–3634.

32. Barlow PN, Steinkasserer A, Norman DG, et al. Solution structure of a pair of complement modules by nuclear magnetic resonance. J Mol Biol 1993;232:268–284.

33. Wiles AP, Shaw G, Bright J, et al. NMR studies of a viral protein that mimics the regulators of complement activation. J Mol Biol 1997;272:253–265.

34. Henderson CE, Bromek K, Mullin N, et al. Solution structure and dynamics of the central CCP module pair of a poxvirus complement control protein. J Mol Biol 2001;307:323–339.
35. Schwarzenbacher R, Zeth K, Diederichs K, et al. Structure of human beta2- glycoprotein I: implications for phospholipid binding and the antiphospholipid syndrome. EMBO J 1999;18:6228–6239.
36. Bouma B, de Groot PG, van den Elsen JM, et al. Adhesion mechanism of human beta(2)-glyco-protein I to phospholipids based on its crystal structure. EMBO J 1999;18:5166–5174.
37. Gaboriaud CG, Rossi V, Bally I, Arlaud GJ, Fontecilla-Camps JC. Crystal structure of the cat-alytic domain of human complement C1s: a serine protease with a handle. EMBO J 2000;19:1755–1765.
38. Seya T, Ballard LL, Bora NS, et al. Distribution of membrane cofactor protein of complement on human peripheral cells. An altered form is found in granulocytes. Eur J Immunol 1988;18:1289–1294.
39. McNearney T, Ballard L, Seya T, Atkinson JP. Membrane cofactor protein of complement is pre-sent on human fibroblast, epithelial, and endothelial cells. J Clin Invest 1989;84:538–545.
40. Purcell DFJ, Clark GJ, Brown MA, et al. HuLy- m5, an antigen sharing epitopes with envelope gp70 molecules of primate retroviruses has a structural relationship with complement regulatory molecules. In: Knapp W (ed.). Leukocyte Typing IV. Oxford: Oxford University Press, 1989, pp. 653–655.
41. McLaughlin PJ, Holland SJ, Taylor CT, et al. Soluble CD46 (membrane cofactor protein, MCP) in human reproductive fluids. J Reprod Immunol 1996;31:209–219.
42. Christiansen D, Milland J, Thorley BR, et al. Engineering of recombinant soluble CD46: an inhibitor of complement activation. Immunology 1996;87:348–354.
43. Christiansen D, Milland J, Thorley BR, McKenzie IFC, Loveland BE. A functional analysis of recombinant soluble CD46 in vivo and a comparison with recombinant soluble forms of CD55 and CD35 in vitro. Eur J Immunol 1996;26:578–585.
44. Thorley BR, Milland J, Christiansen D, et al. Transgenic expression of a CD46 (membrane cofactor protein) minigene: studies of xenotransplantation and measles virus infection. Eur J Immunol 1997;27:726–734.
45. Seya T, Kurita M, Hara T, et al. Blocking measles virus infection with a recombinant soluble form of, or monoclonal antibodies against, membrane cofactor protein of complement (CD46). Immunology 1995;84:619–625.
46. Seya T, Turner J, Atkinson JP. Purification and characterization of a membrane protein (gp45–70) that is a cofactor for cleavage of C3b and C4b. J Exp Med 1986;163:837–855.
47. Tatsuo H, Ono N, Tanaka K, Yanagi Y. SLAM (CDw150) is a cellular receptor for measles virus. Nature 2000;406:893–896.
48. Yanagi Y. The cellular receptor for measles virus—elusive no more. Rev Med Virol 2001;11:149–156.
49. Manchester M, Valsamakis A, Kaufman R, et al. Measles virus and C3 binding sites are distinct on membrane cofactor protein. Proc Natl Acad Sci USA 1995;92:2303–2307.
50. Iwata K, Seya T, Yanagi Y, et al. Diversity of sites for measles virus binding and for inactivation of complement C3b and C4b on membrane cofactor protein CD46. J Biol Chem 1995;270:15148–15152.
51. Nussbaum O, Broder CC, Moss B, et al. Functional and structural interactions between measles virus hemagglutinin and CD46. J Virol 1995;69:3341–3349.
52. Manchester M, Gairin JE, Patterson JB, et al. Measles virus recognizes its receptor, CD46, via two distinct binding domains within SCR1-2. Virology 1997;233:174–184.
53. Kallstrom H, Blackmer Gill D, Albiger B, et al. Attachment of *Neisseria gonorrhoeae* to the cel-lular pilus receptor CD46: identification of domains important for bacterial adherence. Cell Microbiol 2001;3:133–143.

54. Manchester M, Naniche D, Stehle T. CD46 as a measles virus receptor: form follows function. Virology 2000;274:5–10.

55. Maisner A, Alvarez J, Liszewski MK, et al. The N-glycan of the SCR2 region is essential for membrane cofactor protein (CD46) to function as a measles virus receptor. J Virol 1996;70:4973–4977.

56. Adams EM, Brown MC, Nunge M, Krych M, Atkinson JP. Contribution of the repeating domains of membrane cofactor protein (CD46) of the complement system to ligand binding and cofactor activity. J Immunol 1991;147:3005–3011.

57. Liszewski MK, Leung MK, Atkinson JP. Membrane cofactor protein: importance of N- and O-glycosylation for complement regulatory function. J Immunol 1998;161:3711–3718.

58. Liszewski MK, Leung M, Cui W, et al. Dissecting sites important for complement regulatory activity in membrane cofactor protein (MCP; CD46). J Biol Chem 2000;275:37692–37701.

59. Fearon DT. The complement system and adaptive immunity. Semin Immunol 1998;10:355–361.

60. Iida K, Nadler L, Nussenzweig V. Identification of the membrane receptor for the complement fragment C3d by means of a monoclonal antibody. J Exp Med 1983;158:1021–1033.

61. Aubry JP, Pochon S, Graber P, Jansen KU, Bonnefoy JY. CD21 is a ligand for CD23 and regulates IgE production. Nature 1992;358:505–507.

62. Aubry JP, Pochon S, Gauchat JF, et al. CD23 interacts with a new functional extracytoplasmic domain involving N-linked oligosaccharides on CD21. J Immunol 1994;152:5806–5813.

63. Nemerow GR, Houghten RA, Moore MD, Cooper NR. Identification of an epitope in the major envelope protein of Epstein-Barr virus that mediates viral binding to the B-lymphocyte EBV receptor (CR2). Cell 1989;56:369–377.

64. Molina H, Perkins SJ, Guthridge JM, et al. Characterization of a complement receptor 2 (CR2, CD21) ligand binding site for C3. An initial model of ligand interaction with two linked short consensus repeat modules. J Immunol 1995;154:5426–5435.

65. Prodinger WM, Schwendinger MG, Schoch J, et al. Characterization of C3dg binding to a recess formed between short consensus repeats 1 and 2 of complement receptor type 2 (CR2; CD21). J Immunol 1998;161:4604–4610.

66. Nagar B, Jones RG, Diefenbach RJ, Isenman DE, Rini JM. X-ray crystal structure of C3d: a C3 fragment and ligand for complement receptor 2. Science 1998;280:1277–1281.

67. Clemenza L, Isenman DE. Structure-guided identification of C3d residues essential for its binding to complement receptor 2 (CD21). J Immunol 2000;165:3839–3848.

68. Kotarsky H, Hellwage J, Johnson E, et al. Identification of a domain in human factor H and factor H-like protein-1 required for the interaction with streptococcal M proteins. J Immunol 1998;160:3349–3354.

69. Lubinski J, Nagashunmugam T, Friedman HM. Viral interference with antibody and complement. Semin Cell Dev Biol 1998;9:329–337.

70. Rosengard AM, Ahearn JM. Viral complement regulatory proteins. Immunopharmacology 1999;42:99–106.

71. Kotwal GJ, Moss B. Vaccinia virus encodes a secretory polypeptide structurally related to complement control proteins. Nature 1988;335:176–178.

72. Kotwal GJ, Isaacs SN, McKenzie R, Frank MM, Moss B. Inhibition of the complement cascade by the major secretory protein of vaccinia virus. Science 1990;250:827–830.

73. Kirkitadze MD, Henderson C, Price NC, et al. Central modules of the vaccinia virus complement control protein are not in extensive contact. Biochem J 1999;344:167–175.

74. Krych M, Hauhart R, Atkinson JP. Structure-function analysis of the active sites of complement receptor type 1. J Biol Chem 1998;273:8623–8629.

75. Smith SA, Mullin NP, Parkinson J, et al. Conserved surface-exposed K/R-X-K/R motifs and net positive charge on poxvirus complement control proteins serve as putative heparin binding sites and contribute to inhibition of molecular interactions with human endothelial cells: a novel mechanism for evasion of host defense. J Virol 2000;74:5659–5666.

76. Lin HH, Stacey M, Saxby C, et al. Molecular analysis of the epidermal growth factor-like short consensus repeat domain-mediated protein-protein interactions: dissection of the CD97-CD55 complex. J Biol Chem 2001;276:24160–24169.

77. Xiong JP, Li R, Essafi M, Stehle T, Arnaout MA. An isoleucine-based allosteric switch controls affinity and shape shifting in integrin CD11b A-domain. J Biol Chem 2000;275:38762–38767.

78. Zhukov I, Jaroszewski L, Bierzynski A. Conservative mutation Met8 → Leu affects the folding process and structural stability of squash trypsin inhibitor CMTI-I. Protein Sci 2000;9:273–279.

79. Wu H, Kwong PD, Hendrickson WA. Dimeric association and segmental variability in the structure of human CD4. Nature 1997;387:527–530.

80. Casasnovas JM, Stehle T, Liu J, Wang J, Springer T. A dimeric crystal structure for the N-terminal two domains of intercellular adhesion molecule-1. Proc Natl Acad Sci USA 1998;95:4134–4139.

81. Bella J, Kolatkar PR, Marlor CW, Greve JM, Rossmann MG. The structure of the two amino-terminal domains of human ICAM-1 suggests how it functions as a rhinovirus receptor and as an LFA-1 integrin ligand. Proc Natl Acad Sci USA 1998;95:4140–4145.

82. Jones TA, Zhou JY, Cowan SW, Kjeldgaard M. Improved methods for building protein models in electron density maps and the location of errors in these models. Acta Crystallographica 1991;A47:110–119.

83. Carson M. Ribbon models of macromolecules. J Mol Graph 1987;5:103–106.

84. Nicholls A, Sharp KA, Honig B. Protein folding and association: insights from the interfacial and thermodynamic properties of hydrocarbons. Proteins 1991;11:281–296.

14
Lipopolysaccharide-Binding Protein and CD14

Peter S. Tobias

1. INTRODUCTION

If one role of the innate immune system is to act as a sentinel for infection, then sensitive detection of pathogens is surely important. Whatever other roles they may play, lipopolysaccharide binding protein (LBP) and CD14 serve to enhance sensitivity to the surface structures of pathogens. LBP is resitricted to enhancing sensitivity to LPS and perhaps a few other glycolipids. CD14 has a much broader spectrum of activity, acting with LBP to enhance sensitivity to LPS but also functioning with components of Gram-positive organisms, mycobacteria, yeast, and at least one virus. As described elsewhere in this volume, these functions are critical for immediate inflammatory responses as well as activation of adaptive immune responses. Other functions of LBP and CD14 are not as well documented. LBP and CD14 may serve as opsonins to clear infectious organisms as well as inflammatory bacterial components via pathways that do not initiate inflammation. CD14 may also be important in the clearance of apoptotic cells via noninflammatory pathways. These are principally acute roles for the proteins. Recent epidemologic studies also suggest that CD14 may play a role in more chronic situations that result in allergy and cardiovascular disease. Several recent reviews of LBP and CD14 have been published; therefore this review presents only an overview of the older work and highlights the newer findings. Since the previous reviews, knowledge concerning LBP seems to have advanced primarily in the details. On the other hand, information about CD14 has advanced into several new areas, perhaps most surprisingly with respect to CD14 polymorphisms and disease as well as discovery of ligands for CD14 of unexpected types. Finally, fluorescence methods have suggested new views of the organization of CD14 and other molecules on the cell surface.

2. THE PARADIGM

Several key papers led to the basic paradigm for the major role of LBP and CD14 illustrated in Fig. 1 *(1–4)*. This is the LBP-mediated complexation of LPS with CD14 followed by the interaction of LPS-CD14 complexes with a receptor capable of initiating signaling that leads to inflammatory mediator production. This paradigm was basically known by 1990, but it was not until 10 years later that the signaling receptor for LPS was identified as Toll-like receptor 4 (TLR4), and only in 2001 was a direct inter-

From: *Infectious Disease: Innate Immunity*
Edited by: R. A. B. Ezekowitz and J. A. Hoffmann © Humana Press Inc., Totowa, NJ

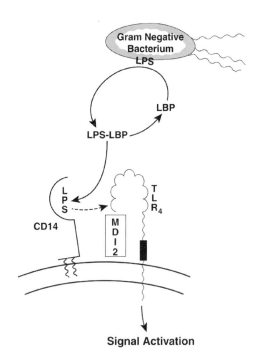

Fig. 1. Lipopolysaccharide binding protein (LBP) mediates LPS binding to CD14. The LPS-CD14 complex then interacts with Toll-like receptor (TLR4)-MD2 to initiate signaling.

action between LPS and TLR4-MD2 demonstrated. Several workers have shown that LBP and CD14 are not absolutely necessary for presentation of ligands to TLR4 *(5,6)*. However, many papers show that the sensitivity of the system is dramatically enhanced when they are present and functional, *(1,2,5,7)*. Although Fig. 1 shows the membrane-anchored form of CD14 (mCD14), as it is in myeloid cells, the soluble form of CD14 (sCD14) functions in a fundamentally similar manner *(4,8)*.

3. LIPOPOLYSACCHARIDE BINDING PROTEIN

LBP is a member of the lipid transferase family with a unique ability to shuttle LPS from bacterial membrane fragments or LPS aggregates to CD14. Other members of the family include bactericidal/permeability-increasing protein (BPI), cholesterol ester transfer protein (CETP), and phospholipase transfer protein (PLTP). These all bind LPS but have no ability to interact with CD14. The two functions of LBP, LPS binding and transfer of LPS to CD14, appear to reside in different domains of the molecule. The fragment comprised of residues 1–197 avidly binds LPS but has no ability to transfer LPS to CD14 *(9,10)*. One assumes therefore that the 198–456 fragment should interact with CD14, but this has not been specifically shown. An LPS binding motif has been described that encompasses four basic amino acid residues shown to interact with the phosphate moiety of LPS in its complex with the outer membrane protein FhuA from *E. coli (11)*. The significance of one of the motif residues in LBP was previously shown by site-directed mutation *(12)*. Unfortunately, although crystallization of LBP has not been successful enough to provide crystals suitable for structural elucidation, the X-ray structure of its congener, BPI, has been successful and this provides some basis for thinking about the three-dimensional structure of LBP *(13)*. The structure is roughly banana-shaped, with some fair degree of symmetry between the two ends of the banana. The charged LPS binding motif is arrayed at one tip of the banana. Upon interpretation of the electron density map, some nonprotein density was observed, which turned out to be 2 mol of glycerol phospholipid. In subsequent experiments carried out with Alan Hunt at the University of Southampton and Luc Teyton at Scripps Research Institute, we have found that purified LBP also carries phospholipid. The role of the phospholipid is as yet undetermined.

It is tempting to imagine that the site of phospholipid binding is related to the LPS binding site, but the phosphate moieties of the glycerol lipid are not in direct contact with the residues of the LPS binding motif. Although comparison of the structures of BPI and LBP is provocative, some care should be taken in drawing conclusions because LBP is capable of disaggregating LPS and presenting it to CD14, whereas BPI does not present LPS to CD14 and seems to have a condensing effect on LPS aggregates *(14)*. Altering the structure of LPS aggregates, as in the outer membranes of Gram-negative bacteria, may be important to the antibiotic effects of BPI. Interestingly, LBP enhances the antibiotic effects of BPI *(15)*. The association of LBP with planar phospholipid membranes has been investigated by Gutsmann et al. *(16)*. These workers found that LBP inserts through a planar bilayer in an oriented fashion, yet it can bind LPS offered from either side. Further work with this model comparing BPI and LBP could be quite interesting.

LBP was first detected as an acute-phase reactant *(17)*, and many papers have subsequently documented a rise in LBP concentration following an inflammatory stimulus. Observations published to date suggest that LBP is elevated following every possible sort of inflammatory stimulus and in any possible anatomic site [burn *(18)*, pancreatitis *(19)*, sepsis *(20,21)*, tuberculosis *(22)*, peritonitis *(23)*, labor *(24,25)*, arthritis *(26)*, chemical stimulus *(27,28)*, lung *(29–32)*]. Studies of the regulation of LBP expression showed that cytokines interleukin-6 (IL-6), IL-1, and tumor necrosis factor (TNF) as well as dexamethasone were important regulators of LBP expression in HepG2 cells *(33)*. Further study of LBP expression showed that signal transducer and activator of transcription-3 (STAT-3), activator protein (AP)-1, and CCAAT-enhancer binding protein (C/EBPβ) are important transcriptional regulators and that both transcriptional and translational mechanisms were important in regulating expression *(34,34a)*. As described in greater detail below, LBP catalytically transfers LPS to CD14. Furthermore, observations with cells in culture suggest that there is ample LBP in serum to serve as a catalyst for LPS-dependent cellular activation, and thus the role of LBP as a strong acute-phase reactant suggested that it may have some other role as well. Consistent with the observation that LBP is an opsonin, we have found that LBP is co-internalized with LPS in tissue culture, and others have shown that high levels of LBP are protective in vivo *(35–37)*.

It is now abundantly clear, as noted above, that LBP enhances sensitivity to LPS. Recent experiments with LBP knockout mice confirm in vivo the validity of this conclusion that was originally based on ex vivo experiments on cytokine release *(1,38,39)*. Two versions of LBP$^{-/-}$ mice have been made. The first to appear focused on challenges of mice with LPS or *Salmonella typhimurium* and made the point that inflammation was beneficial for resolution of an infection *(40)*. Thus, these workers showed that LBP$^{-/-}$ mice were hyporesponsive to LPS when that response was measured in a lethality model that reflects the LPS-stimulated expression of TNF, but that the mice were hyperesponsive to death by bacteremia. The second report of LBP$^{-/-}$ mice observed that whole blood from LBP$^{-/-}$ mice was hyporespospsonsive to LPS but that the mice themselves were normoresponsive to LPS *(41)*. As far as I am aware, this difference between the two strains of LBP$^{-/-}$ mice remains unexplained. Further experiments with the second strain of mice to look at airway reactivity relevant to asthma with LBP$^{-/-}$ mice showed hyporeactivity in OVA-immunized LBP$^{-/-}$ mice to a methacholine challenge *(42)*. This result suggests that the LBP$^{-/-}$ mice are hyporesponsive to inflammatory stimuli. The nature of the stimulus in this instance remains unclear, but the usual suspect is endotoxin from some source. Several workers recently showed that LPS preparations may contain agonists capable of stimulating cells through TLR2 in addition to TLR4 *(43,44)*. It is possible that differences in the LPS preparations used to initiate inflammatory responses in the two strains of LBP$^{-/-}$ mice could explain the different results obtained. Other recent work *(45)* tends to support the view that LBP is critical for sensitive detection of LPS.

The mechanism by which LBP enhances cellular LPS responses has not advanced significantly since previous reviews. The essence of the matter is that LBP acts catalytically as a transferase delivering LPS from aggregates or bacterial membranes to CD14. The most useful tool to observe the details has been fluorescently labeled LPS. Fluorescein or bodipy labeled LPS is self-quenched because it is highly aggregated. Upon disaggregation, the fluorescence is enhanced, and the kinetics of transfer from the LPS aggregate to the acceptor can thereby be readily observed. Consistent with the recognition of LBP as a member of the lipid transferase family, LBP has also been shown to mediate the transfer of glycerol lipids into lipoproteins. This finding led to the speculation that LBP might function in vivo as a glycerol lipid transferase like its congener, PLTP. However, studies of LBP$^{-/-}$ mice do not support such a role for LBP. Glycolipids from *Treponema* and a component from *Bacillus subtilis* may also be recognized by LBP *(46,47)*. Kitchens et al. *(48,49)* have continued to explore the abilities of LBP to transfer LPS among various compartments, showing that LBP will actually remove LPS from monocytes *(48,49)*. This would be consistent with the principle of microscopic reversibility, whereby a catalyst catalyzes a given reaction in both directions *(50)*. Recent reviews relevant to LBP include refs. *51–58*.

4. CD14

Unlike LBP, CD14 has no near relatives. Structurally, it has 10 leucine-rich repeats, but this feature does not help much as an aid to understanding its function except to indicate that CD14 interacts with other proteins *(59)*. CD14 is both a membrane-bound receptor, bound via a glycosylphosphatidyl inositol (GPI) tail, and a soluble plasma glycoprotein, functioning similarly in both environments to enhance activation of cells by LPS *(2,8,60,61)*. Structure function studies of CD14 mutants lead to three conclusions: (1) the posttranslationally added GPI tail is not required for its function with TLRs *(62)*; (2) amino acid residues beyond 152, which eliminates all but three of the leucine-rich repeats, are not required for LPS or peptidoglycan binding by CD14 *(63,64)*; and (3) within the 1–152-fragment, different residues are important for LPS binding and peptidoglycan binding *(65–69)*. There is no LPS binding motif of the sort defined in LBP. Soluble CD14 may be generated from membrane-bound CD14 or secreted without posttranslational modification *(70)*. Unfortunately, no three-dimensional structure for CD14 has been published, although crystallization studies are ongoing and "promising" (Luc Teyton, Scripps Research Institute, personal communication). Probably the most unusual feature concerning the activity of CD14 is its ability to enhance cellular activation by a large variety of agonists. Stelter *(71)* recently enumerated some of the pathogen-derived materials that CD14 recognizes. In addition to these ligands are several protein ligands, including heat shock protein 60 (HSP60), HSP70, and the fusion glycoprotein from respiratory syncytial virus *(72–75)*. It would be interesting if someone would go back to the available CD14 mutants and determine whether all this huge diversity of agonists uses the same small region of CD14 for binding. Beyond even these agonists, CD14 recognizes apoptotic cells, which leads to cellular activation of a very different sort than that activated by microbial ligands *(76)*.

How do all the different agonists get sorted out at the cell surface to activate the appropriate receptors? The obvious but uninformative answer is that the bound agonists are only recognized by the appropriate receptors. The possibility that CD14 is surrounded by a host of receptors is suggested by results with fluorescence resonance energy transfer experiments *(77)*. These authors present evidence implying that HSP70 and-90, chemokine receptor 4, and growth differentiation factor 5 are the main mediators of activation by bacterial LPS. Whether this idea will stand up to the evidence for TLR4 as the signaling receptor for LPS is unclear, but the concept that CD14 is in a cluster with a variety of receptors and that these receptors mediate various agonist-dependent phenomena is attractive. It is possible that all the molecules are gathered in lipid rafts *(78)*. GPI-tailed proteins such as CD14 are known to associate with such rafts. The only problematic observation in this regard is that CD14 anchored to the membrane by means of a peptide tail that does not target the CD14 to a lipid raft functions perfectly well as far as LPS is concerned *(62,79)*. At this juncture, nothing is known about the structural features that enable CD14 to interact with TLR4, TLR2, or any other signaling receptor.

The relevance of CD14 to acute disease mediated by Gram-negative organisms is by now well established from models involving CD14-deficient mice as well as models wherein CD14 function is blocked by antibodies. Blockade of inflammation is essentially universally observed *(80,81)*, although some cytokine responses persist *(82)*. However, the consequences for responses to whole bacteria are quite varied *(81,83–85)*. This may represent species variations in the bacteria as well as the host and obviously will take some time to sort out fully.

In a somewhat different vein, a relationship between CD14 polymorphisms and the chronic conditions of asthma and heart disease has recently emerged that promises to be most interesting. The CD14 promoter has a polymorphism at an Sp1 site that leads to allelic variation in the levels of soluble CD14 produced *(86,87)*. Because inflammation alters levels of cytokines and Th2 responses, the altered CD14 levels may be related to a potential for allergic sensitization *(88)*. Thus it is possible that CD14 is involved in the so-called hygiene hypothesis whereby exposure to environmental LPS or higher CD14 levels leads to a diminished tendency to allergic responses *(89,90)*. In this connection Arias et al. *(91)* have observed that soluble CD14 interacts with B cells to lower IgE production. Other studies suggest that the same CD14 allele protecting against allergy may predispose to myocardial infarction *(92)* and to atherosclerosis *(93,94)*, but not to ischemic cerebral disease *(95)*. Recent reviews of CD14 include those found in refs. *96–102*.

ACKNOWLEDGMENTS

This work was supported by NIH grants AI32021, GM37696, and HL23584. This is publication number 14584-IMM from the Scripps Research Institute.

REFERENCE

1. Schumann RR, Leong SR, Flaggs GW, et al. Structure and function of lipopolysaccharide (LPS) binding protein; a plasma protein that controls the response of macrophages to LPS. Science 1990;249:1429–1431.
2. Wright SD, Ramos RA, Tobias PS, Ulevitch RJ, Mathison JC. CD14 serves as the cellular receptor for complexes of lipopolysaccharide with lipopolysaccharide binding protein. Science 1990;249:1431–1433.
3. Poltorak A, He X, Smirnova I, et al. Defective LPS signaling in C3H/HeJ and C57BL/10ScCr mice: mutations in Tlr4 gene. Science 1998;282:2085–2088.
4. da Silva CJ, Soldau K, Christen U, Tobias PS, Ulevitch RJ. Lipopolysaccharide is in close proximity to each of the proteins in its membrane receptor complex: transfer from CD14 to TLR4 and MD-2. J Biol Chem 2001;.
5. Lee J-D, Kato K, Tobias PS, Kirkland TN, Ulevitch RJ. Transfection of CD14 into 70Z/3 cells dramatically enhances the sensitivity to complexes of lipopolysaccharide (LPS) and LPS binding protein. J Exp Med 1992;175:1697–1705.
6. Lynn WA, Liu Y, Golenbock DT. Neither CD14 nor serum is absolutely necessary for activation of mononuclear phagocytes by bacterial lipopolysaccharide. Infect Immun 1993;61:4452–4461.
7. Mathison JC, Tobias PS, Wolfson E, Ulevitch RJ. Plasma lipopolysaccharide (LPS)-binding protein: a key component in macrophage recognition of Gram-negative LPS. J Immunol 1992;149:200–206.
8. Pugin J, Schurer-Maly C-C, Leturcq D, et al. Lipopolysaccharide activation of human endothelial and epithelial cells is mediated by lipopolysaccharide-binding protein and soluble CD14. Proc Natl Acad Sci USA 1993;90:2744–2748.
9. Han J, Mathison J, Ulevitch R, Tobias P. Lipopolysaccharide (LPS) binding protein, truncated at Ile-197, binds LPS but does not transfer LPS to CD14. J Biol Chem 1994;269:8172–8175.
10. Theofan G, Horwitz A, Williams R, et al. An amino-terminal fragment of human lipopolysaccharide-binding protein retains lipid A binding but not CD14-stimulatory activity. J Immunol 1994;152:3623–3629.
11. Ferguson AD, Welte W, Hofmann E, et al. A conserved structural motif for lipopolysaccharide recognition by procaryotic and eucaryotic proteins. Structure Fold Des 2000;8:585–592.
12. Lamping N, Hoess A, Yu B, et al. Effects of site-directed mutagenesis of basic residues (Arg 94, Lys 95, Lys 99) of lipopolysaccharide (LPS)-binding protein on binding and transfer of LPS and subsequent immune cell activation. J Immunol 1996;157:4648–4656.
13. Beamer LJ, Carroll SF, Eisenberg D. Crystal structure of human BPI and two bound phospholipids at 2.4 angstrom resolution. Science 1997;276:1861–1864.
14. Tobias PS, Soldau K, Iovine NM, Elsbach P, Weiss J. Lipopolysaccharide (LPS)-binding proteins BPI and LBP form different types of complexes with LPS. J Biol Chem 1997;272:18682–18685.

15. Horwitz AH, Williams RE, Nowakowski G. Human lipopolysaccharide-binding protein potentiates bactericidal activity of human bactericidal/permeability-increasing protein. Infect Immun 1995;63:522–527.

16. Gutsmann T, Haberer N, Carroll SF, Seydel U, Wiese A. Interaction between lipopolysaccharide (LPS), LPS-binding protein (LBP), and planar membranes. Biol Chem 2001;382:425–434.

17. Tobias PS, Soldau K, Ulevitch RJ. Isolation of a lipopolysaccharide-binding acute phase reactant from rabbit serum. J Exp Med 1986;164:777–793.

18. Klein RD, Su GL, Aminlari A, et al. Skin lipopolysaccharide-binding protein and IL-1beta production after thermal injury. J Burn Care Rehabil 2000;21:345–352.

19. Erwin PJ, Lewis H, Dolan S, et al. Lipopolysaccharide binding protein in acute pancreatitis. Crit Care Med 2000;28:104–109.

20. Opal SM, Palardy JE, Marra MN, et al. Relative concentrations of endotoxin-binding proteins in body fluids during infection. Lancet 1994;344:429–431.

21. Opal SM, Scannon PJ, Vincent JL, et al. Relationship between plasma levels of lipopolysaccharide (LPS) and LPS-binding protein in patients with severe sepsis and septic shock. J Infect Dis 1999;180:1584–1589.

22. Juffermans NP, Verbon A, van Deventer SJ, et al. Serum concentrations of lipopolysaccharide activity-modulating proteins during tuberculosis. J Infect Dis 1998;178:1839–1842.

23. Schafer K, Schumann RR, Stoteknuel S, Schollmeyer P, Dobos GJ. Lipopolysaccharide-binding protein is present in effluents of patients with Gram-negative and Gram-positive CAPD peritonitis. Nephrol Dial Transplant 1998;13:969–974.

24. Gardella C, Hitti J, Martin TR, Ruzinski JT, Eschenbach D. Amniotic fluid lipopolysaccharide-binding protein and soluble CD14 as mediators of the inflammatory response in preterm labor. Am J Obstet Gynecol 2001;184:1241–1248.

25. Roos T, Martin TR, Ruzinski JT, et al. Lipopolysaccharide binding protein and soluble CD14 receptor protein in amniotic fluid and cord blood in patients at term. Am J Obstet Gynecol 1997;177:1230–1237.

26. Heumann D, Bas S, Gallay P, et al. Lipopolysaccharide binding protein as a marker of inflammation in synovial fluid of patients with arthritis: correlation with interleukin 6 and C-reactive protein. J Rheumatol 1995;22:1224–1229.

27. Tobias PS, Soldau K, Ulevitch RJ. Isolation of a lipopolysaccharide-binding acute phase reactant from rabbit serum. J Exp Med 1986;164:777–793.

28. Ramadori G, Meyer zum Buschenfelde KH, Tobias PS, Mathison JC, Ulevitch RJ. Biosynthesis of lipopolysaccharide-binding protein in rabbit hepatocytes. Pathobiology 1990;58:89–94.

29. Ishii Y, Wang Y, Haziot A, et al. Lipopolysaccharide binding protein and CD14 interaction induces tumor necrosis factor-alpha generation and neutrophil sequestration in lungs after intratracheal endotoxin. Circ Res 1993;73:15–23.

30. Klein RD, Su GL, Aminlari A, Alarcon WH, Wang SC. Pulmonary LPS-binding protein (LBP) upregulation following LPS-mediated injury. J Surg Res 1998;78:42–47.

31. Dentener MA, Vreugdenhil AC, Hoet PH, et al. Production of the acute-phase protein lipopolysaccharide-binding protein by respiratory type II epithelial cells: implications for local defense to bacterial endotoxins. Am J Respir Cell Mol Biol 2000;23:146–153.

32. Martin TR. Recognition of bacterial endotoxin in the lungs. Am J Respir Cell Mol Biol 2000;23:128–132.

33. Grube BJ, Cochrane CG, Ye RD, et al. Lipopolysaccharide binding protein expression in primary human hepatocytes and HepG2 hepatoma cells. J Biol Chem 1994;269:8477–8482.

34. Kirschning CJ, Unbehaun A, Fiedler G, et al. The transcriptional activation pattern of lipopolysaccharide binding protein (LBP) involving transcription factors AP-1 and C/EBP beta. Immunobiology 1997;198:124–135.

34a. Kirschning C, Unbehaun A, Lamping N, Pfeil D, Herrmann F, and Schumann RR. Control of transcriptional activation of the lipopolysaccharide binding protein (LBP) gene by proinflammatory cytokines. Cytokines Cell Mol Ther 1997;3:59–62.

35. Gegner JA, Ulevitch RJ, Tobias PS. LPS signal transduction and clearance. Dual roles for LBP and mCD14. J Biol Chem 1995;270:5320–5325.

36. Tapping RI, Tobias PS. Cellular binding of soluble CD14 requires lipopolysaccharide (LPS) and LPS-binding protein. J Biol Chem 1997;272:23157–23164.

37. Lamping N, Dettmer R, Schroder NW, et al. LPS-binding protein protects mice from septic shock caused by LPS or gram-negative bacteria. J Clin Invest 1998;101:2065–2071.

38. Mathison JC, Tobias PS, Wolfson E, Ulevitch RJ. LPS-induced adaptive responses in macrophages (MO): reversal by LPS binding protein (LBP). In: Powanda MC, Oppenheim JJ, Kluger MJ, Dinarello CA (eds.). Molecular and Cellular Biology of Cytokines. Wiley-Liss, New York, 1989, pp. 75–80.

39. Mathison JC, Ulevitch RJ, Tobias PS. Control of TNF secretion from rabbit peritoneal exudate macrophages by lipopolysaccharide and lipopolysaccharide binding protein. In: Marchalonis J, Reinisch C (eds.). Defense Molecules: UCLA Symposia on Molecular and Cellular Biology, New Series. New York: Alan R. Liss, 1989.

40. Heinrich JM, Bernheiden M, Minigo G, et al. The essential role of lipopolysaccharide-binding protein in protection of mice against a peritoneal *Salmonella* infection involves the rapid induction of an inflammatory response. J Immunol 2001;167:1624–1628.

41. Wurfel MM, Monks BG, Ingalls et al. Targeted deletion of the lipopolysaccharide (LPS)-binding protein gene leads to profound suppression of LPS responses ex vivo, whereas in vivo responses remain intact. J Exp Med 1997;186:2051–2056.

42. Strohmeier GR, Walsh JH, Klings ES, et al. Lipopolysaccharide binding protein potentiates airway reactivity in a murine model of allergic asthma. J Immunol 2001;166:2063–2070.

43. Hirschfeld M, Ma Y, Weis JH, Vogel SN, Weis JJ. Cutting edge: repurification of lipopolysaccharide eliminates signaling through both human and murine toll-like receptor 2. J Immunol 2000;165:618–622.

44. Tapping RI, Akashi S, Miyake K, Godowski PJ, Tobias PS. Toll-like receptor 4, but not toll-like receptor 2, is a signaling receptor for *Escherichia* and *Salmonella* lipopolysaccharides. J Immunol 2000;165:5780–5787.

45. Heumann D, Adachi Y, Le Roy D, et al. Role of plasma, lipopolysaccharide-binding protein, and CD14 in response of mouse peritoneal exudate macrophages to endotoxin. Infect Immun 2001;69:378–385.

46. Fan X, Stelter F, Menzel R, et al. Structures in *Bacillus subtilis* are recognized by CD14 in a lipopolysaccharide binding protein-dependent reaction. Infect Immun 1999;67:2964–2968.

47. Schroder NW, Opitz B, Lamping N, et al. Involvement of lipopolysaccharide binding protein, CD14, and Toll-like receptors in the initiation of innate immune responses by *Treponema* glycolipids. J Immunol 2000;165:2683–2693.

48. Kitchens RL, Wolfbauer G, Albers JJ, Munford RS. Plasma lipoproteins promote the release of bacterial lipopolysaccharide from the monocyte cell surface. J Biol Chem 1999;274:34116–34122.

49. Vesy CJ, Kitchens RL, Wolfbauer G, Albers JJ, Munford RS. Lipopolysaccharide-binding binding protein and phospholipid transfer protein release lipopolysaccharides from gram-negative bacterial membranes. Infect Immun 2000;68:2410–2417.

50. Espenson JH. Chemical Kinetics and Reaction Mechanisms. New York:McGraw-Hill, 1981.

51. Schutt C. Fighting infection: the role of lipopolysaccharide binding proteins CD14 and LBP. Pathobiology 1999;67:227–229.

52. Schumann RR, Latz E. Lipopolysaccharide-binding protein. Chem Immunol 2000;74:42–60.

53. Schumann RR, Zweigner J. A novel acute-phase marker: lipopolysaccharide binding protein (LBP). Clin Chem Lab Med 1999;37:271–274.

54. Tobias PS, Tapping RI, Gegner JA. Endotoxin interactions with lipopolysaccharide-responsive cells. Clin Infect Dis 1999;28:476–481.
55. Fenton MJ, Golenbock DT. LPS-binding proteins and receptors. J Leukoc Biol 1998;64:25–32.
56. Kirschning C, Unbehaun A, Lamping N, et al. Control of transcriptional activation of the lipopolysaccharide binding protein (LBP) gene by proinflammatory cytokines. Cytokines Cell Mol Ther 1997;3:59–62.
57. Su GL, Simmons RL, Wang SC. Lipopolysaccharide binding protein participation in cellular activation by LPS. Crit Rev Immunol 1995;15:201–214.
58. Ulevitch RJ, Tobias PS. Receptor-dependent mechanisms of cell stimulation by bacterial endotoxin. Annu Rev Immunol 1995;13:437–457.
59. Kobe B, Deisenhofer J. A Structural basis of the interactions between leucine-rich repeats and protein ligands. Nature 1995;374:183–186.
60. Simmons DL, Tan S, Tenen DG, Nicholson Weller A, Seed B. Monocyte antigen CD14 is a phospholipid anchored membrane protein. Blood 1989;73:284–289.
61. Frey EA, Miller DS, Jahr TG, et al. Soluble CD14 participates in the response of cells to lipopolysaccharide. J Exp Med 1992;176:1665–1671.
62. Lee J-D, Kravchenko V, Kirkland TN, et al. Glycosylphosphatidylinositol-anchored or integral membrane forms of CD14 mediate identical cellular responses to endotoxin. Proc Natl Acad Sci USA 1993;90:9930–9934.
63. Juan TS, Kelley MJ, Johnson DA, et al. et al. Soluble CD14 truncated at amino acid 152 binds lipopolysaccharide (LPS) and enables cellular response to LPS. J Biol Chem 1995;270:1382–1387.
64. Viriyakosol S, Kirkland TN. The N-terminal half of membrane CD14 is a functional cellular lipopolysaccharide receptor. Infect Immun 1996;64:653–656.
65. Juan TS-C, Hailman E, Kelley MJ, Wright SD, Lichenstein HS. Identification of a domain in soluble CD14 essential for lipopolysaccharide (LPS) signaling but not LPS binding. J Biol Chem 1995;270:17237–17242.
66. Juan TS-C, Hailman E, Kelley MJ, et al. Identification of a lipopolysaccharide binding domain in CD14 between amino acids 57 and 64. J Biol Chem 1995;270:5219–5224.
67. Viriyakosol S, Kirkland TN. A region of human CD14 required for lipopolysaccharide binding. J Biol Chem 1995;270:361–368.
68. Stelter F, Bernheiden M, Menzel R, et al. Mutation of amino acids 39–44 of human CD14 abrogates binding of lipopolysaccharide and *Escherichia coli*. Eur J Biochem 1997;243:100–109.
69. Dziarski R, Viriyakosol S, Kirkland TN, Gupta D. Soluble CD14 enhances membrane CD14-mediated responses to peptidoglycan: structural requirements differ from those for responses to lipopolysaccharide. Infect Immun 2000;68:5254–5260.
70. Labeta MO, Durieux JJ, Fernandez N, Herrmann R, Ferrara P. Release from a human monocyte-like cell line of two different soluble forms of the lipopolysaccharide receptor, CD14. Eur J Immunol 1993;23:2144–2151.
71. Stelter F. Structure/function relationships of CD14. Chem Immunol 2000;74:25–41.
72. Asea A, Kraeft SK, Kurt-Jones EA, et al. HSP70 stimulates cytokine production through a CD14-dependent pathway, demonstrating its dual role as a chaperone and cytokine. Nat Med 2000;6:435–442.
73. Kol A, Lichtman AH, Finberg RW, Libby P, Kurt-Jones EA. Cutting edge: heat shock protein (HSP) 60 activates the innate immune response: CD14 is an essential receptor for HSP60 activation of mononuclear cells. J Immunol 2000;164:13–17.
74. Haynes LM, Moore DD, Kurt-Jones EA, et al. Involvement of toll-like receptor 4 in innate immunity to respiratory syncytial virus. J Virol 2001;75:10730–10737.
75. Kurt-Jones EA, Popova L, Kwinn L, et al. Pattern recognition receptors TLR4 and CD14 mediate response to respiratory syncytial virus. Nat Immunol 2000;1:398–401.

76. Devitt A, Moffatt OD, Raykundalia C, et al. Human CD14 mediates recognition and phagocytosis of apoptotic cells. Nature 1998;392:505–509.
77. Triantafilou K, Triantafilou M, Dedrick RL. A CD14-independent LPS receptor cluster. Nat Immunol 2001;2:338–345.
78. Galbiati F, Razani B, Lisanti MP. Emerging themes in lipid rafts and caveolae. Cell 2001;106:403–411.
79. Pugin J, Kravchenko VV, Lee JD, et al. Cell activation mediated by glycosylphosphatidylinositol-anchored or transmembrane forms of CD14. Infect Immun 1998;66:1174–1180.
80. Haziot A, Ferrero E, Xing YL, Stewart CL, Goyert SM. CD14-deficient mice are exquisitely insensitive to the effects of LPS. In: Levin J, Alving CR, Munford RS, Redl H (eds.). Bacterial Endotoxins. From Genes to Therapy. New York: Wiley-Liss, 1994, pp. 349–351.
81. Moore KJ, Andersson LP, Ingalls RR, et al. Divergent response to LPS and bacteria in CD14-deficient murine macrophages. J Immunol 2000;165:4272–4280.
82. Haziot A, Lin XY, Zhang F, Goyert SM. The induction of acute phase proteins by lipopolysaccharide uses a novel pathway that is CD14-independent. J Immunol 1998;160:2570–2572.
83. Frevert CW, Matute-Bello G, Skerrett SJ, et al. Effect of CD14 blockade in rabbits with *Escherichia coli* pneumonia and sepsis. J Immunol 2000;164:5439–5445.
84. Wenneras C, Ave P, Huerre M, et al. Blockade of CD14 increases *Shigella*-mediated invasion and tissue destruction. J Immunol 2000;164:3214–3221.
85. Haziot A, Hijiya N, Gangloff SC, Silver J, Goyert SM. Induction of a novel mechanism of accelerated bacterial clearance by lipopolysaccharide in CD14-deficient and Toll-like receptor 4-deficient mice. J Immunol 2001;166:1075–1078.
86. Le Van TD, Bloom JW, Bailey TJ, et al. A common single nucleotide polymorphism in the CD14 promoter decreases the affinity of Sp protein binding and enhances transcriptional activity. J Immunol 2001;167:5838–5844.
87. Zhang DE, Hetherington CJ, Tan S, et al. Sp1 is a critical factor for the monocytic specific expression of human CD14. J Biol Chem 1994;269:11425–11434.
88. Vercelli D, Baldini M, Stern D, et al. CD14: a bridge between innate immunity and adaptive IgE responses. J Endotoxin Res 2001;7:45–48.
89. Williams H, Robertson C, Stewart A, et al. Worldwide variations in the prevalence of symptoms of atopic eczema in the International Study of Asthma and Allergies in Childhood. J Allergy Clin Immunol 1999;103:125–138.
90. Strachan D, Sibbald B, Weiland S, et al. Worldwide variations in prevalence of symptoms of allergic rhinoconjunctivitis in children: the International Study of Asthma and Allergies in Childhood (ISAAC). Pediatr Allergy Immunol 1997;8:161–176.
91. Arias MA, Rey Nores JE, Vita N, et al. Cutting edge: human B cell function is regulated by interaction with soluble CD14: opposite effects on IgG1 and IgE production. J Immunol 2000;164:3480–3486.
92. Shimada K, Watanabe Y, Mokuno H, et al. Common polymorphism in the promoter of the CD14 monocyte receptor gene is associated with acute myocardial infarction in Japanese men. Am J Cardiol 2000;86:682–684.
93. Unkelbach K, Gardemann A, Kostrzewa M, et al. A new promoter polymorphism in the gene of lipopolysaccharide receptor CD14 is associated with expired myocardial infarction in patients with low atherosclerotic risk profile. Arterioscler Thromb Vasc Biol 1999;19:932–938.
94. Hubacek JA, Rothe G, Pit'ha J, et al. C(−260) → T polymorphism in the promoter of the CD14 monocyte receptor gene as a risk factor for myocardial infarction. Circulation 1999;99:3218–3220.
95. Ito D, Murata M, Tanahashi N, et al. Polymorphism in the promoter of lipopolysaccharide receptor CD14 and ischemic cerebrovascular disease. Stroke 2000;31:2661–2664.

96. Landmann R, Muller B, Zimmerli W. CD14, new aspects of ligand and signal diversity. Microbes Infect 2000;2:295–304.

97. Gregory CD. CD14-dependent clearance of apoptotic cells: relevance to the immune system. Curr Opin Immunol 2000;12:27–34.

98. Antal-Szalmas P. Evaluation of CD14 in host defence. Eur J Clin Invest 2000;30:167–179.

99. Tapping RI, Tobias PS. Soluble CD14-mediated cellular responses to lipopolysaccharide. Chem Immunol 2000;74:108–121.

100. Dziarski R, Ulmer AJ, Gupta D. Interactions of CD14 with components of gram-positive bacteria. Chem Immunol 2000;74:83–107.

101. Kitchens RL. Role of CD14 in cellular recognition of bacterial lipopolysaccharides. Chem Immunol 2000;74:61–82.

102. Stelter F. Structure/function relationships of CD14. Chem Immunol 2000;74:25–41.

Section IV

Mammalian Host Defenses:
Links Between Innate and Adaptive Immunity

Section Editor: Steven L. Kunkel

It is becoming increasingly clear that the successful operation of the human host defense system is the culmination of a number of interactive processes, which places constant pressure on eliminating a foreign antigen or pathogen. Various levels of immune sophistication dictate the interactive processes of an immune/inflammatory response, ranging from the nonspecific preprogrammed reaction to pattern recognition molecules to the exquisitely specific cell-mediated response to a single antigen. Innate immunity constitutes the former reaction and is triggered within minutes of exposure to a foreign agent, while the latter response is a characteristic of an acquired or adaptive immune response and requires a number of days to imprint its effect on the host. The importance of innate over acquired immunity or vice versa is an illogical argument, as a concerted and interactive innate and adaptive immune reaction is key for an automatic, dynamic, sustained, and regulated response. Thus, it is imperative that the in vivo concept of innate and acquired immunity be considered a continuum within a system-wide assault on a foreign agent and not two different modes totally independent of each other.

In this section on *Mammalian Host Defenses: Links Between Innate and Adaptive Immunity*, the various authors present information that addresses different aspects of linking these diverse facets of host defense. Investigations into the biology of chemokines during innate and acquired immune reactions have clearly demonstrated that this class of mediators are important to the natural progression of host defense. Chemokines make an important contribution to both innate and acquired immunity via the ability to recruit specific subpopulations of leukocytes to an area of inflammation, thereby insuring the arrival of the most appropriate leukocyte populations needed to respond to the foreign challenge. In addition, chemokines can regulate the systemic traf-

From: *Infectious Disease: Innate Immunity*
Edited by: R. A. B. Ezekowitz and J. A. Hoffmann © Humana Press Inc., Totowa, NJ

ficking of leukocytes between lymphoid and nonlymphoid tissue during normal immune surveillance. This phenomenon is likely attributable to the ability of all nucleated cells in the body to generate chemokines rapidly upon exposure to a foreign antigen or pathogen, resulting in a chemokine phenotype tailored to the specific outside threat.

Antimicrobial peptides and proteins generated during the activation of the complement cascade are additional mediators that bridge innate and acquired immunity. At high concentrations the antimicrobial peptides, such as defensins, act as either membrane disruptive agents or lipopolysaccharide binding molecules, while at lower concentrations they possess chemotactic activity for the recruitment of leukocyte populations. When the host is exposed to a pathogen, these antimicrobial peptides are rapidly released and contribute to the initial resistance to the pathogen and facilitate the evolution of distal humoral and cell-mediated immunity. In a similar fashion, activation of the complement system may result in an antimicrobial effect via either targeting the pathogen for destruction by the establishment of a lytic membrane attack complex pathway or targeting the pathogen for phagocytosis. This latter aspect of immunity is one of the fundamental underpinnings of an effective host response, as a deficiency in phagocytosis would result in an immunosuppressed host. In addition, activation of the complement pathway generates chemotactic split complement product, such as C5a, which is important to leukocyte trafficking and the transition of innate to acquired immunity.

While a number of molecular signals are key to the initiation of an innate response and the subsequent transition into an acquired response, there are also a number of cells that actively link innate and acquired immunity. Neutrophils, fixed macrophages, and natural killer cells have received attention for their roles in innate immune reactions and their activity in the transition toward adaptive immunity. However, less recognized cells, such as mast cells and CD-1 restricted T cells, also contribute to these host defense processes. The contribution of mast cells via the production of histamine, proteases, proteoglycans, eicosanoids, cytokines, and chemokines are important in the initiation and maintenance of various aspects of host defense. Furthermore, these cells are recognized as key participants in wound repair, angiogenesis, and tissue remodeling. CD-1 restricted T cells are an additional subset of leukocytes that bridge the innate and acquired immune spectrum. Interestingly, CD-1 restricted T cells can have either a limited T cell receptor repertoire and react to a small number of foreign antigens that possess a conserved molecular pattern or can respond to a limited spectrum of antigens via clonally varied receptors.

The information presented in this section supports the link between innate and acquired immunity and underscores the various systems that are important to the success of each immune response. Diverse cells and mediators are key to the progression of innate immunity to adaptive immunity and their integration allows for a rapid and dynamic host response to foreign antigens and pathogens.

Steven L. Kunkel

15

The Role of Chemokines in Linking Innate and Adaptive Immunity

Cory M. Hogaboam and Steven L. Kunkel

1. INTRODUCTION

Of the myriad of immune defense systems that exist in nature, the mammalian defense system is clearly the most sophisticated and successful. This immune sophistication arises from the fact that immune events in mammals involve a progression of detailed events leading to exquisite specificity toward a bacterial, viral, or fungal byproduct, or a nonself protein. On its simplest level, the immune response in mammals is divided into two major components: the nonspecific innate and the adaptive or acquired immune systems *(1)*. When examined phylogenetically, the innate immune system appears to be more ancient than its acquired counterpart, and, historically, it was thought that the innate response was nonselectively directed toward microorganisms. However, the distinctions between the innate and acquired immune responses are now widely viewed as somewhat artificial, as it has been shown that both arms of the immune response share several common features including amazing degrees of specificity for pathogens and foreign antigens *(2)*. Indeed, there is increasing evidence that the induction of different types of effector adaptive responses is directed by the innate immune system after its highly selective recognition of particular groups of pathogens through pattern recognition molecules (i.e., the Toll-like receptor family) and the elaboration of soluble protein signals that activate the relevant lymphoid cell population. The aim of this review is to highlight the role that the soluble protein molecules known as chemotactic cytokines or chemokines exert in the bidirectional communication between the innate and acquired immune responses during host defense.

2. THE INTERLINKED INNATE AND ACQUIRED IMMUNE SYSTEMS

Innate immunity typically serves as the rapid, first-line defense against invading pathogens and foreign antigens. Phagocytes, including neutrophils and macrophages, and natural killer (NK) cells are critical participants in the innate response because of their ability to neutralize and clear a wide array of micro- and macroorganisms.

From: *Infectious Disease: Innate Immunity*
Edited by: R. A. B. Ezekowitz and J. A. Hoffmann © Humana Press Inc., Totowa, NJ

Although phagocytes can be found in various tissue sites throughout the body, the successful containment and destruction of most infectious foci typically require the influx of freshly activated leukoctyes from the circulation. The migratory events that leukocytes follow in moving from the circulation to the extravascular space are well orchestrated and involve critical cell-associated and soluble proteins. The recruitment of leukocytes into inflamed tissue is regulated by interactions between the circulating leukocytes and endothelial cells. Integrins expressed by leukocytes have a pivotal role in leukocyte adhesion to endothelial cells, and the activation of integrins by chemokines is essential for integrin-mediated adhesion: the chemokine signal transduced in the leukocyte converts the functionally inactive integrin to an active adhesive configuration *(3)*.

The innate response is normally short lived, given its propensity to destroy invader and tissue indiscriminately *(4)*. However, before terminating its activity, the innate response can induce key costimulatory molecules on antigen-presenting cells (APCs), largely owing to the generation of potent adjuvants; APCs then direct the antigen-driven clonal expansion of T-and B-cells and other antigen-specific cells of the acquired immune response *(5)*. The subsequent involvement of the adaptive immunity appears to provide two major advantages: first, it provides another avenue of defense against primary infection, and, second, it provides immunologic memory, thereby providing the host with resistance to reinfection *(6)*. It can be argued that neither arm is more efficient than the other, but through their concerted efforts the mammalian immune system is able to gauge accurately the magnitude of the threat that a given pathogen or foreign antigen poses to the host. Furthermore, the concert of innate and acquired immune responses ensures that self antigens are clearly discriminated from nonself antigens, thereby avoiding inappropriate autoimmune events *(7)*. Thus, the complex integration of innate and adaptive immune responses allows for both rapid responses and dynamic regulation of inflammation in vivo *(8)*.

3. CHEMOKINES

Chemokines belong to a supergene family of 8–10-kDa protein mediators widely known as soluble factors that attract and activate specific leukocyte populations in the context of inflammatory and immune events *(9,10)*. However, recent evidence suggests that chemokines also play a wider role in the development and homeostasis of inflammatory and immune responses *(11,12)*. Chemokines, owing to their differing effects on the recruitment of specific leukocytes, ultimately determine which cells will regulate and participate in localized innate and adaptive immune responses. However, nearly half of the currently described chemokines have the capacity to suppress the proliferation of myeloid progenitor cells *(13)*, and several recently described chemokines also exquisitely regulate the systemic trafficking of inflammatory and immune cells between lymphoid and nonlymphoid tissues for surveillance and effector purposes *(14,15)*. Nearly every mammalian cell appears to have the ability to respond to factors associated with pathogens through the production of chemokines, and this production is carefully regulated on several levels so that the kinetics and phenotype of the localized inflammatory response is tailored to the specific pathogen threat. This form of regulation ensures that only the appropriate inflammatory cells are attracted to the target tissue. Given the direct association between chemokine expression and the severity of inflammatory and immune responses in several tissues, blocking the actions of chemokines is viewed as a novel therapeutic strategy for the treatment of diseases precipitated by excessive immune activation *(16)*.

4. CHEMOKINE NOMENCLATURE

Bioinformatic-based analysis of nucleotide databases has enormously increased the number of chemokines to at least 50 members in four distinct structural families *(17)*. The chemokine families are distinguished by the relative positioning of cysteines at the amino terminus in these proteins. The two largest families encompass the C-C and the C-X-C chemokines, which tend to promote preferentially the chemotaxis of mononuclear and polymorphonuclear cells, respectively, although exceptions to this rule exist in both families.

C-C chemokines include monocyte chemoattractant proteins (MCP) 1–5, eotaxin, eotaxin-2, regulated on T-cell activation, normal T-cell expressed and secreted (RANTES) proteins, macrophage inflammatory protein-1α and -β (MIP-1α and -β), macrophage-derived chemokine (MDC), and C10 chemokine. C-X-C chemokines can be divided into two subsets. The first subset is comprised of C-X-C chemokines that possess the amino acid residues Glu-Leu-Arg (abbreviated ELR) such as interleukin-8 (IL-8.) epithelial neutrophil-activating factor-78 (ENA-78), the growth-related oncogene proteins (GROs), and murine MIP-2, a murine chemokine. The second subset, the non-ELR C-X-C chemokines, lacks the ELR motif and includes interferon-inducible protein-10 (IP-10) and monokine induced by interferon-γ (MIG). Lymphotactin, a C chemokine lacking the first and third cysteine but structurally homologous to the C-C chemokines *(18,19)*, and fractalkine, a membrane-bound C-X$_3$-C chemokine, presently represent the only members of their respective families.

Chemokine nomenclature has been standardized to mirror the sequential classification scheme presently used for the chemokine receptors *(20)*. Thus, chemokines are numbered consecutively as C-C ligand (CCL), C-X-C ligand (CXCL), C ligand (XCL), and C-X$_3$-C ligand (CX3CL), eliminating the confusion that surrounds the use of multiple names for a single chemokine. Subsequent reference to chemokines in this review will include both the old and the new nomenclatures for these factors.

5. CHEMOKINE RECEPTOR NOMENCLATURE

The chemokine superfamily of leukocyte chemoattractants coordinates the development and deployment of the immune system by signaling through a family of distinct rhododopsin-like GTP-binding protein-coupled receptors *(21)*. A further layer of complexity within the arena of chemokine biology is the fact that most of the chemokine receptors are not selective for a single chemokine. C-C chemokines interact with at least 11 distinct receptors designated CCR1–CCR11. Whereas the promiscuity of chemokine receptors sometimes obscures the relative importance of each chemokine in immune responses, the selectivity of chemokine effects in these responses appears to be tightly regulated at the level of chemokine receptor expression and the cell distribution of these receptors.

Differences in chemokine ligand specificity for chemokine receptors exist between the murine and human system. Generally, CCR1 binds RANTES/CCL5, MCP-3/CCL7, and MIP-1α/CCL3. CCR2 binds MCP-1/CCL21, -2/CCL8, -3/CCL7 and -4/CCL13 *(22)*, whereas CCR3 binds MCP-3/CCL7, MCP-4/CCL13, eotaxin/CCL11, and eotaxin-2/CCL24 *(23)*. CCR4 binds TARC/CCL17 and MDC/CCL22, and CCR5 binds RANTES/CCL5, MIP-1α/CCL3, and MIP-1β/CCL4 *(24)*. Some of the more recently discovered C-C chemokine receptors appear to bind C-C ligands in a more selective fashion, as in the case of CCR6, which only binds MIP-3α/CCL20 *(25)*, CCR7, which binds MIP-3β/CCL19 and 6Ckine/CCL21, CCR8, which binds TCA-3/CCL1 *(20)*, and CCR10, which binds CTACK/CCL27 *(26)*. C-X-C chemokines interact with at least six distinct CXCRs, of which the first two bind the prototypical human C-X-C chemokine, IL-8/CXCL8. CXCR2 binds IL-8/CXCL8, ENA-78/CXCL5, growth-related GROs (CXCL1–3), and MIP-2, and CXCR3 binds induced by interferon-γ (IFN-γ)-inducible non-ELR CXC chemokines such as IP-10/CXCL10 and MIG/CXCL9. The primary chemokine that binds CXCR4 is stromal cell-derived factor-1 (SDF-1/CXCL12), and CXCR5 binds BLC/CXCL13. Finally, lymphotactin/XCL1 binds specifically to XCR1, and fractalkine/CX3CL1 binds exclusively to CX3CR1 *(11)*.

6. CHEMOKINES LINK CELLS OF THE INNATE AND ACQUIRED IMMUNE SYSTEMS

In the sections that follow, published data is highlighted providing clear evidence that chemokines link the innate with adaptive immune responses. As shown in Table 1, a variety of cytokines, including the chemokines, provide important communication links between innate and acquired immunity. However, one of the more specific cytokines, which appears to be restricted to the acquired immune response, is IL-2. The manner in which chemokines coordinate both arms of the immune response is described first in a cell-specific fashion.

6.1. Neutrophils

Because of their ability to perform a series of aggressive effector functions, neutrophils are key cellular innate immune elements in inflammatory responses against injury and infection. The contribution of neutrophils to host defense and innate immunity extends beyond their traditional role as professional phagocytes. In particular, neutrophils can be induced to express a variety of chemokines such as IL-8/CXCL8, GRO/CXCL1-3, MIP-1α/CCL3, MIP-1β/CCL4, IP-10/CXCL10, and MIG/CXCL9 *(27)*. Through its ability to elaborate these chemokines, it is conceivable that neutrophils can subsequently orchestrate the chemotaxis of other leukocyte subsets including monocytes, immature dendritic cells (DCs), and T-lymphocyte subsets. The manner in which neutrophils regulate mononuclear cell recruitment to sites of infection of inflammation is presently unknown.

6.2. Dendritic Cells

To date, the best evidence for chemokines linking the innate and acquired immune responses is derived from studies of DC activation and migration *(28)*. DCs are an heterogeneous family of cells that function as sentinels of the immune system and are critical for moving antigens from peripheral sites to regional lymph nodes, to allow appropriate transmission of antigenic specificity to T-cells *(29)*. Under homeostatic

Table 1
Cytokines and Chemokines Involved in the Evolution of Both Innate and Acquired Immunity[a]

Cell	Mediator
Innate	
NK cells	IL-12, IL-14, IFN-γ, CC chemokines
Mast cells	IL-4, IL-13, CC chemokines
Monocytes	IL-1, IL-10, IL-12, TNF, CXC, CC chemokines
Macrophages	IL-13, IL-12, IL-18, CXC, CC chemokines
Acquired	
T-cells (Th-1)	IFN-γ, **IL-2,** cc chemokines
T-cells (Th-2)	IL-4, IL-5, IL-6, IL-10, IL-13, CC chemokines
T-cells (Th-3)	TGF-β
Macrophages	IL-12, IL-18 CXC, CC chemokines

[a] Interestingly, the cellular source of these various mediators is quite diverse. IFN, interferon; IL, interleukin; TGF, transforming growth factor; TNF, tumor necrosis factor.

conditions, DCs typically fulfill a surveillance function in all tissues, but following a pathogenic or injurious cue, these cells capture antigens, migrate from the tissues, and move to the draining lymphoid organs *(30)*. In lymphoid organs, DCs undergo a maturation process that temporarily positions them within the lymphoid organ such that they can prime naive T-cells. The fact that DC migration is an integral component of their sentinel function has led to a number of studies of the responsiveness of various DC populations to chemokines *(31)*. Immature DCs respond to a number of CC and CXC chemokines including MIP-1α/CCL3, MIP-1β/CCL4, MIP-3α/CCL20, MCP-3/CCL7, MCP-4/CCL13, RANTES/CCL5, TECK/CCL25, and SDF-1/CXCL12, but each immature DC population appears to respond to a particular subset of chemokines. Examples include Langerhans cells, which express CCR6 and migrate selectively to MIP-3α/CCL20, blood CD11c+ DCs, which express CCR2 and migrate to MCP-1/CCL2, and monocyte-derived-DCs, which express CCR1 and CCR5 and migrate to MIP-1α/CCL3 or MIP-1β/CCL4 *(28)*.

Conversely, mature DCs in the lymphoid tissue lose their responsiveness to most of these inflammatory chemokines through receptor downregulation or desensitization. These cells subsequently acquire responsiveness to MIP-3β/CCL19 and SLC/CCL21 (via CCR7 upregulation) *(32–34)*. This change in responsiveness ensures that mature DCs (also referred to as interdigitating DCs) home to the T-cell-rich areas in the lymphoid tissue where MIP-3β/CCL19 and SLC/CCL21 are specifically expressed *(35)*. Furthermore, because DCs are the major APCs in the induction of cellular responses to intracellular pathogens, such as mycobacteria, these cells directly control the development of a Th1-type protective immunity *(36)*. Accordingly, chemokines are responsible for the rapid movement of DCs during the first wave of cells into inflamed tissue *(37)*, and these cells in turn participate in the further elaboration of chemokines necessary for the recruitment and activation of other inflammatory cells *(38)*. Macrophage-derived DCs regulate the generation of Th1-type cells, in part through their generation of CCR5 agonists such as MIP-1α/CCL3, MIP-1β/CCL4, and RANTES/CCL5, and not Th1-type cytokines such as IL-12 *(39)*. Conversely, elaboration of MDC/CCL22 by DCs results in the attraction of CCR4-positive polarized Th2 and Tc2 cells *(40)*, thereby serving as an amplification loop for polarized Th2 responses *(41)*. Clearly, chemokines have a major impact on the involvement of DCs in the link between the innate and acquired immune response.

6.3. NK Cells

NK cells are unique lymphocytes that exhibit cytotoxic activity and produce high levels of certain cytokines and chemokines; as such, these cells are important in innate and adaptive immune responses to a number of different infectious agents, including viruses *(42)*. The regulation of NK cell migration to inflammatory sites and subsequent activation has been the subject of intense research. For example, MIP-3α/CCL20, SLC/CCL21, and MIP-3β/CCL19 did not induce detectable chemotaxis of resting peripheral blood NK cells, but the latter two chemokines stimulated the migration of various types of activated peripheral blood NK cells *(43)*. Because of their ability to respond to these unique chemokines (normally expressed in defined lymphoid tissues), NK cells may be able to interact directly with T-cells in defined lymphoid organs.

6.4. T-Cells

The adaptive immune response is initiated by the interaction of T-cell antigen receptors with MHC molecule-peptide complexes *(5)*. Although the interaction between chemokines and their receptors is an important step in the control of T-cell migration into sites of inflammation (an adaptive immune response against intracellular pathogens requires the recruitment of effector T-cells to sites of infection), it has become apparent that chemokines also have a major role in determining T-cell cytokine generation. Activated T-cells differentiate into two major effector subtypes, namely, Th1 and Th2 cells, which secrete cytokines that enhance cell-mediated (IFN-γ) and humoral immunity (IL-4 and IL-13), respectively. These cytokines, which define either a type 1 or type 2 inflammatory phenotype, have the ability to induce a set of either IFN-γ-inducible chemokines or a set of IL-4/IL-13-inducible chemokines (Table 2). MCP-1/CCL2 produced by APCs *(44)* and fibroblasts *(45)* can regulate IL-4 synthesis by isolated CD4-positive T-cells, and its overexpression is associated with defects in cell-mediated immunity *(46)*, indicating that it might be involved in the polarization of Th2 responses. MCP-1 influences both innate immunity *(47)* through effects on monocytes, and acquired immunity through control of T-helper cell polarization *(48,49)*.

Chemokines also mediate a variety of effects independent of chemotaxis, including induction and enhancement of Th1- and Th2-associated cytokine responses *(50)*. Recent studies have shown that human Th1 and Th2 clones, activated under polarizing conditions with polyclonal stimuli in vitro, display distinct patterns of chemokine receptor expression: Th1 clones preferentially express CCR5 and CXCR3 *(51)*, whereas many Th2 clones express CCR4, CCR8 *(52,53)*, and, to a lesser extent, CCR3. These differential patterns of chemokine receptor expression suggest a mechanism for selective induction of migration and activation of Th1- and Th2-type cells during inflammation and (perhaps) normal immune homoeostasis *(54)*. For example, IP-10/CXCL10 appears to have a broad role in the localization and function of effector T-cells at sites of Th1 inflammation *(55)*. Finally, the differentiation of T-cell effectors

Table 2
Cytokine Control of Specific Chemokine Expression[a]

Cytokine type	Chemokine
Interferon-γ inducible	IP-10, MIG, ITAC
IL-4/IL-13-inducible	MCP-1, MDC, C10

[a] The cytokines define either a type 1 or 2 phenotype. IL, interleukin; IP-10, interferon-inducible protein-10; ITAC, interferon inducible T-cell alpha chemoattractant; MCP, monocyte chemoattractant protein; MDC, macrophage-derived chemokine; MIG, monokine induced by interferon-γ.

allows for further regulation of local inflammation since the cytokines they generate also affect chemokine production *(56)*.

6.5. Epithelial Cells

Although not normally associated with either the innate or acquired immune systems, epithelial cells from various tissues have been shown to respond to innate immune signals and consequently secrete an array of chemokines that participate in both arms of the immune response. The epithelial cell layer is ideally located at the interface between the host and its environment, and thus it is an immediate-early warning system in the host, particularly when breached by invasive microbial pathogens *(57)*. One recent example of the significant role that epithelial cells may play in the transition between innate and acquired immunity is suggested in the studies of Izadpanah et al. *(58)*, who showed that MIP-3α/CCL20 was constitutively expressed by human intestinal epithelium and that the levels of this CCR6 ligand (expressed on DCs, T-cells, and NK cells) could be markedly upregulated by inflammatory cytokines such as tumor necrosis factor-α (TNF-α) and IL-1β (Fig. 1). RANTES/CCL5 is another chemokine that is produced by lymphoid and epithelial cells at several mucosal sites in response to various external stimuli; it is chemotactic for T-cells. Evidence that RANTES/CCL5 can serve as a link between the initial innate signals of the host and the adaptive immune system is derived from the fact that this CC chemokine enhances mucosal and systemic humoral antibody responses through help provided by Th1- and select Th2-type cytokines *(59)*. RANTES/CCL5 can also induce the expression of costimulatory molecules and cytokine receptors on T-cells *(59)*.

6.6. Fibroblasts

As in the case of epithelial cells, fibroblasts are not normally given any consideration in discussions of innate or acquired immune responses, but these cells are an excellent source of chemokines during inflammatory reactions in several tissues. Fibroblasts are a major source of constitutive and cytokine-induced MCP-1/CCL2, MIP-1α/CCL3, RANTES/CCL5, IP-10/CXCL10, and eotaxin/CCL11 *(60)*, but in their capacity as sentinel cells *(61)* they are able to produce different patterns of chemokines in response to different alarm stimuli. Xia and colleagues *(62)* have shown that an important regulator of chemokine production by fibroblasts appears to be RelB, a transcription factor that is rapidly increased following the activation of fibroblasts with inflammatory stimuli such as IL-1β, TNF-α, and lipopolysaccharide (LPS). When RelB gene expression was deleted in mice (RelB$^{-/-}$), fibroblasts (but not macrophages)

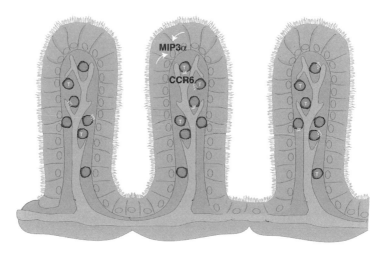

Fig. 1. The trafficking of T-cells in the epithelium of the gut involves the expression of macrophage inflammatory protein (MIP)-3α from the epithelial cells, which binds to CCR6 on the T-cells.

exhibited NF-κB activity that remained unchecked, and chemokine generation continued unabated. Interestingly, RelB$^{-/-}$ mice exhibited a syndrome of multiorgan inflammation characterized by a predominant interstitial infiltrate of neutrophils, monocytes, and macrophages *(62)*. These studies demonstrate that the fibroblast appears to be uniquely involved in regulating the nature of the inflammatory response in its environment and that the unique molecular mechanisms fibroblasts employ to regulate chemokine synthesis suggest that these cells have an important surveillance role in many tissues.

7. CHEMOKINES LINK INNATE AND ACQUIRED IMMUNE RESPONSES DURING DISEASE

The sections that follow provide relevant in vivo examples of the manner in which chemokines link the innate and acquired immune responses during HIV infection and in models of pulmonary disease and septic shock syndrome.

7.1. Chemokines, HIV, and Other Viruses

Since the discovery that RANTES/CCL5, MIP-1α/CCL3, and MIP-1β/CCL4 inhibit the binding of M-trophic HIV to macrophages *(63)* and that numerous herpesviruses and poxviruses encode chemokine mimics able to block chemokine action *(64)*, the relationship between viruses and chemokines has been a hot topic of research. HIV infection affects the innate as well as the acquired immune systems because it targets macrophages (via a CCR5 co-receptor) and T-cells (via a CXCR4 co-receptor) during its dissemination *(65,66)*, but HIV infection also changes the phagocytic function of macrophages *(67)*. This latter effect is manifest in the fact that HIV patients have a reduced capacity to deal with subsequent pathogen exposure, and many suffer from chronic pulmonary infections such as mycobacteria *(68)*. Considerable excitement surrounds the clinical application of inhibitors of chemokine receptors such as CCR5 in the treatment of HIV-infected individuals *(66)*, but it is clear that HIV has had considerable time to develop strategies that circumvent the need for exclusive chemokine receptor usage during infection *(65)*.

Recent engaging findings also suggest that therapeutic potential may lie in the use of molecular piracy and mimicry tactics that viruses have evolved to elude the normal host defense response. For example, the Kaposi sarcoma-associated herpesvirus (KSHV) or human herpesvirus 8 encodes C-C chemokine-like molecules such as KSHV vMIP-I *(69,70)* and vMIP-II *(71)*, which have potent agonist effects on CCR8 (a C-C chemokine receptor that regulates the chemotaxis of Th2-type lymphocytes *(71)*. However, vMIP-II and vMMC-I also exhibit potent in vitro antagonistic activities against CCRs, CXCRs, and CX3CR1 *(72)*. The antiinflammatory activity of recombinant vMIP-II was recently documented in a rat model of experimental glomerulonephritis, and this viral chemokine potently inhibited leukocyte infiltration to the glomeruli and markedly attenuated proteinuria *(73)*. Although viruses presumably use chemokines and chemokine receptors to ensure their survival or create a tissue environment that facilitates dissemination *(74)*, it is conceivable that viral chemokines could be modified to benefit humans undergoing an inflammatory or immune event.

7.2 Chemokine Regulation of Pulmonary Inflammatory and Immune Responses

To facilitate adequate gas exchange, the lung contains the largest epithelial surface area of the body. Via its contact with the external environment, the upper and lower airways of the lung are repeatedly exposed to a multitude of potentially harmful airborne particles and microorganisms. This constant exposure necessitates an elaborate system of defense mechanisms to prevent overgrowth and tissue destruction by the invading pathogens. The initial clearance of microorganisms from the lung is mediated by a dual phagocytic system involving both alveolar macrophages and polymorphonuclear leukocytes. The cellular source of chemokines has been under intense investigation, and they appear to be derived from multiple sources. As shown in Fig. 2, when the host is challenged with a pathogen, a number of systems are set in motion aimed at the appropriate productions of chemokines. Tissue macrophages, such alveolar macrophages in the lung, can generate early response cytokines, IL-1 and TNF, when challenged with pathogens. These early response cytokines can network with surrounding cells in the lung tissue and generate a set of chemokines that are involved in moving leukocytes from the lumen of the vasculature to the site of inflammation.

The rapid establishment of chemokine gradients has been shown to be critical for the recruitment and activation of inflammatory cells such as neutrophils into the lung, and the nature of the chemokine response can fundamentally alter the types of leukocytes that are recruited to the lungs, as well as the ultimate resolution of the inflammatory response *(75)*. Studies by Itakura et al. *(76)* provide an excellent example of the manner in which chemokine actions in the lung affect not only the acute inflammatory response but also the much later acquired response. These investigators examined the role of MIP-2 and SLC/CCL21 in the development of acute pulmonary inflammation induced by an intratracheal injection of *Propionibacterium acnes* in mice. Immunoneutralization of MIP-2 and CXCR2 (neutrophil-specific chemokine and chemokine receptor) was shown to alleviate the *P. acnes*-induced pulmonary inflammation, as has been shown for a number of acute infectious-type insults in the lung *(77)* including

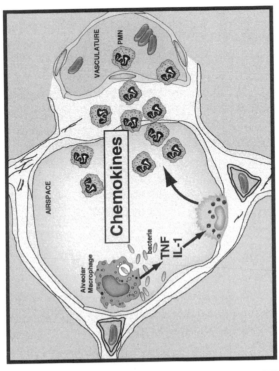

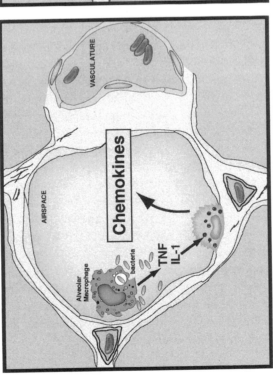

Fig. 2. A variety of immune, inflammatory, and resident tissue cells are capable of expressing different chemokines. The ability of lung epithelial cells to express chemokines is dependent on a cytokine network that is established between the early response cytokines, such as interleukin-1 (IL-1) and tumor necrosis factor (TNF), produced by activated resident macrophages (alveolar macrophages) and resident lung epithelial cells. PMN, polymorphonuclear neutrophil.

pneumonia *(78)*. However, in the same study, the immunoneutralization of SLC/CCL21 exacerbated the pulmonary inflammation owing to a marked increase in the numbers of mature DCs, macrophages, and neutrophils but decreased CD4+ T-cell counts in the *P. acnes*-challenged lungs. These findings were attributed to the fact that DCs were detained in the lungs of *P. acnes*-challenged mice, thus preventing the development of antigen-specific T-cell response in regional lymph nodes.

Certain chemokine receptors also appear to be involved in linking the innate with the acquired immune response. Pulmonary challenge of CCR2$^{-/-}$ mice with purified protein derivative (PPD) of *Mycobacterium bovis* is associated with a marked impairment in the recruitment of macrophages to sites of inflammation and a concomitant decrease in IFN-γ synthesis in draining lymph nodes *(79)*. The defect in IFN-γ synthesis was recently shown to be a direct result of impaired trafficking of APCs in the CCR2 $(^{-/-})$ mice *(80)*, but other studies have shown that this defect can be overcome during a state of persistent antigen stimulation (or chronic infection) *(81)*. Similarly, a deficiency of CCR2, but not CCR5 or MIP-1-α/CCL3, has also been shown to lead to major, but reversible, defects in Langerhans cell (skin DC) function and the localization of splenic DCs from the marginal zone to the T-cell areas during a *Leishmania major* infection *(82)*. Thus, chemokines and chemokine receptors have a clear role in modulating the subsequent development of acquired immunity through its regulation of the trafficking of DCs and other APCs necessary to elicit the adaptive response.

Relatively little is known about the role of chemokines in the evolution of immune responses, but the early and marked expression of chemokines during an immune response appear to participate in determining the intensity and type of the developing immune response. Systemic overexpressing MCP-1/CCL2 via an adenoviral vector during the sensitization phase of Th1 (PPD-induced)- and Th2 [*Schistosoma* egg antigen (SEA)-induced]-type pulmonary granulomatous responses had a major impact on the overall phenotype associated with these lesions *(50)*. Systemic overexpression of MCP-1 during the sensitization phase of the Th1 model significantly reduced the granulomatous response, whereas increased MCP-1 during the sensitization phase of the Th2 model enhanced granulomatous reaction *(50)*. Restimulation of splenocytes ex vivo from both models revealed an altered cytokine profile in which IFN-γ and IL-12 levels were significantly reduced in the Th1 model, and IL-10 and IL-13 levels were increased in the Th2 model *(50)*.

In another adenovirus-mediated gene transfer study, the overexpression of the Th1-affiliated, CXC chemokine IP-10/CXCL10 in the airways of mice undergoing a dominant Th2-polarized mucosal sensitization regimen was shown to reduce all parameters of allergic airway disease *(83)*. These findings appeared to demonstrate that localized (i.e., lung) expression of the IP-10/CXCL10 promoted a Th1-type response that prevented the development of a Th2 response *(83)*. The manner in which chemokines subvert the development of acquired Th1 and Th2 responses in the lung is currently unknown, but it is the subject of considerable investigation.

7.3. Chemokines and Sepsis

Sepsis is quite common: as more than 100,000 people develop the syndrome annually in the United States alone *(84)*. Despite significant advances in the antibiotic arsenal and in intensive care unit technology (including mechanical ventilation), sepsis-related morbidity and mortality remain unacceptably high. Ultimately 25–50% of all septic episodes end in death. Although microorganisms and microorganism-derived products are important inciters of the disease state, the clinicopathologic manifestations and ultimate mortality associated with sepsis largely stem from the intense cellular and molecular interactions that contribute to the systemic inflammatory state [systemic inflammatory response syndrome (SIRS)] *(85)*. A number of strategies have been used to curb the progression of SIRS with immune or inflammatory modulating therapies, but to date none of these interventions has resulted in significant improvement in survival; some have proved to be deleterious *(86)*. However, recent progress has been made in the context of experimental sepsis suggesting that certain chemokines have the ability to activate the innate response effectively to clear the offending pathogen without inducing significant collateral damage or dampening the acquired immune response. Septic patients often develop nosocomial infections because their immune system has succumbed to a global anergic state *(87)*.

In a murine model of septic peritonitis induced by cecal ligation and puncture (CLP), MCP-1/CCL2 appears to have a prominent role in the recruitment of leukocytes, including neutrophils, necessary for the containment of bacteria that have leaked into the peritoneal cavity *(47)*. As demonstrated in Fig. 3, this insult to the gut establishes a system of organ-to-organ communication whereby pathogens and host cell-derived products enter the blood vessels of the gut and interact with cells of the next vascular bed, the liver. Products from the liver in turn impact on the next vascular bed, the lung. This chain of events results in the production of high chemokines levels via superimposing cell-to-cell communication on organ-to-organ communication, with the lung being targeted as the terminal downstream organ. Interestingly, MCP-1/CCL2 has also a marked effect on the systemic cytokine profile associated with CLP-*(88)* and LPS- *(89)* induced septic responses. Specifically, in both experimental septic conditions, MCP-1/CCL2 shifted the immune balance in favor of antiinflammatory cytokine expression and away from the production of proinflammatory cytokines.

More recently, MDC/CCL22 and C10 chemokine have been shown to share key characteristics with MCP-1/CCL2 during septic responses, but some notable differences between these chemokines and MCP-1/CCL2 were observed. First, in contrast to MCP-1/CCL2, either exogenous MDC/CCL22 or C10 chemokine could be administered to mice after the induction of CLP sepsis to achieve a clear survival benefit *(90,91)*. Second, both chemokines have a distinct effect on the phagocytic activities of resident peritoneal macrophages (through upregulation of TNF-α), but these macrophage-activating effects appeared to be confined to the peritoneal cavity. The best evidence for this temperance was that there was no spillover of the inflammatory response from the peritoneal cavity into the systemic circulation. This lack of spillover meant that liver, lung, and kidney functions remained almost normal in MDC/CCL22- or C10-treated mice undergoing CLP-induced sepsis, corresponding with decreased levels of proinflammatory mediators such as TNF-α, MIP-1α/CCL3, MIP-2, and KC in these organs *(90)*.

Finally, it appeared that C10 therapy significantly reduced the amount of material that leaked from the damaged gut, suggesting that this chemokine had a direct effect on structural cells necessary to maintain the gut's epithelial barrier *(91)*, coinciding with direct proliferative effects of C10 on epithelial cells (M.J.S., unpublished findings).

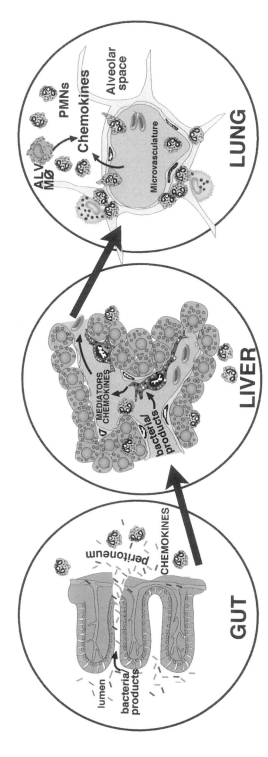

Fig. 3. During the development of systemic inflammatory response syndrome, communications networks are established whereby cytokine-directed organ-to-organ communication is superimposed on local tissue cell-to-cell communication. ALVM, alveolar macrophage; PMNs, polymorphonuclear neutrophil.

Collectively, these results indicate that chemokines such as MDC/CCL22 and C10 have important, novel regulatory activities in the innate response during sepsis and suggest that chemokines are important modulators of the overall outcome following sepsis *(90)*. Studies are currently under way to determine whether exogenous MDC/CCL22 or C10 chemokine therapy hampers subsequent immune responses to nosocomial infections.

8. CONCLUSIONS

Since the discovery of chemokines approx 14 years ago, their biologic sphere has expanded exponentially. Although initially described as soluble factors that regulate recruitment of neutrophils and monocytes during acute inflammatory events, chemokines have been shown to affect nearly all aspects of innate and acquired immunity. With the recognition that the innate and acquired immune systems are interrelated, it has become clear that the actions of chemokines in various cells and during a number of disease events contribute to the interrelatedness of these two arms of the immune system. Some of these chemokine-mediated events are poorly understood, such as the manner in which neutrophils regulate T-cell recruitment, whereas the involvement of chemokines in other events such as DC activation, migration, and maturation has received considerable research consideration. The overall excitement regarding the investigation of chemokines stems from the fact that these mediators link complex immune events that clearly contribute to cardiovascular disease, allergic inflammatory disease, transplantation, neuroinflammation, cancer, and HIV-associated disease *(12)*.

ACKNOWLEDGMENTS

This work was supported in part by NIH grants HL35276, and HL 31237.

REFERENCES

1. Alam R. A brief review of the immune system. Prim Care 1998;25:727–738.
2. Palucka K, Banchereau J. Linking innate and adaptive immunity. Nat Med 1999;5:868–870.
3. Tanaka Y. T cell integrin activation by chemokines in inflammation. Arch Immunol Ther Exp (Warsz) 2000;48:443–450.
4. Flesch IE, Collins H, Hess J, Kaufmann SH. Checkpoints in antibacterial immunity. Res Immunol 1998;149:693–697.
5. Bromley SK, Burack WR, Johnson KG, et al. The immunological synapse. Annu Rev Immunol 2001;19:375–396.
6. Wiedle G, Dunon D, Imhof BA. Current concepts in lymphocyte homing and recirculation. Crit Rev Clin Lab Sci 2001;38:1–31.
7. Parish CR, O'Neill ER. Dependence of the adaptive immune response on innate immunity: some questions answered but new paradoxes emerge. Immunol Cell Biol 1997;75:523–527.
8. Lo D, Feng L, Li L, et al. Integrating innate and adaptive immunity in the whole animal. Immunol Rev 1999;169:225–239.
9. Moser B, Loetscher P. Lymphocyte traffic control by chemokines. Nat Immunol 2001;2:123–128.
10. Thelen M. Dancing to the tune of chemokines. Nat Immunol 2001;2:129–134.
11. Yoshie O. Immune chemokines and their receptors: the key elements in the genesis, homeostasis and function of the immune system. Springer Semin Immunopathol 2000;22:371–391.
12. Gerard C, Rollins BJ. Chemokines and disease. Nat Immunol 2001;2:108–115.

13. Youn BS, Mantel C, Broxmeyer HE. Chemokines, chemokine receptors and hematopoiesis. Immunol Rev 2000;177:150–174.
14. Cyster JG. Chemokines and cell migration in secondary lymphoid organs. Science 1999;286:2098–2102.
15. Cyster JG, Ngo VN, Ekland EH, et al. Chemokines and B-cell homing to follicles. Curr Top Microbiol Immunol 1999;246:87–92; discussion 93.
16. Matsukawa A, Hogaboam CM, Lukacs NW, Kunkel SL. Chemokines and innate immunity. Rev Immunogenet 2000;2:339–358.
17. Kunkel SL. Through the looking glass: the diverse in vivo activities of chemokines. J Clin Invest 1999;104:1333–1334.
18. Kelner GS, Kennedy J, Bacon KB, et al. Lymphotactin: a cytokine that represents a new class of chemokine. Science 1994;266:1395.
19. Bianchi G, Sozzani S, Zlotnick A, Mantovani A, Allavena P. Migratory response of human NK cells to lymphotactin. Eur. J. Immunol. 1996;26:3238.
20. Zlotnik A, Yoshie O. Chemokines: a new classification system and their role in immunity. Immunity 2000;12:121–127.
21. Rossi D, Zlotnik A. The biology of chemokines and their receptors. Annu Rev Immunol 2000;18:217–242.
22. Frade JM, Mellado M, del Real G, Gutierrez-Ramos JC, Lind P, Martinez AC. Characterization of the CCR2 chemokine receptor: functional CCR2 receptor expression in B cells. J Immunol 1997;159:5576–5584.
23. Gao JL, Sen AI, Kitaura M, et al. Identification of a mouse eosinophil receptor for the C-C chemokine eotaxin. Biochem Biophys Res Commun 1996;223:679–684.
24. Raport CJ, Gosling J, Schweickart VL, Gray PW, Charo IF. Molecular cloning and functional characterization of a novel human CC chemokine receptor (CCR5) for RANTES, MIP-1beta, and MIP-1alpha. and MIP-1alpha. J Biol Chem 1996;271:17161–17166.
25. Baba M, Imai T, Nishimura M, et al. Identification of CCR6, the specific receptor for a novel lymphocyte-directed CC chemokine LARC. J Biol Chem 1997;272:14893–14898.
26. Homey B, Wang W, Soto H, et al. Cutting edge: the orphan chemokine receptor G protein-coupled receptor-2 (GPR-2, CCR10) binds the skin-associated chemokine CCL27 (CTACK/ALP/ILC). J Immunol 2000;164:3465–3470.
27. Scapini P, Lapinet-Vera JA, Gasperini S, et al. The neutrophil as a cellular source of chemokines. Immunol Rev 2000;177:195–203.
28. Yoshie O. Role of chemokines in trafficking of lymphocytes and dendritic cells. Int J Hematol 2000;72:399–407.
29. Clark GJ, Angel N, Kato M, et al. The role of dendritic cells in the innate immune system. Microbes Infect 2000;2:257–272.
30. Stockwin LH, McGonagle D, Martin IG, Blair GE. Dendritic cells: immunological sentinels with a central role in health and disease. Immunol Cell Biol 2000;78:91–102.
31. Foti M, Granucci F, Aggujaro D, et al. Upon dendritic cell (DC) activation chemokines and chemokine receptor expression are rapidly regulated for recruitment and maintenance of DC at the inflammatory site. Int Immunol 1999;11:979–986.
32. Caux C, Ait-Yahia S, Chemin K, et al. Dendritic cell biology and regulation of dendritic cell trafficking by chemokines. Springer Semin Immunopathol 2000;22:345–369.
33. Gunn MD, Kyuwa S, Tam C, et al. Mice lacking expression of secondary lymphoid organ chemokine have defects in lymphocyte homing and dendritic cell localization [see comments]. J Exp Med 1999;189:451–460.
34. Chan VW, Kothakota S, Rohan MC, et al. Secondary lymphoid-tissue chemokine (SLC) is chemotactic for mature dendritic cells. Blood 1999;93:3610–3616.

35. Willimann K, Legler DF, Loetscher M, et al. The chemokine SLC is expressed in T cell areas of lymph nodes and mucosal lymphoid tissues and attracts activated T cells via CCR7. Eur J Immunol 1998;28:2025–2034.

36. Demangel C, Britton WJ. Interaction of dendritic cells with mycobacteria: where the action starts. Immunol Cell Biol 2000;78:318–324.

37. McWilliam AS, Napoli S, Marsh AM, et al. Dendritic cells are recruited into the airway epithelium during the inflammatory response to a broad spectrum of stimuli. J Exp Med 1996;184:2429–2432.

38. Rescigno M, Granucci F, Ricciardi-Castagnoli P. Molecular events of bacterial-induced maturation of dendritic cells. J Clin Immunol 2000;20:161–166.

39. Zou W, Borvak J, Marches F, et al. Macrophage-derived dendritic cells have strong Th1-polarizing potential mediated by beta-chemokines rather than IL-12. J Immunol 2000;165:4388–4396.

40. Mantovani A, Gray PA, Van Damme J, Sozzani S. Macrophage-derived chemokine (MDC). J Leukoc Biol 2000;68:400–404.

41. Yoneyama H, Kawasaki S, Matsushima K. Regulation of Th1 and Th2 immune responses by chemokines. Springer Semin Immunopathol 2000;22:329–344.

42. Biron CA, Nguyen KB, Pien GC, Cousens LP, Salazar-Mather TP. Natural killer cells in antiviral defense: function and regulation by innate cytokines. Annu Rev Immunol 1999;17:189–220.

43. Robertson MJ, Williams BT, Christopherson K, Brahmi Z, Hromas R. Regulation of human natural killer cell migration and proliferation by the exodus subfamily of CC chemokines. Cell Immunol 2000;199:8–14.

44. Lukacs NW, Chensue SW, Karpus WJ, et al. C-C chemokines differentially alter interleukin-4 production from lymphocytes. Am J Pathol 1997;150:1861–1868.

45. Hogaboam CM, Lukacs NW, Chensue SW, Strieter RM, Kunkel SL. Monocyte chemoattractant protein-1 synthesis by murine lung fibroblasts modulates CD4+ T cell activation. J Immunol 1998;160:4606–4614.

46. Gunn MD, Nelken NA, Liao X, Williams LT. Monocyte chemoattractant protein-1 is sufficient for the chemotaxis of monocytes and lymphocytes in transgenic mice but requires an additional stimulus for inflammatory activation. J Immunol 1997;158:376–383.

47. Matsukawa A, Hogaboam CM, Lukacs NW, et al. Endogenous monocyte chemoattractant protein-1 (MCP-1) protects mice in a model of acute septic peritonitis: cross-talk between MCP-1 and leukotriene B4. J Immunol 1999;163:6148–6154.

48. Karpus WJ, Lukacs NW, Kennedy KJ, et al. Differential CC chemokine-induced enhancement of T helper cell cytokine production. J Immunol 1997;158:4129–4136.

49. Gu L, Tseng S, Horner RM, et al. Control of Th2 polarization by the chemokine monocyte chemoattractant protein-1. Nature 2000;404:407–411.

50. Matsukawa A, Lukacs NW, Standiford TJ, Chensue SW, Kunkel SL. Adenoviral-mediated overexpression of monocyte chemoattractant protein-1 differentially alters the development of Th1 and Th2 type responses in vivo. J Immunol 2000;164:1699–1704.

51. Odum N, Bregenholt S, Eriksen KW, et al. The CC-chemokine receptor 5 (CCR5) is a marker of, but not essential for the development of human Th1 cells. Tissue Antigens 1999;54:572–577.

52. D'Ambrosio D, Iellem A, Bonecchi R, et al. Selective up-regulation of chemokine receptors CCR4 and CCR8 upon activation of polarized human type 2 Th cells. J Immunol 1998;161:5111–5115.

53. Zingoni A, Soto H, Hedrick JA, et al. The chemokine receptor CCR8 is preferentially expressed in Th2 but not Th1 cells. J Immunol 1998;161:547–551.

54. Campbell JD, HayGlass KT. T cell chemokine receptor expression in human Th1- and Th2-associated diseases. Arch Immunol Ther Exp (Warsz) 2000;48:451–456.

55. Khan IA, MacLean JA, Lee FS, et al. IP-10 is critical for effector T cell trafficking and host survival in *Toxoplasma gondii* infection. Immunity 2000;12:483–494.

56. Lukacs NW, Hogaboam C, Campbell E, Kunkel SL. Chemokines: function, regulation and alteration of inflammatory responses. Chem Immunol 1999;72:102–120.

57. Naumann M. Nuclear factor-kappa B activation and innate immune response in microbial pathogen infection. Biochem Pharmacol 2000;60:1109–1114.

58. Izadpanah A, Dwinell MB, Eckmann L, Varki NM, Kagnoff MF. Regulated MIP-3alpha/CCL20 production by human intestinal epithelium: mechanism for modulating mucosal immunity. Am J Physiol Gastrointest Liver Physiol 2001;280:G710–G719.

59. Lillard JW, Boyaka PN, Taub DD, McGhee JR. RANTES potentiates antigen-specific mucosal immune responses. J Immunol 2001;166:162–169.

60. Hogaboam CM, Smith RE, Kunkel SL. Dynamic interactions between lung fibroblasts and leukocytes: implications for fibrotic lung disease. Proc Assoc Am Physicians 1998;110:313–320.

61. Smith RS, Smith TJ, Blieden TM, Phipps RP. Fibroblasts as sentinel cells. Synthesis of chemokines and regulation of inflammation. Am J Pathol 1997;151:317–322.

62. Xia Y, Pauza ME, Feng L, Lo D. RelB regulation of chemokine expression modulates local inflammation. Am J Pathol 1997;151:375–387.

63. Cocchi F, DeVico AL, Arya SK, Gallo RC, Lusso P. Identification of RANTES, MIP-1 alpha, and MIP-1 beta as the major HIV-suppressive factors produced by CD8+ T cells. Science 1995;270:1811–1815.

64. Murphy PM. Viral exploitation and subversion of the immune system through chemokine mimicry. Nat Immunol 2001;2:116–122.

65. Scarlatti G, Tresoldi E, Bjorndal A, et al. In vivo evolution of HIV-1 co-receptor usage and sensitivity to chemokine-mediated suppression. Nat Med 1997;3:1259–1265.

66. Simmons G, Reeves JD, Hibbitts S, et al. Co-receptor use by HIV and inhibition of HIV infection by chemokine receptor ligands. Immunol Rev 2000;177:112–126.

67. Howie S, Ramage R, Hewson T. Innate immune system damage in human immunodeficiency virus type 1 infection. Implications for acquired immunity and vaccine design. Am J Respir Crit Care Med 2000;162:S141–S145.

68. Holland SM. Host defense against nontuberculous mycobacterial infections. Semin Respir Infect 1996;11:217–230.

69. Dairaghi DJ, Fan RA, McMaster BE, Hanley MR, Schall TJ. HHV8-encoded vMIP-I selectively engages chemokine receptor CCR8. Agonist and antagonist profiles of viral chemokines. J Biol Chem 1999;274:21569–21574.

70. Endres MJ, Garlisi CG, Xiao H, Shan L, Hedrick JA. The Kaposi's sarcoma-related herpesvirus (KSHV)-encoded chemokine vMIP-I is a specific agonist for the CC chemokine receptor (CCR)8. J Exp Med 1999;189:1993–1998.

71. Sozzani S, Luini W, Bianchi G, et al. The viral chemokine macrophage inflammatory protein-II is a selective Th2 chemoattractant. Blood 1998;92:4036–4039.

72. Kledal TN, Rosenkilde MM, Coulin F, et al. A broad-spectrum chemokine antagonist encoded by Kaposi's sarcoma-associated herpesvirus. Science 1997;277:1656–1659.

73. Chen S, Bacon KB, Li L, et al. In vivo inhibition of CC and CX3C chemokine-induced leukocyte infiltration and attenuation of glomerulonephritis in Wistar-Kyoto (WKY) rats by vMIP-II. J Exp Med 1998;188:193–198.

74. Penfold ME, Dairaghi DJ, Duke GM, et al. Cytomegalovirus encodes a potent alpha chemokine. Proc Natl Acad Sci USA 1999;96:9839–9844.

75. Zhang P, Summer WR, Bagby GJ, Nelson S. Innate immunity and pulmonary host defense. Immunol Rev 2000;173:39–51.

76. Itakura M, Tokuda A, Kimura H, et al. Blockade of secondary lymphoid tissue chemokine exacerbates *Propionibacterium acnes*-induced acute lung inflammation. J Immunol 2001;166:2071–2079.

77. Standiford TJ. Cytokines and pulmonary host defenses. Curr Opin Pulm Med 1997;3:81–88.

78. Standiford TJ, Huffnagle GB. Cytokines in host defense against pneumonia. J Invest Med 1997;45:335–345.
79. Boring L, Gosling J, Chensue SW, et al. Impaired monocyte migration and reduced type 1 (Th1) cytokine responses in C-C chemokine receptor 2 knockout mice. J Clin Invest 1997;100:2552–2561.
80. Peters W, Dupuis M, Charo IF. A mechanism for the impaired IFN-gamma production in C-C chemokine receptor 2 (CCR2) knockout mice: role of CCR2 in linking the innate and adaptive immune responses. J Immunol 2000;165:7072–7077.
81. Sato N, Kuziel WA, Melby PC, et al. Defects in the generation of IFN-gamma are overcome to control infection with *Leishmania donovani* in CC chemokine receptor (CCR) 5-, macrophage inflammatory protein-1 alpha-, or CCR2-deficient mice. J Immunol 1999;163:5519–5525.
82. Sato N, Ahuja SK, Quinones M, et al. CC chemokine receptor (CCR)2 is required for Langerhans cell migration and localization of T helper cell type 1 (Th1)-inducing dendritic cells. Absence of CCR2 shifts the *Leishmania major*-resistant phenotype to a susceptible state dominated by Th2 cytokines, B cell outgrowth, and sustained neutrophilic inflammation. J Exp Med 2000;192:205–218.
83. Wiley R, Palmer K, Gajewska B, et al. Expression of the Th1 chemokine IFN-gamma-inducible protein 10 in the airway alters mucosal allergic sensitization in mice. J Immunol 2001;166:2750–2759.
84. Brun-Buisson C. The epidemiology of the systemic inflammatory response. Intensive Care Med 2000;26:S64–S74.
85. Fry DE. Sepsis syndrome. Am Surg 2000;66:126–132.
86. Glauser MP. Pathophysiologic basis of sepsis: considerations for future strategies of intervention. Crit Care Med 2000;28:S4–S8.
87. Deitch EA, Goodman ER. Prevention of multiple organ failure. Surg Clin North Am 1999;79:1471–1488.
88. Matsukawa A, Hogaboam CM, Lukacs NW, et al. Endogenous MCP-1 influences systemic cytokine balance in a murine model of acute septic peritonitis. Exp Mol Pathol 2000;68:77–84.
89. Zisman DA, Kunkel SL, Strieter RM, et al. MCP-1 protects mice in lethal endotoxemia. J Clin Invest 1997;99:2832–2836.
90. Matsukawa A, Hogaboam CM, Lukacs NW, et al. Pivotal role of the CC chemokine, macrophage-derived chemokine, in the innate immune response. J Immunol 2000;164:5362–5368.
91. Steinhauser ML, Hogaboam CM, Matsukawa A, et al. Chemokine C10 promotes disease resolution and survival in an experimental model of bacterial sepsis. Infect Immun 2000;68:6108–6114.

16
Antimicrobial Peptides

Tomas Ganz and Robert I. Lehrer

1. INTRODUCTION

This review centers on the endogenous antimicrobial polypeptides of humans. Such molecules, which typically contain fewer than 100 amino acids, occur in many types of cells and secretions and are increasingly recognized as ancient and integral components of the innate immune systems of all living organisms. They are generally cationic (positively charged) and amphipathic, an overall configuration that facilitates their binding and insertion into the anionic cell walls and phospholipid membranes of microbes. Analogous peptides exist in vertebrates, invertebrates, plants, and protozoa. For example, several antimicrobial molecules structurally related to granulysin (an α-helical antimicrobial peptide of human T-cells) *(1)* have been purified from amoebae, including the parasite *Entamoeba histolytica (2)* and the free-living slime mold *Dictyostelium discoides (3)*. Antimicrobial peptides are also produced by some prokaryotes *(4)* and even by archaea *(5)*. Microbe-made antimicrobial peptides often contain extensive posttranslational modifications or "exotic" amino acids not found in the antimicrobial peptides of animals.

2. ANTIMICROBIAL MECHANISMS

Most (probably all) antimicrobial peptides initially bind to microbial membranes and then increase the membrane's permeability in a general or specific manner. Even peptides whose ultimate target is intracellular must do something to traverse microbial membrane barriers, because the porin channels of *E. coli* and *Salmonella typhimurium* normally exclude macromolecules larger than 600–800 Da *(6)*. Several mechanisms have been invoked to explain how various antimicrobial peptides interact with biologic membranes, and readers interested in the field will encounter unfamiliar terms, including "self-promoted uptake" *(7)*, "carpet mechanism" *(8)*, "wormhole" (toroidal) pores *(9)*, "barrel stave pores" *(10)*, and "supramolecular complex pore accompanied with lipid flip-flop and peptide translocation" *(11)*. This multiplicity probably signals (1) that different peptides have different mechanisms of action; (2) that peptide interactions with membranes may go through multiple phases as the peptide concentration increases and as they successively penetrate the various layers of the microbial cell wall; and (3) that there is yet much to be learned about the subject.

From: *Infectious Disease: Innate Immunity*
Edited by: R. A. B. Ezekowitz and J. A. Hoffmann © Humana Press Inc., Totowa, NJ

An early mechanistic study was performed with human neutrophil peptide (HNPs) α-defensins and *E. coli (12)*. Under conditions that supported bactericidal activity, HNP-1 sequentially permeabilized the outer and inner membranes of *E. coli*. Coincident with these events, bacterial DNA, RNA, and protein synthesis ceased, and the colony count fell. Although these events were closely coupled under standard assay conditions, if outer membrane permeabilization was partially dissociated from inner membrane permeabilization, bacterial death closely paralleled the loss of inner membrane integrity. *E. coli* killed by defensins manifested striking electron-dense deposits ("funereal warts") within their periplasmic space and on their outer membrane.

Disruption of microbial membrane integrity has been shown with many, but not all, antimicrobial peptides. Such changes can interfere with bacterial metabolism, homeostasis, and proton-motive force. If sufficiently severe, they can cause leakage of cellular contents and allow noxious or injurious molecules (including the peptides themselves) to enter the bacterial cytoplasm. Pores formed by human defensin HNP-2 in model membranes—liposomes composed of palmitoyloleoylphosphatidyl glycerol (POPG)—had an estimated maximum diameter of approx 25 Å *(13)*. If similar sized pores form in the outer membranes of Gram-negative bacteria, they could allow the passage of lysozyme (muramidase), whose hydrodynamic radius is approx 20 Å *(14)* and whose target—the peptidoglycan layer—affords crucial protection against potentially lethal osmotic distension.

Microbial damage may be exacerbated by osmotic stresses resulting from excessive entry of water or by displacing the bacterium's autolytic enzymes from their cell wall docking sites, thereby inducing inappropriate cell wall remodeling. Other host defense substances, including oxidants, lytic enzymes, pore-forming proteins, and binders of essential nutrients may act concomitantly to potentiate the damage to the target. In addition to acting on cell wall structures (outer membrane, peptidoglycan, plasma membrane), antimicrobial peptides may enter the cytoplasm through pores or by flip-flop movements through phospholipid membranes *(15)*. Within the cytoplasm, antimicrobial peptides have been shown to inhibit certain enzymes, but the contribution of such interactions to the ultimate fate of the cell remains to be established.

3. CLASSIFICATION OF VERTEBRATE ANTIMICROBIAL PEPTIDES

The structures of antimicrobial peptides are diverse, but amphipathic peptides that assume α-helical conformations in membrane-mimetic environments and disulfide-stabilized β-sheet-rich peptides are particularly common. Also represented are peptides with repetitive motifs (often containing prolines) and peptides with a high percentage of tryptophan. In mammals, the two major peptide families are defensins, characterized by a β-sheet-rich structure stabilized by three disulfides, and cathelicidins, characterized by a conserved precursor motif (the "cathelin" domain) joined to a highly variable C-terminal mature peptide. In addition, there are histidine-rich peptides (histatins) produced by the salivary glands, and several peptides (lactoferricin, buforin, and so on.) generated by partial hydrolysis of macromolecular precursors (lactoferrin and histone H2A).

4. DEFENSINS

4.1. Structure

Human defensins *(16,17)* belong to a widely distributed family of microbicidal peptides with a characteristic three-dimensional fold and a six-cysteine/three-disulfide pattern. Depending on the spacing and connectivity of the cysteines, the peptides are classified as α- or β-defensins. In addition, cyclic minidefensin peptides (θ-defensins) that are posttranslationally circularized from two demidefensin segments were recently discovered in rhesus leukocytes *(18)*. No human counterpart(s) of circular defensins have yet been reported.

The crystal structures of human α-defensin HNP-3 *(19)* and human β-defensin (HBD)-2 *(20)* are available, as well as the solution structures of human α-defensin HNP-1, rabbit α-defensins NP-1 and NP-5, human β-defensin HBD-2, and bovine β-defensin (BNBD)-12 *(21–24)*; they indicate that α- and β-defensins have a similar three-dimensional structure that is rich in antiparallel β-sheet. Although human β-defensin-2 generally conforms to this pattern, its solution structure was recently reported to contain an α-helical segment near the N-terminus *(24)*. Some defensins form stable dimers in solution, whereas others are monomeric. Differences in activity may be largely caused by variations in charge and its distribution, as well as differences in the length and composition of the N-terminal segment. Many or perhaps even all defensins may form assemblies in membranes as part of their pore-forming process.

4.2. Distribution and Tissue-Specific Forms

Defensins were first recognized in the 1960s by Zeya and Spitznagel *(25,26)*, who described the presence of antimicrobial components ("lysosomal cationic proteins") in rabbit and guinea pig granulocytes. Because oxidative antimicrobial mechanisms related to reduced nicotinamide adenine dinucleotide phosphate (NADPH) oxidase and myeloperoxidase occupied the center stage in this area of leukocyte research for the next 15 years, it was not until 1983 that the first α-defensins (purified from rabbit alveolar macrophages) were sequenced *(27)*. Although naming the human representatives of this peptide family "defensins" when they were described in 1985 *(28)* may have represented a leap of faith, the term has since gained widespread usage by the repeated finding of defensin homologs and analogs in cell types involved in host defense.

Three closely related defensins, HNP-1, -2 and -3, are major components of the myeloperoxidase-containing azurophil granules of neutrophils. A fourth α-defensin, HNP-4, is found in the same location but is much less abundant *(28–30)*. When neutrophils that ingested *S. typhimurium* were assayed by radioiodination and subcellular fractionation, defensins appeared to be the most abundant neutrophil-derived polypeptides within phagocytic vacuoles *(31)*. The secretory granules of Paneth cells contain two human defensins, HD-5 and -6 *(32–35)*. Paneth cells are long-lived, granule-rich secretory epithelial cells positioned at the bottom of small intestinal crypts. They also contain lysozyme and secretory phospholipase A2 and are thought to be involved in local host defense *(36)*. It was recently reported that α-defensins are expressed by certain populations of human T-lymphocytes and natural killer (NK) cells *(37)*.

The three well-characterized human β-defensins, HBD-1, -2, and -3, *(38–41)*, differ slightly from the classical α-defensins in the placement and connectivity of their cysteines. Their mRNAs were expressed in epithelial cells and some glands. HBD-1 was highly expressed in the genitourinary tract epithelia. In the kidney, HBD-1 mRNA was localized to the loops of Henle, distal tubules, and collecting ducts. Normal urine contained low levels (10–100 μg/L) of HBD-1 forms containing 36–47 amino acids *(42)*.

Since many of these forms displayed salt-sensitive antimicrobial activity, renal β-defensins may act preferentially where they occur in the greatest concentration—the Henle's loop/distal convoluted tubule complex, whose free-water generating properties can provide the low salt environments conducive to defensin-mediated antimicrobial activity *(43)*. In females, prominent expression of HBD-1 was present in the vagina, ectocervix, endocervix, uterus, and fallopian tubes. In addition to these high-expressing tissues, lower levels of HBD-1 expression were noted in many organs, including the salivary gland, trachea, prostate, and placenta *(39)*.

Although HBD-2 is not expressed constitutively by skin keratinocytes, its synthesis is induced by inflammation, probably by a transcriptional control mechanism analogous to that described for bovine epithelial defensins in the trachea and tongue *(44–46)*. Exposing human monocytes in vitro for 18 hours to lipopolysaccharide (LPS) or interferon-γ increased their expression of HBD-2 mRNA in a dexamethasone-insensitive manner *(47)*. In addition to inflamed skin *(41)*, the expression of HBD-3 is prominent in the tonsils and also occurs in airway epithelial cells. HBD-3 is remarkably cationic, and its broad-spectrum antimicrobial activity may be less susceptible than that of other human defensins to inhibition by salt.

The fascinating human EP2 gene contains two promoters, eight exons, and seven introns. It codes at least nine putative message variants—all encoding small secretory proteins specifically expressed within the epididymis. Not only do exons 3 and 6 of this gene encode protein sequences homologous to those of β-defensins, it is located near the defensin gene cluster on chromosome 8p23, separated by only 100 kb or less from DEFB2, the gene for β-defensin-2 *(48)*. An epididymis-specific β-defensin gene was recognized recently in the rat *(49)*. *(50)*. Defense of the male genital tract by antimicrobial peptides may be a widespread phenomenon. A 47-residue antimicrobial peptide (seminalplasmin) is present in bovine seminal plasma *(51)*, and the male reproductive tract of *Drosophila* is defended by several tissue-specific antimicrobial peptides *(52)* that are transferred to female fruit flies during or before mating.

Although defensins have been found in the granulocytes and epithelial cells of an ever increasing number of vertebrate species, to date the substantial production of α-defensins by mononuclear phagocytes appears to be a tissue-specific peculiarity of the rabbit alveolar macrophage *(53)*. Constitutive expression of four β-defensins, especially BNBD-4 and -5, was reported in bovine alveolar macrophages *(54)*.

4.3. Biologic Activity

In vitro, under low salt conditions (e.g., 10 mM sodium phosphate), defensins are microbicidal at micromolar (µg/mL) concentrations against many Gram-positive and Gram-negative bacteria, yeasts fungi, and certain enveloped viruses *(12,28,55–57)*. Increasing salt concentrations competitively inhibit defensin activity *(58,59)*, but the inhibitory effect is modulated by the properties of the target microbe. For example, in the salt concentrations prevalent in extracellular fluid, HD-5 (100 µg/mL) killed more than 90% of an inoculum of *Listeria monocytogenes* in 3 hours but showed little activity against *S. typhimurium* *(33)*. Estimates of defensin concentrations in the phagocytic vacuoles of neutrophils are in the milligram/milliliter range, a concentration that could be sufficient to overcome inhibition by intravacuolar ion concentrations (which are not known). A more detailed understanding of the phagosomal fluid composition may be required before the specific contribution of defensins to phagocytic killing can be assessed. Similar considerations also apply to the activity of defensins in the narrow (5–10-μm diameter) intestinal crypts into which Paneth cells secrete their defensin-containing granules. It should be noted that some defensins manifest additional in vitro activities that may contribute to inflammation and repair, including inhibition of adrenocorticotropic hormone (ACTH)-stimulated cortisol production, inhibition of fibrinolysis, and a mitogenic effect on fibroblasts *(60–63)*.

The microbicidal and cytotoxic activity of defensins is thought to involve several steps *(12,59,64–66)*. Initially, defensins bind to target cell membranes and make them permeable to small molecules such as trypan blue (mol wt 960.8), various β-lactams, or β-galactosides. Both electrostatic interaction and transmembrane electromotive force play a role in defensin-mediated permeabilization of biologic membranes *(12,13,64,65,67–69)*. Studies in model systems of planar lipid bilayers showed that defensin-mediated pore formation requires an application of electromotive force to drive cationic defensin molecules into the membrane.

In anionic phospholipid liposomes (but not zwitterionic or mixed liposomes), human defensin HNP-2 induced leakage of vesicle contents through stable pores large enough to pass dextran molecules of several kDa mass, yielding an estimated pore size of 25 Å. A model of a defensin pore consisting of a ring of six homodimers has been proposed based on the measurement of pore size, steric considerations, and the expected interactions of HNP-2 with the hydrophobic and charged regions of the bilayer membrane. It is of interest that rabbit defensins permeabilized phospholipid vesicles in a graded, rather than in an all-or-none fashion.

4.4. Genes

Human defensins are encoded by a cluster of genes *(34,35,70–72)* on chromosome band 8p23 (the *def* locus) that includes all the known defensin genes. The adjacent genomic location of the structurally distinct α- and β-defensins supports the notion that these genes diverged from a common precursor. A curious (and still unexplained) property of defensins is that the precursor's signal sequence can be more highly conserved than the domain containing the mature peptide. Just as the fossilized feathered dinosaurs *Archaeopteryx* and *Confuciusornis* provide hard evidence of the reptilian origins of birds, the conserved signal sequences of avian defensins and snake venom toxins provide additional evidence of this historical linkage *(73)*. Defensins have not yet been found in amphibians or in fish, perhaps because their tissues have only been examined selectively for antimicrobial peptides. Similar, but less obviously related peptides (insect and plant defensins) exist in insects, molluscs, and plants, in which their synthesis is often induced by microbial invasion.

4.5. Interspecies Variation

There is impressive interspecies variation in the expression of defensins (as well as other antimicrobial polypeptides). Thus neutrophil defensins have been found in rabbit, guinea pig, hamster, rat, and cow but appear to be lacking in the inbred mouse *(74)*. Wild mice have not been studied to determine whether the loss of neutrophil defensins is recent or related to laboratory husbandry. Any potential host defense deficit suffered by the mouse as a result of its naturally "knocked-out" neutrophil defensins appears to be compensated for by other systems, including the inducible nitric oxide synthase of murine macrophages, the more than a dozen α-defensin genes expressed in the murine small intestine, and the several (at least four) murine β-defensins *(75–78)*. The high redundancy of host defense systems presumably reflects (1) the low cost of genetic experimentation and the high cost (i.e., extinction) of failing to experiment; and (2) the continuously changing selection pressures exerted by the coevolving pathogenic microbes characteristic to each animal species.

4.6. Signaling Effects

At nanomolar concentrations, lower than those required for microbicidal activity, some defensins act as signaling molecules. Rabbit neutrophil defensin NP-3a and human neutrophil defensin HNP-4 have been shown to inhibit the response of adrenal cells to ACTH *(79)* by binding to the ACTH receptor and acting as competitive antagonists ("corticostatins") *(80)*. If such binding also occurs in vivo, it could influence the immune system in at least two ways: (1) by decreasing the production of endogenous cortisol by blocking access of ACTH to its receptor on adrenal cells; or (2) by affecting NK cells and lymphocytes via their melanocortin 5 receptors, which bind ACTH 1–24 with high affinity *(81,82)*.

Human neutrophil α-defensins have chemotactic effects on naive T-lymphocytes and immature dendritic cells *(83)*, whereas human β-defensins attract memory T-cells and immature dendritic cells *(84)*. The latter effect is at least in part mediated by the CCR6 chemokine receptor and is likely to be important in the initiation of adaptive immune response by infected and inflamed mucosal epithelia and the epidermis.

4.7. Evidence for a Biologic Role In Vivo

The idea that defensins have a primary role in host defense was originally based on their in vitro antimicrobial activity and on their predominant site of expression: in the phagocytic granules of neutrophils and in epithelia exposed to microbes or inflammatory stimuli. It was reassuring that the conservatively estimated concentration of defensin in the neutrophil phagosomes (several milligrams/milliliter) was sufficient to exert antimicrobial activity under a variety of assumptions about the composition of the intraphagosomal milieu. Additional evidence for the proposed role has been accumulating. In a rare human genetic disease, specific granule deficiency, neutrophil defensins are present at 10% of the normal amount *(85)*. The affected patients suffer from frequent bacterial infections, and their neutrophils are defective in killing bacteria *(86)*. However, because multiple other components of neutrophil granules are also deficient, including human cationic antimicrobial peptide of 18kDa (hCAP-18) and bactericidal/permeability-increasing protein (BPI) *(87)*, the phenotype (frequent infections) cannot be attributed solely to the lack of defensins.

The mouse, currently the only experimental mammal in which gene ablation experiments can be routinely performed, naturally lacks neutrophil defensins but has a large number of Paneth cell α-defensin genes and epithelial β-defensin genes. Individual murine β-defensin genes were selectively disrupted in several laboratories, but the characterization of their phenotypes is complex and still ongoing. An indirect strategy proved more fruitful when it was observed that mice with disruption of the gene for matrilysin [matrix metalloproteinase (MMP-6)] did not activate their Paneth cell prodefensins to mature defensins and showed increased suspectibility to intestinal infections *(88)*. Matrilysin colocalized with defensins in Paneth cell granules and correctly cleaved prodefensin to mature defensin in vitro, suggesting that it is the prodefensin convertase of the Paneth cells. The antibacterial activity of isolated intestinal crypts could be neutralized with anti-defensin antibodies, showing that it depends primarily on defensins. Isolated crypts from matrilysin-deficient mice failed to generate normal antibacterial activity when stimulated with bacteria *(89)*. Assuming that matrilysin is not also involved in the processing of other antimicrobial peptides, these findings are consistent with the proposed primary role of Paneth cell defensins as antimicrobial effectors in the small intestinal crypt.

In further support of the proposed antimicrobial effector role of defensins, peptides structurally similar to defensins (and possessing similar antibacterial and antifungal properties) have been detected as abundant molecules in host defense settings in mussels *(90)*, insects *(91–93)*, and plants *(94)*. The defensin-like molecule drosomycin is the most abundant peptide in the hemolymph of microbially challenged *Drosophila* and accounts for most of its antifungal activity *(95,96)*.

If defensins function primarily as antimicrobial molecules, their transgenic overexpression would be expected to increase the resistance to infection. Indeed, overexpression of defensins in macrophage-like cell lines *(97)* or primary human macrophages *(98)* increased their ability to restrict the multiplication of intracellular *Histoplasma capsulatum* and *Mycobacterium tuberculosis*, respectively. Similarly, transgenic expression of rabbit alveolar macrophage defensins (NP-1) in tomato plants enhanced their resistance to the tomato wilt fungus *Fusarium oxysporum (99)*.

5. CATHELICIDINS

5.1. Diversity

The cathelicidins *(100)* comprise a large family of microbicidal *pro*peptides with a conserved N-terminal precursor cathelin domain of about 100 amino acid residues and an antimicrobial C-terminal domain that is typically 10–40 amino acid residues long. In many cases, their antimicrobial domains end in a C-terminal glycine that is later converted to an amide *(101)*. Some cathelicidin propeptides have a very short antimicrobial domain. For example, bovine cyclic bactenecins have 12 amino acids *(102)*, bovine indolicidin has 13 *(103)*, and the porcine protegrins have 16–18 *(104)*. Proline-rich cathelicidin peptides are considerably larger. For example, bovine Bac-5 has 43 residues, and Bac-7 has 59. Of these, approx 45% are proline, 20% are arginine, and the remaining residues are mainly hydrophobic—isoleucine, leucine, and phenylalanine *(105)*. Many cathelicidin propeptides, including hCAP-18, have antimicrobial domains that comprise α-helical peptides, typically containing 23–37 residues. Among these, rabbit CAP-18 (37 residues) and ovine Smap-29 (29 residues) were considerably more potent than human LL-37 *(106)*. Unlike defensins, the α-helical cathelicidin peptides generally retain strong, broad-spectrum antimicrobial activity in the presence of physiologic concentrations of NaCl and divalent cations *(107)*.

Most mammalian cathelicidins undergo an extracellular proteolytic cleavage that frees the active C-terminal antimicrobial peptide from cathelin domain of the precursor

(100,108–110). In contrast, a few members of the family appear to be active in the uncleaved form *(111,112)*.

5.2. Species Differences

Whereas the neutrophils of cattle, pigs, sheep, and goats may contain 10 or more different cathelicidin molecules, only one cathelicidin (hCAP-18/LL-37) is known to exist in humans. The human peptide was discovered by several groups that followed different paths to its discovery. Larrick and associates had been studying the LPS-binding properties *(113)* of rabbit CAP-18. After finding and cloning its human counterpart *(114)*, they named it "human CAP-18". A similar name (hCAP-18) was bestowed by Borregaard et al. *(115)*. A third group *(116)* was seeking human relatives of PR-39, a 39-residue porcine peptide with a cathelin-containing precursor. When they described its cDNA, gene, and peptide forms *(117)*, they called it "FALL-39," to reflect the length (39 residues) and the initial four residues (Phe, Ala, Leu, Leu) of its postulated mature peptide domain *(118)*. However, when they later isolated the "mature" peptide and found it to contain 37 residues starting with Leu-Leu, its name became LL-37. The term *hCAP-18/LL-37* is used here, with its first part denoting the propeptide and its second part the antimicrobial peptide after it has been processed by human neutrophils. It remains to be determined whether hCAP-18 is converted to LL-37 or to other antimicrobial peptides in other tissues, such as skin or secretions.

5.3. Tissue-Specific Expression of hCAP-18/LL-37, the Human Cathelicidin

Unlike defensins, which are stored within the neutrophil's primary (azurophil) granules in a fully processed form, hCAP-18/LL-37 is found in the specific (secretory) granules of neutrophils in its 17-kDa (140-amino acid), cathelin-containing hCAP-18 proform. hCAP-18/LL-37 was about one-third as abundant as lactoferrin or lysozyme, the two major proteins of specific granules *(119)*. During or after its secretion, the stored propeptide can undergo processing *(117)* to the mature 5-kDa (37-amino acid) peptide, LL-37. Processing may be mediated by proteinase 3, a neutrophil enzyme closely related to neutrophil elastase *(119a)*. The processing of the cathelicidins proBac5 and proBac7 by bovine neutrophils, and of proprotegrins by porcine neutrophils, is mediated by trace amounts of neutrophil elastase *(108,109)*.

Although hCAP-18/LL-37 was initially recognized as a constitutive component of the human neutrophil, it is also expressed in other cells and by nonmyeloid tissues. Normal skin keratinocytes do not express hCAP-18, but the peptide is induced in psoriasis, injury, and various inflammatory conditions *(120)*. hCAP-18 mRNA and protein is also expressed by squamous epithelia of the mouth, tongue, esophagus, cervix, and vagina *(121)*. High levels of LL-37/hCAP-18 RNA were observed in surface epithelial cells and submucosal glands of the conducting airway, and LL-37/hCAP-18 peptide was partially purified from human lung airway surface fluid *(122)*.

hCAP-18 is also produced within the epididymis and could play a prominent role in host defense of the genitourinary tract. Normal human seminal plasma was reported to contain 86.5± 12.0 µg/mL (mean ± SEM) of hCAP-18, a level 70-fold higher than was found in blood plasma *(123)*. Much of this was attached to spermatozoa, which carried, on average, over 6 million hCAP-18 molecules each. Most of the hCAP-18 in circulating blood is bound to apolipoproteins A-I and B via its antibacterial C-terminal domain, and it circulates as a high molecular weight complex *(124)*. Whether this affinity plays a role in safely clearing LPS from sites of infection remains to be ascertained.

It was recently observed that early in *Shigella* spp. infections and other dysenteries, rectal expression of the antibacterial peptides LL-37 (and human β-defensin-1) was reduced or turned off for up to several weeks. When the phenomenon was studied in *Shigella*-infected epithelial and monocyte cultures, it appeared that *Shigella* plasmid DNA could mediate the effect. The authors suggested that downregulation of these endogenous antimicrobial peptides might promote both bacterial adherence and their invasion of host epithelium *(125)*.

5.4. Conformation and Activities

Whereas micromolar concentrations of LL-37 displayed a largely disordered structure in saline *(126)*, the addition of 15 m*M* bicarbonate (the principal buffer of blood and tissue fluids), induced the peptide to assume an α-helical conformation, whose extent was correlated with its antibacterial activity. However, the addition of serum greatly diminished the peptide's antimicrobial (and cytotoxic) activity *(126)*. Biophysical measurements in model systems revealed that LL-37 was predominantly α-helical and oriented nearly parallel with the surface of zwitterionic-lipid membranes—a result interpreted to be consistent with a detergent-like (rather than a pore-forming) mechanism *(127)*.

In vitro, human LL-37 displays LPS binding *(128)* and antimicrobial properties *(118)*. Its binding of *E. coli* 0111:B4 LPS was of relatively high affinity and showed positive cooperativity *(107)*. The LPS binding domain(s) of LL-37 have not yet been identified. In addition to these properties, LL-37 is chemotactic for human neutrophils, monocytes, and T-lymphocytes, apparently acting via the formyl peptide receptor-like-1 (FPRL1) receptor. Consequently, LL-37 may also contribute to adaptive immunity by recruiting monocytes and T-cells *(129)*.

5.5. Evidence for an In Vivo Role of Cathelicidins

In porcine skin wounds, the most active antimicrobial peptides are protegrins, secreted from neutrophils as proprotegrins and activated by proteolytic cleavage by neutrophil elastase *(108)*. In vitro, inhibition of neutrophil elastase by specific inhibitors blocked the conversion of proprotegrins to protegrins and largely ablated the stable antimicrobial activity secreted by porcine neutrophils *(130)*. The application of neutrophil elastase inhibitor to porcine wounds decreased the concentration of mature protegrin in wound fluid and impaired the clearance of bacteria from wounds. The deficit could be restored by supplementing the wound fluid with synthetic protegrin in vitro or in vivo *(131)*. In this system, neutrophil elastase by itself had no direct antimicrobial activity. Thus, protegrins act as natural antibiotics that contribute to the clearance of microbes from wounds. This role is unlikely to be exclusive, as the pig is equipped with many other antimicrobial peptides of the cathelicidin family.

Mice with elastase-deficient neutrophils show impaired resistance to infection by fungi *(132)* and Gram-negative bacteria *(133,134)*. Although this has been attributed to loss of the direct antimicrobial effects of neutrophil elastase on *E. coli,* the possibility of impaired processing of cathelicidins such as cathelin-related antimicrobial peptide (CRAMP), the murine homologue of hCAP-18/LL-37 *(135)*, was not excluded.

Respiratory epithelia of cystic fibrosis (CF) patients are abnormally susceptible to bacterial infection. Overexpression of hCAP18/LL-37 by recombinant adenovirus in CF respiratory epithelial cell culture increased epithelial resistance to infection with *Pseudomonas aeruginosa* and *Staphylococcus aureus (136)*. Moreover, the adenovirus construct also augmented the resistance of mice against airway challenge with *P. aeruginosa (137)*. The effect of CAP18/LL-37 may be partly mediated by its ability to bind LPS, since systemic administration of the adenovirus construct also protected against systemic challenge with LPS.

6. SUMMARY AND CONCLUSIONS

Antimicrobial peptides, when expressed at high concentrations (approx. 10^{-3}–10^{-6} M) in epithelia and phagocytes of multicellular animals, act predominantly as antimicrobial and LPS-binding effector molecules. The former activity depends largely on their ability to form membrane-disruptive configurations. At lower concentrations (approx. 10^{-6}–10^{-8} M), certain mammalian antimicrobial peptides have chemokine-like activity that attracts cells involved in the initiation of primary or recall adaptive responses. In some cases, this activity results from the interaction of antimicrobial peptides with known chemotactic receptors, but in other situations specific receptors have not yet been pinpointed. In tissues under attack by pathogens, induction and release of these endogenous peptides may not only contribute to intial antimicrobial resistance but may also facilitate the later development of humoral and cell-mediated immunity.

REFERENCES

1. Krensky AM, Okada S, Clayberger C, Kumar J. Granulysin: a novel antimicrobial. Expert Opin Invest Drugs 2001;10:321–329.
2. Leippe M. Antimicrobial and cytolytic polypeptides of amoeboid protozoa–effector molecules of primitive phagocytes. Dev Comp Immunol 1999;23:267–279.
3. Zhai Y, Saier MH Jr. The amoebapore superfamily. Biochim Biophys Acta 2000;1469:87–99.
4. Sablon E, Contreras B, Vandamme E. Antimicrobial peptides of lactic acid bacteria: mode of action, genetics and biosynthesis. Adv Biochem Eng Biotechnol 2000;68:21–60.
5. Haseltine C, Hill T, Montalvo-Rodriguez R, et al. Secreted eutyarchaeal microhalocins kill hyperthermophilic crenarchaea. J Bacteriol 2001;183:287–291.
6. Benz R. Porin from bacterial and mitochondrial outer membranes. CRC Crit Rev Biochem 1985;19:145–190.
7. Hancock RE, Bell A. Antibiotic uptake into gram-negative bacteria. Eur J Clin Microbiol Infect Dis 1988;7:713–720.
8. Shai Y. Mechanism of the binding, insertion and destabilization of phospholipid bilayer membranes by alpha-helical antimicrobial and cell non-selective membrane-lytic peptides. Biochim Biophys Acta 1999;1462:55–70.
9. Ludtke SJ, He K, Heller WT, et al. Membrane pores induced by magainin. Biochemistry 1996;35:13723–13728.
10. Higashimoto Y, Kodama H, Jelokhani-Niaraki M, Kato F, Kondo M. Structure-function relationship of model Aib-containing peptides as ion transfer intermembrane templates. J Biochem (Tokyo) 1999;125:705–712.
11. Hara T, Kodama H, Kondo M, et al. Effects of peptide dimerization on pore formation: antiparallel disulfide-dimerized magainin 2 analogue. Biopolymers 2001;58:437–446.

12. Lehrer RI, Barton A, Daher KA, Harwig SS, Ganz T, Selsted ME. Interaction of human defensins with *Escherichia coli*. Mechanism of bactericidal activity. J Clin Invest 1989;84:553–561.

13. Wimley WC, Selsted ME, White SH. Interactions between human defensins and lipid bilayers: evidence for formation of multimeric pores. Protein Sci 1994;3:1362–1373.

14. Wilkins DK, Grimshaw SB, Receveur V, et al. Hydrodynamic radii of native and denatured proteins measured by pulse field gradient NMR techniques. Biochemistry 1999;38:16424–16431.

15. Kobayashi S, Takeshima K, Park CB, Kim SC, Matsuzaki K. Interactions of the novel antimicrobial peptide buforin 2 with lipid bilayers: proline as a translocation promoting factor. Biochemistry 2000;39:8648–8654.

16. Ganz T, Lehrer RI. Defensins. Pharmacol Ther 1995;66:191–205.

17. Lehrer RI, Lichtenstein AK, Ganz T. Defensins: antimicrobial and cytotoxic peptides of mammalian cells. Annu Rev Immunol 1993;11:105–128.

18. Tang YQ, Yuan J, Osapay G, et al. A cyclic antimicrobial peptide produced in primate leukocytes by the ligation of two truncated alpha-defensins [see comments]. Science 1999;286:498–502.

19. Hill CP, Yee J, Selsted ME, Eisenberg D. Crystal structure of defensin HNP-3, an amphiphilic dimer: mechanisms of membrane permeabilization. Science 1991;251:1481–1485.

20. Hoover DM, Rajashankar KR, Blumenthal R, et al. The structure of human beta-defensin-2 shows evidence of higher-order oligomerization. J Biol Chem 2000;275:32,911–32,918.

21. Pardi A, Zhang XL, Selsted ME, Skalicky JJ, Yip PF. NMR studies of defensin antimicrobial peptides.2. Three-dimensional structures of rabbit NP-2 and human HNP-1. Biochemistry 1992;31:11357–11364.

22. Skalicky JJ, Selsted ME, Pardi A. Structure and dynamics of the neutrophil defensins NP-2, NP-5, and HNP-1: NMR studies of amide hydrogen exchange kinetics. Proteins 1994;20:52–67.

23. Zimmermann GR, Legault P, Selsted ME, Pardi A. Solution structure of bovine neutrophil beta-defensin-12: the peptide fold of the beta-defensins is identical to that of the classical defensins. Biochemistry 1995;34:13663–13671.

24. Sawai MV, Jia HP, Liu L, et al. The NMR structure of human beta-defensin-2 reveals a novel alpha-helical segment. Biochemistry 2001;40:3810–3816.

25. Zeya HI, Spitznagel JK. Antibacterial and enzymic basic proteins from leukocyte lysosomes: separation and identification. Science 1963;142:1085–1087.

26. Zeya HI, Spitznagel JK. Arginine-rich proteins of polymorphonuclear leukocyte lysosomes. Antimicrobial specificity and biochemical heterogeneity. J Exp Med 1968;127:927–941.

27. Selsted ME, Brown DM, DeLange RJ, Lehrer RI. Primary structures of MCP-1 and MCP-2, natural peptide antibiotics of rabbit lung macrophages. J Biol Chem 1983;258:14485–14489.

28. Ganz T, Selsted ME, Szklarek D, et al. Defensins. Natural peptide antibiotics of human neutrophils. J Clin Invest 1985;76:1427–1435.

29. Selsted ME, Harwig SS, Ganz T, Schilling JW, Lehrer RI. Primary structures of three human neutrophil defensins. J Clin Invest 1985;76:1436–1439.

30. Gabay JE, Scott RW, Campanelli D, et al. Antibiotic proteins of human polymorphonuclear leukocytes. Proc Natl Acad Sci USA 1989;86:5610–5614.

31. Joiner KA, Ganz T, Albert J, Rotrosen D. The opsonizing ligand on *Salmonella typhimurium* influences incorporation of specific, but not azurophil, granule constituents into neutrophil phagosomes. J Cell Biol 1989;109:2771–2782.

32. Porter EM, Liu L, Oren A, Anton PA, Ganz T. Localization of human intestinal defensin 5 in Paneth cell granules. Infect Immun 1997;65:2389–2395.

33. Porter EM, vanDam E, Valore EV, Ganz T. Broad-spectrum antimicrobial activity of human intestinal defensin 5. Infect Immun 1997;65:2396–2401.

34. Jones DE, Bevins CL. Defensin-6 mRNA in human Paneth cells: implications for antimicrobial peptides in host defense of the human bowel. FEBS Lett 1993;315:187–192.

35. Jones DE, Bevins CL. Paneth cells of the human small intestine express an antimicrobial peptide gene. J Biol Chem 1992;267:23216–23225.

36. Ouellette AJ. Paneth cells and innate immunity in the crypt microenvironment. Gastroenterology 1997;113:1779–1784.

37. Agerberth B, Charo J, Werr J, et al. The human antimicrobial and chemotactic peptides LL-37 and alpha-defensins are expressed by specific lymphocyte and monocyte populations. Blood 2000;96:3086–3093.

38. Bensch KW, Raida M, Magert HJ, Schulz-Knappe P, Forssmann WG. hBD-1: a novel beta-defensin from human plasma. FEBS Lett 1995;368:331–335.

39. Zhao CQ, Wang I, Lehrer RI. Widespread expression of beta-defensin HBD-1 in human secretory glands and epithelial cells. FEBS Lett 1996;396:319–322.

40. Harder J, Bartels J, Christophers E, Schroeder J-M. A peptide antibiotic from human skin. Nature 1997;387:861–862.

41. Harder J, Bartels J, Christophers E, Schroder JM. Isolation and characterization of human beta-defensin-3, a novel human inducible peptide antibiotic. J Biol Chem 2001;276:5707–5713.

42. Valore EV, Park CH, Quayle AJ, et al. Human beta-defensin-1: an antimicrobial peptide of urogenital tissues. J Clin Invest 1998;101:1633–1642.

43. Bartoli E, Romano G. Measurement of reabsorption by single segments of the human nephron. J Nephrol 1999;12:275–287.

44. Diamond G, Russell JP, Bevins CL. Inducible expression of an antibiotic peptide gene in lipopolysaccharide-challenged tracheal epithelial cells. Proc Natl Acad Sci USA 1996;93:5156–5160.

45. Schonwetter BS, Stolzenberg ED, Zasloff MA. Epithelial antibiotics induced at sites of inflammation. Science 1995;267:1645–1648.

46. Diamond G, Zasloff M, Eck H, et al. Tracheal antimicrobial peptide, a cysteine-rich peptide from mammalian tracheal mucosa: peptide isolation and cloning of a cDNA. Proc Natl Acad Sci USA 1991;88:3952–3956.

47. Dutis LA, Rademaker M, Ravensbergen B, et al. Inhibition of hBD-3, but not hBD-1 and hBD-2, mRNA expression by corticosteroids. Biochem Biophys Res Commun 2001;280:522–525.

48. Frohlich O, Po C, Young LG. Organization of the human gene encoding the epididymis-specific ep2 protein variants and its relationship to defensin genes. Biol Reprod 2001;64:1072–1079.

49. Li P, Chan HC, He B, et al. An antimicrobial peptide gene found in the male reproductive system of rats. Science 2001;291:1783–1785.

50. Lung O, Kuo L, Wolfner MF. *Drosophila* males transfer antibacterial proteins from their accessory gland and ejaculatory duct to their mates. J Insect Physiol 2001;47:617–622.

51. Sitaram N, Subbalakshmi C, Krishnakumari V, Nagaraj R. Identification of the region that plays an important role in determining antibacterial activity of bovine seminalplasmin. FEBS Lett 1997;400:289–292.

52. Samakovlis C, Kylsten P, Kimbrell DA, Engstrom A, Hultmark D. The andropin gene and its product, a male-specific antibacterial peptide in *Drosophila melanogaster.* EMBO J 1991;10:163–169.

53. Ganz T, Rayner JR, Valore EV, et al. The structure of the rabbit macrophage defensin genes and their organ-specific expression. J Immunol 1989;143:1358–1365.

54. Ryan LK, Rhodes J, Bhat M, Diamond G. Expression of beta-defensin genes in bovine alveolar macrophages. Infect Immun 1998;66:878–881.

55. Ogata K, Linzer BA, Zuberi RI, et al. Activity of defensins from human neutrophilic granulocytes against *Mycobacterium avium-Mycobacterium intracellulare.* Infect Immun 1992;60:4720–4725.

56. Miyasaki KT, Bodeau AL, Ganz T, Selsted ME, Lehrer RI. In vitro sensitivity of oral, gram-negative, facultative bacteria to the bactericidal activity of human neutrophil defensins. Infect Immun 1990;58:3934–3940.

57. Daher KA, Selsted ME, Lehrer RI. Direct inactivation of viruses by human granulocyte defensins. J Virol 1986;60:1068–1074.

58. Lehrer RI, Ganz T, Szklarek D, Selsted ME. Modulation of the in vitro candidacidal activity of human neutrophil defensins by target cell metabolism and divalent cations. J Clin Invest 1988;81:1829–1835.

59. Lehrer RI, Szklarek D, Ganz T, Selsted ME. Correlation of binding of rabbit granulocyte peptides to *Candida albicans* with candidacidal activity. Infect Immun 1985;49:207–211.

60. Higazi AA, Barghouti II, Abu-Much R. Identification of an inhibitor of tissue-type plasminogen activator-mediated fibrinolysis in human neutrophils. A role for defensin. J Biol Chem 1995;270:9472–9477.

61. Murphy CJ, Foster BA, Mannis MJ, Selsted ME, Reid TW. Defensins are mitogenic for epithelial cells and fibroblasts. J Cell Physiol 1993;155:408–413.

62. Singh A, Bateman A, Zhu QZ, et al. Structure of a novel human granulocyte peptide with anti-ACTH activity. Biochem Biophys Res Commun 1988;155:524–529.

63. Zhu QZ, Singh AV, Bateman A, Esch F, Solomon S. The corticostatic (anti-ACTH) and cytotoxic activity of peptides isolated from fetal, adult and tumor-bearing lung. J Steroid Biochem 1987;27:1017–1022.

64. Lehrer RI, Barton A, Ganz T. Concurrent assessment of inner and outer membrane permeabilization and bacteriolysis in *E. coli* by multiple-wavelength spectrophotometry. J Immunol Methods 1988;108:153–158.

65. Lichtenstein AK, Ganz T, Nguyen TM, Selsted ME, Lehrer RI. Mechanism of target cytolysis by peptide defensins. Target cell metabolic activities, possibly involving endocytosis, are crucial for expression of cytotoxicity. J Immunol 1988;140:2686–2694.

66. Lichtenstein A, Ganz T, Selsted ME, Lehrer RI. In vitro tumor cell cytolysis mediated by peptide defensins of human and rabbit granulocytes. Blood 1986;68:1407–1410.

67. White SH, Wimley WC, Selsted ME. Structure, function, and membrane integration of defensins. Curr Opin Struct Biol 1995;5:521–527.

68. Fujii G, Selsted ME, Eisenberg D. Defensins promote fusion and lysis of negatively charged membranes. Protein Sci 1993;2:1301–1312.

69. Kagan BL, Selsted ME, Ganz T, Lehrer RI. Antimicrobial defensin peptides form voltage-dependent ion-permeable channels in planar lipid bilayer membranes. Proc Natl Acad Sci USA 1990;87:210–214.

70. Liu L, Zhao C, Heng HHQ, Ganz T. The human β-defensin-1 and α-defensins are encoded by adjacent genes: two peptide families with differing disulfide topology share a common ancestry. Genomics 1997;43:316–320.

71. Linzmeier R, Michaelson D, Liu L, Ganz T. The structure of neutrophil defensin genes. FEBS Lett 1993;321:267–273.

72. Sparkes RS, Kronenberg M, Heinzmann C, et al. Assignment of defensin gene(s) to human chromosome 8p23. Genomics 1989;5:240–244.

73. Zhao C, Nguyen T, Liu L, et al. Gallinacin-3, an inducible epithelial beta-defensin in the chicken. Infect Immun 2001;69:2684–2691.

74. Eisenhauer PB, Lehrer RI. Mouse neutrophils lack defensins. Infect Immun 1992;60:3446–3447.

75. Huttner KM, Kozak CA, Bevins CL. The mouse genome encodes a single homolog of the antimicrobial peptide human beta-defensin 1. FEBS Lett 1997;413:45–49.

76. Morrison GM, Davidson DJ, Dorin JR. A novel mouse beta defensin, Defb2, which is upregulated in the airways by lipopolysaccharide. FEBS Lett 1999;442:112–116.

77. Bals R, Wang X, Meegalla RL, et al. Mouse beta-defensin 3 is an inducible anitimicrobial peptide expressed in the epithelia of multiple organs. Infect Immun 1999;67:3542–3547.

78. Jia HP, Wowk SA, Schutte BC, et al. A novel murine beta-defensin expressed in tongue, esophagus, and trachea [In Process Citation]. J Biol Chem 2000;275:33314–33320.

79. Zhu QZ, Hu J, Mulay S, et al. Isolation and structure of corticostatin peptides from rabbit fetal and adult lung. Proc Natl Acad Sci USA 1988;85:592–596.

80. Tominaga T, Fukata J, Naito Y, et al. Effects of corticostatin-I on rat adrenal cells in vitro. J Endocrinol 1990;125:287–292.

81. Masera RG, Bateman A, Muscettola M, Solomon S, Angeli A. Corticostatins/defensins inhibit in vitro NK activity and cytokine production by human peripheral blood mononuclear cells. Regul Pept 1996;62:13–21.

82. Akbulut S, Byersdorfer CA, Larsen CP, et al. Expression of the melanocortin 5 receptor on rat lymphocytes. Biochem Biophys Res Commun 2001;281:1086–1092.

83. Yang D, Chen Q, Chertov O, Oppenheim JJ. Human neutrophil defensins selectively chemoattract naive T and immature dendritic cells. J Leukoc Biol 2000;68:9–14.

84. Yang D, Chertov O, Bykovskaia SN, et al. Beta-defensins: linking innate and adaptive immunity through dendritic and T cell CCR6 [see comments]. Science 1999;286:525–528.

85. Ganz T, Metcalf JA, Gallin JI, Boxer LA, Lehrer RI. Microbicidal/cytotoxic proteins of neutrophils are deficient in two disorders: Chediak-Higashi syndrome and "specific" granule deficiency. J Clin Invest 1988;82:552–556.

86. Gallin JI, Fletcher MP, Seligmann BE, et al. Human neutrophil-specific granule deficiency: a model to assess the role of neutrophil-specific granules in the evolution of the inflammatory response. Blood 1982;59:1317–1329.

87. Gombart AF, Shiohara M, Kwok SH, A et al. Neutrophil-specific granule deficiency: homozygous recessive inheritance of a frameshift mutation in the gene encoding transcription factor CCAAT/enhancer binding protein-epsilon. Blood 2001;97:2561–2567.

88. Wilson CL, Ouellette AJ, Satchell DP, et al. Regulation of intestinal alpha-defensin activation by the metalloproteinase matrilysin in innate host defense. Science 1999;286:113–117.

89. Ayabe T, Satchell DP, Wilson CL, et al. Secretion of microbicidal α-defensins by intestinal Paneth cells in response to bacteria. Nature Immunology 2000;1:113–118.

90. Charlet M, Chernysh S, Philippe H, et al. Innate immunity. Isolation of several cysteine-rich antimicrobial peptides from the blood of a mollusc, *Mytilus edulis*. J Biol Chem 1996;271:21808–21813.

91. Hoffmann JA, Hetru C. Insect defensins: inducible antibacterial peptides. Immunol Today 1992;13:411–415.

92. Hoffmann JA. Innate immunity of insects. Curr Opin Immunol 1995;7:4–10.

93. Meister M, Lemaitre B, Hoffmann JA. Antimicrobial peptide defense in *Drosophila*. Bioessays 1997;19:1019–1026.

94. Brokaert WF, Terras FR, Cammune BP, Osborn RW. Plant defensins: novel antimicrobial peptides as components of the host defense system. Plant Physiol 1995;108:1353–1358.

95. Fehlbaum P, Bulet P, Michaut L, et al. Insect immunity. Septic injury of *Drosophila* induces the synthesis of a potent antifungal peptide with sequence homology to plant antifungal peptides. J Biol Chem 1994;269:33159–33163.

96. Bulet P, Hetru C, Dimarcq JL, Hoffmann D. Antimicrobial peptides in insects; structure and function. Dev Comp Immunol 1999;23:329–344.

97. Couto MA, Liu L, Lehrer RI, Ganz T. Inhibition of intracellular *Histopasma capsulatum* replication by murine macrophages that produce human defensin. Infect Immun 1994;62:2375–2378.

98. Kisich KO, Heifets L, Higgins M, Diamond G. Antimycobacterial agent based on mRNA encoding human beta-defensin 2 enables primary macrophages to restrict growth of *Mycobacterium tuberculosis*. Infect Immun 2001;69:2692–2699.

99. Zhang XH, Guo DJ, Zhang LM, Li WB, Sun YR. [The research on the expression of rabbit defensin (NP-1) gene in transgenic tomato]. Yi Chuan Xue Bao 2000;27:953–958.

100. Zanetti M, Gennaro R, Romeo D. Cathelicidins: a novel protein family with a common proregion and a variable C-terminal antimicrobial domain. FEBS Lett 1995;374:1–5.

101. Prige ST, Mains RE, Eipper BA, Amzel LM. New insights into copper monooxygenases and peptide amidation: structure, mechanism and function. Cell Mol Life Sci 2000;57 :1236–1259.

102. Romeo D, Skerlavaj B, Bolognesi M, Gennaro R. Structure and bactericidal activity of an antibiotic dodecapeptide purified from bovine neutrophils. J Biol Chem 1988; 263: 9573–9575.

103. Selsted ME, Novotny MJ, Morris WL, et al. Indolicidin, a novel bactericidal tridecapeptide amide from neutrophils. J Biol Chem 1992;267:4292–4295.

104. Kokryakov VN, Harwig SS, Panyutich EA, et al. Protegrins: leukocyte antimicrobial peptides that combine features of corticostatic defensins and tachyplesins. FEBS Lett 1993;327:231–236.

105. Gennaro R, Skerlavaj B, Romeo D. Purification, composition, and activity of two bactenecins, antibacterial peptides of bovine neutrophils. Infect Immun 1989;57:3142–3146.

106. Travis SM, Anderson NN, Forsyth WR, et al. Bactericidal activity of mammalian cathelicidin-derived peptides. Infect Immun 2000;68:2748–2755.

107. Turner J, Cho Y, Dinh NN, Waring AJ, Lehrer RI. Activites of LL-37, a cathelin-associated antimicrobial peptide of human neutrophils. Antimicrob Agents Chemother 1998;42:2206–2214.

108. Panytich A, Shi J, Boutz PL, Zhao C, Ganz T. Porcine polymorphonuclear leukocytes generate extracellular microbicidal activity by elastase-mediated activation of secreted proprotegrins. Infect Immun 1997;65:978–985.

109. Scocchi M, Skerlavaj B, Romeo D, Gennaro R. Proteolytic cleavage by neutrophil elastase converts inactive storage proforms to antibacterial bactenecins. Eur J Biochem 1992;209:589–595.

110. Zanetti M, Litteri L, Griffiths G, Gennaro R, Romeo D. Stimulus-induced maturation of probactenecins, precursors of neutrophil antimicrobial polypeptides. J Immunol 1991;146:4295–4300.

111. Levy O, Weiss J, Zarember K, Ooi CE, Elsbach P. Antibacterial 15-kDa protein isoforms (p15s) are members of a novel family of leukocyte proteins. J Biol Chem 1993;268:6058–6063.

112. Zarember K, Elsbach P, Shin-Kim K, Weiss J. p15s (15-kD antimicrobial proteins) are stored in the secondary granules of rabbit granulocytes: implications for antibacterial synergy with the bactericidal/permeability-increasing protein in inflammatory fluids. Blood 1997;89:672–679.

113. Hirata M, Shimomura Y, Yoshida M, et al. Characterization of a rabbit cationic protein (CAP18) with lipopolysaccharide-inhibitory activity. Infect Immun 1994;62:1421–1426.

114. Larrick JW, Hirata M, Balint RF, et al. Human CAP18: a novel antimicrobial lipopolysaccharide-binding protein. Infect Immun 1995;63:1291–1297.

115. Cowland JB, Johnsen AH, Borregaard N. hCAP-18, a cathelin/pro-bactenecin-like protein of human neutrophil specific granules. FEBS Lett 1995;368:173–176.

116. Gudmundsson GH, Magnusson KP, Chowdhary BP, et al. Structure of the gene for porcine peptide antibiotic PR-39, a cathelin gene family member: comparative mapping of the locus for the human peptide antibiotic FALL-39. Proc Natl Acad Sci USA 1995;92:7085–7089.

117. Gudmundsson GH, Agerberth B, Odeberg J, et al. The human gene FALL39 and processing of the cathelin precursor to the antibacterial peptide LL-37 in granulocytes. Eur J Biochem 1996;238:325–332.

118. Agerberth B, Gunne H, Odeberg J, Kogner P, Boman HG, Gudmundsson GH. FALL-39, a putative human peptide antibiotic, is cysteine-free and expressed in bone marrow and testis. Proc Natl Acad Sci USA 1995;92:195–199.

119. Borregaard N, Sehested M, Nielsen BS, Sengelov H, Kjeldsen L. Biosynthesis of granule proteins in normal human bone marrow cells. Gelatinase is a marker of terminal neutrophil differentiation. Blood 1995;85:812–817.

119a. Sorensen OE, Follin P, Johnsen AH, et al. Human cathelicidin, hCAP-18, is processed to the antimicrobial peptide LL-37 by extracellular cleavage with proteinase 3. Blood 2001;97:3951–3959.

120. Frohm M, Agerberth B, Ahangari G, et al. The expression of the gene coding for the antibacterial peptide LL-37 is induced in human keratinocytes during inflammatory disorders. J Biol Chem 1997;272:15258–15263.

121. Frohm NM, Sandstedt B, Sorensen O, et al. The human cationic antimicrobial protein (hCAP18), a peptide antibiotic, is widely expressed in human squamous epithelia and colocalizes with interleukin-6. Infect Immun 1999;67:2561–2566.

122. Bals R, Wang X, Zasloff M, Wilson JM. The peptide antibiotic LL-37/hCAP-18 is expressed in epithelia of the human lung where it has broad antimicrobial activity at the airway surface. Proc Natl Acad Sci USA 1998;95:9541–9546.

123. Malm J, Sorensen O, Persson T, et al. The human cationic antimicrobial protein (hCAP-18) is expressed in the epithelium of human epididymis, is present in seminal plasma at high concentrations, and is attached to spermatozoa. Infect Immun 2000;68:4297–4302.

124. Sorensen O, Bratt T, Johnsen AH, Madsen MT, Borregaard N. The human antibacterial cathelicidin, hCAP-18, is bound to lipoproteins in plasma. J Biol Chem 1999;274:22445–22451.

125. Islam D, Bandholtz L, Nilsson J, et al. Downregulation of bactericidal peptides in enteric infections: a novel immune escape mechanism with bacterial DNA as a potential regulator. Nat Med 2001;7:180–185.

126. Johansson J, Gudmundsson GH, Rottenberg ME, Berndt KD, Agerberth B. Conformation-dependent antibacterial activity of the naturally occurring human peptide LL-37. J Biol Chem 1998;273:3718–3724.

127. Oren Z, Lerman JC, Gudmundsson GH, Agerberth B, Shai Y. Structure and organization of the human antimicrobial peptide LL-37 in phospholipid membranes: relevance to the molecular basis for its non-cell-selective activity. Biochem J 1999;341:501–513.

128. Hirata M, Zhong J, Wright SC, Larrick JW. Structure and functions of endotoxin-binding peptides derived from CAP18. Prog Clin Biol Res 1995;392:317–326.

129. De Y, Chen Q, Schmidt AP, et al. LL-37, the neutrophil granule- and epithelial cell-derived cathelicidin, utilizes formyl peptide receptor-like 1 (FPRL1) as a receptor to chemoattract human peripheral blood neutrophils, monocytes, and T cells. J Exp Med 2000;192:1069–1074.

130. Shi J, Ganz T. The role of protegrins and other elastase-activated polypeptides in the bactericidal properties of porcine inflammatory fluids. Infect Immun 1998;66:3611–3617.

131. Cole AM, Shi J, Ceccarelli A, et al. Inhibition of neutrophil elastase prevents cathelicidin activation and impairs clearance of bacteria from wounds. Blood 2001;97:297–304.

132. Tkalcevic J, Novelli M, Phylactides M, et al. Impaired immunity and enhanced resistance to endotoxin in the absence of neutrophil elastase and cathepsin G. Immunity 2000;12:201–210.

133. Belaaouaj A, McCarthy R, Baumann M, et al. Mice lacking neutrophil elastase reveal impaired host defense against gram negative bacterial sepsis. Nat Med 1998;4:615–618.

134. Belaaouaj A, Kim KS, Shapiro SD. Degradation of outer membrane protein A in *Escherichia coli* killing by neutrophil elastase. Science 2000;289:1185–1188.

135. Gallo RL, Kim KJ, Bernfield M, et al. Identification of CRAMP, a cathelin-related antimicrobial peptide expressed in the embryonic and adult mouse. J Biol Chem 1997;272:13088–13093.

136. Bals R, Weiner DJ, Meegalla RL, Wilson JM. Transfer of a cathelicidin peptide antibiotic gene restores bacterial killing in a cystic fibrosis xenograft model. J Clin Invest 1999;103:1113–1117.

137. Bals R, Weiner DJ, Moscioni AD, Meegalla RL, Wilson JM. Augmentation of innate host defense by expression of a cathelicidin antimicrobial peptide. Infect Immun 1999;67:6084–6089.

17
The Role of Complement in Innate and Adaptive Immunity

Mihaela Gadjeva, Admar Verschoor, and Michael C. Carroll

1. INTRODUCTION

Early complement factors can be found among arthropods that evolved as early as 500 million years ago. The early complement proteins are limited to components of the alternative pathway, which is regarded as the most ancient pathway of complement activation. Traits of adaptive immunity arise with the appearance of vertebrates. The molecules of the classical pathway of complement activation appeared later, with the development of adaptive immunity *(1)*. Over the course of vertebrate evolution, the complement system has become closely associated with the humoral immune response. Recent studies elucidate how innate and adaptive immunity support each other. Complement serves not only as an *effector* of adaptive immunity but also participates in the *instruction* of the B-lymphocyte response. The bidirectional relationship exemplifies a complex linkage between innate and adaptive immunity, a connection we describe in this chapter.

2. OVERVIEW OF COMPLEMENT ACTIVATION

One strength of the complement response lies in its capacity to target its accumulative activation toward foreign substances while (under normal circumstances) being tightly controlled on self-surfaces. The stages of complement activation can be divided into early and late events. Early events are initiated by one of three distinct pathways (Table 1 and Fig. 1) and consist of a series of proteolytic steps leading to the formation of C3 convertase. Split-products resulting from activation of the cascade mediate inflammation by recruiting and activating phagocytes. Moreover, assembly of the terminal complement components in the membrane of pathogens induces cell lysis. Complement component C3 plays a central role in the complement system, at the point where the initiating pathways converge.

A key event following complement activation is covalent attachment of C3 to the pathogen surface. C3 and C4 possess an internal thioester that enables the molecules to form either ester or amide linkages with acceptor sites on the pathogen surface *(2,3)*. Once it is covalently bound onto nonself surfaces, C3 can become part of its own con-

Table 1
Initiators of Complement Activation

Pathway	Substances activated
Classical	IgM and IgG immune complexes
	Apoptotic material
	Certain viruses and Gram-negative bacteria
	C-reactive protein
Lectin	Microorganisms with terminal mannose,
	glucose, fucose, or N-acetylglucosamine
Alternative	IgG
	Many bacteria, viruses, fungi, and tumor cells

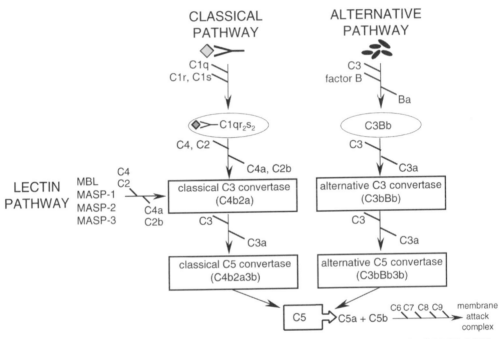

Fig. 1. Overview of the complement system. MBL, mannan-binding leotin; MASP, MBL-associated serine protease.

vertase, creating an amplification loop that activates and then deposits increasing amounts of C3. The deposition of C3 on foreign substances targets them for destruction by the lytic pathway or for uptake by phagocytes through various specific complement receptors. Although they are generated through different pathways that have their origins in various stages of evolution, C3 convertases of each pathway are homologous and support the same late events. Late events are initiated by the formation of C5-convertase and ultimately lead to the formation of a membrane attack complex (MAC) that damages the membranes of pathogens.

The activation of complement is tightly controlled by several mechanisms: (1) the convertases are covalently attached to foreign surfaces to ensure that complement activation only takes place in close proximity to the nonself substance; (2) fast hydrolysis of the activated thioester bond of C3 (or C4) prevents attachment far beyond its site of activation, keeping deposition localized; and (3) regulatory proteins found on cell surfaces and in circulation protect host cells from opsonization and lysis.

2.1. Classical Pathway

Antigen-bound antibody initiates complement activation through binding of the first component (C1) of the classical complement cascade (see also Table 1 and Fig. 1). Activation of C1 exposes a serine protease that activates C4 and C2 *(4)*. In this process, C4 becomes cleaved to C4a and C4b, with C4a functioning as a weak anaphylatoxin and C4b as an opsonin. The latter has only a weak effect as an opsonin, since it does not establish an amplification loop with specific convertase typical for C3. Reminiscent of C4, C2 is split by C1 to form the activated fragments C2a and C2b, thereby forming the classical C3-convertase, which then generates C3a and C3b. C3a functions as a potent anaphylatoxin, while C3b acts as an opsonin.

Classical C5-convertase (C4b2b3b) generates C5a and C5b from C5. C5b initiates the lytic pathway, whereas C5a is the strongest inflammatory mediator generated in the classical pathway. Like C3a, and to a lesser extent C4a, C5a stimulates smooth muscle contraction, vasodilation, chemoattraction of leukocytes to sites of infection, and activation of phagocytic cells.

2.2. Alternative Pathway

The alternative pathway can be initiated in the absence of antigen-specific antibody. Spontaneous hydrolysis of C3, or activation through specific sugar groups on pathogen surfaces, start a continuous cycle of C3 activation *(5)*. This mode of C3 "self-activation" is commonly referred to as "tick-over." The spontaneously activated C3 may be rapidly inactivated by hydrolysis or may bind covalently to nearby surfaces *(6)*. Noncovalent interaction of serum factor B with C3b *(7)* and cleavage by factor D leads to the formation of C3 converatase (C3bBb). This complex, stabilized by factor P, is reminiscent of the C4b2b complex of the classical pathway. It is noteworthy that C4b and C3b, as well as C2b and factor Bb, are homologous proteins, accounting for their similar functional properties.

2.3. Lectin Pathway

Mannan-binding lectin (MBL) binds to an array of carbohydrate structures on the surfaces of microorganisms and activates early classical complement components. Three serine proteases are known to associate with MBL: MBL-associated serine protease (MASP)-1, -2, and -3 (Fig. 1). The C4 cleaving activity can be attributed to the MASP-2 in the MBL-MASP-2 complexes *(8)*, whereas the MBL-MASP-1 complexes are thought to be capable of direct activation of C3 *(9)*. The function of the recently described new components in the MBL lectin pathway, MAp19 and MASP-3 *(10)*, is still unknown. Interestingly, genetic defects in MBL predispose to recurrent childhood infections. This association suggests that the MBL pathway plays an important role in complement activation when the levels of maternal antibody (IgG allotypes capable of activating the classical pathway) diminish while the child's own immune repertoire is still in development *(11)*.

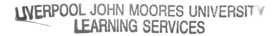

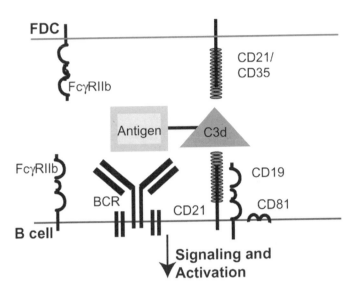

Fig. 2. Coligation of the B-cell receptor (BCR) with CD19/CD21 by antigen coated with C3d regulates essential functions for B-cell activation. C3d-coated antigens are also captured on the surface of the follicular dendritic cells (FDCs) by CD21/CD35, allowing for efficient B-cell stimulation.

2.4. Complement Receptors

Complement receptors play an important role in the uptake and clearance of opsonized antigen, as well as the enhancement of adaptive and innate cellular responses. Several types of complement receptors have been described, differing in their cell distribution and binding specificities. The chemokine-like receptors C3aR and C5aR specifically recognize the anaphylatoxins of C3 and C5, respectively, and are important in the activation of leukocytes. In this chapter we focus on the receptors that bind opsonizing complement fragments.

Complement Receptor 1 (CR1)

CR1 (CD35) *(12,13)* has been described as a receptor for opsonizing activation products of C3 (C3b), C4 (C4b) *(14)*, human C1q *(15)*, and MBL *(16)*. In humans, CR1 on erythrocytes plays an important role in the clearance of immune complexes and microorganisms by targeting them to spleen and liver. Once in the spleen, the complexed antigen can be removed and degraded. CR1 fulfills notable functions on monocytes by promoting phagocytosis. On dendritic and B-cells, it serves to internalize antigen for processing and presentation. CR1 on follicular dendritic cells (FDCs) plays a role in retaining antigen in native form, discussed in more detail below. In addition, CR1 regulates C3 convertase deposited on host cells.

Complement Receptor 2 (CR2)

CR2 (CD21) fulfills a key function in directly linking adaptive and innate immunity. It has a binding specificity for C3d, C3dg, and iC3b. In mice, both CR1 and CR2 are encoded at the *Cr2* locus, and alternative splicing generates the distinct receptors. On B-cells, CR2 forms in conjunction with CD19 and CD81, a co-receptor for the antigen-specific B-cell receptor (BCR) (Fig. 2). Coligation of the BCR and co-receptor by complement-decorated antigen lowers the activation threshold of the naive B-cell by as much as 10,000-fold compared with antigen alone. Expression of CR2 on FDCs, like CR1, is important in antigen trapping, which is critical for clonal selection of B-cells *(17,18)*.

Complement Receptors 3 (CR3) and 4 (CR4)

CR3 (CD11b/CD18, Mac-1) and CR4 (CD11c/CD18) share a number of characteristics that justify their joint discussion. Both have considerable structural homology and consist of two noncovalently associated type I membrane glycoproteins referred to as subunits α (CD11b or c, respectively) and β (CD18). As adhesion molecules on phagocytes, CR3 and CR4 aid migration through the vascular endothelium into sites of inflammation. Expression of CR3 and CR4 is detected mainly on cells of the myeloid lineage. Other nonmyeloid cells positive for CR3 include natural killer (NK) cells and CD5+ B-lymphocytes. High levels of CR4 are found on tissue macrophages and dendritic cells (DCs). Both CR3 and CR4 bind iC3b, a proteolytic breakdown product of antigen-bound C3b *(19)*. Opsonization by complement greatly enhances phagocytosis by neutrophils and mononuclear phagocytes, often via combined interaction with Fc-receptors and CD14. Indirect evidence suggests an important role for CR3 and CR4 on macrophages in the complement-dependent induction of thymus (T)-independent B-cell responses *(20)*.

3. NATURAL ANTIBODY, COMPLEMENT ACTIVATION, AND ANTIGEN PRESENTATION

IgM is the most efficient initiator of classical complement activation, approx 1000 times more efficient than IgG *(21)*. Natural, or preexisting, IgM is an important first line of defense that not only limits pathogen spread in the early onset of infection but also forms a basis for complement-mediated linkage of innate and adaptive immunity. Natural IgM is thought to be secreted independent of immunization or infection; it is constitutively produced by a long-lived, self-renewing population of B-lymphocytes called B1 cells. Natural IgM is primarily encoded by germline V regions and is characterized by an absence of somatic mutations. These antibodies show a broad range of avidities for both foreign and self-antigens *(22)*. Although B1 cells are primarily found in the peritoneal cavity *(23)* of mice, they are also identified in the spleen.

Natural antibody has several important functions in host protection. First, it can form complexes with pathogens or soluble toxins, e.g., endotoxin. In the case of viral infection, the formation of complexes leads to complement-dependent and-independent neutralization, thus limiting disseminated infection. Antigen complexed in this manner is efficiently filtered from circulation by the spleen and liver. Second, natural antibody is an efficient activator of the classical pathway. This property is significant for the linkage of innate and adaptive immunity.

It has been shown that B-cell responses to IgM-antigen-C3 complexes are strongly increased compared with the antigen alone *(24)*. Conversely, in mice lacking the secreted form of IgM, antigen-specific IgG responses are significantly reduced *(22)*. The impairment bears a close resemblance to the one observed in mice deficient in complement components C3 and C4 and in mice with a disrupted *Cr2* locus. The

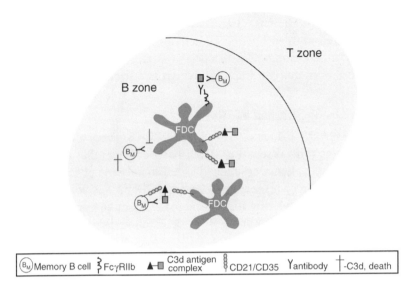

Fig. 3. Trapping of antigen-C3d complex on follicular dendritic cells (FDCs) via CD21/CD35 enhances B-cell activation and allows for long-term B-cell memory development.

impairment can be traced to two sources: a lack of coligation of the CD21/CD19/CD81 co-receptor and BCR, and reduced retention of antigen on FDCs. The former will affect the threshold of B-cell activation, whereas the latter negatively influences the germinal center (GC) reaction, which is important in the response to T-dependent antigens.

4. COMPLEMENT INFLUENCES T-DEPENDENT ANTIBODY RESPONSES

The importance of complement for antibody responses to T-dependent antigen was first demonstrated in the early 1970s. Bianco and Nussenzweig *(25)* postulated a role for complement in humoral immunity based on their observation of complement receptors expressed on B-lymphocytes. Subsequently, it was found that suppression of C3 levels in mice resulted in impairment of humoral immunity *(26)*. The mechanism for complement enhancement of B-cell responses may be explained by two, non-mutually exclusive, hypotheses: (1) co-receptor signaling on B-cells; and/or (2) antigen retention on FDCs. As discussed above, C3 coupled to antigen provides a ligand for the B-cell co-receptor CD21/CD19/CD81. For example, the amount of C3d conjugated hen egg lysozyme (HEL) required to stimulate optimal antibody responses in mice is three to four orders of magnitude less than that required for HEL alone. This effect is probably owing to both co-receptor signaling on B-cells and an increased localization of antigen on FDCs *(27)*. (Fig. 2). Recent experiments have demonstrated that complement-coated antigens stimulate the translocation of the BCR and co-receptor complex into the lipid rafts *(28)*, resulting in prolonged signaling. Complement-dependent retention of antigen on FDCs enhances the generation of antibody responses and the maintenance of immunologic memory by allowing for an efficient presentation of antigen to GC B cells (Fig. 3) *(29)*.

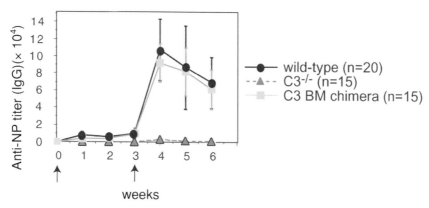

Fig. 4. Reconstitution of C3-deficient mice with wild-type bone marrow (BM) restores the humoral response to protein antigens administered i.v.

4.1. The Phenotype of C3−/− and C4−/− Animals

Humans, dogs, and guinea pigs bearing natural deficiencies in C1q, C4, or C3 have diminished antibody responses to T-dependent antigens. Genetically engineered strains of mice deficient in the early complement components C1q, C3, or C4 also show defective responses to T-dependent antigens. Thus, the classical pathway appears to be important in enhancement of humoral responses. The impaired response of the deficient mice is characterized by a reduction in primary IgM and a failure to switch to IgG *(30)*. Reduction in antibody production correlates with a reduction in size and frequency of GCs. This effect is mediated by complement receptors CD21/CD35, and the phenotype is similar to that observed in mice deficient in Cr2 or mice treated with antibodies against CD21 *(24)*. The defect lies at the B-cell level, as T-cells are stimulated normally.

4.2. Local C3 Synthesis and Response to Inert Protein Antigen in the Circulation

The C3 levels in blood are largely dependent on liver synthesis. Extrahepatic sources of C3 have also been identified and include macrophages, keratinocytes, kidney tubular cells, and endothelial cells. Local C3 production, especially in the secondary lymphoid organs, is important for enhancing responses to T-dependent antigens and might represent the critical source. Evidence in support of the importance of myeloid C3 synthesis comes from studies with bone marrow chimeric mice. Reconstitution of C3−/− mice with wild-type (WT) bone marrow (BM) (WT BM → C3−/−) restores the humoral response to protein antigen injected intravenously. Following immunization, the WT BM → C3−/− chimeric animals switch to IgG and mount normal IgG responses (Fig. 4). The numbers of GCs are comparable in both WT mice and WT BM → C3−/− chimeras, as observed 7 days after secondary immunization. However, plasma C3 levels are negligible in WT BM → C3−/− chimeras. C3 mRNA was identified in the spleens of immunized WT BM → C3−/− mice (Fig. 5), the major source of which appears to be monocyte/macrophage marker (MOMA)-2-positive macrophages. In the splenic tissues of immune WT mice, cells synthesizing C3 mRNA appear to be randomly distributed among the B- and T-cell zones within the white pulp. Immunohistochemical analysis of splenic sections *(31)* reveals that C3 protein colocalizes with antigen on FDCs.

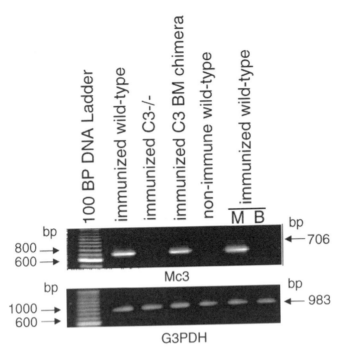

Fig. 5. RT-PCR specific for mC3 in splenic cells from immunized C3 BM chimeras, C3$^{-/-}$ mice, or WT control animals. Splenic mononuclear cells (MNCs) were isolated from WT animals, C3$^{-/-}$ mice, and C3 BM chimeras 7 d after the second immunization, and from nonimmune WT. Alternatively, MOMA-2-positive macrophages (M) and B220+ B cells (B) were isolated by positive magnetic immunoselection from splenic MNCs from immunized WT mice. Total RNA was isolated, reverse transcribed, and amplified with specific primer pairs for mC3 and mG3DPH.

The cytokine milieu within lymphoid organs of immune mice may favor induction of local complement C3 expression. Cytokines such as interferon-α (IFN-γ), tumor necrosis factor-α (TNF-α), interleukin-1 (IL-1), and IL-6 are known to regulate C3 synthesis. For example, IL-6-deficient animals have impaired IgG antibody responses, and it was proposed that these animals failed to induce synthesis of C3 in both serum and secondary lymphoid organs *(32)*. GC B-cells isolated from IL-6- and C3-deficient mice have a comparable defect in IgG2a and IgG2b antibody production. Other regulators of local C3 synthesis are thought to be IFN-γ and TNF-α. Mice deficient for IFN-γ receptor (IFN-R) have decreased titers of hapten-specific IgG2a and IgG3, 12 and 21 days after immunization with haptenated protein. A major source of IFN-γ is T-lymphocytes, which are stimulated following immunization; this could provide a possible stimulus for local synthesis of C3 by splenic myeloid cells. Production of C3 within the lymphoid compartment, and in the presence of early components of complement, could lead to enhanced activation and coupling to antigen. A potential model is discussed further below.

4.3. Complement, Humoral Immunity, and Infection in the Periphery

Dermal infection of mice with herpes simplex virus 1 (HSV-1) induces a T-dependent response, characterized by IFN-γ production and secondary antibody responses.

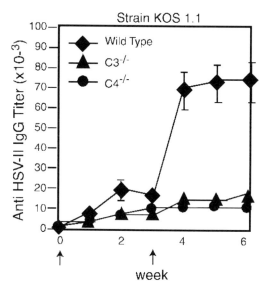

Fig. 6. Humoral response to infectious herpesvirus is complement-dependent.

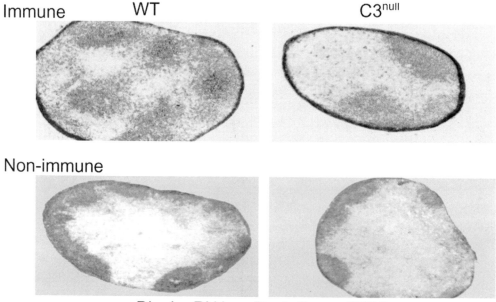

Fig. 7. Germinal center response is impaired in C3[−/−] mice after infection with 2×10^6 pfu of HSV-1 (HD-2 strain). LNs (inguinal and popliteal) were harvested from either WT or C3[−/−] mice 7 d after a third viral challenge (immune) or from those that were unimmunized (nonimmune). Cryosections were prepared and treated with antibody specific for B220 (B cell-specific) (gray) and peanut agglutinin (black). Representative sections identify PNA + GC in LN follicles of immune WT, but not immune C3[−/−] mice. WT, wild type.

Analysis of mice deficient in C3 or C4, following infection with HSV showed an impaired secondary response characterized by a reduction in GCs *(33)* (Figs. 6 and 7). These results suggest that the classical pathway is important in initiating complement

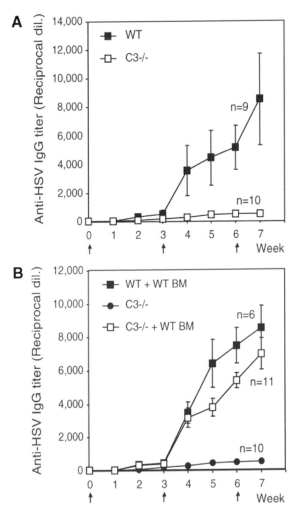

Fig. 8. Reconstitution of C3-deficient mice with wild-type bone marrow (WT BM) restores humoral response to infectious HSV-1.

activation leading to the activation of C3. The effects of C3 are mediated by CD21/CD35, as a similar impairment was observed in $Cr2^{-/-}$ mice *(33)*.

The finding that complement plays an important role in response to peripheral infection with virus raised the question: is serum-derived or locally produced C3 critical for humoral immunity? As discussed above, reconstitution of C3-deficient mice with WT BM restores the humoral response to T-dependent antigen introduced intravenously. Since serum complement might be less than optimal in peripheral lymph nodes and the dermis, it seems likely that macrophage-derived C3 would provide an important source of complement. To test this hypothesis, mice deficient in C3 were reconstituted with WT BM and subsequently challenged intradermally with HSV-1. Reconstitution with BM completely restored the humoral response to the virus (Fig. 8), indicating that adequate amounts of complement are produced on a local level, as serum C3 was virtually

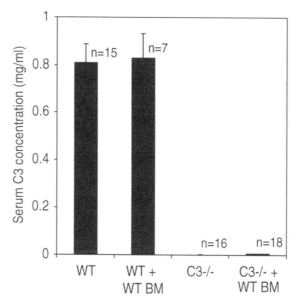

Fig. 9. Serum C3 levels in wild-type (WT) mice and wild-type C3-deficient bone marrow (BM) chimeras.

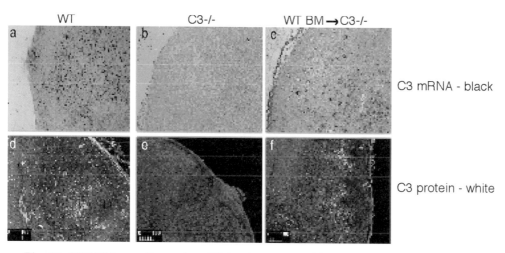

Fig. 10. WT BM engraftment into C3$^{-/-}$ mice restores C3 synthesis and C3 protein deposition in lymph nodes. Representative examples are shown. (**a–d**) *In situ* hybridization detection of C3 mRNA within cryosections of draining inguinal lymph nodes following intradermal HSV-1 infection in the flank. WT BM engraftment of C3$^{-/-}$ animals shows partially restored C3 production in the draining lymph node (**c**), as determined by the intensity and number of localized staining when compared with WT (**a**). C3$^{-/-}$ control mice show no specific C3 mRNA detection in the lymphoid compartment (**b**). (**d**) Detection of C3 protein within lymph node follicles by immunofluorescence. In addition to C3 (white) deposition in the GC, WT animals show abundant C3 at various sites in the lymphoid compartment that presumably represents C3 from circulation (e.g., in the subcapsular sinus and various vessel structures in both B and T cell zones (**d**). C3$^{-/-}$ mice (**e**) are negative for C3 staining. Restored production and retention of C3 in lymph nodes of WT BM-C3$^{-/-}$ mice correlates with restored humoral responses to intradermal infection with HSV-1.

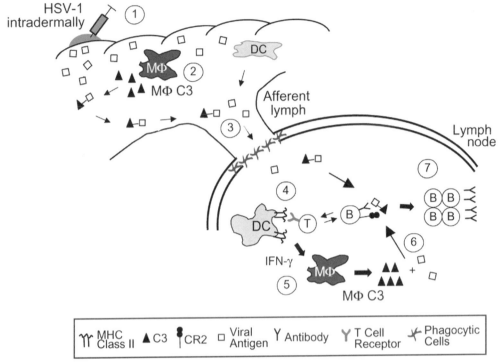

Fig. 11. How locally produced C3 affects the response to infectious herpes simplex virus-1 (HSV-1) (see explanation in the text). DC, dendritic cell; IFN-γ, interferon-γ; MΦ, macrophage.

absent *(34)* (Fig. 9). Moreover, C3 messenger RNA and protein were found in the white pulp of the draining lymph nodes (Fig. 10). These results strongly support the significance of local C3 synthesis in promoting the humoral response to peripheral viral infection. However, it remains unclear whether myeloid production of C3 by infiltrating macrophages at the site of infection is also important. It will also be necessary to determine whether local C3 synthesis is essential for humoral immunity to peripheral infection, or if serum C3 alone is sufficient.

One explanation for the role of local C3 synthesis in the viral model is that upon intradermal infection with the HSV-1 (Fig. 11, step 1), viral replication takes place, and mediators of inflammation are generated. It is conceivable that at this initial stage of infection, dermal-resident or infiltrating macrophages are induced to produce early complement proteins (step 2). Production of complement would allow for early opsonization of viral antigen near the peripheral site of infection. Antigen-presenting cells, such as Langerhans cells or DCs, would be aided in their uptake of antigen through their complement receptors. Subsequently, opsonized or unbound viral antigen drains and/ or is transported into the subcapsular sinus (step 3). Activated DCs stimulate naive T-cells, which provide costimulation to naive B-lymphocytes for response to the T-dependent virus (step 4). Moreover, both activated DC and T-cells produce cytokines, such as IFN-γ, which induce C3 (and possibly C1, C2, and C4) production by macrophages (step 5). The locally produced C3, activated by natural IgM, becomes covalently attached to the viral antigen (step 6). Complement-coated viral antigens activate B-lymphocytes, leading to clonal expansion (step 7). Opsonized and complexed antigen is trapped in GCs on FDCs, ensuring efficient B-cell stimulation, affinity maturation, and maintenance of memory.

5. MACROPHAGES

The observations that local C3 synthesis within secondary lymphoid tissue is sufficient to restore humoral immunity raises a general question regarding the source of other early components of complement. Macrophages are a source of early complement proteins C1 and C4, as well as late components such as C5. Thus, it is very likely that sufficient amounts of each of the early complement components are produced by macrophages to form C3 convertase and activate C3. From an evolutionary point of view, this concept seems reasonable. Given the central protective role of macrophages in innate immunity, it seems logical that they can make each of the necessary complement proteins to induce inflammation and opsonize pathogens. Further studies directed at regulation of macrophage synthesis of complement proteins will be important in addressing this exciting concept.

6. ROLE OF COMPLEMENT IN T-INDEPENDENT IMMUNE RESPONSES

Many bacteria and viruses activate B-cells independently of T-cell help. They can be divided into two classes: type I and II. In T-independent type I responses, antigens activate B-cells without the need for secondary signals in a polyclonal or antigen-specific manner (e.g., endotoxin and viruses such as vesicular stomatitis virus). By contrast, T-independent type II antigens (e.g., bacterial polysaccharide) require residual, noncognate, T-cell help. The involvement of complement in both T-independent type I and II responses has been unraveled recently. T-independent IgM responses against vesicular stomatitis virus are reduced in C3$^{-/-}$ animals *(35)*. In this systemic viral model, complement C3 is responsible for uptake and targeting of viral antigens to the splenic marginal zone. This region of the spleen is located at the junction of the white and red pulp, where it harbors macrophages, DCs, and B-cells. C3-coated virus is targeted efficiently to complement receptor-expressing cells. Deposition of the virus may, therefore, depend on complement receptors 3 and 4 (CR3 and CR4), which are expressed on the surface of the metalophilic marginal zone macrophages.

The response to TNP-Ficoll, a haptenated T-independent type II antigen, can also involve complement C3 activation *(36)*. Guinamard et al. *(36)* observed reduced anti-TNP Ficoll IgM and IgG responses in C3$^{-/-}$ animals. This effect was mediated by CD21/CD35, as Cr2$^{-/-}$ mice also had an impaired response. Interestingly, the impaired response correlated with a reduction in uptake of NP-Ficoll by marginal zone B-cells. Thus, this distinct population of B-cells appears to be critical in complement-dependent uptake of Ficoll antigen and enhancement of the B-cell response.

7. CONCLUSIONS

In summary, the mammalian complement system serves a dual role, acting both to mediate inflammation and to "instruct" the humoral B-lymphocyte response. Covalent attachment of activated C3 to pathogen provides an important "marker" for identification and elimination of foreign antigens by the innate immune system. Moreover, adaptive immunity has utilized this important marker as a mechanism to localize antigen within the lymphoid compartment and significantly enhance activation of antigen-specific B-lymphocytes. Recent studies on the relative importance of locally produced C3 have led to the novel concept that macrophages produce sufficient levels of early classical pathway complement protein to ensure covalent attachment of C3 to antigen. Future studies will be necessary to examine in vivo regulation of complement protein synthesis by macrophages.

ACKNOWLEDGMENTS

This work was supported by NIH grants AI42257, AI39246, HD38749, and GM52585

REFERENCES

1. Fearon DT. The complement system and adaptive immunity. Semin Immunol 1998;10:355–361.
2. Law SK, Dodds AW. The internal thioester and the covalent binding properties of the complement proteins C3 and C4. Protein Sci 1997;6:263–274.
3. Law SK, Lichtenberg NA, Levine RP. Covalent binding and hemolytic activity of complement proteins. Proc Natl Acad Sci USA 1980;77:7194–7198.
4. Kerr MA. The human complement system: assembly of the classical pathway C3 convertase. Biochem J 1980;189:173–181.
5. Pangburn MK, Schreiber RD, Muller-Eberhard HJ. Formation of the initial C3 convertase of the alternative complement pathway. Acquisition of C3b-like activities by spontaneous hydrolysis of the putative thioester in native C3. J Exp Med 1981;154:856–867.
6. Law SK, Lichtenberg NA, Levine RP. Evidence for an ester linkage between the labile binding site of C3b and receptive surfaces. J Immunol 1979;123:1388–1394.
7. Fishelson Z, Pangburn MK, Muller-Eberhard HJ. C3 convertase of the alternative complement pathway. Demonstration of an active, stable C3b, Bb (Ni) complex. J Biol Chem 1983;258:7411–7415.
8. Vorup-Jensen T, Petersen SV, Hansen AG, et al. Distinct pathways of mannan-binding lectin (MBL)- and C1-complex autoactivation revealed by reconstitution of MBL with recombinant MBL-associated serine protease-2. J Immunol 2000;165:2093–2100.
9. Vorup-Jensen T, Jensenius JC, Thiel S. MASP-2, the C3 convertase generating protease of the MBLectin complement activating pathway. Immunobiology 1998;199:348–357
10. Dahl M, Thiel S, Matsushita M, et al. MASP-3 and its association with distinct complexes of the mannan-binding lectin complement activation. Immunity 2001;15:127–135.
11. Walport MJ. Complement. First of two parts. N Engl J Med 2001;344:1058–1066.
12. Fearon DT. Identification of the membrane glycoprotein that is the C3b receptor of the human erythrocyte, polymorphonuclear leukocyte, B lymphocyte, and monocyte. J Exp Med 1980;152:20–30.
13. Carroll MC, Alicot EM, Katzman PJ, et al. Organization of the genes encoding complement receptors type 1 and 2, decay-accelerating factor, and C4-binding protein in the RCA locus on human chromosome 1. J Exp Med 1988;167:1271–1280.
14. Tas SW, Klickstein LB, Barbashov SF, Nicholson-Weller A. C1q and C4b bind simultaneously to CR1 and additively support erythrocyte adhesion. J Immunol 1999;163:5056–5063.
15. Klickstein LB, Barbashov SF, Liu T, Jack RM, Nicholson-Weller A. Complement receptor type 1 (CR1, CD35) is a receptor for C1q. Immunity 1997;7:345–355.

16. Ghiran I, Barbashov SF, Klickstein LB, et al. Complement receptor 1/CD35 is a receptor for mannan-binding lectin. J Exp Med 2000;192:1797–1808.
17. Carroll MC. CD21/CD35 in B cell activation. Semin Immunol 1998;10:279–286.
18. Fearon DT, Carroll MC. Regulation of B lymphocyte responses to foreign and self-antigens by the CD19/CD21 complex. Annu Rev Immunol 2000;18:393–422.
19. Law SK. C3 receptors on macrophages. J Cell Sci Suppl 1988;9:67–97.
20. Ochsenbein AF, Fehr T, Lutz C, et al. Control of early viral and bacterial distribution and disease by natural antibodies. Science 1999;286:2156–2159.
21. Cooper NR. The classical complement pathway: activation and regulation of the first complement component. Adv Immunol 1985;37:151–216.
22. Boes M. Role of natural and immune IgM antibodies in immune responses. Mol Immunol 2000;37:1141–1149.
23. Hamilton AM, Lehuen A, Kearney JF. Immunofluorescence analysis of B-1 cell ontogeny in the mouse. Int Immunol 1994;6:355–361.
24. Heyman B. Regulation of antibody responses via antibodies, complement, and Fc receptors. Annu Rev Immunol 2000;18:709–737.
25. Nussenzweig V, Bianco C, Dukor P, Eden A. Receptors for C3 on B lymphocytes: possible role in the immune response. In: Amos B (ed). Progress in Immunology, vol 59. New York: Academic Press, 1971. p. 73.
26. Pepys MB. Role of complement in induction of the allergic response. Nat New Biol 1972;237:157–159.
27. Dempsey PW, Allison ME, Akkaraju S, Goodnow CC, Fearon DT. C3d of complement as a molecular adjuvant: bridging innate and acquired immunity. Science 1996;271:348–350.
28. Cherukuri A, Cheng PC, Pierce SK. The role of the cd19/cd21 complex in B cell processing and presentation of complement-tagged antigens. J Immunol 2001;167:163–172.
29. Klaus GG, Humphrey JH, Kunkl A, Dongworth DW. The follicular dendritic cell: its role in antigen presentation in the generation of immunological memory. Immunol Rev 1980;53:3–28.
30. Fischer MB, Ma M, Goerg S, et al. Regulation of the B cell response to T-dependent antigens by classical pathway complement. J Immunol 1996;157:549–556.
31. Fischer MB, Ma M, Hsu NC, Carroll MC. Local synthesis of C3 within the splenic lymphoid compartment can reconstitute the impaired immune response in C3-deficient mice. J Immunol 1998;160:2619–2625.
32. Kopf M, Herren S, Wiles MV, Pepys MB, Kosco-Vilbois MH. Interleukin 6 influences germinal center development and antibody production via a contribution of C3 complement component. J Exp Med 1998;188:1895–1906.
33. Da Costa XJ, Brockman MA, Alicot E, et al. Humoral response to herpes simplex virus is complement-dependent. Proc Natl Acad Sci USA 1999;96:12708–12712.
34. Verschoor A, Brockman MA, Knipe DM, Carroll MC. Cutting edge: myeloid complement c3 enhances the humoral response to peripheral viral infection. J Immunol 2001;167:2446–2451.
35. Ochsenbein AF, Pinschewer DD, Odermatt B, et al. Protective T cell-independent antiviral antibody responses are dependent on complement. J Exp Med 1999;190:1165–1174.
36. Guinamard R, Okigaki M, Schlessinger J, Ravetch JV. Absence of marginal zone B cells in Pyk-2-deficient mice defines their role in the humoral response. Nat Immunol 2000;1:31–36.

18

The Role of Natural Killer Cells in Innate Immunity to Infection

Wayne M. Yokoyama

1. INTRODUCTION

Natural killer (NK) cells comprise the third major lymphocyte population *(1,2)* and can be distinguished from other lymphocytes by the absence of B- and T-cell antigen receptors, i.e., sIg and T-cell receptor (TCR), respectively. Although freshly isolated NK cells express the ζ-chain of the TCR/CD3 complex *(3,4)*, they do not display other components of the complex, do not express mRNA for mature TCR chains, and do not rearrange TCR genes *(5)*. Indeed, they are present in mice with defects in the antigen receptor recombination pathway, such as *scid* mice and mice with Rag-1 or -2 deficiency *(6)*. They typically display a large, granular morphology and are found in peripheral lymphoid tissues and blood.

Although initial studies focused on the capacity of NK cells to kill tumor targets and their role in tumor surveillance *(7)*, NK cells also participate in the normal host response to microbial infections *(8)*. A role for NK cells in controlling infections is dramatically illustrated by the case of an adolescent woman with a selective deficiency in NK cells in whom there were frequent, recurrent septicemic episodes caused by uncontrolled herpes viral infections, including cytomegalovirus (CMV), varicella, and herpes simplex virus (HSV) *(9)*. Importantly, this and other case reports reveal that human NK cell-deficient patients have in common a propensity to severe and/or recurrent herpesvirus infections *(10)*.

NK cell activity is also significantly diminished in AIDS patients *(11,12)* by infection with herpesvirus 6, inducing cytopathic changes and *de novo* expression of CD4, a cellular receptor for HIV-1 not normally expressed by NK cells *(13)*. This renders NK cells susceptible to infection by HIV-1, resulting in an NK cell deficiency, perhaps accounting, in part, for the increased susceptibility of patients to other infections, such as CMV, which may be particularly severe.

The NK cell compartment is not fully developed at birth, as indicated by lower natural killing by cord blood lymphocytes and corroborated by studies on the ontogeny of splenic NKR-P1 expression in rodents *(14,15)*. Interestingly, in the classic TORCH syndrome, birth defects and severe fetal anomalies are associated with maternal *Toxo-*

From: *Infectious Disease: Innate Immunity*
Edited by: R. A. B. Ezekowitz and J. A. Hoffmann © Humana Press Inc., Totowa, NJ

plasma, rubella, cytomegalovirus, and herpesvirus infections *(16).* Since NK cells are generally active against these organisms, the relative immaturity of NK cells during the neonatal period may be clinically relevant.

Like other lymphocytes, NK cells therefore appear to provide clinically significant host antimicrobial responses. In this chapter we relate the functions of NK cells to their in vivo capacity to resist certain infections. The emphasis is on experimental studies that have yielded important principles in terms of the role of NK cells in innate immunity to infections.

1.1. General Comments on the Study of NK Cells in Infections

Although there has yet to be a consensus on how to define NK cells in molecular terms, such as by expression of a specific function-defining receptor akin to the TCR on T-cells, most workers in the field generally consider the following phenotypes for NK cells. In humans, NK cells are usually CD56$^+$, CD3$^-$, whereas in C57BL/6 mice, they are NK1.1$^+$, CD3$^-$ *(2,5).* Both human and mouse NK cells also express the low-affinity Fc receptor for IgG, FcγRIII (CD16) *(17).* Human NK cells specifically express the FcγRIIIA transmembrane isoform, whereas there is only one FcγRIII isoform in mice; it is recognized by the anti-mouse FcγRIII monoclonal antibody (MAb) 2.4G2, which recognizes both FcγRII and FcγRIII. Although NK cells use their Fc receptors to mediate antibody-dependent cellular cytotoxicity (ADCC) against antibody-coated targets, the role of these receptors in innate immunity is unclear, since specific antibody production implies a previous specific immune encounter.

NK cells from mouse strains other than C57BL/6 or C57BL/10 often do not express the NK1.1 (NKR-P1c) molecule and instead can be detected with the DX5 MAb (Pharmingen, La Jolla, CA). In the older literature, antisera against asialo-GM1 was also used frequently, although this marker is now known to be more widely expressed. Thus, the NK cell phenotype in humans (CD56$^+$ FcγRIII$^+$ CD3$^-$) and mice [NK1.1$^+$ (or DX5$^+$ or asialo-GM1$^+$) FcγRII/III$^+$ CD3$^-$] can be used to isolate NK cells for in vitro analysis.

In mice, experimental approaches to determine an NK cell-dependent effect frequently use administration of polyclonal rabbit anti-asialo-GM1 antiserum or the anti-NK1.1 MAb (PK136) for effective NK cell depletion. However, anti-asialo-GM1 also reacts with activated T-cells and perhaps other cells, and anti-NK1.1 reacts with NK/T cells. To date, there is less experience with the DX5 MAb in vivo. Nevertheless, the NK cell-specific effect of these antibodies may be confirmed when they are used in combination with studies on *scid* or RAG$^{-/-}$ mice that express no T-cells or CD1$^{-/-}$ mice that express no NK/T cells. Since the anti-NK1.1 MAb is highly effective for NK cell depletion, and reacts with the best serologic determinant on mouse NK cells *(18),* the anti-NK1.1 MAb has become essentially the standard for NK cell depletion in C57BL/6 and related mouse strains.

A number of targeted mutant mice have been described that have been useful in terms of beginning to define NK cell development. In addition, these mice are helpful in studies of NK cells in innate immunity. Targeted mutations in several genes affect the development of CD3$^-$ NK cells [(i.e., Ikaros, interleukin-2 receptor γ (IL-2Rγ), IL-2Rβ, interferon regulatory factor-1 (IRF-1), IL-15, and IL-15Rα) *(19–26).* However, these mice have defects in other lymphoid compartments and, of course, the deficient factor.

Mutant mice with defects in NK cell effector mechanisms are also helpful in the dissection of innate immunity. NK cell-mediated killing, i.e., natural killing, of targets, is severely impaired in mice with mutations in molecules involved in this effector function, i.e., perforin or granzyme B *(27–31)*. However, all these mice have other non-NK cell abnormalities, affecting cytotoxic T-cells, for example. Mutant beige mice also fit in this latter category and were frequently used in the older literature. These mice and the corresponding human disease, Chédiak-Higashi syndrome, have abnormal granules owing to mutations in Lyst, a molecule expressed in lysosomes. Since the function of Lyst is as yet uncharacterized, beige mice are better thought of a "model for vesicle formation, fusion or trafficking" *(32)*, affecting all granulated immune cells rather than being NK cell-specific.

Among transgenic mice with NK cell defects, the transgenic Tgε26 mouse has been useful owing to an absolute deficiency in NK cells by virtue of overexpression of a human CD3ε transgenic construct. However, it also has a prominent defect in T-cell development *(33,34)*. Recent studies also indicated that mice transgenic for a granzyme A-Ly49A construct appear to have a selective NK cell deficiency, but these mice are less well characterized *(35)*. Therefore, it has been particularly challenging to study NK cells *in vivo* because there is no clear-cut animal model in which CD3⁻ NK cells are genetically and selectively deficient. Nevertheless, abnormalities in infection control in antibody-treated mice or in any of the above-mentioned targeted or spontaneously mutant mice would be consistent with NK cell-dependent resistance to infection that can be corroborated by experiments involving complementary approaches.

In vitro assays for NK cell function may support a role for NK cells in pathogen resistance. However, it should be noted that NK cells are generally propagated, especially in mice, in high concentrations of IL-2, which has several effects. First, IL-2-stimulated NK cells kill a broader panel of targets than freshly isolated NK cells for reasons that are as yet unknown. This is related to the phenotype of lymphokine-activated killer (LAK) cells *(36)*. In the high-dose IL-2 cultures, there are usually contaminating T-cells that are also "promiscuous killers" *(37)*. The CD3⁻ NK cells adhere better to plastic, so adherent LAK (A-LAK) cells are enriched for NK cells *(38)*. However, *in vitro* expansion is usually limited, so these primary cultures need to be regenerated frequently.

The *in vitro* NK cell proliferative response to high concentrations of IL-2 is unlikely to be related to a physiologically important role for IL-2 *in vivo*. However, the IL-2R shares two subunits, IL-2Rβ and IL-2Rγ, with IL-15R, which also contains the IL-15 binding subunit, IL-15Rα. It is likely that IL-15 plays a more important physiologic role in NK cell responses *in vivo,* since mice deficient in IL-15 or IL-15Rα fail to develop NK cells *(25,26)*.

Finally, NK cells are not homogeneous and are best considered to be a "polyclonal" population. In humans, NK cell clones can be generated and were instrumental in dissecting the molecular basis for NK cell tumor target recognition, but mouse NK cell clones have been difficult to produce unless they are made in relatively unusual circumstances, such as from p53-deficient mice or from fetal organs *(39,40)*. Whereas NK cell clones, particularly from humans, have been instrumental in the molecular definition of NK cell receptors for tumor targets, this approach has not yet been as successful to date in mice. Hence, there may be differences between the *in vivo* characterization of an NK cell contribution to pathogen resistance and the apparent *in vitro* correlate.

2. ROLE OF NK CELLS IN INFECTIONS

NK cell responses against many different viruses have been studied (summarized in ref. *41*). In addition, NK cells can apparently respond to a variety of Gram-positive, Gram-negative, and intracellular bacteria and protozoan parasites (summarized in ref. *8*). Analysis of the NK cell responses against many of these organisms has been limited. However, detailed and ongoing evaluation of NK cell responses, especially against *Listeria* and certain viral infections, have been informative and may be revealing of general principles that may be applicable to other organisms.

In mouse models, there is abundant experimental *in vivo* evidence supporting a role for NK cells in resisting certain infections. Shellam and colleagues *(42)* found that beige mice are susceptible to murine cytomegalovirus (MCMV) infections. Furthermore, Welsh and co-workers *(43–45)* eliminated NK cells *in vivo* by administration of the anti-NK1.1 MAb, or other anti-NK cell antibodies. When mice were then infected with MCMV, the infection resulted in marked viral replication in internal organs (spleen, liver), as evidenced by significantly higher viral titers in these organs, and lethality. A similar phenotype was observed in the Tgε26 mouse, which lacks NK and T-cells *(46)*. Interestingly, antibody studies further showed that if the anti-NK cell antibody administration was delayed, there was no untoward effect, indicating that NK cells are important in the early phases of host immune responses against MCMV *(44)*. Thus, NK cells are significant in early, innate immunity.

3. NK CELL EFFECTOR RESPONSES

To appreciate NK cell responses in innate immunity to infections, it is helpful to consider the responses with respect to their two major effector mechanisms, cytokine production and target killing.

3.1. Cytokine-Induced Production of Other Cytokines

NK cells can respond to several different cytokines, resulting in production of other cytokines. In the context of infection, the best studied have been induction of NK cell production of interferon-γ (IFN-γ) by IL-12 and the type I interferons.

In listeriosis, the classic model for T-cell-dependent resistance, it was noted that *scid* mice achieved partial control of the infection despite the absence of T-cells *(47)*. Neutralization of IFN-γ or elimination of NK cells by anti-NK cell antibodies (against NK1.1 and other NK cell receptors or anti-asialo-GM1) abrogated control of infection *(48)*. Furthermore, IFN-γ production was also markedly reduced with administration of the anti-NK cell antibodies, indicating that NK cells were responsible for early production of IFNγ. Interestingly, NK cells do not appear to respond directly to *Listeria* infection; rather, macrophage production of IL-12 is required for production of IFN-γ by NK cells as well as infection control *(49,50)*. Furthermore, tumor necrosis factor-α (TNF-α) can synergize with IL-12 to induce NK cell production of IFN-γ, whereas IL-10 is an antagonist *(49)*. Studies with mutant mice have indicated the increased susceptibility of mice lacking IL-12 receptor, IFN-γ, IFN-γ receptor or the IFN-γ receptor signaling pathway *(51–54)*, consistent with this model of *Listeria* infection inducing macrophage production of IL-12 that stimulates IFN-γ secretion by NK cells.

On the other hand, this macrophage IL-12-NK cell IFN-γ pathway is more complex. In immunocompetent mice, CD8$^+$, T-cells can also produce IFN-γ in response to bacterial infection. Whereas NK cells produce IFN-γ shortly (5 hours) after infection, T-cells produce IFN-γ after 15 hours and represent the dominant source. In addition, IL-18 also contributes to stimulation of IFN-γ by both populations. A role for IL-18 may explain the capacity of IL-12-deficient mice to survive low but not high inoculi of *Listeria* organisms *(51)*. *Listeria monocytogenes* can also induce CD8α$^+$ dendritic cells to produce IFN-γ in an IL-12-dependent manner *(55)*. Thus, as a variety of new experimental conditions, new mediators, and cellular participants are tested in listeriosis, the intricacies of the IL-12-IFN-γ pathway will be revealed and the relative contribution of NK cells will be more evident.

A similar IL-12-IFN-γ pathway is also operational in MCMV infections *(41)*. As already mentioned above, elimination of NK cells by administration of MAbs results in susceptibility of mice to MCMV *(43–45)*. As in listeriosis, one component of the NK cell response is the production of IFN-γ stimulated by IL-12 because antibody elimination of NK cells abrogates IFN-γ production in response to MCMV *(46,56)*. Furthermore, anti-IFN-γ increases susceptibility, whereas administration of IL-12 has a protective effect, which is abrogated by NK cell elimination or IFN-γ neutralization. As with listeriosis, IL-18 also contributes somewhat, although IL-12 appears to be more important (especially in the liver) for IFN-γ responses *(57)*.

Importantly, not all viral infections are controlled by NK cells. The best studied virus illustrating this point is lymphocytic choriomeningitis virus (LCMV) *(41,43,58)*. Elimination of NK cells has little effect on systemic LCMV infections, such as survival or viral replication. Interestingly, Biron and colleagues *(46)* have shown that LCMV infection does not induce IL-12-dependent IFN-γ production. Furthermore, neutralization of IL-12 had no effect on LCMV replication. However, NK cells are stimulated by LCMV infection.

During viral infections, including LCMV, the cytotoxicity of NK cells is enhanced, and proliferation ensues. These events constitute some of the systemic effects directly or indirectly mediated by the type I interferons *(59)*. Although the type I interferons also stimulate IFN-γ production that is independent of IL-12, IFN-γ production is not seen in LCMV infections *(46,60)*. Furthermore, administration of IL-12 does not promote NK cell production of IFN-γ. This apparent paradox was recently shown to be caused by an inhibitory effect of the type I interferons on IL-12-dependent IFN-γ production *(60)*. Inhibition by IFN-α/β is mediated through the STAT1 signaling pathway. In the absence of STAT1, IL-12 responsiveness is restored, and IFN-α/β induces IFN-γ production. Although it remains to be determined how the type I interferon response to LCMV differs from that to MCMV, these elegant studies indicate that the NK cell cytokine response to infection varies with the pathogen, even though the responses are similar superficially.

An emerging area of investigation is the role of IL-15 in NK cell responses *in vivo* *(61)*. This is a challenging area of study since mice deficient in IL-15 or IL-15Rα lack NK cells *(25,26)*. Nevertheless, a series of studies indicate that NK cells are stimulated during the course of infection by IL-15 *(61–65)*. As expected from studies of IL-2-activated NK cells (LAK cells), IL-15-stimulated NK cells have increased killing potential against tumor targets *(62)*. However, the IL-15-stimulated NK cells also have increased activity against virus-infected cells, which may be physiologically more relevant in innate immunity. Interestingly, several viruses can stimulate human peripheral blood mononuclear cells to secrete IL-15 and induce NK cell activity, resulting in *in vitro* control of viral replication *(63,64)*. This appears to be physiologically important in vivo since IL-15 can have a protective effect in herpes simplex viral infections in mice *(65)*.

NK cell responses to cytokines are also regulated by other innate lymphocytes. In TCRδ$^{-/-}$ mice, *Listeria* organism growth at day 1 after infection is significantly enhanced compared with TCRβ$^{-/-}$ mice. This is associated with diminished production of IFN-γ by NK cells and TNF-α production in TCRδ$^{-/-}$ mice, whereas comparable amounts of IL-12 were made, suggesting that γ/δT-cells regulate NK cell responses. Similarly, NK/T cells contribute to IFN-γ production by NK cells *(66)*. Administration of α-galactosylceramide, a potent ligand for the TCR on NK/T-cells, results in nearly concomitant activation of NK cells, possibly owing to release of IFN-γ by the NK/T-cell. Inasmuch as NK/T-cells can recognize glycolipid antigens in mycobacteria *(67,68)*, these studies indicate a potential physiologically important mechanism for NK cell activation in innate immunity to these organisms.

NK cells can also produce several other cytokines that have been less well studied in the context of infection. Also, early NK cell responses appear to be relatively nonspecific with polyclonal activation. Analysis of activation markers that are absent on resting NK cells reveals that all NK cells display these activation markers during MCMV infection *(69)*. Although this requires further study, presumably such activation reflects stimulation from a variety of cytokines that are induced upon infection.

Hence, the pathways involving NK cell cytokine responses with resultant production of other cytokines, such as IL-12-stimulated NK cell production of IFN-γ, are likely to be more complex than currently appreciated. Nevertheless, the perceptive studies defining these pathways in the context of *in vivo* infections have already yielded important principles that will continue to guide our understanding of NK cell cytokine responses to infections.

3.2. Target Killing

Classically, NK cells kill their targets by the triggered release of preformed cytoplasmic granules containing perforin and granzymes, a process termed granule exocytosis *(70)*. Conventionally, it has been thought that perforin polymerizes in the target cell plasma membrane, producing a pore through which the granzymes enter and are then activated to trigger target cell apoptosis. Although recent studies suggest that granzymes may enter the cell via the mannose-6-phosphate receptor, rather than through the perforin-formed pore *(71)*, it is nevertheless clear that both perforin and granzymes are required for the full apoptotic "hit" from granule exocytosis. Recent studies also suggest that NK cells can kill certain targets through other means, including Fas and TNFα-related apoptosis-inducing ligand (TRAIL), but the functional significance of these pathways to *in vivo* infections is not yet clear *(72)*. In addition, resting NK cells apparently do not express Fas ligand on their cell surface, and therefore must be triggered to mediate Fas-induced death *(73)*. Thus, NK cell activation by their targets remains a critical element in the function of NK cells, raising the issue that NK cell receptors specific for infected cells may be important in infection control.

3.2.1. Molecular Basis for NK Cell Recognition of Cellular Targets

To understand how infected cells could trigger NK cells, it is useful to review their spontaneous capacity to kill certain tumor targets, a phenomenon termed *natural killing*. Early studies described an inverse correlation between target cell expression of MHC class I and susceptibility to NK cells *(74)*. Targets that do not express MHC class I are killed by NK cells, whereas MHC class I-bearing targets are generally resistant *(75)*. These studies provided major insights into NK cell recognition, particularly with a teleologic explanation, termed the *missing-self hypothesis*. Kärre *(76)* postulated that NK cells survey tissues for normal expression of MHC class I that is ubiquitously expressed. If a cell lacks expression of MHC class I, such as in tumorigenesis or viral infection, thereby evading MHC class I-restricted T cells, the chronic inhibitory influence of MHC class I is lost, permitting NK cells to lyse the target. This hypothesis suggested a potential rationale for why the inhibitory influence of MHC class I should be a physiologically relevant phenomenon for NK cell function.

3.2.1.1. INHIBITORY RECEPTORS

It is now appreciated that NK cells express MHC class I-specific inhibitory receptors, as first shown by studies on the mouse receptor Ly49A *(77)*. The inhibitory NK cell receptors fall into two general structural types (reviewed in ref. 78). Human killer Ig-like receptors (KIRs) are type I integral membrane proteins with Ig-like domains encoded in the leukocyte receptor complex. By contrast, human and rodent CD94/NKG2A and rodent Ly49 receptors have type II orientation and are disulfide-linked dimers with domains that are distantly related to the C-type lectins and encoded in the NK gene complex (NKC). Despite their structural differences, the inhibitory receptors have several shared features. In addition to relatively restricted expression on NK cells (and NK/T-cells for the C-type lectins), the receptors generally belong to families of highly related molecules. Importantly, all inhibitory receptors to date contain immunoreceptor tyrosine-based inhibitory motifs (ITIMs) in their cytoplasmic domains (reviewed in ref. 79). Upon receptor crosslinking and subsequent ITIM phosphorylation, the ITIMs recruit and activate the cytoplasmic tyrosine phosphatase SHP-1. This recruitment then presumably leads to dephosphorylation of molecules involved in cellular activation, particularly pathways involving immunoreceptor tyrosine-based activation motif (ITAM)-containing signaling chains. These general mechanisms are now appreciated as being applicable to a large number of other inhibitory receptors that are expressed on a wide variety of hematopoietic cells *(79)*.

In contrast to T-cells, NK cell receptors for MHC class I have different requirements for MHC-associated peptides. Some receptors appear to have no peptide selectivity. For example, Ly49A binds its MHC class I ligand regardless of bound peptide, although it does not appear to recognize "empty" MHC class I *(80,81)*. On the other hand, other NK cell receptors have an apparent peptide selectivity *(82,83)*. An appreciation for how peptides could alter recognition is now beginning to be recognized with the crystallization of NK cell receptor-ligand complexes. *(84,85)*, indicating that the NK cell receptors engage MHC class I in a manner distinct from TCR binding.

3.2.1.2. ACTIVATION RECEPTORS

The inhibitory receptors, however, do not explain all aspects of NK cell specificity. NK cell recognition also appears to involve activation receptors, compatible with a two-receptor model for the mechanism of NK cell activation *(86)*. This model predicts that the fate of a target cell is determined by the engagement (or not) of both activation and inhibitory receptors on the NK cell by their target cell ligands and the integration of signals transduced by such receptors. In other words, inhibitory receptors appear to regulate activation receptors (or *vice versa*) that may have their own specificity for ligands on targets. The nature and specificity of putative activation receptors are less well understood.

A number of receptors resembling the inhibitory receptors were identified that do not contain cytoplasmic ITIMs *(87,88)*. Although the cytoplasmic domains of these molecules do not contain obvious signaling motifs, such as ITAMs, crosslinking of several of these molecules appears to stimulate NK cells *(89)*. Interestingly, these ITAM-and ITIM-less molecules generally have charged residues in their transmembrane domains, implying co-association with other molecules. Indeed, co-immunoprecipitation experiments have shown that such receptors are noncovalently associated with proteins that are phosphorylated upon receptor crosslinking or upon pervanadate stimulation *(90)*. Furthermore, a number of candidate activation receptors were identified because of their ability to stimulate NK cell activities when crosslinked by their specific MAbs. For example, crosslinking of the rat NKR-P1 molecule results in NK cell killing of targets that are not usually killed *(91)*.

Recently, Lanier et al. *(92)* identified DAP12 as a signaling chain that is associated with several ITIM-less NK cell receptors with charged transmembrane residues. Like the contribution of the CD3ζ chain to the assembly and signaling of the TCR/CD3 complex, DAP12 is required for efficient expression of putative NK cell activation receptors, such as CD94/NKG2C, Ly49D, and Ly49H *(93,94)*. Moreover, DAP12 is phosphorylated when the associated receptor is crosslinked *(92,95)*. Furthermore, NK cells also express other ITAM-associated signaling chains, including CD3ζ, and FcεRIγ. These signaling chains provide similar functions as DAP12 but they are associated with different ligand-binding receptors, such as CD16 or NKR-P1C *(3,4,96)*.

The downstream signaling consequences of activation receptor engagement have not yet been fully described *(97)*. However, it is likely that the pathway will resemble but be distinct from the tyrosine kinase activation cascade in T- and B-cells. The proximal Syk family tyrosine kinases, ζ-associated protein of 70 kDa (ZAP-70) and Syk itself, are expressed in NK cells and can be phosphorylated upon crosslinking of activation receptors *(95,98)* or exposure to sensitive targets *(99)*. Many of the subsequent downstream effector and adapter molecules are also present, but their contribution to NK cell activities may differ from that in other lymphocytes *(100,101)*. On the other hand, recent studies indicate a role for the phosphoinositide-3-kinase (PI-3-kinase) and mitogen-activated protein kinase (MAPK) pathway in NK cell cytotoxicity against tumor targets *(102)*. In this regard, the C-type lectin-like NK cell receptor NKG2D deserves special mention because it is coupled to DAP10, which has a PI-3-kinase docking site instead of ITAMs *(103,104)*. NKG2D can trigger target lysis by NK cells and also stimulate T-cells that co-express it *(105)*, suggesting that it is an activation receptor that uses a distinct signaling pathway or perhaps is a costimulatory receptor.

Importantly, the ligands for NKG2D are related to MHC class I molecules *(106)*. In humans, these ligands include mononuclear inflammatory cell A (MICA), MICB, and UL binding protein (ULBP) 1, -2, and -3 molecules whereas in mice, they include the RAE1 isoforms and H60 molecules *(107–110)*. With respect to innate immunity, these ligands are particularly notable because they appear to be inducible, and human CMV has evolved molecules that block ligand recognition by NKG2D (see below).

The ligand specificity of other activation receptors is an area under intense investigation. Certainly, some of the activation receptors appear to be responsible for target specificity *(88,111)*. Some of the receptors appear to be specific for MHC class I molecules *(88,112,113)*, although their relationship to inhibitory receptor binding of the same ligand is incompletely understood.

The function of these activation receptors is regulated by the inhibitory receptors. In general, simultaneous engagement of activation and inhibitory receptors is associated with inhibition, indicating that inhibition dominants over activation *(114,115)*. However, the outcome of activation or inhibition is likely to result from a balance between the kinases and phosphatases activated by respective ligand interactions, as revealed by earlier studies demonstrating that NK cell inhibition can be directly correlated to the level of MHC class I expression on the targets *(116)*.

Thus, there is abundant evidence that NK cells express activation receptors that can trigger through their associated signaling chains and that the action of these receptors is regulated by the inhibitory receptors. These activation receptors, originally defined in terms of tumor killing, may be important in NK cell responses in innate immunity.

3.2.2. Evidence for Involvement of NK Cell Activation Receptors in Viral Resistance

Although the role of NK cell activation receptors in NK cell-mediated resistance to infections is just beginning to be understood, several important observations indicate that such receptors are likely to be important in this context. Probably the most significant are from studies of viral evasion tactics. Whereas viruses have evolved numerous strategies to downregulate MHC class I molecules on infected cells to avoid MHC class I-restricted cytotoxic T-lymphocytes *(117)*, this should lead to enhanced susceptibility to NK cell lysis. However, viruses encode proteins that interfere with natural killing *(118–124)*.

In many cases, this interference is caused by enhanced function of inhibitory MHC class I-specific NK cell receptors. For example, human CMV (HCMV) encodes an MHC class I-like molecule (UL18) that interacts with long intergenic region (LIR)-1, inhibitory receptor Ig-like-transcript (ILT)-2, an Ig-SF inhibitory receptor on NK cells. HCMV also encodes a peptide that binds HLA-E, an MHC class Ib molecule that usually binds only leader peptides derived from MHC class Ia molecules. The HCMV peptide permits enhanced expression of HLA-E, which in turn binds CD94/NKG2A, a C-type lectin-like NK cell-inhibitory receptor. Another elegant example of viral evasion of NK cells is the selective downregulation of MHC class I by the human immunodeficiency virus HIV-1 *(118)*. In this case, the virus downregulates HLA-A and B but not HLA-C or E. In HCMV and HIV, therefore, the viruses have evolved mechanisms that result in inhibition owing to selective engagement of both structural types of inhibitory receptors.

Importantly, the inhibitory receptors should not block NK responses to inflammatory cytokines because the inhibitory receptors generally do not affect cytokine receptor signaling; rather, as described above in natural killing of tumors, NK cell inhibitory receptors prevent *in vitro* killing by blocking signals from activation receptors that are coupled to ITAM-containing molecules *(79,125)*, and the transfected expression of the HCMV molecules blocks killing of tumor targets *(121–123)*. These data suggest that viral strategies have evolved to limit NK cell activation receptors involved in target killing.

Consistent with this explanation, viruses have evolved mechanisms to block triggering of NK cell activation receptors directly. In one recent example, the human CMV open reading frame UL16 was seen to bind molecules termed ULBP1, -2, and -3, which are expressed on human tissues *(110)*. In turn, the ULBP molecules bound human NKG2D. Thus UL16 expression on an infected cell may mask recognition of ULBP (Rael) on the same cell and prevent killing by an NKG2D-expressing NK cell *(106)*.

More generally, the Kaposi's sarcoma-associated herpesvirus (KSHV) has also been shown to have a mechanism to avoid NK cells *(124)*. In this case, the KSHV protein K5 downregulates expression of intracellular adhesion molecule (ICAM)-1 and B7-2, which are ligands for NK cell receptors involved in cytotoxicity. Indeed, the interaction of leukocyte function-associated antigen-1 (LFA-1) on the NK cell with ICAM-1 on the target was one of the first receptor-ligand interactions important in NK cell killing of targets to be recognized *(126)*. In contrast to the limited distribution of most NK cell activation and inhibitory receptors, LFA-1 in particular is broadly expressed, and its function is required for target cytotoxicity.

The *in vivo* advantage to the virus of enhancing inhibition or blocking activation is obvious. Conversely, these observations strongly suggest that NK cells should mediate *in vivo* antiviral defense with activation receptors that are functionally related to those used in tumor killing.

3.2.3. An NK Cell Activation Receptor Critical to Viral Resistance

Recent studies indicate that the Ly49H NK cell activation receptor is vital to resistance to MCMV. A genome-wide scan identified that autosomal dominant *Cmvl* resistance gene as being responsible for the genetically determined resistance of certain strains of mice to MCMV *(127)*. Two alleles were identified, resistant and susceptible, or *Cmvl^r* and *Cmvl^s*, respectively. Abundant genetic mapping data from three different approaches (recombinant inbred, backcross panels, and congenic strains) indicated that *Cmvl* maps to the NKC on mouse chromosome 6 *(128–130)*, which contains clusters of genes encoding the C-type lectin-like NK cell receptors *(131)*. These studies implicated NK cell involvement in the resistant phenotype *(131)*. Indeed, when NK cells are depleted with anti-NK1.1 MAB, resistant C57BL/6 *(Cmvl^r)* mice became susceptible *(132)*.

The successful isolation of the *Cmvl^r* allele depended on genetic evidence that the BXD-8 recombinant inbred mouse strain, derived from C57BL/6 and susceptible DBA/2 *(Cmvl^s)* inbred strains, appeared to have inherited the entire NKC and flanking genomic segments from its resistant C57BL/6 progenitor but displayed the susceptible phenotype *(132)*. These mice were subsequently found to lack expression of Ly49H specifically, whereas other NKC-encoded molecules were expressed normally. Furthermore, when resistant C57BL/6 mice were injected with an anti-Ly49H MAb, they became susceptible, as measured by viral titers in the spleen and lethality. These studies suggest that Ly49H is an activation receptor that responds to MCMV-infected cells.

The identification of Ly49H as a resistance factor for MCMV infections also suggests that it may be involved in defense against other pathogens, such as mouse pox (ectromelia) virus and HSV, for which resistance loci have also been genetically mapped to the NKC *(133,134)*. These loci are termed *Rmp1* and *Rhs1*, respectively, and C57BL/6 mice are resistant. However, recent studies have reported that *Rhs1* appears to be segregated independently from *Cmv1 (134)*. Nevertheless, the parallel phenotypes with *Cmv1* strongly suggest that further studies are required to evaluate these phenotypes and determine whether they are related to *Ly49h*.

One hallmark of innate immunity is the involvement of *pattern recognition receptors* (PRRs) on innate immune cells that can discriminate among patterns shared by microbes *(135)* and utilize signaling pathways that are distinct from the Syk family tyrosine kinase pathway stimulated by ITAM-coupled T- and B-cell antigen receptors. For example, the Toll-like receptors recognize pathogen-associated molecular patterns on bacteria; by way of their IL-1R-like cytoplasmic domains, they signal through myeloid differentiation factor 88 (MyD88) and ultimately NF-κB *(136)*. Ly49H, by virtue of DAP12 association and ITAM signaling, does not have an apparent relationship to the PRRs.

Instead, Ly49H more closely resembles antigen receptors on T- and B-cells because of coupling to the Syk family tyrosine kinase (Syk itself and ZAP-70) pathway via ITAM-containing signaling chains. Despite their distinct features, NK cells therefore resemble T- and B-cells in a manner not previoulsy appreciated. In many respects, then, Ly49H has TCR-like properties but is involved in innate host pathogen responses. Furthermore, Ly49H and other NK cell receptors do not require somatic gene rearrangement for receptor expression and are normally expressed and functional in mice with mutations in the recombination machinery *(6)*. In addition, individual NK cells do not express clonally restricted activation receptors but rather express a multitude of receptors such that overlapping subsets of cells express the same receptor *(137)*. This preformed, widely expressed repertoire of receptors appears to confer upon NK cells the capacity for immediate innate response, in contrast to the days required for clonal expansion of antigen receptor-specific T- and B-cells. In this way, like other innate immune cells (macrophages, neutrophils), NK cells can control pathogen invasion during the time in which specific immunity develops. Although this suggests that NK cells do not need to undergo clonal expansion, it is possible that specific NK cell activation may occur along with their more generic, nonspecific activation in response to proinflammatory cytokines.

3.3.3. Specific Stimulation of Cytokine Production

Note that the mechanism presumably triggered by Ly49H engagement has not been elucidated even though the NK cell activation receptors were discussed in this chapter in the context of target killing. Also, NK cells produce cytokines (in response to crosslinking of their activation receptors) and IFN-γ (in response to inflammatory cytokines). It has long been known that crosslinking of NK cell activation receptors such as CD16 leads to cytokine production *(138)*. In addition, whereas engagement of the NK1.1 molecule with an immobilized anti-NK1.1 MAb also results in NK cell production of IFN-γ, TNF-α, and granulocyte/macrophage colony-stimulating factor *(139)*, cytokine production through this receptor can be blocked by engagement of an inhibitory receptor. The contribution of this pathway of cytokine secretion to NK cell function in infection is currently unknown.

3.3. NK Cell Trafficking and Infection

For NK cells to effect target killing, they obviously must be in the physical proximity of their targets. Interestingly, NK cells have a relatively restricted distribution, being predominantly located in the peripheral blood and spleen. In solid organs such as the liver, they appear to be recruited. In the course of MCMV infection, Biron and colleagues *(140,141)* have shown that this recruitment is dependent on the chemokine macrophage inflammatory protein-1α (MIP-1α). In MIP-1α-deficient mice, NK cell migration into the liver and NK cell-dependent IFN-γ production was markedly impaired, whereas spleen NK cell responses were less affected.

The distribution of NK cells and recruitment may be related to organ-specific differences in the NK cell effector mechanism controlling MCMV replication *(142)*. Interestingly, IFN-γ receptor-deficient mice displayed high viral titers in the liver but not the spleen. Conversely, viral replication in the spleen was uncontrolled in perforin-deficient mice, whereas liver MCMV replication was unaffected. The latter phenotype is reminiscent of the effect of *Cmv1* (Ly49H) *(127)*. Since NK cells must be recruited to the liver, and this takes time, antiviral effector responses that do not require precise physical proximity, such as IFN-γ secretion, may be more effective at earlier time points.

4. SUMMARY

Thus far, a number of different infections have been shown to trigger similar cytokine secretion pathways in NK cells, whereas killing of infected targets is still poorly understood. However, recent observations suggest that NK cells use specific activation receptors in resisting infection that resemble the NK cell receptors involved in tumor target killing and are more closely related to the T-cell receptor than receptors on other innate immune cells. The relative contributions of these mechanisms in any given infection remain to be elucidated. The emerging picture suggests that NK cells counter infection by both nonspecific cytokine and specific activation responses.

REFERENCES

1. Trinchieri G. Biology of natural killer cells. Adv Immunol 1989;47:187–376.
2. Yokoyama WM. Natural killer cells. In: Paul WE (ed.). Fundamental Immunology. New York: Lippincott-Raven, 1999, pp. 575–603.
3. Anderson P, Caligiuri M, Ritz J, Schlossman SF. CD3-negative natural killer cells express zeta TCR as part of a novel molecular complex. Nature 1989;341:159–162.
4. Lanier LL, Yu G, Phillips JH. Co-association of CD3 zeta with receptor (CD16) for IgG Fc on human natural killer cells. Nature 1989;342:803–805.
5. Lanier LL, Phillips JH, Hackett J Jr, Tutt M, Kumar V. Natural killer cells: definition of a cell type rather than a function. J Immunol 1986;137:2735–2739.

6. Hackett J Jr, Bosma GC, Bosma MJ, Bennett M, Kumar V. Transplantable progenitors of natural killer cells are distinct from those of T and B lymphocytes. Proc Natl Acad Sci USA 1986;83:3427–3431.

7. Herberman R. NK Cells and Other Natural Effector Cells. New York Academic, 1982.

8. Bancroft GJ. The role of natural killer cells in innate resistance to infection. Curr Opin Immunol 1993;5:503–510.

9. Biron CA, Byron KS, Sullivan JL. Severe herpesvirus infections in an adolescent without natural killer cells. N Engl J Med 1989;320:1731–1735.

10. Jawahar S, Moody C, Chan M, et al. Natural killer (NK) cell deficiency associated with an epitope-deficient Fc receptor type IIIA (CD16-II). Clin Exp Immunol 1996;103:408–413.

11. Rook AH, Masur H, Lane HC, et al. Interleukin-2 enhances the depressed natural killer and cytomegalovirus-specific cytotoxic activities of lymphocytes from patients with the acquired immune deficiency syndrome. J Clin Invest 1983;72:398–403.

12. Bonavida B, Katz J, Gottlieb M. Mechanism of defective NK cell activity in patients with acquired immunodeficiency syndrome (AIDS) and AIDS-related complex. I. Defective trigger on NK cells for NKCF production by target cells, and partial restoration by IL 2. J Immunol 1986;137:1157–1163.

13. Lusso P, Malnati MS, Garzino-Demo A, et al. Infection of natural killer cells by human herpesvirus 6. Nature 1993;362:458–462.

14. Seki H, Ueno Y, Taga K, et al. Mode of in vitro augmentation of natural killer cell activity by recombinant human intereukin 2: a comparative study of Leu-11+ and Leu-11– cell populations in cord blood and adult peripheral blood. J Immunol 1985;135:2351–2356.

15. Cook JL, Ikle DN, Routes BA. Natural killer cell ontogeny in the athymic rat. Relationship between functional maturation and acquired resistance to E1A oncogene-expressing sarcoma cells. J Immunol 1995;155:5512–5518.

16. Greenough A. The TORCH screen and intrauterine infections. Arch Dis Child Fetal Neonatal Ed 1994;70:F163–F165.

17. Ravetch JV, Kinet JP. Fc receptors. Annu Rev Immunol 1991;9:457–491.

18. Hackett J Jr, Tutt M, Lipscomb M, et al. Origin and differentiation of natural killer cells. II. Functional and morphologic studies of purified NK-1.1+ cells. J Immunol 1986;136:3124–131.

19. Georgopoulos K, Bigby M, Wang JH, et al. The Ikaros gene is required for the development of all lymphoid lineages. Cell 1994;79:143–156.

20. DiSanto JP, Muller W, Guy-Grand D, Fischer A, Rajewsky K. Lymphoid development in mice with a targeted deletion of the interleukin 2 receptor gamma chain. Proc Natl Acad Sci USA 1995;92:377–381.

21. Suzuki H, Duncan GS, Takimoto H, Mak TW. Abnormal development of intestinal intraepithelial lymphocytes and peripheral natural killer cells in mice lacking the IL-2 receptor beta chain. J Exp Med 1997;185:499–505.

22. Duncan GS, Mittrucker HW, Kagi D, Matsuyama T, Mak TW. The transcription factor interferon regulatory factor-1 is essential for natural killer cell function in vivo. J Exp Med 1996;184:2043–2048.

23. Ohteki T, Yoshida H, Matsuyama T, et al. The transcription factor interferon regulatory factor 1 (IRF-1) is important during the maturation of NK1.1+ T cell receptor-ab+ (NK1+ T) cells, natural killer cells, and intestinal intraepithelial T cells. J Exp Med 1998;187:967–972.

24. Ogasawara K, Hida S, Azimi N, et al. Requirement for IRF-1 in the microenvironment supporting development of natural killer cells. Nature 1998;391:700–703.

25. Kennedy MK, Glaccum M, Brown SN, et al. Reversible defects in natural killer and memory CD8 T cell lineages in interleukin 15-deficient mice. J Exp Med 2000;191:771–780.

26. Lodolce JP, Boone DL, Chai S, et al. IL-15 receptor maintains lymphoid homeostasis by supporting lymphocyte homing and proliferation. Immunity 1998;9:669–676.

27. Kagi D, Ledermann B, Burki K, et al. Cytotoxicity mediated by T cells and natural killer cells is greatly impaired in perforin-deficient mice. Nature 1994;369:31–37.

28. Walsh CM, Matloubian M, Liu CC, et al. Immune function in mice lacking the perforin gene. Proc Natl Acad Sci USA 1994;91:10854–10858.

29. Lowin B, Beermann F, Schmidt A, Tschopp J. A null mutation in the perforin gene impairs cytolytic T lymphocyte- and natural killer cell-mediated cytotoxicity. Proc Natl Acad Sci USA 1994;91:11571–11575.

30. Ebnet K, Hausmann M, Lehmann-Grube F, et al. Granzyme A-deficient mice retain potent cell-mediated cytotoxicity. EMBO J 1995;14:4230–4239.

31. Heusel JW, Wesselschmidt RL, Shresta S, Russell JH, Ley TJ. Cytotoxic lymphocytes require granzyme B for the rapid induction of DNA fragmentation and apoptosis in allogeneic target cells. Cell 1994;76:977–987.

32. Introne W, Boissy RE, Gahl WA. Clinical, molecular, and cell biological aspects of Chédiak-Higashi syndrome. Mol Genet Metab 1999;68:283–303.

33. Wang B, Biron C, She J, et al. A block in both early T lymphocyte and natural killer cell development in transgenic mice with high-copy numbers of the human CD3E gene. Proc Natl Acad Sci USA 1994;91:9402–9406.

34. Wang BP, Hollander GA, Nichogiannopoulou A, et al. Natural killer cell development is blocked in the context of aberrant T lymphocyte ontogeny. Int Immunol 1996;8:939–949.

35. Kim S, Iizuka K, Aguila HL, Weissman IL, Yokoyama WM. In vivo natural killer cell activities revealed by natural killer cell-deficient mice. Proc Natl Acad Sci USA 2000;97:2731–2736.

36. Grimm EA, Mazumder A, Zhang HZ, Rosenberg SA. Lymphokine-activated killer cell phenomenon. Lysis of natural killer-resistant fresh solid tumor cells by interleukin 2-activated autologous human peripheral blood lymphocytes. J Exp Med 1982;155:1823–1841.

37. Brooks CG, Holscher M, Urdal D. Natural killer activity in cloned cytotoxic T lymphocytes: regulation by interleukin 2, interferon, and specific antigen. J Immunol 1985;135:1145–1152.

38. Gunji Y, Vujanovic NL, Hiserodt JC, Herberman RB, Gorelik E. Generation and characterization of lymphokine-activated killer cells in mice. J Immunol 1989;142:1748–1754.

39. Karlhofer FM, Orihuela MM, Yokoyama WM. Ly-49-independent natural killer (NK) cell specificity revealed by NK cell clones derived from p53-deficient mice. J Exp Med 1995;181:1785–1795.

40. Manoussaka MS, Smith RJ, Conlin V, Toomey JA, Brooks CG. Fetal mouse NK cell clones are deficient in Ly49 expression, share a common broad lytic specificity, and undergo continuous and extensive diversification in vitro. J Immunol 1998;160:2197–21206.

41. Biron CA, Nguyen KB, Pien GC, Cousens LP, Salazar-Mather TP. Natural killer cells in antiviral defense: function and regulation by innate cytokines. Annu Rev Immunol 1999;17:189–220.

42. Shellam GR, Allan JE, Papadimitriou JM, Bancroft GJ. Increased susceptibility to cytomegalovirus infection in beige mutant mice. Proc Natl Acad Sci USA 1981;78:5104–5108.

43. Bukowski JF, Woda BA, Habu S, Okumura K, Welsh RM. Natural killer cell depletion enhances virus synthesis and virus-induced hepatitis in vivo. J Immunol 1983;131:1531–1538.

44. Bukowski JF, Woda BA, Welsh RM. Pathogenesis of murine cytomegalovirus infection in natural killer cell-depleted mice. J Virol 1984;52:119–128.

45. Welsh RM, Dundon PL, Eynon EE, et al. Demonstration of the antiviral role of natural killer cells in vivo with a natural killer cell-specific monoclonal antibody (NK 1.1). Natural Immun Cell Growth Regul 1990;9:112–120.

46. Orange JS, Biron CA. An absolute and restricted requirement for IL-12 in natural killer cell IFN-gamma production and antiviral defense. Studies of natural killer and T cell responses in contrasting viral infections. J Immunol 1996;156:1138–1142.

47. Bancroft GJ, Schreiber RD, Unanue ER. Natural immunity: a T-cell-independent pathway of macrophage activation, defined in the scid mouse. Immunol Rev 1991;124:5–24.

48. Dunn PL, North RJ. Early gamma interferon production by natural killer cells is important in defense against murine listeriosis. Infect Immun 1991;59:2892–2900.

49. Tripp CS, Wolf SF, Unanue ER. Interleukin 12 and tumor necrosis factor alpha are costimulators of interferon gamma production by natural killer cells in severe combined immunodeficiency mice with listeriosis, and interleukin 10 is a physiologic antagonist. Proc Natl Acad Sci USA 1993;90:3725–3729.

50. Tripp CS, Gately MK, Hakimi J, Ling P, Unanue ER. Neutralization of IL-12 decreases resistance to *Listeria* in SCID and C.B-17 mice. Reversal by IFN-gamma. J Immunol 1994;152:1883–1887.

51. Brombacher F, Dorfmuller A, Magram J, et al. IL-12 is dispensable for innate and adaptive immunity against low doses of *Listeria monocytogenes* [In Process Citation]. Int Immunol 1999;11:325–332.

52. Harty JT, Bevan MJ. Specific immunity to *Listeria monocytogenes* in the absence of IFN gamma. Immunity 1995;3:109–117.

53. Huang S, Hendriks W, Althage A, et al. Immune response in mice that lack the interferon-gamma receptor. Science 1993;259:1742–1745.

54. Meraz MA, White JM, Sheehan KC, et al. Targeted disruption of the Stat1 gene in mice reveals unexpected physiologic specificity in the JAK-STAT signaling pathway. Cell 1996;84:431–442.

55. Ohteki T, Fukao T, Suzue K, et al. Interleukin 12-dependent interferon gamma production by CD8alpha+ lymphoid dendritic cells [In Process Citation]. J Exp Med 1999;189:1981–1986.

56. Orange JS, Wang B, Terhorst C, Biron CA. Requirement for natural killer cell-produced interferon gamma in defense against murine cytomegalovirus infection and enhancement of this defense pathway by interleukin 12 administration. J Exp Med 1995;182:1045–1056.

57. Pien GC, Satoskar AR, Takeda K, Akira S, Biron CA. Cutting edge: selective IL-18 requirements for induction of compartmental IFN-gamma responses during viral infection. J Immunol 2000;165:4787–4791.

58. Bukowski JF, Warner JF, Dennert G, Welsh RM. Adoptive transfer studies demonstrating the antiviral effect of natural killer cells in vivo. J Exp Med 1985;161:40–52.

59. Guidotti LG, Chisari FV. Noncytolytic control of viral infections by the innate and adaptive immune response. Annu Rev Immunol 2001;19:65–91.

60. Nguyen KB, Cousens LP, Doughty LA, et al. Interferon α/β-mediated inhibition and promotion of interferon-γ: STAT1 resolves a paradox. Nat Immunol 2000;1:70–76.

61. Waldmann TA, Tagaya Y. The multifaceted regulation of interleukin-15 expression and the role of this cytokine in NK cell differentiation and host response to intracellular pathogens. Annu Rev Immunol 1999;17:19–49.

62. Gosselin J, Tomoiu A, Gallo RC, Flamand L. Interleukin-15 as an activator of natural killer cell-mediated antiviral response. Blood 1999;94:4210–4219.

63. Fawaz LM, Sharif-Askari E, Menezes J. Up-regulation of NK cytotoxic activity via IL-15 induction by different viruses: a comparative study. J Immunol 1999;163:4473–4480.

64. Ahmad A, Sharif-Askari E, Fawaz L, Menezes J. Innate immune response of the human host to exposure with herpes simplex virus type 1: in vitro control of the virus infection by enhanced natural killer activity via interleukin-15 induction. J Virol 2000;74:7196–7203.

65. Tsunobuchi H, Nishimura H, Goshima F, et al. A protective role of interleukin-15 in a mouse model for systemic infection with herpes simplex virus. Virology 2000;275:57–66.

66. Carnaud C, Lee D, Donnars O, et al. Cutting edge: Cross-talk between cells of the innate immune system: NKT cells rapidly activate NK cells. J Immunol 1999;163:4647–4650.

67. Moody DB, Reinhold BB, Guy MR, et al. Structural requirements for glycolipid antigen recognition by CD1b-restricted T cells. Science 1997;278:283–286.

68. Moody DB, Ulrichs T, Muhlecker W, et al. CD1c-mediated T-cell recognition of isoprenoid glycolipids in *Mycobacterium tuberculosis* infection. Nature 2000;404:884–888.

69. Wang LL, Chu DT, Dokun AO, Yokoyama WM. Inducible expression of the gp49B inhibitory receptor on NK cells. J Immunol 2000;164:5215–5220.

70. Henkart PA. Lymphocyte-mediated cytotoxicity: two pathways and multiple effector molecules. Immunity 1994;1:343–346.

71. Motyka B, Korbutt G, Pinkoski MJ, et al. Mannose 6-phosphate/insulin-like growth factor II receptor is a death receptor for granzyme B during cytotoxic T cell-induced apoptosis. Cell 2000;103:491–500.

72. Zamai L, Ahmad M, Bennett IM, et al. Natural killer (NK) cell-mediated cytotoxicity: differential use of TRAIL and Fas ligand by immature and mature primary human NK cells. J Exp Med 1998;188:2375–2380.

73. Bradley M, Zeytun A, Rafi-Janajreh A, Nagarkatti PS, Nagarkatti M. Role of spontaneous and interleukin-2-induced natural killer cell activity in the cytotoxicity and rejection of Fas+ and Fas– tumor cells. Blood 1998;92:4248–4255.

74. Karre K, Ljunggren HG, Piontek G, Kiessling R. Selective rejection of H-2-deficient lymphoma variants suggests alternative immune defence strategy. Nature 1986;319:675–678.

75. Ljunggren HG, Karre K. In search of the 'missing self': MHC molecules and NK cell recognition. Immunol Today 1990;11:237–244.

76. Karre K. Role of target histocompatibility antigens in regulation of natural killer activity: a reevaluation and a hypothesis. In: Herberman RB, Callewaert DM (eds.). Mechanisms of Cytotoxicity by NK Cells. Orlandflo, FL: Academic, 1985, pp. 81–92.

77. Karlhofer FM, Ribaudo RK, Yokoyama WM. MHC class 1 alloantigen specificity of Ly-49+ IL-2-activated natural killer cells. Nature 1992;358:66–70.

78. Yokoyama WM. What goes up must come down: the emerging spectrum of inhibitory receptors. J Exp Med 1997;186:1803–1808.

79. Long EO. Regulation of immune responses through inhibitory receptors. Annu Rev Immunol 1999;17:875–904.

80. Correa l, Raulet DH. Binding of diverse peptides to MHC class 1 molecules inhibits target cell lysis by activated natural killer cells. Immunity 1995;2:61–71.

81. Orihuela M, Margulies DH, Yokoyama WM. The natural killer cell receptor Ly-49A recognizes a peptide-induced conformational determinant on its major histocompatibility complex class 1 ligand. Proc Natl Acad Sci USA 1996;93:11792–11797.

82. Michaelsson J, Achour A, Salcedo M, et al. Visualization of inhibitory Ly49 receptor specificity with soluble major histocompatibility complex class I tetramers. Eur J Immunol 2000;30:300–307.

83. Mandelboim O, Wilson SB, Vales-Gomez M, Reyburn HT, Strominger JL. Self and viral peptides can initiate lysis by autologous natural killer cells. Proc Natl Acad Sci USA 1997;94:4604–4609.

84. Tormo J, Natarajan K, Margulies DH, Mariuzza RA. Crystal structure of a lectin-like natural killer cell receptor bound to its MHC class 1 ligand. Nature 1999;402:623–631.

85. Fan QR, Long EO, Wiley DC. Crystal structure of the human natural killer cell inhibitory receptor KIR2DL1-HLA-Cw4 complex. Nat Immunol 2001;2:452–460.

86. Yokoyama WM. Natural killer cell receptors. Curr Opin Immunol 1995;7:110–120.

87. Smith HRC, Karlhofer FM, Yokoyama WM. Ly-49 multigene family expressed by IL-2-activated NK cells. J Immunol 1994;153:1068–1079.

88. Biassoni R, Cantoni C, Falco M, et al. The human leukocyte antigen (HLA)-C-specific "activatory" or "inhibitory" natural killer cell receptors display highly homologous extracellular domains but differ in their transmembrane and intracytoplasmic portions. J Exp Med 1996;183:645–650.

89. Mason LH, Anderson SK, Yokoyama WM, et al. The Ly-49D receptor activates murine natural killer cells. J Exp Med 1996;184:2119–2128.

90. Mason LH, Willettebrown J, Anderson SK, et al. Characterization of an associated 16-KDa tyrosine phosphoprotein required for Ly-49D signal transduction. J Immunol 1998;160:4148–4152.

91. Chambers WH, Vujanovic NL, DeLeo AB, et al. Monoclonal antibody to a triggering structure expressed on rat natural killer cells and adherent lymphokine-activated killer cells. J Exp Med 1989;169:1373–1389.

92. Lanier LL, Corliss B, Wu J, Phillips JH. Association of DAP12 with activating CD94/NKG2C NK cell receptors. Immunity 1998;8:693–701.

93. Smith KM, Wu J, Bakker AB, Phillips JH, Lanier LL. Cutting edge: Ly-49D and Ly-49H associate with mouse DAP12 and form activating receptors. J Immunol 1998;161:7–10.

94. Bakker AB, Hoek RM, Cerwenka A, et al. DAP12-deficient mice fail to develop autoimmunity due to impaired antigen priming. Immunity 2000;13:345–353.

95. Lanier LL, Cortiss BC, Wu J, Leong C, phillips JH. Immunoreceptor DAP12 bearing a tyrosine-based activation motif is involved in activating NK cells. Nature 1998;391:703–707.

96. Arase N, Arase H, Park SY, et al. Association with FcR-γ is essential for activation signal through NKR-P1 (CD161) in natural killer (NK) cells and NK1.1$^+$ T cells. J Exp Med 1997;186:1957–1963.

97. Brumbaugh KM, Binstadt BA, Leibson PJ. Signal transduction during NK cell activation: balancing opposing forces. Curr Top Microbiol Immunol 1998;230:103–122.

98. Viver E, da Silva AJ, Ackerly M, et al. Association of a 70-kDa tyrosine phosphoprotein with the CD16:zeta:gama complex expressed in human natural killer cells. Eur J Immunol 1993;23:1872–1876.

99. Brumbaugh KM, Binstadt BA, Billadeau DD, et al. Functional role for Syk tyrosine kinase in natural killer cell-mediated natural cytotoxicity. J Exp Med 1997;186:1965–1974.

100. Jevremovic D, Billadeau DD, Schoon RA, et al. Cutting edge: a role for the adaptor protein LAT in human NK cell-mediated cytotoxicity. J Immunol 1999;162:2453–2456.

101. Peterson EJ, Clements JL, Ballas ZK, Koretzky GA. NK cytokine secretion and cytotoxicity occur independently of the SLP-76 adaptor protein. Eur J Immunol 1999;29:2223–2232.

102. Jiang K, Zhong B, Gilvary DL, et al. Pivotal role of phosphoinositide-3 kinase in regulation of cytotoxicity in natural killer cells. Nat Immunol 2000;1:419–425.

103. Wu J, Song Y, Bakker AB, et al. An activating immunoreceptor complex formed by NKG2D and DAP10 [see comments]. Science 1999;285:730–732.

104. Wu J, Cherwinski H, Spies T, Phillips JH, Lanier LL. DAP10 and DAP12 form distinct, but functionally cooperative, receptor complexes in natural killer cells [In Process Citation]. J Exp Med 2000;192:1059–1068.

105. Groh V, Rhinehart R, Randolph-Habecker J, et al. Costimulation of CD8alphabeta T cells by NKG2D via engagement by MIC induced on virus-infected cells. Nat Immunol 2001;2:255–260.

106. Yokoyama WM. Now you see it, now you don't! Nat Immunol 2000;1:95–97.

107. Bauer S, Groh V, Wu J, et al. Activation of NK cells and T cells by NKG2D, a receptor for stress-inducible MICA [see comments]. Science 1999;285:727–729.

108. Diefenbach A, Jamieson AM, Liu SD, Shastri N, Raulet DH. Novel ligands for the murine NKG2D receptor: expression by tumor cells and activation of NK cells and macrophages. Nat Immunol 2000;1:119–126.

109. Cerwenka A, Bakker ABH, McClanahan T, et al. Retinoic acid early inducible genes define a ligand family for the activating NKG2D receptor in mice. Immunity 2000;12:721–727.

110. Cosman D, Mullberg J, Sutherland CL, et al. ULBPs, novel MHC class I-related molecules, bind to CMV glycoprotein UL16 and stimulate NK cytotoxicity through the NKG2D receptor. Immunity 2001;14:123–33.

111. Idris AH, Smith HRC, Mason LH, et al. The natural killer cell complex genetic locus, Chok, encodes Ly49D, a target recognition receptor that activates natural killing. Proc Natl Acad Sci USA 1999;96:6330–6335.
112. Nakamura MC, Linnemeyer PA, Niemi EC, et al. Mouse Ly-49D recognizes H-2Dd and activates natural killer cell cytotoxicity. J Exp Med 1999;189:493–500.
113. George TC, Mason LH, Ortaldo JR, Kumar V, Bennett M. Positive recognition of MHC class I molecules by the Ly49D receptor of murine NK cells. J Immunol 1999,162:2035–2043.
114. Karlhofer FM, Ribaudo RK, Yokoyama WM. The interaction of Ly-49 with H-2Dd globally inactivates natural killer cell cytolytic activity. Trans Assoc Am Physicians 1992;105:72–85.
115. Correa I, Corral L, Raulet DH. Multiple natural killer cell-activating signals are inhibited by major histocompatibility complex class I expression in target cells. Eur J Immunol 1994;24:1323–1331.
116. Storkus WJ, Alexander J, Payne JA, Dawson JR, Cresswell P. Reversal of natural killing susceptibility in target cells expressing transfected class I HLA genes. Proc Natl Acad Sci USA 1989;86:2361–2364.
117. Tortorella D, Gewurz BE, Furman MH, Schust DJ, Ploegh HL. Viral subversion of the immune system. Annu Rev Immunol 2000;18:861–926.
118. Cohen GB, Gandhi RT, Davis DM, et al. The selective downregulation of class I major histocompatibility complex proteins by HIV-1 protects HIV-infected cells from NK cells. Immunity 1999;10:661–671.
119. Reyburn HT, Mandelboim O, Vales-Gomez M, et al. The class I MHC homologue of human cytomegalovirus inhibits attack by natural killer cells. Nature 1997;386:514–517.
120. Farrell HE, Vally H, Lynch DM, et al. Inhibition of natural killer cells by a cytomegalovirus MHC class I homologue in vivo. Nature 1997;386:510–514.
121. Cosman D, Fanger N, Borges L, et al. A novel immunoglobulin superfamily receptor for cellular and viral MHC class I molecules. Immunity 1997;7:273–282.
122. Tomasec P, Braud VM, Rickards C, et al. Surface expression of HLA-E, an inhibitor of natural killer cells, enhanced by human cytomegalovirus gpUL40. Science 2000;287:1031.
123. Ulbrecht M, Martinozzi S, Grzeschik M, et al. Cutting edge: the human cytomegalovirus UL40 gene product contains a ligand for HLA-E and prevents NK cell-mediated lysis. J Immunol 2000;164:5019–5022.
124. Ishido S, Choi JK, Lee BS, et al. Inhibition of natural killer cell-mediated cytotoxicity by Kaposi's sarcoma-associated herpesvirus K5 protein. Immunity 2000;13:365–374.
125. Ravetch JV, Lanier LL. Immune inhibitory receptors. Science 2000;290:84–89.
126. Schmidt RE, Bartley G, Levine H, Schlossman SF, Ritz J. Functional characterization of LFA-1 antigens in the interaction of human NK clones and target cells. J Immunol 1985;135:1020–1025.
127. Scalzo AA, Fitzgerald NA, Simmons A, La Vista AB, Shellam GR. Cmv-1, a genetic locus that controls murine cytomegalovirus replication in the spleen. J Exp Med 1990;171:1469–1483.
128. Scalzo AA, Lyons PA, Fitzgerald NA, et al. Genetic mapping of Cmv1 in the region of mouse chromosome 6 encoding the NK gene complex-associated loci Ly49 and musNKR-P1. Genomics 1995;27:435–441.
129. Forbes CA, Brown MG, Cho R, et al. The Cmv1 host resistance locus is closely linked to the Ly49 multigene family within the natural killer cell gene complex on mouse chromosome 6. Genomics 1997;41:406–413.
130. Depatie C, Muise E, Lepage P, Gros P, Vidal SM. High-resolution linkage map in the proximity of the host resistance locus CMV1. Genomics 1997;39:154–163.
131. Brown MG, Scalzo AA, Matsumoto K, Yokoyama WM. The natural killer gene complex—a genetic basis for understanding natural killer cell function and innate immunity. Immunol Rev 1997;155:53–65.

132. Scalzo AA, Fitzgerald NA, Wallace CR, et al. The effect of the Cmv-1 resistance gene, which is linked to the natural killer cell gene complex, is mediated by natural killer cells. J Immunol 1992;149:581–589.

133. Delano ML, Brownstein DG. Innate resistance to lethal mousepox is genetically linked to the NK gene complex on chromosome 6 and correlates with early restriction of virus replication by cells with an NK phenotype. J Virol 1995;69:5875–5877.

134. Pereira RA, Scalzo A, Simmons A. Cutting edge: a NK complex-linked locus governs acute versus latent herpes simplex virus infection of neurons. J Immunol 2001;166:5869–5873.

135. Medzhitov R, Janeway CA Jr. Innate immune recognition and control of adaptive immune responses. Semin Immunol 1998;10:351–353.

136. Aderem A, Ulevitch RJ. Toll-like receptors in the induction of the innate immune response. Nature 2000;406:782–787.

137. Smith HR, Chuang HH, Wang LL, et al. Nonstochastic coexpression of activation receptors on murine natural killer cells. J Exp Med 2000;191:1341–1354.

138. Cuturi MC, Anegon I, Sherman F, et al. Production of hematopoietic colony stimulating factors by human natural killer cells. J Exp Med 1989;169:569.

139. Kim S, Yokoyama WM. NK cell granule exocytosis and cytokine production inhibited by Ly-49A engagement. Cell Immunol 1998;183:106–112.

140. Salazar-Mather TP, Orange JS, Biron CA. Early murine cytomegalovirus (MCMV) infection induces liver natural killer (NK) cell inflammation and protection through macrophage inflammatory protein 1-alpha (MIP-1-alpha)-dependent pathways. J Exp Med 1998;187:1–14.

141. Salazar-Mather TP, Hamilton TA, Biron CA. A chemokine-to-cytokine-to-chemokine cascade critical in antiviral defense. J Clin Invest 2000;105:985–993.

142. Tay CH, Welsh RM. Distinct organ-dependent mechanisms for the control of murine cytomegalovirus infection by natural killer cells. J Virol 1997;71:267–275.

19

Innate Immune Signaling During Phagocytosis

David M. Underhill

1. INTRODUCTION

Phagocytosis of pathogens is a primitive, general, effective innate immune mechanism of host defense in mammals that also initiates the highly specific adaptive immune response *(1)*. Phagocytosis as a mechanism of innate immune defense has been appreciated since the late 19th century, when Eli Metchnikov first proposed that mobile phagocytic cells survey tissues for foreign particles and engage in pitched battles with potential pathogens *(2)*. In our current view of the process, we understand that specialized professional phagocytes including macrophages, neutrophils, and dendritic cells seek out invading pathogens and then bind, internalize, kill, and degrade them *(1)*. During this process, phagocytes are stimulated to produce cytokines and chemokines that influence the recruitment and activation of additonal cells of the innate and adaptive immune systems, and they upregulate cell surface molecules required for efficient presentation of antigenic pathogen-derived peptides. For several decades we have understood that particle internalization and the elicitation of inflammatory responses can be uncoupled, leading to the hypothesis that the two systems function independently. With our current understanding of the molecular mechanisms regulating particle internalization and the induction of inflammatory responses, it is now clear that there is much overlap in the molecules utilized for both processes and that there is likely to be crosstalk between the systems. The aim of this review is to provide an overview of the mechanisms by which macrophages and other phagocytic cells internalize pathogens and how these processes are coupled to the inflammatory responses associated with them.

Phagocytosis is the process by which particles larger than about 0.5 µm diameter are engulfed by the plasma membrane of a cell and internalized into an intracellular membrane-bound phagosome *(1,3,4)*. In its most general case, the process can be described by the following steps (Fig. 1): (1) receptors on the cell surface recognize and bind to a foreign particle; (2) a signal is generated that induces actin polymerization under the membrane at the site of contact; (3) actin-rich membrane extensions reach out around the particle; (4) the membranes fuse behind the particle, pulling it in towards the center of the cell; and (5) the newly formed phagosome matures into an acidic, hydrolytic compartment. Although this model provides a useful framework in which to discuss phago-

From: *Infectious Disease: Innate Immunity*
Edited by: R. A. B. Ezekowitz and J. A. Hoffmann © Humana Press Inc., Totowa, NJ

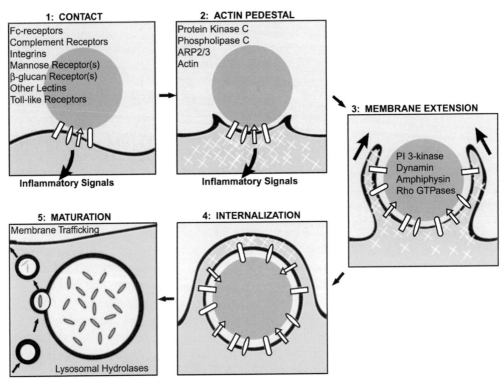

Fig. 1. General steps required for phagocytosis. The model presents features common to internalization mediated by many phagocytic receptors, but many variations on the mechanicm have been observed. PI-3-Kinase, phosphatidyl inositol-3-Kinase.

cytic mechanisms, the precise mechanism of internalization exhibits surprising heterogeneity and depends largely on the type of receptor(s) that participate in particle recognition *(1)*. Thus the above model is largely true for particles internalized via Fc receptors or the mannose receptor, but particles internalized through the complement receptor appear to sink into the cell without significant membrane protrusion and with actin remaining localized to punctate foci around the particle *(5)*. In addition, the immunologic consequences of particle internalization vary; particles internalized by receptors such as the Fc receptor and the mannose receptor evoke potent proinflammatory responses, whereas particles internalized by the complement receptor appear largely silent, and phagocytosis of apoptotic cells induces antiinflammatory responses *(1)*.

The process of phagocytosis lies at the interface of the innate and the adaptive immune systems. Inflammatory responses accompanying pathogen internalization by immune recognition receptors orchestrate the elaboration of the adaptive immune response. Similarly, the adapative immune system utilizes phagocytes as effector cells; antibody-opsonized particles are recognized by Fc receptors on phagocytes, leading to particle internalization and sterilization *(1,6,7)*. Much of the work performed to date on the mechanisms of phagocytosis has focused on Fc receptor-mediated internalization of IgG-opsonized particles, although internalization through innate immune recognition receptors requires many of the same molecules. This review focuses on innate immune phagocytic receptors, the mechanisms by which these receptors trigger particle internalization, and the spatial, temporal, and functional relationship between particle internalization and the nature of the accompanying inflammatory response.

2. RECOGNITION RECEPTORS

Although an extraordinarily broad range of proteins have been implicated in direct recognition of pathogens, relatively few types of innate immune recognition receptors appear to be individually competent to generate signals required for both particle ingestion and inflammatory responses (as is the case for Fc receptors) *(1,4,7)*. Thus, processes accompanying pathogen recognition are likely to be caused by simultaneous engagement of a variety of receptors that together influence phagocyte responses. The principles of pathogen recognition through pattern recognition receptors have been extensively discussed in previous chapters, so the current discussion will remain focused solely on the participation of these receptors in phagocytosis.

2.1. Integrin Receptors

Foreign particles entering the body may be opsonized by a variety of serum proteins including complement iC3b, fibronectin, and vitronection, all of which are recognized by members of the integrin receptor family. Particles coated with iC3b are recognized by the $\alpha_M\beta_2$-integrin (also called complement receptor 3, CD11b/CD18, or Mac1) found on monocytes, macrophages, neutrophils, granulocytes, dendritic cells, and NK cells *(8)*. An additional integrin, $\alpha_X\beta_2$ (also called complement receptor 4, CD11c/CD18, or gp150/95), also binds iC3b-opsonized particles, but this receptor is expressed highly only on tissue macrophages and dendritic cells and has not been as well characterized as $\alpha_M\beta_2$ *(8)*. The extracellular binding domain structure of leukocyte integrins has been extensively studied, and most of the properties of the protein domains have been established. Like other α-integrins, the extracellular domains of α_M and α_X consist of seven tandem repeats that mediate divalent cation binding. Their extracellular domains also contain a 200-amino acid inserted domain (I-domain) that is required by leukocyte β_2-integrins for ligand recognition *(8,9)*. In fact, recombinant α_M I-domain is sufficient for divalent cation-dependent binding to iC3b *(10)*. Proximal to the extracellular face of the membrane, α_M contains a lectin-binding domain that may participate in binding to some types of β-glucan-containing particles *(8,11)* (see discussion below). The extracellular domain of β_2 is shorter than those of the α-chains, consisting of a membrane-proximal cysteine-rich repeat region and a distal region with an insert having some homology to the α-chain I-domain *(8)*.

Leukocyte α- and β-integrins have short 45- and 23-amino acid cytoplasmic tails, respectively, that together mediate intracellular signaling *(12)*. Internalization signaled by $\alpha_M\beta_2$ requires a second activation step (inside-out signaling) that increases the number of receptors at the cell surface *(9,13,14)* and the affinity of the receptors *(15)*, and allows the receptors to trigger phagocytosis *(16–18)*. In vitro, this inside-out signal can be stimulated with phorbol esters and is thus likely to involve protein kinase C (PKC) activation *(1,16)*. Additional evidence presented by Caron et al. *(19)* suggests that activation of Rap1, a small molecular weight GTPase in the Ras family, is required for phorbol myristate acetate (PMA)-stimulated phagocytosis of complement-opsonized particles. Although circulating leukocytes cannot internalize complement-opsonized particles without additional stimulation *(1,9,16)*, the second signal is often likely to be constitutively present in vivo since it can be provided by adhesion to fibronectin-coated surfaces *(16–18)*.

Ligand binding by β_2-integrins including $\alpha_M\beta_2$ induces intracellular signaling that is required for downstream functions including adhesion, migration, and phagocytosis *(12)*. β_2-integrins have been shown to activate intracellular nonreceptor tyrosine kinases such as Syk and the src family of kinases, Fgr, Hck, and Lyn, all kinases extensively implicated in phagocytosis mediated by Fc receptors *(12,20–22)*. β_2-integrins also stimulate directly activation of phosphoinositide-3-kinase (PI-3-kinase), Rho family GTPases, and PKC, all signaling pathways with well-defined roles in phagocytosis *(1,3,4,23)* (see below). During macrophage internalization of complement-opsonized particles, the particles appear to sink into the cell, with little extension of membrane processes, and actin polymerization is stimulated in discrete foci equally spaced around the newly forming phagosome. Additional cytoskeletal proteins including vinculin, α-actinin, and paxillin are recruited to these foci *(5,24)*. This process differs morphologically from Fc receptor-mediated internalization, clearly indicating that mechanistically some differences exist, although ultimately many of the same molecules required for internalization of IgG-opsonized particles are also required for internalization of complement-opsonized particles including F-actin, Arp2/3, PI-3-kinase, and PKC *(5,24–26)*.

Both fibronectin and vitronectin can nonspecifically opsonize pathogens and cell debris, and phagocytes recognize and ingest these particles primarily through $\alpha_5\beta_1$- and $\alpha_v\beta_3$ -integrins *(9)*. Expression of either $\alpha_5\beta_1$ or $\alpha_v\beta_3$ renders cells competent to internalize fibronectin- or vitronectin-coated pathogens, although (as noted for internalization via $\alpha_M\beta_2$) such internalization requires a second signal that can be provided by activation of PKC with phorbol esters *(9,27)*. In a manner that highlights the importance of understanding how multiple simultaneous signals combine to mediate phagocytosis, when $\alpha_5\beta_1$ and $\alpha_v\beta_3$ are expressed together, $\alpha_5\beta_1$ primarily mediates internalization, whereas antibody-mediated ligation of $\alpha_v\beta_3$ blocks internalization by inhibiting the high-affinity function of $\alpha_5\beta_1$ *(9,27)*. This inhibition requires serine phosphorylation of the β_3 cytoplasmic tail, although the precise nature of the signal is not clear *(28)*. The inhibitory signal may be in part owing to the association of $\alpha_v\beta_3$ with CD47 [also called integrin associated protein (IAP)], a G-protein-coupled receptor that has been implicated in thrombospondin-induced inhibition of inflammatory signaling *(29,30)* and, through its ligand CD47-signal regulatory protein-α (SIRP-α), inhibition of both Fc and complement receptor-mediated phagocytosis *(31–33)*. Intriguingly, $\alpha_v\beta_3$ and another vitronectin-binding integrin, $\alpha_v\beta_5$, can interact with CD36, a class B scavenger receptor CD36 (see below), to mediate thrombospondin-facilitated phagocytosis of apoptotic cells, a process that is accompanied by the elicitation of antiinflammatory cytokines *(34,35)*. Thus, integrin engagement activates multiple downstream signaling pathways that can mediate particle internalization and are also likely to be involved in mediating inflammatory responses.

2.2. Mannose Receptor

The macrophage mannose receptor is a type I transmembrane protein with a short, 45-amino acid cytoplasmic tail. The extracellular domain of the receptor consists of eight C-type lectin carbohydrate recognition domains (CRDs) together with a short amino-terminal cysteine-rich region and a fibronectin type II repeat. Expression of mannose receptor in normally nonphagocytic COS cells is sufficient to mediate internalization of zymosan, a yeast cell wall particle made up primarily of α-mannan/mannoproteins and β-glucans *(36,37)*. Importantly, expression of tailless mutant mannose receptor mediated zymosan binding but not internalization *(38)*, expression of a chimeric receptor consisting of the extracellular domain of FcγRI fused to the transmembrane and intracellular domain of the mannose receptor, faciliated uptake of IgG-opsonized particles *(39)*. Together these observations indicate that signals initiated by mannose receptor ligation are sufficient to induce particle internalization. The molecular mechanisms by which mannose receptors activate downstream signals for particle internalization have not yet been described.

2.3. β-Glucan Receptor

Soluble forms of both α-mannan and β-glucan inhibit phagocytosis of zymosan by macrophages, suggesting that receptors for both of these sugars participate in particle recognition and uptake *(40–43)*. Although the mannose receptor almost certainly accounts for the mannose-inhibitable phagocytic activity seen in some types of macrophages, the identity of the β-glucan receptor is less clear. The α_M-chain of complement receptor 3 has a high-affinity (5×10^{-8} M) β-glucan binding site, suggesting that this receptor may also be the functional β-glucan receptor *(8)*. Indeed, antibodies to $\alpha_M\beta_2$ block binding and internalization of unopsonized zymosan *(44)*, and patients with a deficiency in β_2-integrins show defects in phagocytosis of unopsonized zymosan *(45)*. However, it is possible that the effects of $\alpha_M\beta_2$ inhibition on zymosan phagocytosis are owing to signals originating from $\alpha_M\beta_2$ that modulate the affinity, expression, or function of another β-glucan receptor that mediates internalization.

2.4. Scavenger Receptors

The scavenger receptors are a family of receptors defined initally by their ability to bind and internalize modified lipoproteins such as acetylated low-density lipoprotein, although the spectrum of targets recognized by these receptors has grown to include such diverse ligands as polyribonucleotides, lipopolysaccharide (LPS), and silica particles *(46)*. There is ample evidence that several scavenger receptors participate in phagocytosis. Macrophages from mice lacking scavenger receptor A are significantly less efficient at phagocytosing heat-killed *E. coli (47,48)*. An additional member of the class A scavenger receptors, macrophage structure with collagenous structure (MARCO), has been described that is expressed constitutively on certain subpopulations of macrophages such as those in the marginal zone of the spleen *(49)* and can be induced in other macrophage populations by exposure to inflammatory stimuli such as LPS *(50)*. MARCO binds to a variety of particles including Gram-positive, Gram-negative bacteria and artificial particles such as latex, and antibodies to MARCO significantly block internalization of each of these targets *(50,51)*. CD36 (a class B scavenger receptor) is required for phagocytosis of apoptotic cells by macrophages and dendritic cells *(34,35)*. A CD36-related protein, croquemort, is also required for phagocytosis of apoptotic cells in *Drosophila,* suggesting a long evolutionary history for these receptors in mediating particle ingestion *(52)*. Scavenger receptors clearly mediate clearance of soluble ligands such as acetylated low-density lipoprotein by triggering receptor-mediated endocytosis, but there is no evidence that scavenger receptors are capable of generating a phagocytic signal directly. Indeed, as discussed above, expression of the mannose receptor or complement receptor 3 in nonphagocytic cells can make the cells competent to internalize targets, but expression of scavenger receptors mediates binding without notable internalization *(47,49,50)*. Thus, during phagocytosis, it is likely that scavenger receptors participate in holding target particles long enough for other receptors to bind and signal internalization.

3. SIGNALING MECHANISMS FOR PARTICLE INTERNALIZATION

Particle internalization requires activation of a number of signaling pathways that together orchestrate rearrangement of the actin cytoskeleton, extension of the plasma membrane, and fusion to form a phagosome. Although some signaling molecules such as PI-3-kinase appear to be required for internalization mediated by any phagocytic receptor, other proteins such as tyrosine kinases are required for some types of internalization and not others (see below). In addition, many of the same molecules that orchestrate the mechanics of particle ingestion also participate in signaling events leading to gene transcription and protein secretion, alterations in cell morphology, and activation of antimicrobial mechanisms. The extensive overlap in signaling molecules utilized for these different processes and the recruitment of these molecules together to phagosomes makes it likely that the different signaling pathways interact functionally. A number of these signaling molecules are discussed in this section, and a direct discussion of functional interactions between phagocytic and inflammatory signaling follows in the next section.

3.1. Tyrosine Kinases

Tyrosine phosphorylation of phagosome-associated and cytosolic proteins accompanies all types of phagocytosis, suggesting that many types of phagocytic receptors stimulate tyrosine kinase activation *(1,7,9,12)*. However, an absolute requirement for tyrosine kinase activation has been demonstrated only for internalization of IgG-opsonized particles by Fc receptors *(5,24)*. Upon ligation, the immunoreceptor tyrosine-based activation motifs (ITAMs) of Fc receptors are phosphorylated by src family tyrosine kinases, and this probably accounts for the blockade imposed by tyrosine kinase inhibitors. Indeed, macrophages from syk-deficient mice fail to internalize IgG-opsonized particles *(53)*. The requirement for tyrosine kinase activation during internalization through innate immune recognition receptors is less clear. Macrophages from syk-deficient mice internalize complement-opsonized particles, bacteria, and zymosan normally *(53)*. Although general tyrosine kinase inhibitors do not block internalization of particles such as complement-opsonized particles or bacteria, these inhibitors do reduce the efficiency of uptake, suggesting that other tyrosine kinases might be tangentially involved *(5,54)*. In addition, proinflammatory responses initiated during phagocytosis through innate immune recognition receptors require tyrosine kinase activation, and some of this requirement can be attributed to activation of mitogen-activated protein (MAP) kinases *(55)*.

3.2. Protein Kinase C

Of the 12 isoforms of PKC described, at least 5 (PKC-α, -β, -ϵ, -δ, and -ζ) are expressed in macrophages and are recruited to membranes during phagocytosis, where their activities are required for particle internalization *(56–58)*. General inhibitors of PKC activity inhibit internalization of IgG-opsonized, and complement-opsonized particles as well as unopsonized zymosan particles *(56,59)*. PKC is required at the earliest stages of particle internalization since inhibition of PKC blocks the formation of actin filaments beneath the site of particle binding (Fig. 1) *(56)*. Thus, activation of PKC is a general requirement for phagocytosis through a broad variety of receptors. Downstream effects of PKC activation include phosphorylation of myristoylated alanine-rich protein kinase C substrate (MARCKS) family proteins and activation of integrin receptors *(1)*. MARCKS proteins regulate actin cytoskeletal interactions with the plasma membrane and have been associated with phagocytosis and membrane trafficking *(60)*. As discussed above, PKC-mediated activation of integrin receptors like the $\alpha_M\beta_2$ complement receptor is required for phagocytosis through these receptors. Intriguingly, PKCs are also required for cytokine production and antimicrobial activation induced by a variety of stimuli; LPS-induced production of cyclooxygenase-2 (COX-2), tumor necrosis factor-α (TNF-α), and interleukin-1β (IL-1β) and activation of the respiratory burst are blocked by pharmacologic inhibitors of PKC *(61–64)*. Similarly, expression of a dominant-negative negative PKC-α in macrophages inhibits LPS- and Fc receptor-induced cytokine production *(64–66)*. Other PKC isoforms probably mediate particle ingestion, since DN-PKC-α expression and depletion of Ca^{2+} (required for activation of classic PKCs such as PKC-α and PKC-β) do not effect internalization of IgG-opsonized particles *(67)*. The same separation of duties probably applies to internalization through innate immune recognition receptors, since DN-PKC-α expression does not alter internalization of a variety of pathogens including *Leishmania. donovani, Legionella pneumophila,* and *Pseudomonas aeruginosa (66)*.

3.3. Phosphoinositide Signaling

One classic mechanism for activation of PKCs is through phospholipase C (PLC)-mediated cleavage of phosphatidyl inositol-4, 5-biphosphate [PI(4,5)P$_2$] to release inositol triphosphate (IP$_3$) and diacylqlycerol (DAG), second messengers that mobilize intracellular Ca^{2+} stores and activate PKC family members, respectively. PLC is recruited to phagosomes containing IgG-opsonized particles, and inhibition of its activity blocks particle internalization *(68)*. Like PKC inhibitors, PLC inhibitors completely block the formation of actin filaments beneath the site of particle contact (Fig. 1), strongly suggesting that the main role of PLC in particle internalization is to activate PKC *(68)*.

(PI-3-kinase) catalyzes phosphorylation of PI(4,5)P$_2$ to PI(3,4,5)P$_3$, a phospholipid important in recruiting signaling molecules such as the kinase autologous tumor killing (AKT) protein kinase B (PKB) to specific regions of membranes *(69)*. Inhibitors of PI-3-kinase block phagocytosis of a broad spectrum of particles including IgG- and complement-opsonized particles, unopsonized zymosan, and bacteria, clearly demonstrating a universal role for PI-3-kinase activation in particle internalization *(70–73)*. Blockade of PI-3-kinase does not inhibit particle binding or initial actin polymerization beneath the particle (Fig. 1), suggesting that initial phagocytic signaling is intact. Instead, PI-3-kinase is required for membrane extension and fusion behind the particle, perhaps owing to a failure to insert new membrane at the site of particle internalization *(72,73)*.

Although PI-3-kinase and PLC activation are required for the mechanical aspects of particle internalization, they are also implicated in proinflammatory signaling induced by particulate stimuli. Thus, PI-3-kinase is recruited to Toll-like receptors when cells are stimulated with heat-killed *Staphylococcus aureus,* and activation of PI-3-kinase has been implicated in inducing translocation of NF-κB to the nucleus and the induction of cytokine production in macrophages by pathogens *(74)*. Similarly, PLC activity is required for proinflammatory signaling in macrophages, primarily through participation in MAP kinase pathway activation *(75,76)*.

3.4. Rho Family of GTPases

Members of the Rho family of small molecular weight GTPases are key regulators of the actin cytoskeleton, and recent studies demonstrate a central role for these proteins in phagocytosis *(23)*. Like other small molecular weight GTPases, Rho proteins cycle between an inactive GDP-bound state and an active GTP-bound state. Activation is stimulated by GDP-GTP exchange factors, whereas GTPase-activating proteins (GAPs) inactivate the proteins *(23)*. Rho family members Cdc42, Rac, and Rho coordinate actin dynamics during cell adhesion and motility, and they participate in a variety of signaling cascades including activation of MAP kinases and activation of transcription factors such as activator protein (AP)-1 *(23,77)*. The role of Rho family members at the intersection of the actin cytoskeleton and intracellular signaling makes these proteins particularly intriguing candidates for molecules that may couple phagocytosis to inflammatory responses.

Expression of inhibitory mutants of Cdc42 and Rac1 proteins blocks internalization of IgG-opsonized particles by macrophages and mast cells *(78–81)*, demonstrating a role for these proteins in Fc receptor-mediated phagocytosis. Intriguingly, expression of inhibitory Cdc42 and Rac does not inhibit internalization of complement-opsonized particles *(78)*. Rho appears not to be required for Fc receptor-mediated phagocytosis, since expression of C3 transferase, a Rho-specific inhibitor, does not block internalization of IgG-opsonized particles, whereas C3 transferase does block internalization of complement-opsonized particles *(78)*. Although the roles of Rho family proteins in phagocytosis through other specific innate immune recognition receptors has not yet been studied, it is clear that Rho family proteins play a central role in internalization of unopsonized bacteria, since a number of pathogenic bacteria have evolved mechanisms to regulate Rho family GTPases as a means of avoiding immune clearance *(3)*. Thus, *Yersinia* species avoid phagocytosis by host immune cells in part by secreting (via a type III secretion system) a protein called YopE into the cytoplasm of host cells. YopE is a GAP for Cdc42, Rac, and Rho and thus rapidly deactivates these proteins thereby inhibiting the actin rearrangements necessary for phagocytosis *(3,82)*. Similarly, *P. aeruginosa* secretes a protein with Rho family GAP activity called ExoT into host cell cytoplasm to avoid uptake and clearance *(3,83)*.

4. COUPLING INTERNALIZATION TO INFLAMMATORY RESPONSES

Particle internalization by phagocytes is often accompanied by the production of inflammatory mediators and the activation of antimicrobial mechanisms, and the coordination of these responses is crucial for an effective, controlled innate immune response. The molecular mechanisms that mediate particle ingestion share much in common with the mechanisms that mediate many inflammatory responses. Thus, tyrosine kinases, PKC, and Rho family GTPases all have roles in phagocytosis and proinflammatory signaling. However, relatively few phagocytic receptors are themselves capable of eliciting both phagocytic and inflammatory responses. It is clear that ligation of Fc receptors is sufficient to induce both the morphologic rearrangements required for particle internalization and the production and release of inflammatory mediators *(6,7)*. Cytoplasmic tails of activating Fc receptors contain ITAMs that when clustered become phosphorylated by src family kinases, leading to recruitment of syk family kinases, activation of PI-3-kinase, calcium influx, and activation of MAP kinases *(6)*. Different phagocytic receptors often function cooperatively, making it sometimes inappropriate to pin inflammatory responses on individual receptors; thus, despite the above description of Fc receptor-induced responses, it is interesting to note that in patients with leukocyte adhesion deficiency (a deficit in β_2-integrins), IgG-opsonized particles are internalized less efficiently, and the accompanying inflammatory responses are muted *(84,85)*. It is clear that cooperation between receptors involved in phagocytosis occurs both at the level of direct interaction between their downstream signaling components and by their co-association with phagosomes.

4.1. Superoxide Production

Professional phagocytes including monocytes, macrophages, and especially neutrophils kill newly internalized pathogens in part by the production of caustic reactive superoxide ions. Production of superoxide can be induced by soluble stimuli such as PMA, N-formyl-methionyl-leucyl-phenylalanine (FMLP), or calcium ionophores that induce assembly of the reduced nicotinamide adenine dinucleotide phosphate (NADPH) oxidase on plasma membranes, whereas during phagocytosis, assembly of the NADPH oxidase on phagosomal membranes stimulates localized production of superoxide *(86–88)*. This localized production of superoxide during phagocytosis is presumably beneficial since an immune cell would not want to induce this killing mechanism until the pathogen is confined to the phagosome, where locally high superoxide concentrations can be generated with as little collateral damage to the surrounding tissue as possible. The signaling components required to activate the oxidase vary depending on the receptor system activated, but there is remarkable overlap between these components and the signaling molecules required for particle internalization *(88)*. In unstimulated cells, components of the NADPH oxidase are distributed in the membrane (gp91[phox] and p22[phox]) and in the cytosol (p67[phox], p40[phox], p47[phox], and Rac2). Upon stimulation, phosphorylation of p47[phox] induces translocation of a trimeric p67[phox], p40[phox], p47[phox] cytosolic complex to the membrane components (Fig. 2) *(86)*. A number of different kinases including PKC, protein kinase A (PKA), p21-activated kinase (PAK), and PI-3-kinase-stimulated kinases can phosphorylate p47[phox] and are required for activation of the complex *(88)*. Independently Rac2, activated by a GDP-GTP exchange factor, also translocates to the membrane complex, where it is required for electron transfer in the active complex *(89)*. Besides the phox proteins, all these proteins are also important regulators of the actin cytoskeleton, and nearly all stimuli that activate the oxidase also induce profound alterations in the actin

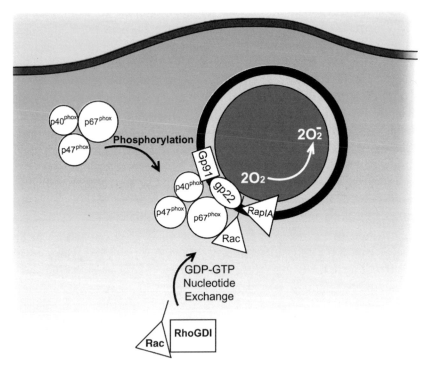

Fig. 2. Assembly of the NADPH oxidase on phagosomal membranes.

cytoskeleton *(86,88)*. In some cases, disruption of the actin cytoskeleton blocks activation of the oxidase by particulate stimuli *(90,91)*. The connection to the actin cytoskeleton is strengthened by the observation that in the cytosol, p40phox and p67phox are associated with coronin, another protein that plays an important role in regulation of the actin cytoskeleton and that strongly localizes to forming phagosomes *(92,93)*.

Despite several shared signaling pathways and a mutual requirement for regulation of the actin cytoskeleton, superoxide production is not inexorably linked to phagocytosis. It has long been known that internalization thought the complement receptor 3 in macrophages is not accompanied by the production of superoxide *(94,95)*. In addition, downregulation of receptor systems required for internalization of nonopsonized zymosan does not block internalization of serum-opsonized zymosan or IgG-opsonized particles, but it does block NADPH oxidase activation by these particles *(96)*. Thus, phagocytosis can clearly occur without inducing superoxide production. Conversely, several soluble stimuli including PMA and FMLP can induce NADPH oxidase activation without concurrent phagocytosis *(86,88)*.

Although crosslinking of Fc receptors is sufficient to induce superoxide production and phagocytosis *(1,88)*, and phagocytosis through complement receptor 3 is not accompanied by NADPH oxidase activation *(94,95)*, it is less clear whether NADPH oxidase activation is stimulated directly by other innate immune phagocytic receptors. It has generally been reported that ligation of the mannose receptor is sufficient to induce a respiratory burst, but these studies have depended on delivery of complex particles to macrophages, making it difficult to be certain which receptors delivered which signals *(97,98)*. In one recent report Maridonneau-Parini and co-workers *(99)* suggest that mannose receptor-mediated phagocytosis does not induce microbicidal mechanisms. They observed that trimannoside-coated latex beads were internalized by human peripheral blood-derived macrophages by a mechanism that was fully inhibitable by soluble mannan but did not induce superoxide production *(99)*. In addition, this group demonstrated that zymosan internalization was partially inhibitable by soluble mannan and soluble β-glucan (laminarin) but that zymosan-induced superoxide production was only inhibited by laminarin, suggesting that whereas the mannose receptor does not activate the oxidase, the β-glucan receptor does.

Integrin ligation can be linked to NADPH oxidase stimulation, but it is highly dependent on the type of integrin, the cell type examined, and whether the cells have been exposed to a priming stimulus. Resting neutrophils challenged with immobilized antibodies to leukocyte function-associated antigen-1 (LFA-1, $\alpha_L\beta_2$) or to CR4 (gp150/95, $\alpha_x\beta_2$) produce superoxide, whereas stimulation through CR3 ($\alpha_M\beta_2$) does not *(90)*. In macrophages, CR3 stimulation does not activate the oxidase *(94,95)* whereas in eosinophils, ligation of LFA-1 and CR3 both do *(100)*. The variability in responses to receptor ligation suggests that in different cell types, integrins signal differently, or that oxidase activation is regulated by the presence or absence of another co-receptor. Interestingly, CD14, a surface molecule required for LPS binding, physically interacts with $\alpha_M\beta_2$ and Toll-like receptor 4 (TLR4, discussed in previous chapters of this volume), and $\alpha_M\beta_2$ is necessary for efficient activation of some LPS-induced responses *(101–103)*. It is possible that in some cases $\alpha_M\beta_2$ ligation might activate TLR4-mediated inflammatory responses.

4.2. Cytokine and Chemokine Production

Activation of gene transcription during phagocytosis is a critical feature of the development of an effective immune response, and in order to detect pathogen-derived products, innate immune recognition receptors must have access to their ligands. Since many pathogen-derived products recognized by the innate immune system such as peptidoglycan or bacterial DNA are presumably not displayed on the surface of pathogens, they become accessible only after killing and lysis of the cell, making phagocytosis and killing an integral part of the recognition mechanism. We have demonstrated that members of the TLR family are actively recruited to phagosomes during pathogen internalization, where they sample the contents of the phagosome to determine the nature of the pathogen being ingested (Fig. 3) *(104,105)*. Recruitment of TLRs to phagosomes provides a mechanism by which phagocytosis and associated inflammatory responses can be linked, although recruitment does not require TLR activation. TLRs are also recruited to phagosomes during internalization of IgG-opsonized particles by Fc receptors, a process that does not require TLR activation, suggesting that TLR recruitment is a general feature of phagocytosis and that TLRs are simply poised to recognize ligands should they become present in the phagosome *(104)*. This mechanism implies that particle internalization and inflammatory responses can be dissociated. Indeed, inhibition of particle internalization with the PI-3-kinase inhibitor wortmannin, or by expression of dominant negative dynamin, does not block TNF-α production induced by zymosan *(73)*. Conversely, inhibition of TLR2, a receptor required for inflammatory responses to zymosan, does not block phagocytosis of zymosan *(105)*.

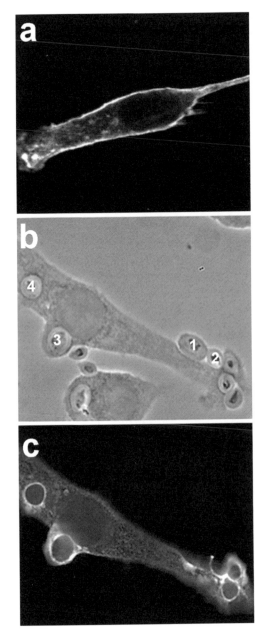

Fig. 3. Toll-like receptor recruitment to phagosomes. **(a)** Epitope-tagged Toll-like receptor 2 expressed in macrophages localizes to the plasma membrane. **(b,c)** During phagocytosis of zymosan particles (numbered), the receptor is recruited to sites of particle contact and is highly enriched on phagosomes. (From Underhill et al., *Nature* 1999, 401:811–815.With permission).

Despite the ability to dissociate the two processes, there remains a remarkable overlap in the signaling molecules whose activation is required for particle internalization and those activated during proinflammatory signaling; this overlap suggests that at some level it is likely that signaling by phagocytic receptors can influence or modify proinflammatory signaling through other receptors. As noted above, TLR4 functionally interacts with $\alpha_M\beta_2$, and Vogel and co-workers *(103)* have demonstrated that macrophages from mice lacking β_2 integrins respond normally to LPS with respect to induction of some genes such as TNF-α and interferon-inducible protein-10 (IP-10), but are deficient in LPS-induced activation of genes such as COX-2, IL-12 p40, and IL-12 p35. Thus, the two receptors cooperate in generating the ultimate inflammatory response.

The mannose receptor has often been reported to stimulate cytokine production, since zymosan and derived products can stimulate macrophages *(106–108),* although the role of the mannose receptor in these responses is complicated by the ability of zymosan also to interact with a β-glucan receptor. Despite the apparent role for multiple lectin receptors in zymosan binding and internalization, we have demonstrated that macrophage inflammatory responses to zymosan are mediated by cooperative interactions between TLR2 and TLR6 *(104,105)*. Thus, expression of dominant negative TLR2 or TLR6 in macrophages blocks zymosan-induced activation of NF-κB and production of TNF-α *(104,105)*. It is likely that various recognition receptors may cooperate in the ultimate generation of proinflammatory responses, and it is not yet clear how TLRs and lectin receptors interact. It is possible that signals originating from a variety of receptors synergize to produce the observed responses. Alternately, additional receptor signaling pathways could modulate the precise nature of a TLR-mediated signals. Such an interaction may account for the apparent role of the mannose receptor and the β-glucan receptor in the induction of specific inflammatory genes.

5. CONCLUSIONS

Phagocytosis requires activation of complex signaling networks that develop over time to mediate internalization of pathogens. Similarly, proinflammatory signaling requires activation of complex signaling networks that determine the nature of the cellular response. The two processes are intrinsically linked in space and time and utilize many of the same signaling components. As our ability to study complex systems progresses, a complete molecular understanding of the interactions will provide better tools for intervention when innate immunity goes awry or would benefit from strategic activation.

ACKNOWLEDGMENTS

I would like to thank Alan Aderem, Adrian Ozinsky, Tom Hawn, and Adam Rupper for critical reading of the manuscript and Tatiana Gill for assistance with the illustrations. This work was supported by the National Institutes of Health, grant GM62995.

REFERENCES

1. Aderem A, Underhill DM. Mechanisms of phagocytosis in macrophages. Annu Rev Immunol 1999;17:593–623.
2. Stossel TP. The early history of phagocytosis. In: Gordon S (ed.). *Phagocytosis: The Host.* Stamford CT: JAI Press, 1999, pp. 3–18.
3. Ernst JD. Bacterial inhibition of phagocytosis. Cell Microbiol 2000;2:379–386.
4. Greenberg S. Modular components of phagocytosis. J Leukoc Biol 1999;66:712–717.
5. Allen LA, Aderem A. Molecular definition of distinct cytoskeletal structures involved in complement- and Fc receptor-mediated phagocytosis in macrophages. J Exp Med 1996;184:627–637.

6. Ravetch JV, Clynes RA. Divergent roles for Fc receptors and complement in vivo. Annu Rev Immunol 1998;16:421–432.

7. Daeron M. Fc receptor biology. Annu Rev Immunol 1997;15:203–234.

8. Ross GD. Regulation of the adhesion versus cytotoxic functions of the Mac-1/CR3/alphaM-beta2-integrin glycoprotein. Crit Rev Immunol 2000;20:197–222.

9. Blystone SD, Brown EJ. Integrin receptors of phagocytes. In *Phagocytosis: The Host.* S. Gordon, editor. Stamford, CT: JAI Press, 1999;103–147.

10. Ueda T, Rieu P, Brayer J, Arnaout MA. Identification of the complement iC3b binding site in the beta 2 integrin CR3 (CD11b/CD18). Proc Natl Acad Sci USA 1994;91:10680–10684.

11. Xia Y, Ross GD. Generation of recombinant fragments of CD11b expressing the functional beta-glucan-binding lectin site of CR3 (CD11b/CD18). J Immunol 1999;162:7285–7293.

12. Dib K. BETA 2 integrin signaling in leukocytes. Front Biosci 5:D438–D451.

13. Berger M, O'Shea J, Cross AS, et al. Human neutrophils increase expression of C3bi as well as C3b receptors upon activation. J Clin Invest 1984;74:1566–1571.

14. Sengelov H, Kjeldsen L, Diamond MS, Springer TA, Borregaard N. Subcellular localization and dynamics of Mac-1 (alpha m beta 2) in human neutrophils. J Clin Invest 1993;92:1467–1476.

15. Jones SL, Knaus UG, Bokoch GM, Brown EJ. Two signaling mechanisms for activation of alphaM beta2 avidity in polymorphonuclear neutrophils. J Biol Chem 1998;273:10556–10566.

16. Wright SD, Griffin FM, Jr. Activation of phagocytic cells' C3 receptors for phagocytosis. J Leukoc Biol 1985;38:327–339.

17. Wright SD, Craigmyle LS, Silverstein SC. Fibronectin and serum amyloid P component stimulate C3b- and C3bi-mediated phagocytosis in cultured human monocytes. J Exp Med 1983;158:1338–1343.

18. Pommier CG, Inada S, Fries LF, et al. Plasma fibronectin enhances phagocytosis of opsonized particles by human peripheral blood monocytes. J Exp Med 1983;157:1844–1854.

19. Caron E, Self AJ, Hall A. The GTPase Rap1 controls functional activation of macrophage integrin alphaMbeta2 by LPS and other inflammatory mediators. Curr Biol 2000;10:974–978.

20. Lowell CA, Fumagalli L, Berton G. Deficiency of Src family kinases p59/61hck and p58c-fgr results in defective adhesion-dependent neutrophil functions. J Cell Biol 1996;133:895–910.

21. Yan SR, Huang M, Berton G. Signaling by adhesion in human neutrophils: Activation of the p72syk tyrosine kinase and formation of protein complexes containing p72syk and Src family kinases in neutrophils spreading over fibrinogen. J Immunol 1997;158:1902–1910.

22. Fernandez R, Suchard SJ. Sky activation is required for spreading and H_2O_2 release in adherent human neutorphils. J Immunol 1998;160:5154–5162.

23. Chimini G, Chavrier P. Function of Rho family proteins in actin dynamics during phagocytosis and engulfment. Nat Cell Biol 2000;2:E191–196.

24. Allen LA, Aderem A. Mechanisms of phagocytosis. Curr Opin Immunol 1996;8:36–40.

25. May RC, Caron E, Hall A, Machesky LM. Involvement of the Arp2/3 complex in phagocytosis mediated by FcgammaR or CR3. Nat Cell Biol 2000;2:246–248.

26. Cox D, Dale BM, Kashiwada M, Helgason CD, Greenberg S. A regulatory role for Src homology 2 domain-containing inositol 5′-phosphatase (SHIP) in phagocytosis mediated by Fc gamma receptors and complement receptor 3 (alpha(M)beta(2); CD11b/CD18). J Exp Med 2001;193:61–71.

27. Blystone SD, Graham IL, Lindberg FP, Brown EJ. Integrin alpha v beta 3 differentially regulates adhesive and phagocytic functions of the fibronectin receptor alpha 5 beta 1. J Cell Biol 1994;127:1129–1137.

28. Blystone SD, Lindberg FP, LaFlamme SE, Brown EJ. Integrin beta 3 cytoplasmic tail is necessary and sufficient for regulation of alpha 5 beta 1 phagocytosis by alpha v beta 3 and integrinassociated protein. J Cell Biol 1995;130:745–754.

29. Frazier WA, Gao AG, Dimitry J, et al. The thrombospondin receptor integrin-associated protein (CD47) functionally couples to heterotrimeric Gi. J Biol Chem 1999;274:8554–8560.

30. Brown EJ, Frazier WA. Integrin-associated protein (CD47) and its ligands. Trends Cell Biol 2001;11:130–135.

31. Demeure CE, Tanaka H, Mateo V, et al. CD47 engagement inhibits cytokine production and maturation of human dendritic cells. J Immunol 2000;164:2193–2199.

32. Armant M, Avice MN, Hermann P, et al. CD47 ligation selectively downregulates human interleukin 12 production. J Exp Med 1999;190:1175–1182.

33. Oldenborg PA, Gresham HD, Lindberg FP. CD47-signal regulatory protein alpha (SIRPalpha) regulates Fcgamma and complement receptor-mediated phagocytosis. J Exp Med 2001;193:855–862.

34. Albert ML, Pearce SF, Francisco LM, et al. Immature dendritic cells phagocytose apoptotic cells via alphavbeta5 and CD36, and cross-present antigens to cytotoxic T lymphocytes. J Exp Med 1998;188:1359–1368.

35. Fadok VA, Warner ML, Bratton DL, Henson PM. CD36 is required for phagocytosis of apoptotic cells by human macrophages that use either a phosphatidylserine receptor or the vitronectin receptor (alpha v beta 3). J Immunol 1998;161:6250–6257.

36. Di Carlo FJ, Fiore JV. On thecomposition of zymosan Science 1958;127:756–757.

37. Lipke PN, Ovalle R. Cell wall architecture in yeast: new structure and new challenges. J Bacteriol 1998;180:3735–3740.

38. Ezekowitz RA, Sastry K, Bailly P, Warner A. Molecular characterization of the human macrophage mannose receptor: demonstration of multiple carbohydrate recognition-like domains and phagocytosis of yeasts in Cos-1 cells. J Exp Med 1990;172:1785–1794.

39. Kruskal BA, Sastry K, Warner AB, Mathieu CE, Ezekowitz RA. Phagocytic chimeric receptors require both transmembrane and cytoplasmic domains from themannose receptor. J Exp Med 1992;176:1673–1680.

40. Sung SS, Nelson RS, Silverstein SC. Yeast mannans inhibit binding and phagocytosis of zymosan by mouse peritoneal macrophages. J Cell Biol 1983;96:160–166.

41. Goldman R. Characteristics of the beta-glucan receptor of murine macrophages. Exp Cell Res 1988;174:481–490.

42. Janusz MJ, Austen KF, Czop JK. Isolation of soluble yeast beta-glucans that inhibit human monocyte phagocytosis mediated by beta-glucan receptors. J Immunol 1986;137:3270–3276.

43. Giaimis J, Lombard Y, Fonteneau P, et al. Both mannose and beta-glucan receptors are involved in phagocytosis of unopsonized, heat-killed *Saccharomyces cerevisiae* by murine macrophages. J Leukoc Biol 1993;54:564–571.

44. Ross GD, Cain JA, Lachmann PJ. Membrane complement receptor type three (CR3) has lectin-like properties analogous to bovine conglutinin as functions as a receptor for zymosan and rabbit erythrocytes as well as a receptor for iC3b. J Immunol 1985;134:3307–3315.

45. Ross GD, Thompson RA, Walport MJ, et al. Characterization of patients with an increased susceptibility to bacterial infections and a genetic deficiency of leukocyte membrane complement receptor type 3 and the related membrane antigen LFA-1. Blood 1985;66:882–890.

46. Platt N, Haworth R, da Silva RP, Gordon S. Scavenger receptors and phagocytosis of bacteria and apoptotic cells. In *Phagocytosis: The Host.* S. Gordon, editor. Stamford, CT: JAI Press. 1999;71–85.

47. Peiser L, Gough PJ, Kodama T, Gordon S. Macrophage class A scavenger receptor-mediated phagocytosis of *Escherichia coli:* role of cell heterogeneity, microbial strain, and culture conditions in vitro. Infect Immun 2000;68:1953–1963.

48. Thomas CA, Li Y, Kodama T, et al. Protection from lethal gram-positive infection by macrophage scavenger receptor-dependent phagocytosis. J Exp Med 2000;191:147–156.

49. Elomaa O, Kangas M, Sahlberg C, et al. Cloning of a novel bacteria-binding receptor structurally related to scavenger receptors and expressed in a subset of macrophages. Cell 1995;80:603–609.

50. van der Laan LJ, Dopp EA, Haworth R, et al. Regulation and functional involvement of macrophage scavenger receptor MARCO in clearance of bacteria in vivo. J Immunol 1999;162:939–947.

51. Placecanda A, Paulauskis J, Al-Mutairi E, et al. Role of the scavenger receptor MARCO in alveolar macrophage binding of unopsonized environmental particles. J Exp Med 1999;189:1497–1506.

52. Franc NC, Heitzler P, Ezekowitz RA, White K. Requirement for croquemort in phagocytosis of apoptotic cells in *Drosophila.* Science 1999;284:1991–1994.

53. Crowley MT, Costello PS, Fitzer-Attas CJ, et al. A critical role for Syk in signal transduction and phagocytosis mediated by Fcgamma receptors on macrophages. J Exp Med 1997;186:1027–1039.

54. Kusner DJ, Hall CF, Schlesinger LS. Activation of phospholipase D is tightly coupled to the phagocytosis of *Mycobacterium tuberculosis* or opsonized zymosan by human macrophages. J Exp Med 1996;184:585–595.

55. Ip YT, Davis RJ. Signal transduction by the c-Jun N-terminal kinase (JNK)—from inflammation to development. Curr Opin Cell Biol 1998;10:205–219.

56. Allen LH, Aderem A. A role for MARCKS, the alphs isozyme of protein kinase C and myosin I in zymosan phagocytosis by macrophages. J Exp Med 1995;182:829–840.

57. Melendez AJ, Harnett MM, Allen JM. Differentiation-dependent switch in protein kinase C isoenzyme activation by FcgammaRI, the human high-affinity receptor for immunoglobulin G. Immunology 1999;96:457–464.

58. Zheng L, Zomerdijk TP, Aarnoudse C, van Furth R, Nibbering PH. Role of protein kinase C isozymes in Fc gamma receptor-mediated intracellular killing of *Staphylococcus aureus* by human monocytes. J Immunol 1995;155:776–784.

59. Zheleznyak A, Brown EJ. Immunoglobulin-mediated phagocytosis by human monocytes requires protein kinase C activation. Evidence for protein kinase C translocation to phagosomes. J Biol Chem 1992;267:12042–12048.

60. Aderem A. The MARCKS brothers: a family of protein kinase C substrates. Cell 1992;71:713–716.

61. Shapira L, Takashiba S, Champagne C, Amar S, Van Dyke TE. Involvement of protein kinase C and protein tyrosine kinase in lipopolysaccharide-induced TNF-alpha and IL-1 beta production by human monocytes. J Immunol 1992;153:1818–1824.

62. Kovacs EJ, Radzioch D, Young HA, Varesio L. Differential inhibition of IL-1 and TNF-alpha mRNA expression by agents which block second messenger pathways in murine macrophages. J Immunol 1988;141:3101–3105.

63. Huwiler A, Pfeilschifter J. A role for protein kinase C-alpha in zymosan-stimulated eicosanoid synthesis in mouse peritoneal macrophages. Eur J Biochem 1993;217:69–75.

64. Giroux M, Descoteaux A. Cyclooxygenase-2 expression in macrophages: modulation by protein kinase C-alpha J Immunol 2000;165:3985–3991.

65. St-Denis A, Chano F, Tremblay P, St-Pierre Y, Descoteaux A. Protein kinase C-alpha modulates lipopolysaccharide-induced functions in a murine macrophage cell line. J Biol Chem 1998;273:32787–32792.

66. St-Denis A, Caouras V, Gervais F, Descoteaux A. Role of protein kinase C-alpha in the control of infection by intracellular pathogens in macrophages. J Immunol 1999;163:5505–5511.

67. Larsen EC, DiGennaro JA, Saito N, et al. Differential requirement for classic and novel PKC isoforms in respiratory burst and phagocytosis in RAW 264.7 cells. J Immunol 2000;165:2809–2817.

68. Botelho RJ, Teruel M, Dierckman R, et al. Localized biphasic changes in phosphatidylinositol-4,5-bisphosphate at sites of phagocytosis. J Cell Biol 2000;151:1353–1368.

69. Chan TO, Rittenhouse SE, Tsichlis PN. AKT/PKB and other D3 phosphoinositide-regulated kinases: kinase activation by phosphoinositide-dependent phosphorylation. Annu Rev Biochem 1999;68:965–1014.

70. Lennartz MR. Phospholipases and phagocytosis: the role of phospholipid-derived second messengers in phagocytosis. Int J Biochem Cell Biol 1999;31:415–430.

71. Celli J, Oliver M, Finlay BB. Enteropathogenic *Escherichia coli* mediates antiphagocytosis through the inhibition of PI 3-kinase-dependent pathways. EMBO J 2001;20:1245–1258.

72. Araki N, Johnson MT, Swanson JA. A role for phosphoinositide 3-kinase in the completion of macropinocytosis and phagocytosis by macrophages. J Cell Biol 1996;135:1249–1260.

73. Gold ES, Underhill DM, Morrissette NS, et al. Dynamin 2 is required for phagocytosis in macrophages. J Exp Med 1999;190:1849–1856.

74. Arbibe L, Mira JP, Teusch N, et al. Toll-like receptor 2-mediated NF-kappa B activation requires a Rac1-dependent pathway. Nat Immunol 2000;1:533–540.

75. Buscher D, Hipskind RA, Krautwald S, Reimann T, Baccarini M. Ras-dependent and -independent pathways target the mitogen-activated protein kinase network in macrophages. Mol Cell Biol 1995;15:466–475.

76. Monick MM, Carter AB, Gudmundsson G, et al. A phosphatidylcholine-specific phospholipase C regulates activation of p42/44 mitogen-activated protein kinases in lipopolysaccharide-stimulated human alveolar macrophages. J Immunol 1999;162:3005–3012.

77. Schmitz AA, Govek EE, Bottner B, Van Aelst L. Rho GTPases: signaling, migration, and invasion. Exp Cell Res 2000;261:1–12.

78. Caron E, Hall A. Identification of two distinct mechanicms of phagocytosis controlled by different Rho GTPases. Science 1998;282:1717–1721.

79. Massol P, Montcourrier P, Guillemot JC, Chavrier P. Fc receptor-mediated phagocytosis requires CDC42 and Racl. EMBO J 1998;17:6219–6229.

80. Guillen N, Boquet P, Sansonetti P. The small GTP-binding protein RacG regulates uroid formation in the protozoan parasite *Entamoeba histolytica.* J Cell Sci 1998;111:1729–1739.

81. Cox D, Chang P, Zhang Q, et al. Requirements for both Racl and Cdc42 in membrane ruffling and phagocytosis in leukocytes. J Exp Med 1997;186:1487–1494.

82. Von Pawel-Rammingen U, Telepnev MV, Schmidt G, et al. GAP activity of the *Yersinia* YopE cytotoxin specifically targets the Rho pathway: a mechanism for disruption of actin microfilament structure. Mol Microbiol 2000;36:737–748.

83. Goehring UM, Schmidt G, Pederson KJ, Aktories K, Barbieri JT. The N-terminal domain of *Pseudomonas aeruginosa* exoenzyme S is a GTPase- activating protein for Rho GTPases. J Biol Chem 1999;274:36369–36372.

84. Gresham HD, Graham IL, Anderson DC, Brown EJ. Leukocyte adhesion-deficient neutrophils fail to amplify phagocytic function in response to stimulation. Evidence for CD11b/CD18-dependent and -independent mechanisms of phagocytosis. J Clin Invest 1991;88:588–597.

85. Graham IL, Lefkowith JB, Anderson DC, Brown EJ. Immune complex-stimulated neutrophil LTB4 production is dependent on beta 2 integrins. J Cell Biol 1993;120:1509–1517.

86. Leusen JHW, Verhoeven AJ, Roos D. Interactions between the components of the human NADPH oxidase: a review about the intrigues in the phox family. Front Biosci 1996;1:72–90.

87. DeLeo FR, Allen LA, Apicella M, Nauseef WM. NADPH oxidase activation and assembly during phagocytosis. J Immunol 1999;163:6732–6740.

88. Segal AW, Wientjes F, Stockely RW, Dekker LV. Components and organization of the NADPH oxidase of phagocytic cells. In *Phagocytosis: The Host.* S. Gordon, editor. Stamford CT: JAI Press, 1999;441–483.

89. Diebold BA, Bokoch GM. Molecular basis for Rac2 regulation of phagocyte NADPH oxidase. Nat Immunol 2001;2:211–215.

90. Berton G, Laudanna C, Sorio C, Rossi F. Generation of signals activating neutrophil functions by leukocyte integrins: LFA-1 and gp150/95, but not CR3, are able to stimulate the respiraroty burst of human neutrophils. J Cell Biol 1992;116:1007–1017.

91. Serrander L, Larsson J, Lundqvist H, et al. Particles binding beta(2)-integrins mediate intracellular production of oxidative metabolites in human neutrophils independently of phagocytosis. Biochim Biophys Acta 1999;1452:133–144.

92. Morrissette NS, Gold ES, Guo J, et al. Isolation and characterization of monoclonal antibodies directed against novel components of macrophage phagosomes. J Cell Sci 1999;112:4705–4713.

93. Grogan A, Reeves E, Keep N, et al. Cytosolic phox proteins interact with and regulate the assembly of coronin in neutrophils. J Cell Sci 1997;110:3071–3081.

94. Wright SD, Silverstein SC. Receptors for C3b and C3bi promote phagocytosis but not the release of toxic oxygen from human phagocytes. J Exp Med 1983;158:2016–2023.

95. Yamamoto K, Johnston RB, Jr. Dissociation of phagocytosis from stimulation of the oxidative metabolic burst in macrophages. J Exp Med 1984;159:405–416.

96. Berton G, Gordon S. Modulation of macrophage mannosyl-specific receptors by cultivation on immobilized zymosan. Effects on superoxide-anion release and phagocytosis. Immunology 1983;49:705–715.

97. Stahl PD, Ezekowitz RA. The mannose receptor is a pattern recognition receptor involved in host defense. Curr Opin Immunol 1998;10:50–55.

98. Fraser IP, Ezekowitz RA. Mannose receptor and phagocytosis. In *Phagocytosis: The Hose.* S. Gordon, editor. Stamford, CT: JAI Press, 1999;87–101.

99. Astarie-Dequeker C, N'Diaye EN, Le Cabec V, et al. The mannose receptor mediates uptake of pathogenic and nonpathogenic mycobacteria and bypasses bactericidal responses in human macrophages. Infect Immun 1999;67:469–477.

100 Laudanna C, Melotti P, Bonizzato C, et al. Ligation of members of the beta 1 or the beta 2 subfamilies of integrins by antibodies triggers eosinophil respiratory burst and spreading. Immunology 1993;80:273–280.

101. Jiang Q, Akashi S, Miyake K, Petty HR. Lipopolysaccharide induces physical proximity between CD14 and toll- like receptor 4 (TLR4) prior to nuclear translocation of NF-kappa B. J Immunol 2000;165:3541–3544.

102 Zarewych DM, Kindzelskii AL, Todd RF. 3rd, and Petty HR. LPS induces CD14 association with complement receptor type 3, which is reversed by neutrophil adhesion. J Immunol 1996;156:430–433.

103. Perera PY, Mayadas TN, Takeuchi O, et al. CD11b/CD18 acts in concert with CD14 and Toll-like receptor (TLR) 4 to elicit full lipopolysaccharide and taxol-inducibel gene expression. J Immunol 2001;166:574–581.

104. Ozinsky A, Underhill DM, Fontenot JD, et al. The repertoire for pattern recognition of pathogens by the innate immune system is defined by cooperation between toll-like receptors. Proc Natal Acad Sci USA 2000;97:13766–13771.

105. Underhill DM, Ozinsky A, Hajjar AM, et al. The Toll-like receptor 2 is recruited to macrophage phagosomes and discriminates between pathogens. Nature 1999;401:811–815.

106. Yamamoto Y, Klein TW, Friedman H. Involvement of mannose receptor in cytokine interleukin-1beta (IL- 1beta), IL-6, and granulocyte-macrophage colony-stimulating factor responses, but not in chemokine macrophage inflammatory protein 1beta (MIP-1beta), MIP-2, and KC responses, caused by attachment of *Candida albicans* to macrophages. Infect Immun 1997;65:1077–1082.

107. Shibata Y, Metzger WJ, Myrvik QN. Chitin particle-induced cell-mediated immunity is inhibited by soluble mannan: mannose receptor-mediated phagocytosis initiates IL-12 production. J Immunol 1997;159:2462–2467.
108. Garner RE, Rubanowice K, Sawyer RT, Hudson JA. Secretion of TNF-alpha by alveolar macrophages in response to *Candida albicans* mannan. J Leukoc Biol 1994;55:161–168.

20

The Role of Mast Cells in Innate Immunity

Joshua A. Boyce and K. Frank Austen

1. INTRODUCTION

Mast cells (MCs) are bone marrow-derived tissue-dwelling immune effector cells that are recognizable by virtue of their distinctive metachromatically staining secretory granules. They are prominent in the tissues and organs that are in contact with the external environment *(1)*. MCs respond to both immunologic and nonimmunologic stimulation with an effector repertoire that includes preformed granule-associated inflammatory mediators such as histamine and protease/proteoglycan complexes, newly formed eicosanoid products of arachidonic acid metabolism (cysteinyl leukotrienes, prostaglandin D_2) and induced expression of several proinflammatory cytokines and chemokines. The diverse effector functions of MCs, their ability to respond to a variety of nonimmune stimuli, and their anatomic distribution are all compatible with a role as initiators of innate immune responses. Furthermore, experimental evidence provides strong support for such a role. This review details the evidence supporting a key role for MCs in innate immunity and the potential mechanisms by which this occurs.

2. MC DEVELOPMENT

2.1. Characterization of MC Progenitors

The fact that MCs normally reside in various tissues implies a constitutive pathway for their development. Current understanding of MC development derives largely from studies of naturally occurring strains of mice that are deficient in MCs. The *W/Wv (2)* strain of mouse has a profound MC deficiency resulting from a mutation at the white-spotting (W) locus that encodes the membrane receptor tyrosine kinase, c-*kit (3)*. The ligand for c-*kit*, stem cell factor (SCF, also known as KIT ligand or Steel factor) *(4)*, is a growth factor that is constitutively and abundantly expressed by fibroblasts and stromal cells and that exists as both a membrane-bound and secretory form. The S1 locus that encodes SCF *(5)* is mutated in a second strain of mast cell-deficient mice (*Sl/Sld* strain) *(6)*. Early studies demonstrated that transplantation of normal bone marrow cells from a histocompatible strain provided progenitor cells that resulted in normal-appearing MCs in the tissues of the *W/Wv* mice *(2)*, thereby establishing the hematopoietic origin of MCs. These studies also indicated that the intact functions of both the c-*kit* receptor and

From: *Infectious Disease: Innate Immunity*
Edited by: R. A. B. Ezekowitz and J. A. Hoffmann © Humana Press Inc., Totowa, NJ

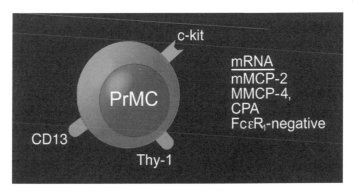

Fig. 1. Characteristics of circulating committed progenitor mast cells (PrMCs). Mouse PrMCs from fetal blood express high levels of c-*kit,* low levels of Thy-1, and mRNA encoding the mast cell-specific proteases mMCP-2, mMCP-4, and CPA, but not FcεRI. Human PrMCs are found within a circulating population of mononuclear cells expressing CD34 and CD13 but not FcεRI. CPA, carboxypeptidase A; mMCP, murine mast cell protease.

its ligand, SCF, are each absolutely required for normal MC development in vivo in mice. The observation that recombinant soluble SCF stimulates the growth of MCs from mouse bone marrow cells in vitro *(7)* and from a variety of human progenitor cell sources including bone marrow *(8),* fetal liver *(9)* cord blood *(10),* and peripheral blood *(11)* in vitro reflects the role of the SCF/c-*kit* interaction in MC development from both rodent and human hematopoietic precursors. The constitutive expression of the c-*kit* receptor by early hematopoietic precursors and the provision of SCF by stromal cells under basal conditions provide a constitutive ligand/receptor pair that is essential for the presence of MCs as an innate characteristic of tissues.

In both rodents and humans, MCs develop from c-*kit*-bearing committed progenitor cells (PrMCs) that transit via the systemic circulation from the bone marrow to the tissues (Fig. 1). PrMCs lack the distinctive secretory granules of their mature counterparts and thus cannot be reliably distinguished from other peripheral blood mononuclear cells based on morphology alone. Nevertheless, PrMCs can be distinguished from other circulating mononuclear cells based on distinct cytofluorographic characteristics and colony-forming capability. Mouse fetal blood contains a population of rare cells with the exclusive colony-forming characteristics of PrMCs (designated *promastocytes*). These PrMCs possess high-level membrane expression of c-*kit* and low-level expression of the thymocyte marker thy-1 *(12).* Mouse fetal blood PrMCs have sparse granules and express steady-state levels of mRNA encoding MC-specific proteases, but not FcεRI (Fig. 1). Although an equivalent pure committed PrMC has not yet been isolated from human blood, cells with MC colony-forming activity in vitro are found in human blood and bone marrow, among a cell population expressing c-*kit* along with the pan-progenitor marker CD34 and the membrane aminopeptidase CD13 *(11).* When purified by flow cytometry and cultured in the presence of recombinant SCF and interleukin (IL)-6, human CD34+/c-*kit*+/CD13+ cells give rise to only three colony types; pure MCs, pure macrophages, and mixed MC/macrophage colonies. It is thus likely that the human equivalent of the mouse promastocyte exists within this pool of cells expressing these surface markers.

2.2. Homing Determinants of PrMC

As with all circulating leukocytes, the movement of PrMCs from blood into tissues requires the function of both chemoattractants and adhesion receptors. Because MCs populate tissues under baseline conditions, the receptors and ligands responsible for PrMC homing are likely to be constitutively expressed. In the absence of markers that unequivocally define PrMC in tissues, their constitutive homing can only be assessed at present by MC colony-forming assays for PrMC numbers in limiting dilution cultures of enzymatically dispersed mouse tissues. Such analyses reveal that normal mouse small intestine contains especially large numbers of PrMCs, exceeding the numbers found in the bone marrow when expressed as the number of MC colony-forming units per million mononuclear cells *(13,14)*. By comparison, much smaller numbers of PrMCs are found in the normal mouse lung *(14)*, suggesting that the two organs differ in their expression of the necessary ligands and receptors for PrMC homing under basal conditions. Indeed, the numbers of PrMCs in the small intestine were profoundly deficient in mice with a targeted disruption of the gene encoding the β_7-integrin, whereas the numbers of PrMCs in the lung were normal. The β_7-integrin pairs with two distinct α-subunits to form the $\alpha_4\beta_7$ and the $\alpha_E\beta_7$ heterodimers, which serve as receptors in lymphocytes for mucosal addressin cellular adhesion molecule (MadCAM)-1 or E-cadherin, respectively. Blockade of the α_4- and β_7-integrin subunits with specific antibodies each resulted in a diminished reconstitution of intestinal PrMCs following sublethal irradiation and reconstitution with normal congenic bone marrow. Anti-Mad-CAM-1 antibodies similarly blocked intestinal PrMC homing, while anti-α_E and anti-β_1 antibodies were inactive. These observations thus indicate a critical requirement for the $\alpha_4\beta_7$/MadCAM-1 adhesion pathway in the maintenance of the normal constitutive small intestinal pool of PrMCs (Fig. 2). These PrMCs probably serve as a reservoir that permits the development of intestinal mucosal MC hyperplasia, which is an essential feature of the normal immune response to helminth infections (see below).

Although $\alpha_4\beta_7$ is critical for PrMC homing to the small intestine, it is likely that other adhesion pathways dictate constitutive PrMC homing and localization of mature MCs in other tissues. The targeted deletion of the α_M (CD11b) integrin subunit, which pairs with β_2 to form a heterodimeric counterligand for intracellular adhesion molecule (ICAM)-1, was associated with a baseline deficit in MCs in the peritoneal cavity and dorsal skin. In contrast, the numbers of mature MCs appearing in response to helminth infection were unaffected *(15)* in this model, and small intestine PrMCs were not enumerated. Human PrMCs derived in vitro from cord blood-associated CD34$^+$ hematopoietic progenitor cells expressed another member of the β_2-integrin family, $\alpha_L\beta_2$, which decreases in its level of expression with increasing maturation of the cultured MC *(16)*. β_2-integrins may thus serve as homing receptors for PrMCs in certain tissues, but they may not be essential to normal localization of mature MCs. This notion is supported by the observation that mature MCs purified from various dispersed human tissues lack β_2-integrins *(17)*, with the exception of uterine MCs, which express CD11c/CD18 *(18)*. In contrast, all human tissue MCs reported to date express the $\alpha_3\beta_1$, $\alpha_4\beta_1$, and $\alpha_5\beta_1$ heterodimers *(16,17,19)*, which probably mediate interactions with extracellular matrix proteins in vivo. Immature mouse MCs derived in vitro from bone marrow (BMMCs) express P-selectin glycoprotein ligand (PSGL-1), which mediates

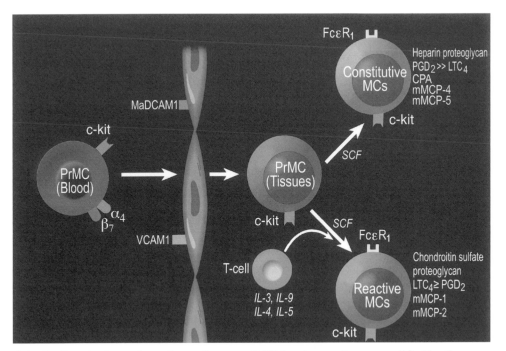

Fig. 2. Constitutive and reactive pathways of MC development as exemplified by the mouse intestine. Circulating progenitor mast cells (PrMCs) home to the intestine using $\alpha_4\beta_7$, which binds both mucosal addressin cellular adhesion molecule (MadCAM-1) and vascular cell adhesion molecule (VCAM-1). The resultant constitutive PrMC pool in the intestine is capable of giving rise to constitutive MCs found within the connective tissues. The same pool permits the T-cell-dependent expansion and differentiation of a reactive intraepithelial MC population that is essential for the elimination of some helminthic parasites. Both MC populations require stem cell factor (SCF) and c-*kit* for their derivation and maintenance. CPA, carboxypeptidase A; IL, interleukin; LTC_4, leukotriene C_4; mMCP, murine mast cell protease; PGD_2, prostaglandin D_2.

rolling to P-selectin in vitro *(20)* and in vivo *(21)*. Thus PrMCs utilize several pathways for recruitment to different tissues, which probably accounts for differences in MC numbers under baseline conditions and under conditions of chronic inflammation, in which MC numbers may increase substantially *(22–24)*.

Although adhesion receptors are necessary for transendothelial movement of leukocytes including PrMCs, chemoattractants are also required to govern directed migration and to ensure activation of the integrins. Recombinant soluble SCF is a chemoattractant for both mouse MCs and a transformed human MC line in vitro *(25,26)*. The absence of constitutive populations of PrMCs in the lungs and intestines of mice in the c-*kit*-deficient *W/Wv* strain, even though PrMCs can be identified in their bone marrow *(14)*, could reflect the in situ function of SCF as a chemoattractant for PrMC in vivo, in addition to its function in maintaining normal PrMC viability and differentiation. Additionally, several chemokines, a large family of structurally homologous low molecular weight chemoattractive cytokines, are active on human or mouse MCs. Human PrMCs derived in vitro from cord blood mononuclear cells expressed the receptors for IL-8 (CXCR2), eotaxins-1, -2, and -3 (CCR3), stromal cell-derived factor-1 (SDF-1; CXCR4), and macrophage inflammatory proteins-1α (MIP-1α) and -β (CCR5) *(27)*. Each of these receptors was functional based on calcium flux and chemotaxis in response to the corresponding recombinant ligand. Of these chemokines, the ligands for CXCR2, CCR3, and CCR5 are each associated with inflammatory responses in vivo, whereas SDF-1α is constitutively expressed in multiple tissues in vivo. Subsequent studies have confirmed the function of SDF-1α/CXCR4 in mediating the chemotaxis of both rodent and human MCs in vitro *(28,29)*. It is reasonable to speculate that CXCR4, along with c-*kit,* may provide receptors involved in the constitutive homing behavior of PrMCs, although the importance of the chemokine receptors as homing determinants for PrMC has not yet been addressed in vivo.

2.3. Anatomic and Functional Heterogeneity of MCs

Although the prevailing evidence holds that all MCs arise from a single PrMC population, the resultant mature MCs are heterogeneous in their anatomic distributions, their biochemical properties, their fixation characteristics, and their functional capabilities. Under baseline conditions, cytologically mature MCs are found in the muscularis and lamina propria of the rodent jejunum, and a few are also present within the normal intestinal mucosal epithelial surfaces *(30,31)*. Analogous groups of cytologically and anatomically distinct MCs exist in human intestines *(32)*. The MCs in the jejunal connective tissues of rodents contain heparin proteoglycans, stain strongly with toluidine blue dye, and retain their staining characteristics in formalin-fixed tissues. These connective tissue-associated MCs are histologically and functionally similar to other MCs found constitutively in the peritoneum and skin. It is noteworthy that these constitutive MCs serve as sentinels of innate immune responses to bacteria in the peritoneum *(33,34),* and similar populations may serve this function in other organs and tissues as well. In contrast, the MCs in the intestinal epithelial compartment lack heparin, stain weakly with toluidine blue, and are rendered invisible in formalin-fixed tissues.

Rodent models of intestinal immune responses to helminthic infections suggest important functional differences between these two groups of MCs. Mucosal intraepithelial MCs sharply and selectively increase in numbers in response to infection with helminthic parasites in mice (reactive hyperplasia), without concomitant changes in the numbers of MCs in the adjacent submucosal connective tissues *(35)*. This reactive hyperplasia, which results from in situ proliferation and differentiation of the constitutive pool of intestinal PrMCs (Fig. 2), is required for normal worm expulsion and resolves once the worm expulsion is complete. The ability to mount a reactive MC hyperplasia depends not only on the innate pool of PrMCs, but also on normal T-cell function, as both athymic nude mice and mice with a targeted deletion of their IL-3 gene fail to mount a reactive hyperplasia and are impaired in their ability to eliminate adult helminths *(36,37)*. In striking contrast, neither a lack of T-cells nor a selective deficiency of IL-3 alters the numbers of MCs that reside constitutively in the submucosa or muscularis of the intestine. The fact that the *W/Wv* and *Sl/Sld* mice lack both the "constitutive" and the "reactive" intestinal MC populations supports the essential functions of c-*kit* and SCF in all MC development in vivo, indicates that they are sufficient alone to support the development of the constitutive MC populations associated with submucosal connective tissues, and supports the innate nature of the PrMC pool.

In contrast to these SCF-driven constitutive MCs, the reactive MCs of the intestinal mucosa require not only the input of SCF and c-*kit*, but additional factors derived from T-lymphocytes, including IL-3, for their derivation and function as effectors in adaptive immunity to helminths. The fact that several additional T-cell-derived cytokines (IL-4, IL-9, and IL-5) can also support proliferation of either human or mouse PrMCs (or MCs) when combined with SCF in vitro suggests parallel signals by which T-cells can support an expansion of MCs at epithelial surfaces in adaptive immunity, representing an interface between the innate and adaptive immune responses *(27)*.

3. MC-ASSOCIATED MEDIATORS AND EFFECTOR FUNCTIONS

3.1. Preformed Mediators

3.1.1. Histamine

The cationic amine histamine is stored in the secretory granules of both human and rodent MCs in all tissue compartments *(38,39)*. Following exocytosis, histamine dissociates from the carboxyl groups of proteoglycans in MC granules at neutral pH and acts throught at least three classes of receptors *(40,41)*. The actions of histamine in vivo include bronchial and gastrointestinal smooth muscle contraction, vasodilation and vasopermeability, secretion of gastric acid, and induction of cutaneous pruritus. Histamine also exerts both stimulatory and inhibitory effects on immune cells in vitro, including enhancement of natural killer (NK) cell activation; stimulation of IL-6 synthesis by B-cells; inhibition of mitogen- and antigen-mediated T-cell proliferation; inhibition of neutrophil activation; and inhibition of tumor necrosis factor (TNF)-α, IL-1, interferon-γ, and IL-2 production by monocytes and T-cells (for review, see ref. *41*). Thus, histamine has both proinflammatory and immunomodulatory functions potentially germane to both innate and adaptive immunity (Fig. 3).

3.1.2. Mast Cell Proteases

MCs are abundantly and uniquely endowed with proteolytic enzymes with both trypsin-like (tryptases) *(42)* and chymotrypsin-like (chymases) *(43)* substrate specificity. Human tryptase genes reside on chromsome 16 *(44)*, and at least four of these [(tryptases-α, -βII, and -γ and the murine mast cell protease-7 (mMCP-7)-like tryptase)] are transcribed by MCs. The homologous mouse genes for the tryptases designated mMCP-6, mMCP-7, and tryptase-γ, are on mouse chromosome 17 *(45–47)*. Although mouse MCs express multiple chymases that arise from distinct genes on chromosome 14 (for review, see ref. *48*), only one MC-specific human chymase gene has been identified to date *(49)*. Human MCs also express a cathepsin G-like chymase that is similar to, if not identical to, neutrophil cathepsin G *(50)*. Both mouse and human MCs also express an exopeptidase, carboxypeptidase (CP)A *(51,52)*. Although the repertoire of chymase genes in mice permits a wide diversity of expression patterns in different tissues, only two distinct patterns of protease composition are generally reported in human MCs. MCs in the skin and submucosa of the small intestine are immunoreactive for tryptase, chymase, cathepsin G, and CPA, whereas those in the intestinal and bronchial mucosa and in the alveoli of the lung express tryptase but lack immunoreactivity for the other proteases *(53)*. MCs expressing tryptase but not chymase are depleted at the gastrointestinal tract mucosal surface in humans with acquired

0

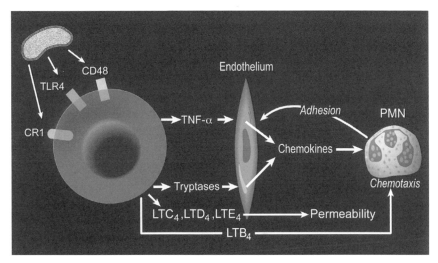

Fig. 3. Effector mechanisms of MCs implicated in innate immunity. Receptor-mediated MC activation results in the release of both preformed and newly formed tumor necrosis factor-α (TNF-α) and granule-associated tryptases that act on endothelial cells to promote neutrophil chemotaxis and adhesion. Newly formed eicosanoids promote venular permeability (the cysteinyl leukotrienes (cys-LTs) LTC$_4$, LTD$_4$, and LTE$_4$), and elicit polymorphonuclear leukocyte (PMN) chemotaxis (LTB$_4$). Chemotaxis also results from chemokines (IL-8 and its homologs) generated by activated endothelial cells after stimulation with TNF-α and probably with tryptases as well. TLR4, Toll-like receptor 4; CR1, complement receptor 1.

T-cell immunodeficiencies, whereas the numbers of submucosal MCs expressing both tryptase and chymase were normal in the same specimens *(32)*. This finding suggests that the latter subset is analogous to the constitutive, SCF-dependent MC populations observed in rodents, whereas the former probably represents the human analog of the T-cell-dependent subpopulation of MCs in the rodent intestinal mucosa.

The homologous mouse tryptases mMCP-6 and mMCP-7 *(54,55)* differ in their proteoglycan binding sites and their substrate specificity. When released by exocytosis in IgE-induced anaphylaxis, mMCP-7 diffuses into the circulation *(56)*, where it selectively degrades plasma fibrinogen, even in the presence of plasma protease inhibitors *(57)*. In contrast, mMCP-6 is retained along with the exocytosed secretory granule core in connective tissues *(56)*. Although mMCP-6 does not degrade fibrinogen, it does elicit a marked, selective, and sustained influx of neutrophils when instilled as a recombinant protein into the peritoneal cavity of mice *(58)*. Furthermore, both mMCP-6 and human tryptase-II/β elicit IL-8 production from endothelial cells in vitro *(59)*. Human tryptase-II/β also stimulates vascular tube formation *(60)* in vitro, as well as the proliferation of both fibroblasts and epithelial cells *(61,62)*. Thus tryptases may function in both early (neutrophil recruitment) and late (tissue remodeling) events in circumstances of host defense and tissue injury, possibly through interactions with the protease-activated receptors that are expressed by multiple stromal cell types *(63,64)*.

All chymases cleave angiotensin I to form angiotensin II *(65,66)*, which may permit MCs to participate in the homeostasis of local vascular tone and perfusion. The cleavage and activation of a 92-kDa gelatinase *(67,68)* by a dog MC chymase implies a role in both leukocyte penetration of tissues and tumor metastasis. MC chymases also cleave and activate various angiogenic factors *(69)* and initiate collagen fibril formation by cleaving type 1 procollagen *(70)*. Human MC chymase cleaves SCF *(71)*, yielding a product that retains activating and mitogenic functions *(72)*. Human MC chymase stimulates secretion by bronchial mucous glands *(73)*. Although these biochemical findings suggest that chymase may be involved in wound repair, extracellular matrix turnover, angiogenesis, mucous secretion, and the local modulation of vascular caliber and tone, none of these have been specifically addressed in vivo.

Two of the mouse MC chymases, mMCP-1 and mMCP-2, are selectively expressed by the MCs that arise in the intestinal mucosal compartment during helminth infections *(74)* (Fig. 2). Mice with a targeted deletion of the mMCP-1 gene have a delayed expulsion of *Trichinella spiralis* and an increased larval burden compared with wild-type controls, whereas expulsion of *Nippostrongylus brasiliensis* was unaffected *(75)*. Although human counterparts for these mucosal MC-associated chymases have not been identified, these observations do suggest that the evolution of diverse chymase genes in mice reflected selective pressures, including specific microbial infections.

3.1.3. Mast Cell Proteoglycans

MCs have proteoglycans in their secretory granules with a peptide core common to cells of hematopoietic lineage *(76–78)*, called serglycin for its repetitive serine and glycine residues that allow negatively charged glycosaminoglycans to polymerize at every second and/or third serine residue. This structure probably accounts for the resistance of proteoglycans to degradation by bound proteases that are freed from their activating peptide. MC secretory granules contain biochemically distinct species of proteoglycans that differ in sulfation of their respective glycosaminoglycan side chains. Both heparin-rich and chondroitin sulfate E-rich proteoglycan species are identified in MCs obtained from various dispersed human tissues *(79–82)*. Rodent MCs also contain both species of proteoglycans, with the MCs of their connective tissue being especially rich in heparin proteoglycans *(83)*. Conversely, the MCs of the rat intestinal mucosa contain lesser amounts of heparin, and chondroitin sulfate E or di-B proteoglycans predominate *(84)*. These differences in proteoglycan content account for striking histochemical differences between these two MC populations in rodents. The heparin-rich content of rat connective tissue MCs permits their uptake of safranin or berberin sulfate dyes. In contrast, the relative lack of heparin in intestinal mucosal MCs renders them safranin-negative.

An intracellular function of proteoglycans is the storage and packaging of MC granule constituents. The negatively charged proteoglycans form the basic structural components of large macromolecular complexes that are stored by and released from MC granules during exocytosis *(85–87)*. These acidic proteoglycans associate with basically charged proteases, as well as histamine and β-hexosaminidase. With exocytosis and release into the extracellular environment at neutral pH, histamine and β-hexosaminidase dissociate from the complex along with mMCP-7, ionically linked by histidine rather than lysine or arginine, which serves to retain many of the proteases. The mouse chymase mMCP-1, which is expressed by the intraepithelial MCs arising in the jejunum during helminthic infection *(88)*, diffuses from the chondroitin sulfate E proteoglycan (which lacks the charges of *N*-sulfation) that predominates in these MCs. In human MCs, chymase and CPA (which are expressed in the same subset of MCs) are complexed with a proteoglycan subspecies (probably heparin-containing) that is different from the subspecies complexed with tryptase (probably chondroitin sulfate E) *(89)*. The recent targeted disruption of the *N*-acetyl/*N*-sulfotransferase-2 (NDST-2) gene, an enzyme required for heparin biosynthesis, revealed that heparin proteoglycans are required for connective tissue-associated MCs to express immunoreactive mMCP-4, mMCP-5, and CPA *(90,91)*, even though steady-state levels of mRNA for these proteases were comparable in the MCs from the knockouts to the MCs of the wild-type controls. Expression of the immunoreactive tryptases mMCP-6 and mMCP-7 was unaffected in these NDST-2 knockout mice. It thus appears that heparin proteoglycan synthesis is absolutely required for the normal expression of chymases and CPA but not tryptases.

3.2. Eicosanoids

When activated either through crosslinkage of FcεRI or through engagement of the c-*kit* receptor, MCs rapidly synthesize the eicosanoid inflammatory mediators leukotriene (LT)C_4 and LTB$_4$, and prostaglandin (PG)D_2 from endogenous membrane arachadonic acid (AA) stores *(92–95)*. Eicosanoid synthesis is initiated by a calcium-dependent cytosolic phospholipase (PL)A$_2$ (cPLA$_2$) that liberates AA from perinuclear membrane phospholipids *(96)*. AA is converted sequentially to 5-hydroperoxyeicosatetraenoic acid (5-HPETE) and then to LTA$_4$ by the actions of 5-lipoxygenase (5-LO) following its reversible translocation from the cytosol to the perinuclear envelope *(97)*, where it requires the cooperation of an integral membrane protein, 5-lipoxygenase-activating protein (FLAP) *(98)*, for its metabolic function. LTA$_4$ is then either converted by a cytosolic LTA$_4$ hydrolase to LTB$_4$ *(99)* or is conjugated to reduced glutathione by LTC$_4$ synthase (LTC$_4$S) *(100)*, an integral perinuclear membrane protein with homology to FLAP, to form LTC$_4$. Both LTB$_4$ *(101)* and LTC$_4$ *(102)* are exported to the extracellular space by distinct, energy-dependent steps.

LTB$_4$ acts as a potent neutrophil chemotactic factor *(103)*, acting through at least two 7-transmembrane-spanning G-protein-coupled receptors (GPCRs), a high-affinity receptor termed the BLT1 receptor *(104)* and a low-affinity receptor, termed the BLT2 receptor *(105)*. LTC$_4$ is sequentially converted extracellularly to the receptor-active cysteinyl leukotrienes (cys-LTs) LTD$_4$ and LTE$_4$ *(106)*. The actions of the cys-LTs include bronchoconstriction *(107,108)* and eosinophil recruitment when experimentally instilled into the airways of human subjects in vivo *(109)*. cys-LTs also elicit wheal-and-flare responses when injected intradermally *(110)*. Mice with a targeted disruption of the LTC$_4$S gene exhibit deficits in permeability of the skin microvasculature in a model of passive cutaneous anaphylaxis (PCA) and also show diminished plasma exudation in a model of zymosan A-induced peritonitis *(111)*. Thus cys-LTs probably function at least partly to mediate vasopermeability changes in response to diverse inflammatory stimuli. The cys-LTs act through at least two 7-transmembrane receptors, termed the CysLT1 and CysLT2 receptors, respectively *(112,113)*. The CysLT1 receptor is expressed on bronchial smooth muscle, alveolar macrophages, CD34-bearing progenitor cells, peripheral blood eosinophils, and B-cells, whereas the CysLT2 receptor is expressed by brain and hematopoietic tissues as well as by bronchial smooth muscle and peripheral blood leukocytes. The CysLT1 receptor is also expressed by cultured human MCs *(114)*. Both the CysLT receptors and the BLT receptors bear structural homology to the P2Y receptor family, a group of GPCRs that mediate activation responses to extracellular nucleotides; indeed, a CysLT1-related receptor on cultured human MCs has dual ligand specificity for both cys-LTs and uridine diphosphate (UDP) *(114)*, which is among the products released by bacteria during infections. The generation of both cys-LTs and LTB$_4$ by MCs could facilitate innate immune responses through induction of venular permeability and transudation of plasma proteins, and recruitment of neutrophils, respectively *(111)*.

PGD$_2$ is generated by the conversion of AA through the sequential actions of prostaglandin endoperoxide synthase (PGHS)-1 or -2 and the hematopoietic form of PGD$_2$ synthase *(115)*. PGD$_2$, like the cysteinyl leukotrienes, is a bronchoconstrictor *(116)*, and its active metabolite, 9α, 11β-PGF$_2$, is a potent constrictor of coronary arteries *(117)*. Two receptors for PGD$_2$, termed DP and CRTH2, have been identified and cloned *(118,119)*. Mice with the targeted disruption of the DP receptor have a markedly attenuated capacity for the development of allergic lung inflammation in an experimental model *(120)*. Combined with selective expression of the CRTH2 receptor on human eosinophils, basophils, and Th2 lymphocytes and its selective chemotactic actions on these cell types *(118)*, these observations support a role for PGD$_2$ in inflammatory responses, particularly in circumstances such as helminth infection, in which Th2-dominated inflammation is typical.

As with the profile of MC granule constituents, MC subpopulations differ in their patterns of AA metabolism. Rat peritoneal MCs, a prototypical "constitutive" MC population, respond to IgE-dependent activation with preferred generation of PGD$_2$ and LTB$_4$, whereas MCs from the rat intestinal mucosa generate LTC$_4$ in preference to PGD$_2$ *(121)*. Human MCs from different tissue sites also display heterogeneity of AA metabolism. MCs from human intestine generated a wide range of PGD$_2$ (1–55 ng; mean = 21.3 ng) and cys-LT (0.2–14.2 ng; mean = 4.4 ng) per 10^6 MCs, when stimulated in vitro with anti-IgE *(122)*. MCs obtained from human lung tissue generated levels of LTC$_4$ and PGD$_2$ comparable to their intestinal counterparts *(123,124)*. In contrast, human uterine MCs generated larger quantities of both PGD$_2$ (89 ng/10^6 cells) and LTC$_4$ (45 ng/10^6 cells) *(125)*, whereas human skin MCs generated PGD$_2$ and almost no LTC$_4$ *(126)*. The capacity for human MCs to generate cys-LTs is probably dictated by microenvironmental factors, including local cytokines. A recent study of human MCs derived in vitro revealed that their expression of the terminal biosynthetic enzyme involved in cys-LT generation, LTC$_4$S, depended on induction by exogenous IL-4, whereas IL-3 or IL-5 were required for the import of cytosolic 5-LO stores to the nucleus. Maximal IgE-dependent cys-LT generation was achieved after priming with IL-4 together with IL-3 or IL-5 *(127)*. Thus, both rodent and human MCs exhibit several patterns of AA metabolism based on their tissue locations. The pattern of intertissue heterogeneity of AA metabolism probably reflects the influences of microenvironmental factors, including locally available cytokines, and is likely to be further modified in response to inflammation. The prominence of receptors for MC-derived eicosanoids on hematopoietic cells predicts additional, as yet unrecognized, functions in inflammation.

3.3. Cytokines Produced by MCs

3.3.1. Early-Acting Cytokines

When stimulated through FcεRI, both human and mouse MCs produce a number of cytokines that are associated with the early phases of an inflammatory response. These include TNF-α *(128)*, IL-1 *(129)*, and IL-6 *(130,131)*. Such early-acting cytokines initiate hepatic acute-phase protein production, endothelial cell adhesion molecule expression, and leukocyte recruitment. The immunolocalization of TNF-α to the MCs of human skin *(132)*, nasal mucosa *(133)*, and bronchial submucosa *(134)* implies that some TNF-α is constitutively synthesized and stored by human MCs in vivo. Stimulation of culture-derived human MCs in vitro through FcεRI results in a rapid, transient generation and release of TNF-α that returns to negligible levels by 24 hours *(135)*. Although IgE-dependent TNF-α release by MCs may favor recruitment of cell populations that sustain the allergic response, the capacity for MCs to secrete TNF-α rapidly via non-IgE-dependent mechanisms would normally facilitate a protective role against bacteria *(33)* (see below).

3.3.2. Th2-Type Cytokines/Co-mitogens

The helminth-induced expansion of intestinal mucosal MC populations depends on both the cytoprotective functions of SCF and the co-mitogenic effects of cytokines such as IL-3, IL-4, IL-5, and others. Although Th2 lymphocytes are generally viewed as the major source of these co-mitogens, the capacity for MCs to produce these same cytokines suggests a possible autocrine priming function that may have arisen before the evolution of the adaptive lymphocyte response. IL-4 and IL-5 are each localized by immunohistochemistry to the MCs in lung tissue of patients with asthma *(134)* and to the MCs in the nasal mucosa of patients with allergic rhinitis *(133)*. Another cytokine with co-mitogenic activity on MCs, IL-3, is transcribed *de novo* along with IL-5 when human lung MCs are stimulated with anti-IgE *(27,135)*. Both immunodetectable IL-4 and IL-5 and their corresponding mRNA species were localized to human skin MCs after cutaneous allergen challenge *(136)* and are also detectable, along with IL-6, in nasal mucosal MCs in biopsy specimens from patients with allergic rhinitis *(137)*. Human intestinal MCs respond ex vivo to IL-4 priming with augmented IgE-dependent production of both IL-3 and IL-5 *(138)*. The process of Th2 cytokine generation in MCs probably has some similarity to the same process in T-cells, in that IL-4 is required for optimal production of the Th2 cytokines, at least in vitro *(138,139)*.

3.3.3. Chemokines

The MCs of both mice and humans generate several members of the CC and CXC chemokine families. Human MCs store IL-8, a potent neutrophil-active chemokine *(140,141)*. Although a mouse homolog of IL-8 has yet to be identified, a related CXC chemokine, epithelial neutrophil-activating factor-78 (ENA-78), is produced by mouse MCs in vitro after IgE-dependent activation *(142)*. Human MCs derived from cord blood in vitro generate the CC chemokine macrophage inflammatory protein-1α (MIP-1α) in response to IgE-dependent activation *(143)*, and mouse MCs secrete both MIP-1α and MIP-1β in vivo during experimental contact hypersensitivity *(144)*. Human lung MCs generate the CC chemokine MCP-1 when stimulated in vitro by SCF and anti-IgE *(145)*. Contact between mouse MCs and fibroblasts induces the production of the CC chemokine eotaxin by MCs *(146)*. These induced mediators selectively target neutrophils (IL-8, ENA-78), lymphocytes (MIP-1α, MIP-1β, MCP-1), and eosinophils, respectively, and may act in sequence with preformed exocytosed mediators and newly formed eicosanoids to recruit different leukocyte subsets selectively (Fig. 3).

2.3.4. Fibrogenic and Angiogenic Growth Factors

MCs generate factors that are involved in fibroblast proliferation, extracellular matrix deposition, and angiogenesis, including vascular permeability factor/vascular endothelial cell growth factor *(147)*, transforming growth factor-β (TGF-β) *(148)*, and basic fibroblast growth factor *(149)*. The latter property supports the role of MCs as modulators of tissue repair, fibrosis, and remodeling. Finally, the fact that MCs store and secrete SCF *(150,151)* illustrates another potential autocrine capability for MC survival.

4. EVIDENCE FOR MC INVOLVEMENT IN INNATE MICROBIAL IMMUNITY

The presence of MCs at the interfaces with the external environment has long implicated their involvement in innate immune responses. Such a role for MCs would require that microbes initiate MC activation and that MCs provide direct or indirect mechanisms for microbial clearance. This potential was supported initially by the observation that MCs phagocytize Gram-negative bacteria in vitro at least partly through their complement receptors *(152)*. The role for MCs in the recruitment of neutrophils to a tissue site was confirmed in a model of immune complex-mediated peritonitis, which elicits biphasic peaks of peritoneal fluid TNF-α and subsequent neutrophil recruitment in WBB6/F1 MC-sufficient mice, but not in MC-deficient *W/Wv* mice *(153)*. The *W/Wv* mice lacked the early peak of TNF-α altogether and had a significantly blunted late peak and poor neutrophil recruitment. All parameters were restored by intraperitoneal transfer of congenic BMMCs to the *W/Wv* mice, suggesting that MCs in vivo respond to immune complexes by providing both preformed and newly synthesized TNF-α, leading to neutrophil influx. These findings were subsequently extended to experimental models of acute septic peritonitis. Two original studies demonstrated that *W/Wv* mice subjected to cecal ligation and puncture *(33)* or directly inoculated with a virulent strain of *Klebsiella pneumoniae* intraperitoneally *(34)* each had substantially greater rates of mortality than their congenic, MC-sufficient WBB6/F1 controls *(33,34)*. In both studies, the increased mortality correlated with impaired neutrophil recruitment to the peritoneum. The *W/Wv* mice were also markedly impaired in their ability to clear an experimental pneumonia elicited by instillation of virulent *Klebsiella* in the lung, again with impaired neutrophil recruitment. The defects in peritoneal neutrophilia and bacterial clearance in the cecal ligation and puncture model were corrected by intraperitoneal transfer of BMMCs, which restores the numbers of peritoneal MCs to normal. Moreover, in a separate study, the repeated instillation of recombinant SCF into the peritoneum of normal C57B1/6 mice augmented MC numbers and survival rates following cecal ligation and puncture *(154)*. The protective effect of exogenously administered SCF was not observed in the MC-deficient *W/Wv* mice with a mutated c-*kit* receptor, indicating that its effect was MC-dependent. Taken together, these studies make a strong case that resident, constitutive MCs are essential for the initiation of neutrophil recruitment in response to bacterial infection.

Probably several effector molecules are generated by MCs that account for their observed protective function in the CLP model. MCs store some preformed TNF-α in their secretory granules *(128)* and can also generate TNF-α rapidly through *de novo* transcription and translation *(138,139)*. As in the immune complex-mediated model of peritonitis, a sharp, transient increase in peritoneal fluid-associated TNF-α was observed in MC-sufficient but not MC-deficient mice in the CLP model, presumably reflecting the preformed and rapidly released MC-associated product. As with neutrophil recruitment and survival rates, the defect in TNF-α secretion was reversed in the *W/Wv* mice with intraperitoneal transfer of BMMCs. Furthermore, TNF-α-deficient mice had a defect in their capacity to survive cecal ligation and puncture that was quantitatively and qualitatively similar to that observed in the *W/Wv* strain. Neutralization of TNF-α in normal mice with an antibody eliminated approx 70% of the peritoneal neutrophilia and decreased clearance of the bacteria. Since the pleiotropic effects of TNF-α include the induced expression of multiple chemokine genes and adhesion molecules by endothelial cells, the provision of TNF-α by resident, constitutive MCs is probably an important component of their role in neutrophil recruitment in innate immune responses to Gram-negative pathogens.

Although TNF-α figured prominently in the cecal ligation and puncture model, it is likely that additional MC-derived factors also support neutrophil recruitment to the peritoneum and other tissue sites. Indeed, the augmentative effects of SCF injection on cecal ligation and puncture-induced mortality were observed even in TNF-α-deficient mice, supporting the involvement of these additional factors *(154)*. The mouse tryptase mMCP-6 generates a marked and sustained local neutrophilia when injected into the peritoneal cavity *(58)*. More recently, instillation of purified recombinant human MC-specific human tryptase-β1 was shown to induce a marked neutrophilia in the lungs of mice *(155)* and to protect *W/Wv* mice from mortality in response to experimentally induced *Klebsiella* pneumonitis. Interestingly, despite eliciting profound pulmonary neutrophilia, tryptase-β1 instillation did not adversely affect pulmonary function or produce an enhanced sensitivity to methacholine. Thus MC tryptases are probably among the mediators involved in MC-dependent aspects of innate immunity, and the diversity of tryptase genes may permit selective, tissue-specific responses. In another study, the administration of the 5-LO inhibitor A-63162 decreased neutrophil influx and bacterial clearance in MC-sufficient but not MC-deficient mice *(156)*. Moreover, this same study demonstrated that mouse MCs generate both LTB_4 and LTC_4 in response to exposure to FimH-expressing type 1 fimbriated *Escherichia coli* in vitro. Thus the capacity of MCs to generate the potent neutrophil chemoattractant LTB_4, as well as the cys-LTs that induce venular permeability in vivo *(111)*, provides an additional mechanism by which they may function in innate immunity. Finally, the ability of MCs to generate neutrophil-active chemokines, such as IL-8 *(141)* or ENA-78 *(142)* provides yet another potential pathway for the recruitment of neutrophils. Taken together, the observations from both in vitro and in vivo models are consistent with the hypothesis that MCs are specialized to initiate recruitment of neutrophils and facilitate bacterial clearance in innate immunity. Moreover, this property of MCs probably reflects the composite effects of several effector systems, including those that function directly as chemoattractants (chemokines, LTB_4), those that augment venular permeability (cys-LTs), and those that function indirectly by inducing new genes in resident tissues that mediate chemotaxis (TNF-α, tryptases) (Fig. 3).

Interactions with invading microorganisms could initiate MC responses directly or indirectly. Pathogens could activate MCs through direct contact with activating receptors for their cell wall constituents, or through release of soluble activating substances. Pathogens could also initiate the alternate complement pathway and thereby generate bioactive fragments capable of opsonizing the bacterium, such as C3b, or of activating the MCs, such as C3a or C5a. In vitro studies of BMMCs, human intestinal MCs, and cord blood-derived human MCs confirm that Gram-negative bacteria can elicit TNF-α secretion by MCs directly *(33,157,158)*. *E. coli* organisms bearing the type 1 fimbria protein FimH1 induced degranulation of BMMCs in vitro *(159)* and were processed for antigen presentation through an endocytic pathway (160). In the cecal ligation and puncture model, MC activation and rapid TNF-α secretion occurred in response to infection with an FimH1-expressing strain of *Klebsiella pneumoniae* but did not occur in response to a FimH1-deficient strain, suggesting an essential role for FimH1 in interactions with peritoneal MCs in vivo *(161)*. The requirement for FimH1 was attributed to its binding to CD48, a glycophosphatidylinositol-anchored protein expressed on mouse MCs *(161)*. In vitro, FimH-expressing *E. coli* bound CD48 on MCs, and blockade of the interaction between CD48 and FimH in vivo interfered with bacterial clearance and with rapid TNF-α generation by MCs in response to *E. coli.*

The CD48-mediated secretion of TNF-α by MCs was recently linked to the phosphorylation of Janus kinase 3 (JAK3). Mice lacking JAK3 exhibited markedly lower levels of TNF-α in their peritoneal fluids sampled 1 hour following after cecal ligation and puncture, and both peritoneal neutrophil recruitment and bacterial clearance were similarly impaired. Although BMMCs from JAK3-deficient mice expressed normal levels of membrane CD48 and were able to ingest FimH1-bearing *E. coli* normally, their secretion of TNF-α following a 1-hour challenge with FimH1-bearing E. coli was markedly impaired *(162)*. Importantly, the reconstitution of peritoneal MCs in *W/Wv* mice by adoptive intraperitoneal transfer of JAK3-deficient BMMCs did not restore their capacities for TNF-α release, neutrophil recruitment, or bacterial clearance, whereas each of these were normalized by reconstitution with wild-type BMMCs.

In another recent study, BMMCs stimulated with bacterial lipopolysaccharide (LPS) for 3 hours secreted TNF-α. This response was mediated through the Toll-like receptor 4 (TLR4) *(163)* and, unlike CD48-mediated stimulation, did not provoke MC exocytosis. The TLR4-mediated generation of TNF-α involved NF-κB transcription factors and occurred without involvement of the mitogen-activated kinases. Adoptive transfer of TLR4-deficient BMMCs to the peritoneal cavity of *W/Wv* mice only partly restored their survival curves and neutrophil recruitment, and TNF-α production at 6 hours following cecal ligation and puncture was severely impaired compared with adoptive transfer of TLR4-sufficient BMMCs *(163)*. Several other proinflammatory cytokines (IL-6, IL-1β, and IL-13) were also markedly decreased in the *W/Wv* mice that received TLR4-deficient BMMCs compared with those receiving control BMMCs.

Taken together, these studies suggest at least two receptors through which Gram-negative organisms can directly initiate MC-dependent neutrophil recruitment and TNF-α generation. CD48 and TLR4 signal through distinct pathways. FimH1/CD48-

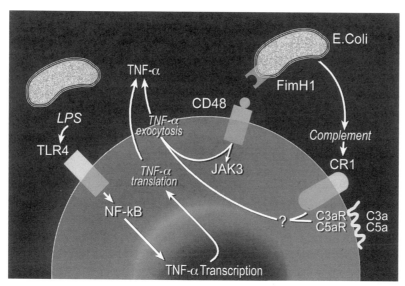

Fig. 4. Receptor-mediated mechanisms of MC activation in Gram-negative bacterial infections as elucidated by the cecal puncture and ligation model or by direct instillation of FimH1-bearing bacteria. FimH1 on both *E. coli* or *Klebsiella* can activate MCs directly through CD48, which leads to both phagocytosis and release of preformed TNF-α through a Janus Kinase-3 (JAK3)-dependent signaling pathway. Bacterial lipopolysaccharide (LPS) activates MCs through Toll-like receptor 4 (TLR4), leading to NF-κB-mediated transcription of tumor necrosis factor-α (TNF-α) and other cytokines. Complement receptors facilitate phagocytosis of bacteria (through CR1) and mediate degranulation (through CR1 and probably the G-protein-coupled C5a and/or C3a receptors) and release of TNF-α in a kinetically similar fashion to CD48-mediated activation.

mediated stimulation involves the JAK3-initiated signal transduction pathway, which is probably necessary for exocytosis and release of preformed TNF-α, but not for CD48 expression or endocytosis. LPS/TLR4-mediated stimulation elicits NF-κB-dependent generation of newly formed TNF-α that is released over several hours independently of exocytosis. Thus the original observation that MC-dependent peritonitis elicits both early and late peaks of TNF-α production is consistent with the involvement of both of these direct receptor-mediated mechanisms of MC activation in vivo (Fig. 4). The likelihood that human MCs respond to bacteria in a similar fashion is suggested by the observation that they ingest both Gram-positive and Gram-negative bacteria ex vivo and secrete TNF-α in response to these organisms *(157)*. Whether MCs possess additional receptors for direct interaction with microorganisms is unknown but such receptors are suggested by a study in which mouse BMMCs released β-hexosaminidase and both preformed and newly formed TNF-α in response to contact with *Leishmania major* or *L. infantum* parasites *(164)*.

In vivo studies also indicate a key role for the complement cascade and complement receptors in MC-mediated defense against Gram-negative pathogens. Mice that were deficient by targeted disruption of the gene in the complement components C3 and C4 were much more susceptible to mortality from cecal ligation and puncture than were congenic controls *(165)*. These complement-null mice also exhibited impaired TNF-α generation and MC degranulation in vivo following cecal ligation and puncture, defects that were restored by the exogenous administration of C3 to the C3-deficient mice *(165)*. Like the complement-null mice, mice deficient in complement receptor (CR)1 (CD35) and CR2 (CD21), which arise from a single gene in mice, or deficient in CD19, which forms a functional heterodimer with CD21, were also shown to be more susceptible to cecal ligation and puncture-induced mortality than were wild-type control mice *(166)*. Compared with wild-type animals, the CR1/2-deficient mice had decreased early-phase TNF-α generation, bacterial clearance, and neutrophil recruitment to the peritoneal cavity. Thus MC activation in septic peritonitis in vivo occurs at least partly through complement pathway activation, perhaps through opsonization and phagocytosis via the CD35/CD21 complex, which replicates the function of the two separate receptors encoded by distinct genes in humans. MCs also express GPCRs that are specific for the "anaphylotoxin" complement protein fragments C3a and C5a. Since stimulation in vitro of MCs through these receptors elicits chemotaxis *(167)* and mediator release *(168)*, these events could parallel the complement-mediated opsonization of bacteria and their phagocytosis in vivo.

Finally, the large pool of PrMCs constitutively residing in the mouse small intestine represents a key feature of innate host defense against helminths. Mice lacking this normal PrMC pool, such as those with a deletion of the β_7-integrin *(14,169)* or with naturally occurring disruptions in either the c-*kit* or SCF genes *(33,34)*, are profoundly impaired in their ability to clear helminthic parasites in vivo. Furthermore, although T-cells are required to provide the cytokines that amplify the development of mucosal MCs from the constitutive PrMC pool, the elimination of helminthic parasites by MCs does not depend on IgE or B-cells. This implies that MC activation in this circumstance also probably occurs by an innate recognition mechanism through an as yet unidentified receptor(s). The observation that MC activation occurs directly in response to *Leishmania* parasites supports such a mechanism.

5. CONCLUSIONS

In summary, MCs possess diverse effector capabilities and are ubiquitously distributed to serve several physiologic functions. Their constitutive localization at interfaces with the external environment fits a role in innate immunity. Mounting evidence holds that the "constitutive" and "reactive" MC developmental pathways reflect evolutionary pressures to serve distinct functions in host defense. Resident peritoneal cavity MCs, a "constitutive" population, are critically required for innate defense against Gram-negative bacteria in mouse models of experimentally induced peritonitis, and these MC-mediated responses probably reflect several activation mechanisms and effector systems (Figs. 3, 4). The ability to augment innate immunity to Gram-negative bacteria in mice by the exogenous administration of SCF *(154)* suggests that MCs could be manipulated to augment their function to therapeutic advantage in immunity, as well as other processes such as revascularization or wound healing. The "reactive" MC component of innate immunity, exemplified by the intestinal pool of PrMCs, represents a unique interface between innate (PrMCs) and adaptive (T-cell cytokines) features of immune responses, both of which are necessary for the elimination of helminths.

REFERENCES

1. McNeil HP, Austen KF. Biology of the mast cell. In: Frank MM, Austen KF, Claman HN, et al. (eds.). Sampter's Immunologic Diseases, 5th ed. Baltimore: Williams & Wilkins, 1995, pp. 185–204.
2. Kitamura Y, Go S, Hatanaka K. Decrease of mast cells in W/Wv mice and their increase by bone marrow transplantation. Blood 1978;52:447–452.
3. Geissler EN, Ryan MA, Housman DE. The dominant-white spotting (W) locus of the mouse encodes the c-*kit* proto-oncogene. Cell 1988;55:185–192.
4. Zsebo KM, Wypych J, McNiece IK, et al. Identification, purification, and biological characterization of hematopoietic stem cell factor from Buffalo rat liver-conditioned medium. *Cell* 1990;63:195–201.
5. Huang E, Nocka K, Beier DR, et al. The hematopoietic growth factor KL is encoded by the SI locus and is the ligand of the c-*kit* receptor, the gene product of the W locus. Cell 1990;63:225–233.
6. Kitamura Y, Go S. Decreased production of mast cells in *Sl/Sld* anemic mice. Blood 1979;53:492–497.
7. de Vries P, Brasel KA, Eisenman JR, et al. The effect of recombinant mast cell growth factor on purified murine hematopoietic progenitor cells. J Exp Med 1991;173:1205–1211.
8. Valent P, Spanblochl E, Sperr WR, et al. Induction of differentiation of human mast cells from bone marrow and peripheral blood mononuclear cells by recombinant human stem cell factor/*kit*-ligand in long-term culture. Blood 1992;80:2237–2245.
9. Irani A-MA, Nillson G, Miettinen U, et al. Recombinant human stem cell factor stimulates differentiation of mast cells from dispersed human fetal liver cells. Blood 1992;80:3009–3021.
10. Mitsui H, Furitsu T, Dvorak AM, et al. Development of human mast cells from umbilical cord blood cells by recombinant human and murine c-*kit* ligand. Proc Natl Acad Sci USA 1993;90:735–739.
11. Kirshenbaum AS, Goff JP, Semere T, et al. Demonstration that mast cells arise from a progenitor cell population that is CD34+, c-*kit*+, and expresses aminopeptidase N (CD13). Blood 1999;94:2333–2342.
12. Rodewald HR, Dessing M, Dvorak AM, et al. Identification of a committed precursor for the mast cell lineage. Science 1996;271:818–822.
13. Guy-Grand D, Dy M, Luffau G, et al. Gut mucosal mast cells: origin, traffic and differentiation. J Exp Med 1984;160:12–28.
14. Gurish MF, Tao H, Abonia JP, et al. Intestinal mast cell progenitors require CD49dβ7 (α4β7) for tissue-specific homing. J Exp Med 2001;194:1243–1252.
15. Rosenkranz AR, Coxon A, Maurer M, et al. Impaired mast cell development and innate immunity in Mac-1 (CD11b/CD18, CR3)-deficient mice. J Immunol 1998;161:6463–6467.
16. Tachimoto H, Hudson SA, Bochner BS. Acquisition and alteration of adhesion molecules during cultured human mast cell differentiation. J Allergy Clin Immunol 2001;107:302–309.
17. Sperr WR, Agis H, Czerwenka K, et al. Differential expression of cell surface integrins on human mast cells and human basophils. Ann Hematol 1992;65:10–16.
18. Guo CB, Kagey-Sobotka A, Lichtenstein LM, Bochner BS. Immunophenotyping and functional analysis of purified human uterine mast cells. Blood 1992;79:708–712.
19. Columbo M, Bochner BS, Marone G. Human skin mast cells express functional β1 integrins that mediate adhesion to extracellular matrix proteins. J Immunol 1995;154:6058–6064.
20. Steegmaier M, Blanks JE, Borges E, Vestweber D. P-selectin glycoprotein ligand-1 mediates rolling of mouse bone marrow-derived mast cells on P-selectin but not efficiently on E-selectin. Eur J Immunol 1997;27:1339–1345.
21. Sriramaro P, Anderson W, Wolitzky BA, Broide DH. Mouse bone marrow-derived mast cells roll on P-selectin under conditions of flow in vivo. Lab Invest 1996;74:634–643.

22. Qu Z, Liebler JM, Powers MR, et al. Mast cells are a major source of basic fibroblast growth factor in chronic inflammation and cutaneous hemangioma. Am J Pathol 1995;147:564–573.

23. Pesci A, Bertorelli G, Gabrielli M, Olivieri D. Mast cells in fibrotic lung disorders. Chest 1993;103:989–996.

24. Gotis-Graham I, McNeil HP. Mast cell responses in rheumatoid synovium. Association of the MCTC subset with matrix turnover and clinical progression. Arthritis Rheum 1997;40:479–489.

25. Nilsson G, Butterfield JH, Nilsson K, Siegbahn A. Stem cell factor is a chemotactic factor for human mast cells. J Immunol 1994;153:3717–3723.

26. Meininger CJ, Yano H, Rottapel R, et al. The c-kit receptor ligand functions as a mast cell chemoattractant. Blood 1992;79:958–963.

27. Ochi H, Hirani WM, Yuan Q, et al. T helper type-2 cytokine-mediated comitogenic responses and CCR3 expression during differentiation of human mast cells in vitro. J Exp Med 1999;190:267–280.

28. Juremalm M, Hjertson M, Olsson N, et al. The chemokine receptor CXCR4 is expressed within the mast cell lineage and its ligand stromal cell-derived factor-1 alpha acts as a mast cell chemotaxin. Eur J Immunol 2000;30:3614–3622.

29. Lin TJ, Issekutz TB, Marshall JS. Human mast cells transmigrate through human umbilical vein endothelial monolayers and selectively produce IL-8 in response to stromal cell-derived factor-1 alpha. J Immunol 2000;165:211–220.

30. Enerback L. Mast cells in rat gastrointestinal mucosa. I. Effects of fixation. Acta Pathol Microbiol Scand 1966;66:289–302.

31. Enerback L. Mast cells in rat gastrointestinal mucosa. II. Dye-binding and metachromatic properties. Acta Pathol Microbiol Scand 1966;66:303–312.

32. Irani AM, Craig S, DeBlois G, et al. Deficiency of the tryptase-positive, chymase-negative mast cell type in gastrointestinal mucosa of patients with defective T lymphocyte function. J Immunol 1987;138:4381–4386.

33. Echtenacher B, Mannel DN, Hultner L. Critical protective role of mast cells in a model of acute septic peritonitis. Nature 1996;381:75–79.

34. Malaviya R, Ikeda T, Ross E, et al. Mast cell modulation of neutrophil influx and bacterial clearance at sites of infection through TNF-alpha. *Nature* 1996;381:77–80.

35. Friend DS, Ghildyal N, Austen KF, et al. Mast cells that reside at different locations in the jejunum of mice infected with *Trichinella spiralis* exhibit sequential changes in their granule ultrastructure and chymase phenotype. J Cell Biol 1996;135:279–290.

36. Ruitenberg EJ, Elgersma A. Absence of intestinal mast cell response in congenitally athymic mice during *Trichinella spiralis* infection. Nature (Lond) 1976;264:258–260.

37. Lantz CS, Boesiger J, Song CH, et al. Role for interleukin-3 in mast cell and basophil development and in immunity to parasites. Nature (Lond) 1998;392:90–93.

38. Schwartz LB, Irani AM, Roller K, et al. Quantitation of histamine, tryptase, and chymase in human T and TC mast cells. J Immunol 1987;138:2611–2615.

39. Benditt EP, Arase M, Roeper ME. Histamine and heparin in isolated rat mast cells. J Histochem Cytochem 1956;4:419.

40. Leino L, Lilius E-M. Histamine receptors on leukocytes are expressed differently in vitro and ex vivo. Int Arch Allergy Appl Immunol 1990;91:30–35.

41. Falus A, Meretey K. Histamine: An early messenger in inflammatory and immune reactions. Immunol Today 1992;13:154–156.

42. Schwartz LB, Lewis RA, Austen KF. Tryptase from human pulmonary mast cells. Purification and characterization. J Biol Chem 1981;256:11939–11943.

43. Schechter NM, Choi JK, Slavin DA, et al. Identification of a chymotrypsin-like proteinase in human mast cells. J Immunol, 1986;137:962–970.

44. Pallaoro M, Fejzo MS, Shayesteh L, et al. Characterization of genes encoding known and novel human mast cell tryptases on chromosome 16p13.3. J Biol Chem 274;3355–3362.

45. Miller JS, Westin EH, Schwartz LB. Cloning and characterization of complementary DNA for human tryptase. J Clin Invest 1989;84:1188–1195.

46. Miller JS, Moxley G, Schwartz LB. Cloning and characterization of a second complementary DNA for human tryptase. J Clin Invest 1990;86:864–870.

47. Wong GW, Tang Y, Feyfant E, et al. Identification of a new member of the tryptase family of mouse and human mast cell proteases which possesses a novel COOH-terminal hydrophobic extension. J Biol Chem 1999;274:30784–30793.

48. Stevens RL. Human and mouse mast cell tryptases. Identification, cloning, expression, function, and metabolism. In: Marone G, Lichtenstein LM, Galli SJ (eds). Mast Cells and Basophils in Physiology, Pathology, and Host Defense, 2002, in press.

49. Urata H, Kinoshita A, Perez DM, et al. Cloning of the gene and cDNA for human heart chymase. J Biol Chem, 1991;266:17173–17179.

50. Schechter NM, Irani AM, Sprows JL, et. al. Identification of a cathepsin G-like proteinase in the MCTC type of human mast cell. J Immunol 1990;145:2652–2661.

51. Reynolds DS, Stevens RL, Gurley DS, et al. Isolation and molecular cloning of mast cell carboxypeptidase A: a novel member of the carboxypeptidase gene family. J Biol Chem 1989;264:20094–20099.

52. Irani AM, Goldstein SM, Wintroub BU, et al. Human mast cell carboxypeptidase. Selective localization to MCTC cells. J Immunol 1991;147:247–253.

53. Irani AA, Schechter NM, Craig SS, et al. Two types of human mast cells that have distinct neutral protease compositions. Proc Natl Acad Sci USA 1986;83:4464–4468.

54. Reynolds DS, Gurley DS, Austen KF, et al. Cloning of the cDNA and gene of the mouse mast cell protease-6. Transcription by progenitor mast cells and mast cells of the connective tissue subclass. J Biol Chem 1991;266:3847–3853.

55. McNeil HP, Reynolds DS, Schiller V, et al. Isolation, characterization, and transcription of the gene encoding mouse mast cell protease 7. Proc Natl Acad Sci USA 1992; 89:11174–11178.

56. Ghildyal N, Friend DS, Stevens RL, et al. Fate of two mast cell tryptases in V3 mastocytosis and normal BALB/c mice undergoing passive systemic anaphylaxis. Prolonged retention of exocytosed mMCP-6 in connective tissues and rapid accumulation of enzymatically active mMCP-7 in the blood. J Exp Med 1996;184:1061–1073.

57. Huang C, Wong GW, Ghildyal N, et al. The tryptase, mouse mast cell protease 7, exhibits anticoagulant activity in vivo and in vitro due to its ability to degrade fibrinogen in the presence of the diverse array of protease inhibitors in plasma. J Biol Chem 1997;272:31885–31893.

58. Huang C, Friend DS, Qiu WT, et al. Induction of a selective and persistent extravasation of neutrophils into the peritoneal cavity by tryptase mouse mast cell protease 6. J Immunol 1998;160:1910–1919.

59. Compton SJ, Cairns JA, Holgate ST, et al. The role of mast cell tryptase in regulating endothelial cell proliferation, cytokine release, and adhesion molecule expression: tryptase induces expression of mRNA for IL-1β and IL-8 and stimulates the selective release of IL-8 from human unbilical vein endothelial cells. J Immunol 1998;161:1939–1946.

60. Blair RJ, Meng H, Marchese MJ, et al. Human mast cells stimulate vascular tube formation. Tryptase is a novel, potent angiogenic factor. J Clin Invest 1997;99:2691–2700.

61. Cairns JA, Walls AF. Mast cell tryptase is a mitogen for epithelial cells. Stimulation of IL-8 production and intercellular adhesion molecule-1 expression. J Immunol 1996;156:275–283.

62. Gruber BL, Kew RR, Jelaska A, et al. Human mast cells activate fibroblasts: tryptase is a fibrogenic factor stimulating collagen messenger ribonucleic acid synthesis and fibroblast chemotaxis. J Immunol 1997;158:2310–2317.

63. Molino M, Barnathan ES, Numerof R, et al. Interactions of mast cell tryptase with thrombin receptors and PAR-2. J Biol Chem 1997;272:4043–4049.
64. Schechter NM, Brass LF, Lavker RM, et al. Reaction of mast cell proteases tryptase and chymase with protease activated receptors (PARs) on keratinocytes and fibroblasts. J Cell Physiol 1998;176:365–373.
65. Chandrasekharan UM, Sanker S, Glynias MJ, et al. Angiotensin II-forming activity in a reconstructed ancestral chymase. Science 1996;271:502–505.
66. Sanker S, Chandrasekharan UM, Wilk D, et al. Distinct multisite synergistic interactions determine substrate specificities of human chymase and rat chymase-1 for angiotensin II formation and degradation. J Biol Chem 1997;272:2963–2968.
67. Fang KC, Raymond WW, Lazarus SC, et al. Dog mastocytoma cells secrete a 92-kD gelatinase activated extracellularly by mast cell chymase. J Clin Invest 1996;97:1589–1596.
68. Fang KC, Raymond WW, Blount JL, et al. Dog mast cell alpha-chymase activates progelatinase B by cleaving the Phe88-Gln89 and Phe91-Glu92 bonds of the catalytic domain. J Biol Chem 1997;272:25628–25635.
69. Coussens LM, Raymond WW, Bergers G, et al. Inflammatory mast cells up-regulate angiogenesis during squamous epithelial carcinogenesis. Genes Dev 1999;13:1382–1397.
70. Kofford MW, Schwartz LB, Schechter NM, et al. Cleavage of type I procollagen by human mast cell chymase initiates collagen fibril formation and generates a unique carboxyl-terminal propeptide. J Biol Chem 272:7127–7131.
71. Longley BJ, Tyrrell L, Ma Y, et al. Chymase cleavage of stem cell factor yields a bioactive, soluble product. Proc Natl Acad Sci USA 1997;94:9017–9021.
72. de Paulis A, Minopoli G, Arbustini E, et al. Stem cell factor is localized in, released from, and cleaved by human mast cells. J Immunol 1999;163:2799–2808.
73. Caughey GH. Roles of mast cell tryptase and chymase in airway function. Am J Physiol 1989;257:L39.
74. Friend DS, Ghildyal N, Gurish MF, et al. Reversible expression of tryptases and chymases in the jejunal mast cells of mice infected with *Trichinella spiralis*. J Immunol 1998;160:5537–5545.
75. Wright SH, Lawrence CE, Paterson YY, Miller HR. Delayed expulsion of the nematode *Trichinella spiralis* in mice lacking the mucosal mast cell-specific granule chymase, mouse mast cell protease-1. J Exp Med 2000;192:1849–1856.
76. Humphries DE, Nicodemus CF, Schiller V, et al. The human serglycin gene. Nucleotide sequence and methylation pattern in human promyelocytic leukemia HL-60 cells and T-lymphoblast Molt-4 cells. J Biol Chem 1992;267:13558–13563.
77. Avraham S, Stevens RL, Gartner MC, et al. Isolation of a cDNA that encodes the peptide core of the secretory proteoglycan of rat basophilic leukemia-1 cells and assessment of its homology to the human analogue. J Biol Chem 1988;263:7292–7296.
78. Avraham S, Stevens RL, Nicodemus CF, et al. Molecular cloning of a cDNA that encodes the peptide core of a mouse mast cell secretory granule proteoglycan and comparison with the analogous rat and human cDNA. Proc Natl Acad Sci USA 1989;86:3763–3767.
79. Metcalfe DD, Soter NA, Wasserman SI, et al. Identification of sulfated mucopolysaccharides including heparin in the lesional skin of a patient with systemic mastocytosis. J Invest Dermatol 1980;74:210–215.
80. Metcalfe DD, Lewis RA, Silbert JE, et al. Isolation and characterization of heparin from human lung. J Clin Invest 1979;64:1537–1543.
81. Stevens RL, Fox CC, Lichtenstein LM, et al. Identification of chondroitin sulfate E proteoglycans in the secretory granules of human lung mast cells. Proc Natl Acad Sci USA 1988;85:2284–2287.

82. Eliakim R, Gilead L, Ligumsky M, et al. Possible presence of E-mast cells in the human colon. Proc Natl Acad Sci USA 1986;83:461–464.

83. Metcalfe DD, Smith JA, Austen KF, Silbert JE. Polydispersity of rat mast cell heparin: implications for proteoglycan assembly. J Biol Chem 1980;255:11753–11758.

84. Stevens RL, Lee TD, Seldin DC, et al. Intestinal mucosal mast cells from rats infected with *Nippostrongylus brasiliensis* contain protease-resistant chondroitin sulfate di-B proteoglycans. J Immunol 1986;137:291–295.

85. Schwartz LB, Riedel C, Caulfield JP, et al. Cell association of complexes of chymase, heparin proteoglycan, and protein after degranulation by rat mast cells. J Immunol 1981;126:2071–2078.

86. Schwartz LB, Riedel C, Schratz JJ, et al. Localization of carboxypeptidase A to the macromolecular heparin proteoglycan-protein complex in secretory granules of rat serosal mast cells. J Immunol 1982;128:1128–1133.

87. Serafin WE, Katz HR, Austen KF, et al. Complexes of heparin proteoglycans, chondroitin sulfate E proteoglycans, and [^{3}H] diisopropyl fluorophosphate-binding proteins are exocytosed from activated mouse bone marrow-derived mast cells. J Biol Chem 1986;261:15017–15021.

88. Knight PA, Wright SH, Lawrence CE, et al. Delayed expulsion of the nematode *Trichinella spiralis* in mice lacking the mucosal mast cell-specific granule chymase, mouse mast cell protease-1. J Exp Med 2000;192:1849–1856.

89. Goldstein SM, Leong J, Schwartz LB, et al. Protease composition of exocytosed human skin mast cell protease-proteoglycan complexes. J Immunol 1992;148:2475–2482.

90. Forsberg E, Pejler G, Ringvall M, et al. Abnormal mast cells in mice deficient in a heparin-synthesizing enzyme. Nature 1999;400:773–776.

91. Humphries DE, Wong GW, Friend DS, et al. Heparin is essential for the storage of specific granule proteases in mast cells. Nature 1999;400:769–772.

92. Paterson NAM, Wasserman SI, Said JW, et al. Release of chemical mediators from partially purified human lung mast cells. J Immunol 1976;117:1356–1362.

93. Heavey DJ, Ernst PB, Stevens RL, et al. Generation of leukotriene C$_4$, leukotriene B$_4$, and prostaglandin D$_2$ by immunologically activated rat intestinal mucosal mast cells. J Immunol 1988;140:1953–1957.

94. Murakami M, Austen KF, Arm JP. The immediate phase of c-*kit* ligand stimulation of mouse bone marrow-derived mast cells elicits rapid leukotriene C$_4$ generation through posttranslational activation of cytosolic phospholipase A$_2$ and 5-lipoxygenase. J Exp Med 1995;182:197–206.

95. Columbo M, Horowitz EM, Botana LM, et al. The human recombinant c-kit receptor ligand, rhSCF, induces mediator release from human cutaneous mast cells and enhances IgE-dependent mediator release from both skin mast cells and peripheral blood basophils. J Immunol 1992;149:599–608.

96. Clark JD, Lin L-L, Kriz RW, et al. A novel arachidonic acid-selective cytosolic PLA$_2$ contains a Ca$_{2+}$-dependent translocation domain with homology to PKC and GAP. Cell 1991;65:1043–1051.

97. Malavia R, Malavia R, Jakschik BA. Reversible translocation of 5-lipoxygenase in mast cells upon IgE/antigen stimulation. J Biol Chem 1993;268:4939–4944.

98. Dixon RAF, Diehl RE, Opas E, et al. Requirement of a 5-lipoxygenase-activating protein for leukotriene biosynthesis. Nature 1990;343:282–284.

99. Evans JF, Dupuis P, Ford-Hutchinson AW. Purification and characterization of leukotriene A$_4$ hydrolase from rat neutrophils. Biochem Biophys Acta 1985;840:43–50.

100. Lam BK, Penrose JF, Freeman GJ, et al. Expression cloning of a cDNA for human leukotriene C$_4$ synthase, an integral membrane protein conjugating reduced glutathione to leukotriene A$_4$. Proc Natl Acad Sci USA 1994;91:7663–7667.

101. Lam BK, Gagnon L, Austen KF, et al. The mechanism of leukotriene B_4 export from human polymorphonuclear leukocytes. J Biol Chem 1990;265:13438–13441.

102. Lam BK, Xu K, Atkins MB, et al. Leukotriene C_4 uses a probenecid-sensitive export carrier that does not recognize leukotriene B_4. Proc Natl Acad Sci USA 1992;89:11598–11602.

103. Lindbom L, Hedqvist P, Dahlen SE, et al. Leukotriene B_4 induces extravasation and migration of polymorphonuclear leukocytes in vivo. Acta Physiol Scand 1982;116:105–108.

104. Yokomizo T, Izumi T, Chang K, Takuwa Y, Shimizu T. A G-protein-coupled receptor for leukotriene B_4 that mediates chemotaxis. Nature 1997;387:620–624.

105. Yokomizo T, Kato K, Terawaki K, Izumi T, Shimizu T. A second leukotriene B(4) receptor, BLT2. A new therapeutic target in inflammation and immunological disorders. J Exp Med 2000;192:421–432.

106. Raulf M, Stuning M, Konig W. Metabolism of leukotrienes by L-gamma-glutamyl-transpeptidase and dipeptidase from human polymorphonuclear granulocytes. Immunology 1985;55:135–147.

107. Davidson AB, Lee TH, Scanlon PD, et al. Bronchoconstrictor effects of leukotriene E_4 in normal and asthmatic subjects. Am Rev Respir Dis 1987;135:333–337.

108. Griffin M, Weiss JW, Leitch AG, et al. Effect of leukotriene D_4 on the airways in asthma. N Engl J Med 1983;308:436–439.

109. Laitinen LA, Laitinen A, Haahtela T, et al. Leukotriene E_4 and granulocytic infiltration into asthmatic airways. Lancet 1993;341:989–990.

110. Soter NA, Lewis RA, Corey EJ, et al. Local effects of synthetic leukotrienes (LTC_4, LTD_4, LTE_4, and LTB_4) in human skin. J Invest Dermatol 1983;80:115–119.

111. Kanaoka Y, Maekawa A, Penrose JF, Austen KF, Lam BK. Attenuated zymosan-induced peritoneal vascular permeability and IgE-dependent passive cutaneous anaphylaxis in mice lacking leukotriene C_4 synthase. J Biol Chem 2001;276:22608–22613.

112. Lynch KR, O'Neill GP, Liu Q, et al. Characterization of the human cysteinyl leukotriene CysLT1 receptor. Nature 1999;399:789–793.

113. Heise CE, O' Dowd BF, Figueroa DJ, et al. Characterization of the human cysteinyl leukotriene 2 receptor. J Biol Chem 2000;275:30531–30536.

114. Mellor EA, Maekawa A, Austen KF, Boyce JA. Cysteinyl leukotriene receptor 1 is also a pyrimidinergic receptor and is expressed by human mast cells. Proc Natl Acad Sci USA 2001;98:7964–7969.

115. Murakami M, Matsumoto R, Urade Y, et al. c-*kit* ligand mediates increased expression of cytosolic phospholipase A_2, prostaglandin endoperoxide synthase 1, and hematopoietic prostaglandin D_2 synthase and increased IgE-dependent PGD_2 generation in immature mouse mast cells. J Biol Chem 1995;270:3239–3246.

116. Liu MC, Bleecker ER, Lichtenstein LM, et al. Evidence for elevated levels of histamine, prostaglandin D_2, and other bronchoconstricting prostaglandins in the airways of subjects with mild asthma. Am Rev Respir Dis 1990;142:126–132.

117. Roberts LJ II, Seibert K, Liston TE, et al. PGD_2 is transformed by human coronary arteries to 9 alpha, 11 beta-PGF_2, which contracts human coronary artery rings. Adv Prostaglandin Thromboxane Leukotr Res 1987;17A:427–429.

118. Hirai H, Tanaka K, Yoshie O, et al. Prostaglandin D_2 selectively induces chemotaxis in T helper type 2 cells, eosinophils, and basophils via seven-transmembrane receptor CRTH2. J Exp Med 2001;193:255–261.

119. Boie Y, Sawyer N, Slipetz DM, Metters KM, Abramovitz M. Molecular cloning and characterization of the human prostanoid DP receptor. J Biol Chem 1995;270:18910–18916.

120. Matsuoka T, Hirata M, Tanaka H, et al. Prostaglandin D_2 as a mediator of allergic asthma. Science 2000;287:2013–2017.

121. Bingham CO, III, Austen KF. Phospholipase A_2 enzymes in eicosanoid generation. Proc Assoc Am Phys 1999;111:516–524.

122. Schulman ES, Kagey-Sobotka A, MacGlashan DW Jr, et al. Heterogeneity of human mast cells. J Immunol 1983;131:1936–1941.

123. MacGlashan DW Jr, Schleimer RP, Peters SP, et al. Generation of leukotrienes by purified lung mast cells. J Clin Invest 1982;70:747–751.

124. Peters SP, MacGlashan DW Jr, Schulman ES, et al. Arachidonic acid metabolism in purified human lung mast cells. J Immunol 1984;132:1972–1979.

125. Massey WA, Guo C-B, Dvorak AM, et al. Human uterine mast cells. Isolation, purification, characterization, ultrastructure, and pharmacology. J Immunol 1991;147:1621–1627.

126. Lawrence ID, Warner JA, Cohan VL, et al. Purification and characterization of human skin mast cells. Evidence for human mast cell heterogeneity. J Immunol 1987;139:3062–3069.

127. Hsieh FH, Lam BK, Penrose JF, Austen KF, Boyce JA. T helper cell type 2 cytokines coordinately regulate IgE-dependent cysteinyl leukotriene production by human cord blood-derived mast cells: profound induction of leukotriene C_4 synthase expression by interleukin 4. J Exp Med 2001 193;123–133.

128. Gordon JR, Galli SJ. Mast cells as a source of both preformed and immunologically inducible TNF-α/cachectin. Nature 1990;346:274–276.

129. Subramanian N, Bray MA. Interleukin 1 releases histamine from human basophils and mast cells in vitro. J Immunol 1987;138:271–275.

130. Lu-Kuo JM, Austen KF, Katz HR. Post-transcriptional stabilization by interleukin-1β of interleukin-6 mRNA induced by c-*kit* ligand and interleukin-10 in mouse bone marrow-derived mast cells. J Biol Chem 1996;271:22169–22174.

131. Gagari E, Tsai M, Lantz CS, et al. Differential release of mast cell interleukin-6 via c-kit. Blood 1997;89:2654–2663.

132. Walsh LJ, Trinchieri G, Waldorf HA, et al. Human dermal mast cells contain and release tumor necrosis factor α, which induces endothelial leukocyte adhesion molecule 1. Proc Natl Acad Sci USA 1991;88:4220–4224.

133. Bradding P, Mediwake R, Feather IH, et al. TNF-α is localized to nasal mucosal mast cells and is released in acute allergic rhinitis. Clin Exp Allergy 1995;25:406–415.

134. Bradding P, Roberts JA, Britten KM, et al. Interleukin-4, -5, and -6 and tumor necrosis factor-α in normal and asthmatic airways: evidence for the human mast cell as a source of these cytokines. Am J Respir Cell Mol Biol 1994;10:471–480.

135. Okayama Y, Semper A, Holgate ST, Church MK. Multiple cytokine mRNA expression in human mast cells stimulated via Fc epsilon RI. Int Arch Allergy Immunol 1995;107:158–159.

136. Barata LT, Ying S, Meng Q, et al. IL-4 and IL-5-positive T lymphocytes, eosinophils, and mast cells in allergen-induced late-phase cutaneous reactions in atopic subjects. J Allergy Clin Immunol 1998;101:222–230.

137. Bradding P, Feather IH, Wilson S, et al. Immunolocalization of cytokines in the nasal mucosa of normal and perennial rhinitic subjects. The mast cell as a source of IL-4, IL-5, and IL-6 in human allergic mucosal inflammation. J Immunol 1993;151:3853–3865.

138. Lorentz A, Schwengberg S, Sellge G, et al. Human intestinal mast cells are capable of producing different cytokine profiles: role of IgE receptor cross-linking and IL-4. J Immunol 2000;164:43–48.

139. Ochi H, De Jesus NH, Hsieh F, Austen KF, Boyce JA. Interleukins 4 and 5 prime human mast cells for different profiles of IgE-dependent cytokine production. Proc Natl Acad Sci USA 2000; 97:10509–10513.

140. Grutzkau A, Kruger-Krasagakes S, Kogel H, et al. Detection of intracellular interleukin-8 in human mast cells: flow cytometry as a guide for immunoelectron microscopy. J Histochem Cytochem 1997;45:935–945.

141. Moller A, Lippert U, Lessmann D, et al. Human mast cells produce IL-8. J Immunol 1993;151:3261–3266.

142. Lukacs NW, Hogaboam CM, Kunkel SL, et al. Mast cells produce ENA-78, which can function as a potent neutrophil chemoattractant during allergic airway inflammation. J Leukoc Biol 1998;63:746–751.

143. Yano K, Yamaguchi M, de Mora F, et al. Production of macrophage inflammatory protein-1 alpha by human mast cells: increased anti-IgE-dependent secretion after IgE-dependent enhancement of mast cell IgE-binding ability. Lab Invest 1997;77:185–193.

144. Tedla N, Wang HW, McNeil HP, et al. Regulation of T lymphocyte trafficking into lymph nodes during an immune response by the chemokines macrophage inflammatory protein (MIP)-1α and MIP-1β. J Immunol 1998;161:5663–5672.

145. Baghestanian M, Hofbauer R, Kiener HP, et al. The c-*kit* ligand stem cell factor and anti-IgE promote expression of monocyte chemoattractant protein-1 in human lung mast cells. Blood 1997;90:4438–4449.

146. Hogaboam C, Kunkel SL, Strieter RM, et al. Novel role of transmembrane SCF for mast cell activation and eotaxin production in mast cell-fibroblast interactions. J Immunol 1998;160:6166–6171.

147. Boesiger J, Tsai M, Maurer M, et al. Mast cells can secrete vascular permeability factor/vascular endothelial cell growth factor and exhibit enhanced release after immunoglobulin E-dependent upregulation of FcεRI expression. J Exp Med 1998;188:1135–1145.

148. Kanbe N, Kurosawa M, Nagata H, et al. Cord blood-derived human cultured mast cells produce transforming growth factor β1. Clin Exp Allergy 1999;29:105–113.

149. Reed JA, Albino AP, McNutt NS. Human cutaneous mast cells express basic fibroblast growth factor. Lab Invest 1995;72:215–222.

150. Zhang S, Anderson DF, Bradding P, et al. Human mast cells express stem cell factor. J Pathol 1998;186:59–66.

151. de Paulis A, Minopoli G, Arbustini E, et al. Stem cell factor is localized in, released from, and cleaved by human mast cells. J Immunol 1999;163:2799–2808.

152. Sher A, Hein A, Moser G, Caulfield JP. Complement receptors promote the phagocytosis of bacteria by rat peritoneal mast cells. Lab Invest 1979;41:490–499.

153. Zhang Y, Ramos BF, Jakschik BA. Neutrophil recruitment by tumor necrosis factor from mast cells in immune complex peritonitis. Science 1992;258:1957–1959.

154. Maurer M, Echtenacher B, Hulktner L, et al. The c-*kit* ligand, stem cell factor, can enhance innate immunity through effects on mast cells. J Exp Med 2001;188:2343–2348.

155. Huang C, De Sanctis GT, O'Brien PJ, et al. Evaluation of the substrate specificity of human mast cell tryptase beta I and demonstration of its importance in bacterial infections of the lung. J Biol Chem 2001;276:26276–26284.

156. Malaviya R, Abraham SN. Role of mast cell leukotrienes in neutrophil recruitment and bacterial clearance in infectious peritonitis. J Leukoc Biol 2000;67:841–846.

157. Arock M, Ross E, Lai-Kuen R, et al. Phagocytic and tumor necrosis factor alpha response of human mast cells following exposure to gram-negative and gram-positive bacteria. Infect Immun 1998;66:6030–6034.

158. Bischoff SC, Sellge G, Manns MP, Lorenz A. Interleukin 4 induces a switch of human intestinal mast cells from proinflammatory cells to Th2-type cells. Int Arch Allergy Immunol 2001;124:151–154.

159. Malaviya R. Ross E. Jakschik BA. Abraham SN. Mast cell degranulation induced by type 1 fimbriated *Escherichia coli* in mice. J Clin Invest 1994;93:1645–1653.

160. Malaviya R, Twesten NJ, Ross EA, Abraham SN, Pfeifer JD. Mast cells process bacterial antigens through a phagocytic route for class I MHC presentation to T cells. J Immunol 1996;156:1490–1496.

161. Malaviya R, Gao Z, Thankavel K, van der Merwe PA, Abraham SN. The mast cell tumor necrosis factor alpha response to FimH-expressing *Escherichia coli* is mediated by the glycosylphosphatidylinositol-anchored molecule CD48. Proc Natl Acad Sci USA 1999;96:8110–8115.

162. Malaviya R, Navara C, Uckun FM. Role of Janus kinase 3 in mast cell-mediated innate immunity against gram-negative bacteria. Immunity 2001;18:313–321.

163. Supajatura V, Ushio H, Nakao A, Okumura K, Ra C, Ogawa H. Protective roles of mast cells against enterobacterial infection are mediated by toll-like receptor 4. J Immunol 2001;167:2250–2256.

164. Bidri M, Vouldoukis I, Mossalayi MD, et al. Evidence for direct interaction between mast cells and *Leishmania* parasites. Parasite Immunol 1997;19:475–483.

165. Prodeus AP, Zhou X, Maurer M, Galli SJ, Carroll MC. Impaired mast cell-dependent natural immunity in complement C3-deficient mice. Nature 1997;390:172–175.

166. Gommerman JL, Oh DY, Zhou X, et al. A role for CD21/CD35 and CD19 in responses to acute septic peritonitis: a potential mechanism for mast cell activation. J Immunol 2000;165:6915–6921.

167. Nilsson G, Johnell M, Hammer CH, et al. C3a and C5a are chemotaxins for human mast cells and act through distinct receptors via a pertussis toxin-sensitive signal transduction pathway. J Immunol 1996;157:1693–1698.

168. el-Lati SG, Dahinden CA, Church MK. Complement peptides C3a- and C5a-induced mediator release from dissociated human skin mast cells. J Invest Dermatol 1994;102:803–806.

169. Artis D, Humphreys NE, Potten CS, et al. β7 integrin-deficient mice: delayed leukocyte recruitment and attenuated protective immunity in the small intestine during enteric helminth infection. Eur J Immunol 2000;30:1656–1664.

21
CD1-Restricted T-Cells

D. Branch Moody

1. INTRODUCTION: *T-CELLS AS EFFECTORS OF INNATE IMMUNITY*

The primary signals for T-cell activation are not generally mediated by soluble antigens. Instead, T-cell receptors (TCRs) interact with antigens complexed to proteins on the surface of antigen-presenting cells (APCs). Until recently, it was thought that peptides bound to MHC-encoded antigen-presenting molecules were the only natural targets of T-cell responses in vivo *(1)*. However, recent studies have shown that T-cells respond to a variety of nonpeptide antigens including lipids bound to CD1 proteins *(2–8)*. This expands our understanding of T-cell function in a number of ways, including those that challenge the traditional paradigms of T-cell function in innate and acquired immunity. In particular, this discovery suggests a fundamentally new function of T-cells involving the recognition of alterations in the lipid content of cellular membranes that result from infection, transformation, or cellular stress.

To explain the roles of these newly discovered lipid-specific T-cells in integrated immune responses, CD1-restricted T-cells have been compared with cells that have established roles in either innate or acquired immunity. In contrast to MHC-restricted T-cells, which express millions of unique TCRs and function in acquired immunity, certain CD1d-restricted NK T-cells have a strikingly limited TCR repertoire and respond to a very limited number of antigens *(7,9–11)*. Therefore, these NK T-cells have been likened to effectors of innate immunity, which use germline-encoded, pattern recognition receptors to interact with foreign antigens *(12,13)*.

However, other CD1-restricted T-cells express clonally varied receptors and recognize a moderately varied spectrum of antigens *(14–17)*. Therefore, it is at least possible that infection could shape the CD1-restricted T-cell repertoire over time. This discussion of the biologic functions of CD1-restricted T-cell function emphasizes criteria that differentiate effectors of innate and acquired immunity: (1) receptor diversity; (2) ligand diversity; (3) precursor frequency; and (4) generation of antigen-specific memory. Overall, CD1-restricted T-cells appear to mediate immunologic functions that are intermediate between classical notions of acquired or innate immunity, leading to a more nuanced understanding of these concepts (Fig. 1).

From: *Infectious Disease: Innate Immunity*
Edited by: R. A. B. Ezekowitz and J. A. Hoffmann © Humana Press Inc., Totowa, NJ

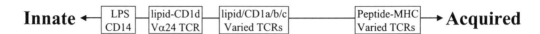

germline encoded pattern recognition receptors   somatically rearranged diverse receptors

antigens of limited diversity and shared patterns   structurally diverse antigens

first antigen exposure mediates response   exposure primes subsequent response

Fig. 1. Receptor-ligand interactions that mediate acquired and innate immune responses. The germline-encoded receptor of the innate immune system, CD14, transmits signals in response to bacterial lipopolysaccharide (LPS). In contrast, MHC-restricted T-cells, which express markedly varied T-cell receptors (TCRs), use clonal selection to acquire increasingly strong response to peptide antigens after multiple exposures. These acquired T-cell responses underlie the therapeutic effects of vaccines against microbial pathogens and tumors. CD1-restricted T-cells use moderately varied TCRs to interact with a moderately varied spectrum of lipid antigens. This suggests that CD1-restricted T-cells have functions that are intermediate between classical notions of acquired and innate immunity.

2. THE CD1 FAMILY OF ANTIGEN-PRESENTING MOLECULES

CD1 genes are present in all mammalian species studied to date, including humans, mice, rats, rabbits, sheep, monkeys, guinea pigs, and dogs *(18–26)*. Humans express five CD1 genes, CD1A, CD1B, CD1C, CD1D, and CD1E, which are encoded outside the MHC on chromosome 1 (Fig. 2) *(3)*. All five of the CD1 genes are now known to be translated into proteins, and four of these, CD1a, CD1b, CD1c, and CD1d, have been shown to function in antigen presentation to T-cells *(7,8,27–31)*. CD1 genes are often described as being nonpolymorphic, since they do not show the high levels of allelic polymorphism that are characteristic of MHC class I and class II antigen presentation molecules *(2,32)*. Shortly after the discovery of the human CD1 locus, the five human CD1 genes were separated into two groups based on their sequence similarities *(27)*. CD1A, CD1B, and CD1C genes have the highest levels of sequence homology to one another and were designated group 1, whereas CD1D was designated group 2, and CD1E had features of both groups. Although this classification was originally based solely on gene structure, subsequent investigations of CD1 protein expression and T-cell function have generally supported the division of CD1 genes into two families, as detailed below (Fig. 2).

CD1 proteins are transmembrane glycoproteins that contain short cytoplasmic domains and three extracellular domains (α_1, α_2, and α_3), which noncovalently associate with β_2-microglobulin (β_2-M) *(33)*. Because of their similar domain organization and β_2-M-dependent expression, CD1 proteins are sometimes referred to as MHC class I-like proteins. However, in terms of amino acid sequence homology, CD1 proteins are similarly related to MHC class I and MHC class II. Therefore, these three families of antigen-presenting molecules are thought to have diverged at similar time point in evolution, and CD1 proteins are more appropriately viewed as a distinct family of antigen-presenting molecules.

3. CD1-GLYCOLIPID ANTIGEN COMPLEXES

Detailed structures of the murine CD1d and CD1b proteins are available from X-ray crystal structure studies (Fig. 3) *(34,35)*. The CD1 α_3-domain has an immunoglobulin-

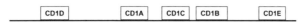

Human Chromosome 1q22-23

Group 2	Group 1
CD1d	CD1a, CD1b, CD1c
α-gal-ceramides and others	varied antigens
TCR conservation	no evidence for TCR conservation
Conserved in all mammals studied	Conserved in mammals except muroid rodents

Fig. 2. Two groups of human CD1 proteins. CD1d mediates presentation of α-galactosyl ceramides and phosphatidylinositols to T cells with a conserved T cell receptor (TCR) repertoire. Group 1 CD1 proteins present a variety of microbial glycolipids to a population of T cells with diverse TCRs.

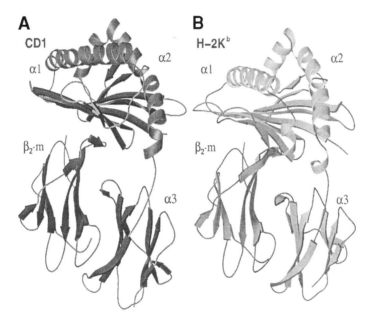

Fig. 3. Murine CD1d (**A**) and MHC class I molecules (**B**) are similar in their overall structure, and both proteins form a groove comprised of a β-sheet floor and α-helices. CD1-antigen complexes are formed by insertion of the alkyl chains into the hydrophobic groove, allowing the hydrophilic portions of the antigen to protrude for direct interactions with the T-cell antigen receptor. β_2-m, β_2-microglobulin. (Reprinted from Zeng Z, Castaño AR, Segelke BW, et al. *Science*, 277:339–344 1997. Copyright 1999 American Association for the Advancement of Science.)

like fold, and the α_1- and α_2 domains form a hollow groove in the distal surface of the protein, which functions as an antigen binding site. The overall architecture of the CD1 grooves are similar to that of MHC-encoded antigen-presenting molecules, insofar as the CD1 grooves are composed of a β-sheet floor that supports antiparallel α-helices that form the lateral margins of the grooves. However, the CD1d has two large pockets, A′ and F′, rather than the seven pockets of a typical MHC class I groove. The groove of human CD1b is much larger and composed of 4 pockets, A', C', F', and T'. Importantly, the amino acids that line the inner surface of the CD1 grooves have predominantly non-polar side chains, providing hydrophobic surfaces for interaction with antigens.

Although it is customary to refer to the CD1 antigen binding structure as a groove, the depth and enclosed nature of this structure can be more readily likened to a pocket or a shallow cave. Interdomain interactions between amino acids in the α_1- and α_2-helices of mCD1d close the groove at both ends and restrict access to the top of the groove, so that the route for entry into the hollow interior of the protein is through a relatively narrow portal above the F' pocket. Thus, the CD1d groove can more fully sequester antigens within the globular head of the protein formed by the α_1- and α_2-domains, in contrast to MHC class I and class II grooves, which are open to solvent over their entire length *(35)*. Thus, the enclosed and hydrophobic nature of the CD1 groove is well suited to bind the antigens that it presents, small amphipathic lipids and glycolipids.

The antigen-presenting function of CD1 proteins was first demonstrated using human T-cell lines that were specifically activated by components of the mycobacterial cell wall *(8)*. Structural characterization of the antigens presented by CD1b molecules indicated that they are lipids or glycolipids including mycolic acid, lipoarabinoman-nan, or glucose monomycolate *(4–6)*. These CD1b-presented microbial lipids, along with CD1c-presented mannosyl phosphoisoprenoids, differ in structure from the gly-colipids that compose mammalian cells and are therefore foreign antigens (Fig. 4) *(36)*. However, self glycolipids of normal structure, including phosphatidylethanolamine, phosphatidylinositol and gangliosides, can also be presented by APCs to CD1-restricted T-cells. *(37–39)* In addition to these naturally occurring foreign and self gly-colipids, synthetic α-galactosyl ceramides, and hydrophobic peptides can bind to CD1d and mediate CD1d-restricted T-cell responses *(7,40)*.

The molecular mechanism of antigen presentation involves the insertion of lipids into the CD1 groove, allowing the aliphatic hydrocarbon chains of the antigens to interact with the hydrophobic interior of the CD1 groove. This binding mechanism allows the carbohydrate portions and other hydrophilic components of the antigen to protrude from the groove into the aqueous solvent, making them available for direct contact with anti-gen-specific TCRs *(6,14,17,35,41)*. This molecular model of antigen presentation is sup-ported by studies of recombinant CD1b and CD1d proteins that directly bind lipid antigens such as lipoarabinomannan, glucose monomycolate, phosphatidylinositol, and α-galac-tosyl ceramide *(42,43)*. Also, phosphatidylinositol-containing compounds have been eluted from cellular CD1d proteins, demonstrating that glycolipids are loaded onto CD1 proteins within cells *(44)*. These data, combined with the reports of CD1d-restricted T-cell binding to CD1d-glycolipid tetramers, provide strong evidence that CD1-glycolipid antigen complexes are the molecular targets of CD1-restricted T-cell responses *(45–47)*.

Early studies of T-cell specificity for glycolipid antigen structure demonstrated that various CD1-restricted T-cell populations recognize individual glycolipid antigens without crossreactivity *(4–6)*. This implied that T-cell activation is mediated by clon-ally distributed receptors expressed on individual T-cells within the CD1-restricted T-cell repertoire. More recently, the introduction of TCRs from CD1-restricted T-cells into the germline of mice or transfection into CD3^{low} lymphoblastoid cells has been shown to transfer antigen recognition, formally demonstrating that CD1-restricted T-cell responses are mediated by TCRs *(7,14)*. There is also evidence that stimulation

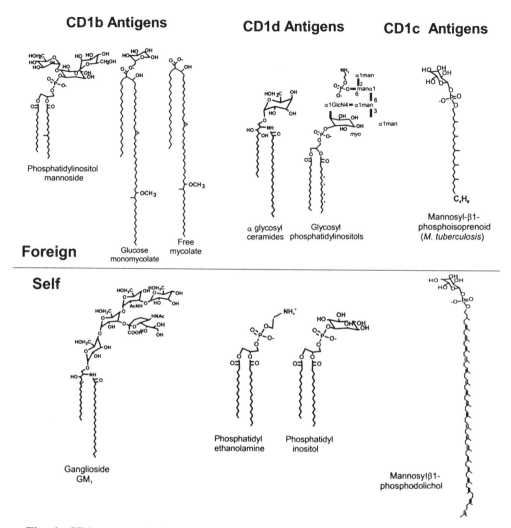

Fig. 4. CD1-presented glycolipid antigens. CD1-presented lipid antigens include foreign lipids derived from the mycobacterial cell wall and self antigens from mammalian cells. Phosphatidylinositol mannoside is depicted with two mannosyl residues, although antigenic forms typically have a larger carbohydrate structure.

through accessory receptors such as natural killer (NK) cell locus-encoded proteins (CD161) or members of the B-7 family of costimulatory proteins can also modulate the activation state of CD1-restricted T-cells, although co-receptors with functions that are analogous to those of CD4 or CD8 are not known *(48–50)*. Thus, T-cell activation by glycolipids occurs by a molecular mechanism that is analogous to the recognition of peptide-MHC complexes, a trimolecular interaction of the variable regions of antigen-specific TCRα- and β-chains with lipid-CD1 complexes *(17)*.

4. CELLULAR PATHWAYS OF LIPID ANTIGEN PRESENTATION

CD1 antigen-presenting molecules are predominantly expressed on hematopoietic cells with specialized immunologic functions, including myeloid dendritic cells,

Langerhans cells, B-cells, and thymocytes *(51)*. Thymocytes and dendritic cells express all four of the known CD1 isoforms with an established function in antigen presentation. Other APCs selectively express only certain CD1 isoforms *(23,51)*. For example, resting human monocytes express only CD1d *(52)*. B-cells generally express only CD1c and CD1d, and epidermal Langerhans cells have been routinely identified in histologic sections by their abundant expression of the CD1a protein *(53,53–55)*. The expression of different human CD1 isoforms on cell types with distinct functions in antigen presentation constitutes one line of evidence that each of the human CD1 isoforms has differing immunologic functions.

In addition, each of the human CD1 proteins differ from one another in their patterns of expression within intracellular compartments of APCs, reflecting their differing patterns of trafficking through secretory, cell surface and endosomal compartments *(54,56–59)*. After translation and folding in the endoplasmic reticulum, CD1 proteins are thought to exit to the cell surface via the secretory pathway. CD1b, CD1c, and CD1d proteins reach the endosomal network by one of two known mechanisms. CD1d proteins associate with invariant chain, which promotes their delivery to late endosomes *(60)*. In addition, cytoplasmic tails of CD1b, CD1c, and CD1d proteins contain a sequence conforming to a tyrosine-based amino acid motif that interacts with clathrin adaptor protein complexes, promoting the trafficking of these CD1 proteins from the cell surface into the endosomal network *(56–61)*. Although CD1b, CD1c, and CD1d are all found in endosomes, CD1b proteins appear to traffic more deeply into the endosomal network, as evidenced by their more extensive colocalization with markers of late endosomes and lysosomes such as LAMP-1 *(58)*. In contrast, CD1a is found almost exclusively at the cell surface, presumably because it has a particularly short cytoplasmic tail, which lacks an endosomal localization motif *(54)*.

These differing trafficking patterns of various human CD1 isoforms suggest that each of the human isoforms functions to survey the glycolipid content of different subcellular locations *(62,63)*. In fact, there is now substantial evidence that the trafficking of CD1b and CD1d proteins through late endosomal compartments influences the development and activation of antigen-specific T-cells. For example, mutation of the tyrosine-containing endosomal targeting motifs in the CD1b or CD1d tails blocks T-cell activation by CD1-presented mycobacterial glycolipids *(8,59,60,64–66)*. Antigen structure can also influence which glycolipids are loaded onto CD1 proteins for T-cell recognition, since CD1b-presented antigens with longer alkyl chains are preferentially presented by myeloid DCs *(67)*. These studies demonstrate the strong influence of cellular pathways of transport of antigens and CD1 proteins on the outcome of antigen-specific T-cell responses.

Since CD1-restricted T-cells are highly specific for lipid antigen structure, cellular mechanisms that control which particular families of lipids are loaded onto CD1 proteins could exert a profound effect on the outcome of immune responses in vivo. These observations have led to growing interest in the cellular pathways of processing glycolipid antigens for recognition by T-cells. However, the precise molecular mechanism of loading glycolipid antigens into the hydrophobic groove of CD1 proteins has not yet been determined. Unlike peptides, glycolipids are not generally soluble in aqueous solution at the concentrations required for activating T-cells. Therefore, antigens will probably be loaded onto CD1 from membranes, lipid-binding proteins, or other aggregated forms. Whether glycolipid antigen processing involves covalent modification of glycolipids, as is known to be the case for peptides, is also an area of ongoing study. Since most natural glycolipids have a lipid moiety that corresponds to the size of the CD1 groove, the molecular trimming of glycolipids prior to loading is probably not a universal requirement for processing *(17)*. However, in some cases, cellular processing reactions involving alterations of lipid chains, glycosylation, or deglycosylation can affect T-cell responses, as has been documented for certain ceramide and mycolyl glycolipids *(68,69)*.

5. CD1D-RESTRICTED T-CELLS

NK T-cells were discovered as a specialized population of $CD4^+$ or $CD4^-/CD8^-$ T-cells that were MHC-unrestricted and expressed receptors encoded in the NK locus, including NK1.1 in the mouse and NKRP-1 in the human (CD161) *(70–72)*. Although NK receptors can modulate the activation state of these cells, studies have now clearly demonstrated that NK T-cell activation is controlled primarily by TCR interactions with lipid-loaded CD1d proteins *(7,45–47,49,73)*.

One striking feature of a major population of NK T-cells in vivo is a marked limitation of TCR gene usage. A large population of NK T-cells expresses an invariant TCR α-chain that pairs with a limited number of Vβ-chains. In mice, this is Vα14Jα281, typically paired with Vβ2, Bβ7, or Vβ8; in humans, the invariant Vα24JαQ usually pairs with Vβ11 *(9,11)*. This limited TCR variability does not result from elements that control the rearrangements of TCR α-chains, but instead results from the positive selection of T-cells bearing these TCRs by CD1d proteins *(74–79)*. This relative lack of complexity of receptor expression distinguishes NK T-cells from the much more complex receptor repertoire of MHC-restricted T-cells, which is shaped by antigen exposure over time (Fig. 1).

The identities of the natural antigenic targets of T-cells are not precisely known. They have been described as autoreactive to CD1d, based on experiments in which T-cell activation requires that APCs express the CD1d heavy chain and β_2-M but does not require addition of an exogenous glycolipid antigen *(73)*. However, this does not imply that these T-cells recognize unliganded CD1d proteins. Instead, it is likely that CD1d binds and presents self or altered self lipids for recognition by T-cells. In support of this hypothesis, phosphatidylinositol-containing compounds have been eluted from cellular CD1d proteins, and lipids of similar structure have been shown to activate T-cells under certain circumstances in vitro *(38,39,44,80,81)*. However, phosphatidylinositol-containing compounds do not stimulate most CD1d-restricted T-cells *(7,44)*. Therefore, it is thought that nonantigenic phosphatidylinositols or other self compounds occupy the CD1d groove, functioning as chaperones prior to insertion of more strongly antigenic lipids into the groove.

The most potent antigens for NK T-cells are a family of structurally related synthetic compounds known as α-galactosyl ceramides. They have been shown to bind CD1d proteins, forming complexes that interact with the invariant TCRs *(45–47,82)*. These antigens, which rapidly activate large populations of CD1d-restricted T-cells both in vitro and in vivo, were discovered in a screen of natural and synthetic compounds for antitumor effects *(7)*. They are naturally produced by marine sponges but are not

known to be made by either mammalian cells or pathogenic microbes (Fig. 4). Therefore, the precise structure of endogenous glycolipids, which control the activation of
CD1d-restricted T-cells in vivo, remains to be defined. One leading hypothesis is that
these antigens are altered self lipids that are related in structure to known synthetic
antigens or natural CD1d ligands.

The functions of CD1d-restricted T-cells in vivo have been investigated by injecting
mice with α-galactosyl ceramides, by germline deletion of CD1d or by deletion of the
the Jα281 gene, which is necessary for expression of the invariant TCR α-chain in
mice *(7,74,79,83)*. Treatment of mice with large doses of α-galactosyl ceramide leads
to strong immunologic effects and systemically detectable levels of interferon-γ, inter-
leukin-4 (IL-4), and other cytokines. However, whether antigen treatment results in
immune activation or immunosuppression in vivo depends on the experimental proto-
col and the disease under study. For example, systemic injections of α-galactosyl
ceramide promote protection against infection by viruses, fungi, and protozoa *(84–88)*.
These effects are typically associated with augmentation of Th1 T-cell responses and
may be mediated in part through interferon-γ secretion by CD1d-restricted T-cells.

On the other hand, treatment of mice with α-galactosyl ceramide also protects
against the development of autoimmune diabetes and allergic encephalomyelitis (EAE)
(86,89–91). These apparent immunosuppressive effects of ceramide antigens have been
confirmed in studies showing that CD1d deletion exacerbates autoimmune diabetes
(92,93). Further confirming the strong, but varied effects of NK T-cells on immune
response, CD1d-restricted T-cells have been shown to promote or inhibit tumor growth
in animal models. For example, mice lacking Jα281 TCRs did not efficiently reject
melanoma cells. In contrast, other studies have shown that CD1d knockout mice were
found to have lower rates of recurrence of virally transformed fibroblast tumors, and
that transfer of NK T-cells promoted growth of skin tumors *(94–96)*.

These studies clearly indicate that selective activation of CD1d-restricted T-cells can
strongly influence the integrated immune response to pathogens, self tissues, and
tumors in vivo, and further studies are aimed at understanding the precise factors that
control whether CD1d-restricted T-cells augment or inhibit immune responses. As in
MHC-restricted T-cells, there is evidence that antigen-mediated signals through the
TCR can lead to activation, apoptotic cell death, or Th1/Th2 polarized responses,
depending on the stimulation conditions *(48,50,86)*. Therefore, to some extent these
varied effects of NK T-cell restriction in vivo may probably result from the specific
aspects of the antigen treatment protocols. In addition, a recent study shows that as NK
T-cells leave the thymus, they switch from a predominantly TH1 to TH2 cytokine profile *(97)*. Thus, the developmental stage at which activation occurs may control whether
NK T-cells promote or inhibit immune responses to pathogens or tumors.

NK T-cells differ from MHC-restricted T-cells in their precursor frequency as well
as their requirements for priming and maturation prior to development of effector functions. For example, peptide-specific MHC-restricted T-cells circulate at very low fre-
quencies, whereas invariant NK T-cells can comprise up to 1% of peripheral blood
T-cells in mice and several percent of the total lymphocytes in certain organs, such as
the liver *(46,97,98)*. Unlike MHC-restricted T-cells this relatively large population of
NK T-cells does not appear to require antigen priming or maturation into a distinct
memory phenotype prior to activation in vivo. In fact, systemic administration of a sin-

gle dose of α-galactosyl ceramide leads to rapid activation of this population in naive animals, which can result in systemically detectable levels of cytokines *(13,99)*.

The high precursor frequency, limited receptor variability, limited antigen variability, and strong activation by a primary immune response suggest that NK T-cells and peptide-specific T-cells may have fundamentally different functions in immune response (Fig. 1). In these respects, NK T-cells have more in common with effector cells of the innate immune system, which use pattern recognition receptors to respond to a limited number of nonself antigens of conserved structure. This model predicts that NK T-cells, like other effectors of innate immunity, play a role early in the immune response, either to combat infection directly or to regulate the other cells, including peptide-specific T-cells.

Recent studies have now demonstrated that not all CD1d-restricted T-cells express the canonical Vα14 in mice and the Vα24 in humans. Certain murine CD1d-restricted T-cell clones express varied α-chains that pair randomly with at least somewhat varied β-chains, producing a large variety of αβ TCRs *(15,100,101)*. Whether these varied CD1d-restricted T-cells mediate recognition of a diverse set of antigens remains to be investigated. However, detection of CD1d-restricted T-cells with varied receptors raises the possibility that this T-cell population has additional functions in immune response that are distinct from invariant NK T-cells.

6. T-CELLS RESTRICTED BY GROUP 1 CD1 PROTEINS

T-cells that recognize glycolipid antigens presented by group 1 CD1 proteins (CD1a, CD1b, CD1c) appear to be somewhat more diverse in their TCR repertoire and range of antigenic targets than NK T-cells. Most of the known antigens for group 1 CD1-restricted T-cells, including mycolic acids, lipoarabinomannans, glucose mono-mycolates, and mannosyl phosphoisoprenoids (Fig. 4), are produced by mycobacteria and related species *(4–6,8,102)*. Since these glycolipids do not have readily identifiable homologs in mammalian cells, they are intrinsically foreign to the mammalian immune system, providing one argument for a role of group 1 CD1 proteins in host defense against infection.

The regulated expression of group 1 CD1 proteins on myeloid dendritic cells (DCs) provides a second line of evidence for group 1 CD1 protein function in host defense. The most extensively studied extrathymic APC that expresses group 1 CD1 proteins is the myeloid DC. DCs undergo a program of differentiation as they migrate from the bone marrow to the peripheral blood, through inflamed tissues and subsequently to secondary lymphoid tissues. Although it has long been appreciated that DCs control the activation of peptide-specific T-cells by acquiring antigen-presenting functions at discrete stages of development, the developmental regulation of group 1 CD1 proteins now provides evidence that this is also the case for glycolipid-specific T-cells *(103)*. Resting peripheral blood monocytes express CD1d, but not group 1 CD1 proteins. Maturation of monocytes into immature or mature DCs can be accomplished by stimulation with granulocyte/macrophage colony-stimulating factor (GM-CSF), IL-4, or other stimuli *(51)*. This process is accompanied by marked upregulation of CD1a, CD1b, and CD1c proteins, whereas changes in CD1d expression, if present, are inconsistent *(52)*. Group 1 CD1 proteins are strongly expressed on myeloid cells in skin biopsies of patients infected with *Mycobacterium leprae,* providing direct evidence for the upregulation of group 1 CD1 proteins on DCs during natural infections *(104)*. These observations suggest that myeloid cells migrate to sites of infection and selectively upregulate group 1 CD1 proteins for antigen presentation during the host response to infection.

CD1a-, CD1b-, and CD1c-restricted T-cells possess effector mechanisms that have established roles in promoting host defense against mycobacteria and other pathogens. In vitro analysis of human group 1 CD1-restricted T-cells has demonstrated that they secrete interferon-γ, synthesize granulysin, and are cytolytic *(105,106)*. Moreover, these mechanisms lead to the killing of target cells that are infected with mycobacteria *(59,105)*. In addition, there is also evidence for the generation of glycolipid-specific T-cell responses during the natural human immune response to *Mycobacterium tuberculosis*, since CD1c-restricted lymphocytes isolated from human tuberculosis patients show greater stimulation by mannosyl phosphoisoprenoid antigens than uninfected patients *(36)*. Although these studies provide evidence for a function of group 1 CD1 proteins in human host defense mechanisms, conclusive evidence for a protective function awaits development of animal models other than mice (which do not express homologs of group 1 CD1 proteins) *(19)*.

In contrast to NK T-cells, analysis of TCR expression in CD1a-, CD1b-, and CD1c-restricted T-cells has failed to find evidence for a conserved TCR structure. Among clones examined to date, the TCRs that mediate recognition of antigens presented by CD1a, CD1b, and CD1c have been found to incorporate varied Vα and Vβ gene segments and apparently random N-region additions *(14)*. These varied TCRs mediate recognition of structurally distinct antigens, and those T-cells that recognize a given antigen do not generally crossreact with structurally related glycolipids or with other known CD1-presented glycolipids *(7,36)*. For example, CD1b-restricted cells, which recognize glucose monomycolate, do not crossreact with mannose monomycolate or free mycolic acid, even though all these antigens contain the lipid moiety that is thought to mediate binding to CD1b proteins (Fig. 3) *(4,6)*.

Although the extent of the structural variability of microbial glycolipid antigens is not known, CD1a, CD1b, and CD1c isoforms present structurally distinct classes of glycolipid antigens, such as mycolyl glycolipids, diacylglycerols, sphingolipids, and polyisoprenoid lipids (Fig. 4). Moreover, the CD1b isoform can bind and present antigens composed of at least three of these classes, mycolates, diacylglycerols, and sphingolipids *(4,5,37)*. Thus, CD1b has some promiscuity for binding chemically varied classes of glycolipid antigens, despite the nonpolymorphic nature of the CD1b antigen binding groove (Fig. 3). Since each of these larger classes contains many different naturally occurring glycosylated derivatives, it is possible that the number of glycolipid antigens recognized by CD1-restricted T-cells is substantially greater than currently known. Thus, with regard to receptor and antigen diversity, group 1 CD1-restricted T-cells appear to be somewhat more complex than invariant CD1d-restricted T-cells. Therefore, the rationale for viewing group 1 CD1-restricted T-cells as typical effectors of innate immunity is less strong than that for NK T-cells restricted by CD1d (Fig. 1).

7. CONCLUSIONS

CD1-restricted T-cells represent a previously unknown arm of the cellular immune system, which is specialized to respond to alterations in the lipid content of cells. Considered as a whole, the CD1-restricted T-cell repertoire represents many populations of

T-cells that respond without crossreactivity to a variety of lipid ligands *(17)*. These lipid antigens differ in their expression among pathogens, vary in their pathways of biosynthesis, and accumulate in different cell types and disease states *(102,107–109)*. Thus, it is unlikely that CD1-restricted T-cells have a single housekeeping function; instead, they likely have diverse functions in immune response to infected, transformed, or otherwise stressed cells *(17,110)*. Given the potential variety of both receptors and ligands used by variable CD1-restricted T-cells, this system has the components necessary to maintain at least a moderately complex repertoire of antigen specificities that could be shaped by immunologic experience. However, the existence of glycolipid antigen-specific memory responses has yet to be experimentally demonstrated, and the phenotype of invariant NK T-cells points to a conserved immunoregulatory function that is not subject to alteration by immunologic experience.

Therefore, understanding where variable and invariant CD1-restricted T-cells fall in the spectrum of innate and acquired immune response is a question of great importance (Fig. 1). If infection or other factors can have long-lasting effects on the repertoire of glycolipid-specific T-cells in humans, then glycolipids, which are easily administered small molecules, will be developed as vaccines. On the other hand, if CD1-restricted T-cells function to activate effector cells of innate immunity rapidly, then CD1-presented glycolipids can be rationally developed as adjuvants or immunomodulatory agents that will augment or polarize the responses to conventional peptide antigens. In either case, CD1-presented self and foreign glycolipids represent a new class of immunomodulatory molecules that are tucked into the membranes of human cells and can be developed for the diagnosis and treatment of human diseases.

REFERENCES

1. Garcia KC, Degano M, Stanfield RL, et al. An alphabeta T cell receptor structure at 2.5 A and its orientation in the TCR-MHC complex. Science 1996;274:209–219.
2. Porcelli SA. The CD1 family: a third lineage of antigen-presenting molecules. Adv Immunol 1995;59:1–98.
3. Calabi F, Milstein C. A novel family of human major histocompatibility complex-related genes not mapping to chromosome 6. Nature 1986;323:540–543.
4. Beckman EM, Porcelli SA, Morita CT, et al. Recognition of a lipid antigen by CD1-restricted alpha beta+ T cells. Nature 1994;372:691–694.
5. Sieling PA, Chatterjee D, Porcelli SA, et al. CD1-restricted T cell recognition of microbial lipoglycan antigens. Science 1995;269:227–230.
6. Moody DB, Reinhold BB, Guy MR, et al. Structural requirements for glycolipid antigen recognition by CD1b- restricted T cells. Science 1997;278:283–286.
7. Kawano T, Cui J, Koezuka Y, et al. CD1d-restricted and TCR-mediated activation of Vα 14 NKT cells by glycosylceramides. Science 1997;278:1626–1629.
8. Porcelli S, Morita CT, Brenner MB. CD1b restricts the response of human CD4(–)8(–) T lymphocyctes to a microbial antigen. Nature 1992;360:593–597.
9. Koseki H, Imai K, Nakayama F, et al. Homogenous junctional sequence of the V14+ T-cell antigen receptor alpha chain expanded in unprimed mice. Proc Natl Acad Sci USA 1990;87:5248–5252.
10. Lantz O, Bendelac A. An invariant T cell receptor alpha chain is used by a unique subset of major histocompatibility complex class I-specific CD4+ and CD4-8– T cells in mice and humans. J Exp Med 1994;180:1097–1106.

11. Procelli S, Gerdes D, Fertig AM, Balk SP. Human T cells expressing an invariant V alpha 24-J alpha Q TCR alpha are CD4- and heterogeneous with respect to TCR beta expression. Hum Immunol 1996;48:63–67.

12. Medzhitov R, Janeway CA Jr. Innate immunity: the virtues of a nonclonal system of recognition. Cell 1997;91:295–298.

13. Park SH, Chiu YH, Jayawardena J, et al. Innate and adaptive functions of the CD1 pathway of antigen presentation. Semin Immunol 1998;10:391–398.

14. Grant EP, Degano M, Rosat JP, et al. Molecular recognition of lipid antigens by T cell receptors. J Exp Med 1999;189:195–205.

15. Cardell S, Tangri S, Chan S, et al. CD1-restricted CD4+ T cells in major histocompatibility complex class II-deficient mice. J Exp Med 1995;182:993–1004.

16. Behar SM, Podrebarac TA, Roy CJ, Wang CR, Brenner MB. Diverse TCRs recognize murine CD1. J Immunol 1999;162:161–167.

17. Moody DB, Besra GS, Wilson IA, Porcelli SA. The molecular basis of CD1-mediated presentation of lipid antigens. Immunol Rev 1999;172:285–296.

18. Moore PF, Schrenzel MD, Affolter VK, Olivry T, Naydan D. Canine cutaneous histiocytoma is an epidermotropic Langerhans cell histiocytosis that expresses CD1 and specific beta 2-integrin molecules. Am J Pathol 1996;148:1699–1708.

19. Dascher CC, Hiromatsu K, Naylor JW, et al. Conservation of a CD1 multigene family in the guinea pig. J Immunol 1999;163:5478–5488.

20. Woo JC, Moore PF. A feline homologue of CD1 is defined using a feline-specific monoclonal antibody. Tissue Antigens 1997;49:244–251.

21. Ichimiya S, Kikuchi K, Matsuura A. Structural analysis of the rat homologue of CD1. Evidence for evolutionary conservation of the CD1D class and widespread transcription by rat cells. J Immunol 1994;153:1112–1123.

22. Calabi F, Belt KT, Yu CY, et al. The rabbit CD1 and the evolutionary conservation of the CD1 gene family. Immunogenetics 1989;30:370–377.

23. Calabi F, Milstein C. A novel family of human major histocompatibility complex-related genes not mapping to chromosome 6. Nature 1986;323:540–543.

24. Bradbury A, Belt KT, Neri TM, Milstein C, Calabi F. Mouse CD1 is distinct from and co-exists with TL in the same thymus. EMBO J. 1988;7:3081–3086.

25. MacHugh ND, Bensaid A, Davis WC, et al. Characterization of a bovine thymic differentiation antigen analogous to CD1 in the human. Scand J Immunol 1988;27:541–547.

26. Dutia BM, Hopkins J. Analysis of the CD1 cluster in sheep. Vet Immunol Immunopathol 1991;27:189–194.

27. Calabi F, Jarvis JM, Martin L, Milstein C. Two classes of CD1 genes. Eur J Immunol 1989;19:285–292.

28. Angenieux C, Salamero J, Fricker D, et al. Characterization of CD1e, a third type of CD1 molecule expressed in dendritic cells. J Biol Chem 2000;275:37757–37764.

29. Mirones I, Oteo M, Parra-Cuadrado JF, Martinez-Naves E. Identification of two novel human CD1E alleles [In Process Citation]. Tissue Antigens 2000;56:159–161.

30. Rosat JP, Grant EP, Beckman EM, et al. CD1-restricted microbial lipid antigen-specific recognition found in the CD8+ alpha beta T cell pool. J Immunol 1999;162:366–371.

31. Beckman EM, Melian A, Behar SM, et al. CD1c restricts responses of mycobacteria-specific T cells. Evidence for antigen presentation by a second member of the human CD1 family. J Immunol 1996;157:2795–2803.

32. Han M, Hannick LI, DiBrino M, Robinson MA. Polymorphism of human CD1 genes. Tissue Antigens 1999;54:122–127.

33. Bauer A, Huttinger R, Staffler G, et al. Analysis of the requirement for beta 2-microglobulin for expression and formation of human CD1 antigens. Eur J Immunol 1997;27:1366–1373.

34. Gadola SD, Zaccai NR, Harlos K, et al. Structure of human CD1b with bound ligands at 2.3 A, a maze for alkyl chains. Nat Immunol 2002;3:721–726.

35. Zeng Z, Castaño AR, Segelke BW et al. Crystal structure of mouse CD1: an MHC-like fold with a large hydrophobic binding groove. Science 1997;277:339–345.

36. Moody DB, Ulrichs T, Muhlecker W, et al. CD1c-mediated T cell recognition of mycobacterial glycolipids in *M. tuberculosis* infection. Nature 2000;404:884–888.

37. Shamshiev A, Donda A, Carena I, et al. Self glycolipids as T-cell autoantigens. Eur J Immunol 1999;29:1667–1675.

38. Gumperz J, Roy C, Makowska A, et al. Murine CD1d-restricted T cell recognition of cellular lipids. Immunity 2000;12:211–221.

39. Schofield L, McConville MJ, Hansen D, et al. CD1d-restricted immunoglobulin G formation to GPI-anchored antigens mediated by NKT cells. Science 1999;283:225–229.

40. Castano AR, Tangri S, Miller JE, et al. Peptide binding and presentation by mouse CD1. Science 1995;269:223–226.

41. Brossay L, Naidenko O, Burdin N, et al. Structural requirements for galactosylceramide recognition by CD1-restricted NK T cells. J Immunol 1998;161:5124–5128.

42. Ernst WA, Maher J, Cho S, et al. Molecular interaction of CD1b with lipoglycan antigens. Immunity 1998;8:331–340.

43. Naidenko O, Maher J, Ernst DN, et al. Binding and antigen presentation of ceramide-containing glycolipids by soluble mound and human CD1d molecules. J Exp Med 1999;190:1069–1079.

44. Joyce S, Woods AS, Yewdell JW, et al. Natural ligand of mouse CD1d1: cellular glycosylphosphatidylinositol. Science 1998;279:1541–1544.

45. Park SH, Weiss A, Benlagha K, et al. The mouse CD1d-restricted repertoire is dominated by a few autoreactive T cell receptor families. J Exp Med 2001;193:893–904.

46. Benlagha K, Weiss A, Beavis A, Teyton L, Bendelac A. In vivo identification of glycolipid antigen-specific T cells using fluorescent CD1d tetramers. J Exp Med 2000;191:1895–1903.

47. Matsuda JL, Naidenko OV, Gapin L, et al. Tracking the response of natural killer T cells to a glycolipid antigen using CD1d tetramers. J Exp Med 2000;192:741–754.

48. Behar SM, Procelli SA, Beckman EM, Brenner MB. A pathway of costimulation that prevents anergy in CD28-T cells: B7-independent costimulation of CD1-restricted T cells. J Exp Med 1995;182:2007–2018.

49. Asea A, Stein-Streilein J. Signalling through NK1.1 triggers NK cells to die but induces NK T cells to produce interleukin-4. Immunology 1998;93:296–305.

50. Pal E, Tabira T, Kawano T, et al. Costimulation-dependent modulation of experimental autoimmune encephalomyelitis by ligand stimulation of V alpha 14 NK T cells. J Immunol 2001;166:662–668.

51. Porcelli SA. The CD1 family: a third lineage of antigen-presenting molecules. Adv Immunol 1995;59:1–98.

52. Spada FM, Borriello F, Sugita M, et al. Low expression level but potent antigen presenting function of CD1d on monocyte lineage cells. Eur J Immunol 2000;30:3468–3477.

53. Small TN, Knowles RW, Keever C, et al. M241 (CD1c) expression on B lymphocytes. J Immunol 1987;138:2864–2868.

54. Sugita M, Grant EP, van Donselaar E, et al. Separate pathways for antigen presentation by CD1 molecules. Immunity 1999;11:743–752.

55. Fithian E, Kung P, Goldstein G, et al. Reactivity of Langerhans cells with hybridoma antibody. Proc Natl Acad Sci USA 1981;78:2541–2544.

56. Sugita M, Jackman RM, van Donselaar E, et al. Cytoplasmic tail-dependent localization of CD1b antigen-presenting molecules to MIICs. Science 1996;273:349–352.

57. Sugita M, van Der W, Rogers RA, Peters PJ, Brenner MB. CD1c molecules broadly survey the endocytic system. Proc Natl Acad Sci USA 2000;97:8445–8450.

58. Briken V, Jackman RM, Watts GF, Rogers RA, Porcelli SA. Human CD1b and CD1c isoforms survey different intracellular compartments for the presentation of microbial lipid antigens. J Exp Med 2000;192:281–288.

59. Jackman RM, Stenger S, Lee A, et al. The tyrosine-containing cytoplasmic tail of CD1b is essential for its efficient presentation of bacterial lipid antigens. Immunity 1998;8:341–351.

60. Jayawardena-Wolf J, Benlagha K, Chiu YH, Mehr R, Bendelac A. CD1d endosomal trafficking is independently regulated by an intrinisic CD1d-encoded tyrosine motif and by the invariant chain. Immunity 2001;15:897–908.

61. Bonifacino JS, Dell'Angelica EC. Molecular bases for the recognition of tyrosine-based sorting signals. J Cell Biol 1999;145:923–926.

62. Briken V, Moody DB, Porcelli SA. Diversification of CD1 proteins: sampling the lipid content of different cellular compartments. Semin Immunol 2000;12:517–525.

63. Sugita M, Peters PJ, Brenner MB. Pathways for lipid antigen presentation by CD1 molecules: nowhere for intracellular pathogens to hide. Traffic 2000;1:295–300.

64. Moody DB, Reinhold BB, Reinhold VN, Besra GS, Porcelli SA. Uptake and processing of glycosylated mycolates for presentation to CD1b-restricted T cells. Immunol Lett 1999;65:85–91.

65. Chiu YH, Jayawardena J, Weiss A, et al. Distinct subsets of CD1d-restricted T cells recognize self-antigens loaded in different cellular compartments. J Exp Med 1999;189:103–110.

66. Spada FM, Koezuka Y, Porcelli SA. CD1d-restricted recognition of synthetic glycolipid antigens by human natural killer T cells. J Exp Med 1998;188:1529–1534.

67. Moody DB, Briken V, Cheng TY, et al. Lipid length controls antigen entry into endosomal and nonendosomal pathways for CD1b presentation. Nat Immunol 2002;3:435–442.

68. Prigozy TI, Naidenko O, Qasba P, et al. Glycolipid antigen processing for presentation by CD1d molecules. Science 2001;291:664–667.

69. Moody DB, Guy MR, Grant E, et al. CD1b-mediated T cell recognition of a glycolipid antigen generated from mycobacterial lipid and host carbohydrate during infection. J Exp Med 2000;192:965–976.

70. Bendelac A, Killeen N, Littman DR, Schwartz RH. A subset of CD4+ thymocytes selected by MHC class I molecules. Science 1994;263:1774–1778.

71. Bendelac A. Mouse NK1+ T cells. Curr Opin Immunol 1995;7:367–374.

72. Beutner U, Launois P, Ohteki T, Louis JA, MacDonald HR. Natural killer-like T cells develop in SJL mice despite genetically distinct defects in NK1.1 expression and in inducible interleukin-4 production. Eur J Immunol 1997;27:928–934.

73. Bendelac A, Lantz O, Quimby ME, et al. CD1 recognition by mouse NK1+ T lymphocytes. Science 1995;268:863–865.

74. Smiley ST, Kaplan MH, Grusby MJ. Immunoglobulin E production in the absence of interleukin-4- secreting CD1-dependent cells. Science 1997;275:977–979.

75. Gapin L, Matsuda JL, Surh CD, Kronenberg M. NKT cells derive from double-positive thymocytes that are positively selected by CD1d. Nat Immunol 2001;2:971–978.

76. Coles MC, Raulet DH. NK1.1+ T cells in the liver arise in the thymus and are selected by interactions with class I molecules on CD4+CD8+ cells. J Immunol 2000;164:2412–2418.

77. Shimamura M, Ohteki T, Beutner U, MacDonald HR. Lack of directed V alpha 14-J alpha 281 rearrangements in NK1+ T cells. Eur J Immunol 1997;27:1576–1579.

78. Mendiratta SK, Martin WD, Hong S, et al. CD1d1 mutant mice are deficient in natural T cells that promptly produce IL-4. Immunity 1997;6:469–477.

79. Chen YH, Chiu NM, Mandal M, Wang N, Wang CR. Impaired NK1+ T cell development and early IL-4 production in CD1-deficient mice. Immunity 1997;6:459–467.

80. Molano A, Park SH, Chiu YH, et al. Cutting edge: the IgG response to the circumsporozoite protein is MHC class II-dependent and CD1d-independent: exploring the role of GPIs in NK T cell activation and antimalarial responses. J Immunol 2000;164:5005–5009.

81. Romero JF, Eberl G, MacDonald HR, Corradin G. CD1d-restricted NK T cells are dispensable for specific antibody responses and protective immunity against liver stage malaria infection in mice. Parasite Immunol 2001;23:267–269.

82. Asou N, Hattori T, Matsuoka M, Kawano F, Takatsuki K. Rearrangements of T-cell antigen receptor delta chain gene in hematologic neoplasms. Blood 1989;74:2707–2712.

83. Kawano T, Nakayama T, Kamada N, et al. Antitumor cytotoxicity mediated by ligand-activated human V alpha24 NKT cells. Cancer Res 1999;59:5102–5105.

84. Gonzalez-Aseguinolaza G, de Oliveira C, Tomaska M, et al. Alpha-galactosylceramide-activated Valpha 14 natural killer T cells mediate protection against murine malaria. Proc Natl Acad Sci USA 2000;97:8461–8466.

85. Kumar H, Belperron A, Barthold SW, Bockenstedt LK. Cutting edge: CD1d deficiency impairs murine host defense against the spirochete, *Borrelia burgdorferi*. J Immunol 2000;165:4797–4801.

86. Miyamoto K, Miyake S, Yamamura T. A synthetic glycolipid prevents autoimmune encephalomyelitis by inducing TH2 bias of natural killer T cells. Nature 2001;413:531–534.

87. Kawakami K, Kinjo Y, Yara S, et al. Activation of Valpha14(+) natural killer T cells by alpha-galactosylceramide results in development of Th1 response and local host resistance in mice infected with *Cryptococcus neoformans*. Infect Immunl 2001;69:213–220.

88. Exley MA, Bigley NJ, Cheng O, et al. CD1d-reactive T-cell activation leads to amelioration of disease caused by diabetogenic encephalomyocarditis virus. J Leukoc Biol 2001;69:713–718.

89. Hong S, Wilson MT, Serizawa I, et al. The natural killer T-cell ligand alpha-galactosylceramide prevents autoimmune diabetes in non-obese diabetic mice. Nat Med 2001;7:1052–1056.

90. Sharif S, Arreaza GA, Zucker P, et al. Activation of natural killer T cells by alpha-galactosylceramide treatment prevents the onset and recurrence of autoimmune type 1 diabetes. Nat Med 2001;7:1057–1062.

91. Shi FD, Flodstrom M, Balasa B, et al. Germ line deletion of the CD1 locus exacerbates diabetes in the NOD mouse. Proc Natl Acad Sci USA 2001;98:6777–6782.

92. Wang B, Geng YB, Wang CR. CD1-restricted NK T cells protect nonobese diabetic mice from developing diabetes. J Exp Med 2001;194:313–320.

93. Wang B, Geng YB, Wang CR. CD1-restricted NK T cells protect nonobese diabetic mice from developing diabetes. J Exp Med 2001;194:313–320.

94. Cui J, Shin T, Kawano T, et al. Requirement for valpha 14 NKT cells in IL-12-mediated rejection of tumors. Science 1997;278:1623–1626.

95. Moodycliffe AM, Nghiem D, Clydesdale G, Ullrich SE. Immune suppression and skin cancer development: regulation by NKT cells. Nat Immunol 2000;1:521–525.

96. Terabe M, Matsui S, Noben-Trauth N, et al. NKT cell-mediated repression of tumor immunosurveillance by IL-13 and the IL-4R-STAT6 pathway. Nat Immunol 2000;1:515–520.

97. Benlagha K, Kyin T, Beavis A, Teyton L, Bendelac A. A thymic precursor to the NK T cell lineage. Science 2002;296:535–555.

98. Eberl G, Lees R, Smiley ST, et al. Tissue-specific segregation of CD1d-dependent and CD1d-independent NK T cells. J Immunol 1999;162:6410–6419.

99. MacDonald HR. NK1.1+ T cell receptor-alpha/beta+ cells: new clues to their origin, specificity, and function. J Exp Med 1995;182:633–638.

100. Park SH, Roark JH, Bendelac A. Tissue-specific recognition of mouse CD1 molecules. J Immunol 1998;160:3128–3134.

101. Behar SM, Podrebarac T, Roy C, Wang CR, Brenner MB. CD1 reactive T cells clones use diverse a TCR repertoire. J Immunol 1999;162:161–167.

102. Barry CE, Lee RE, Mdluli K, et al. Mycolic acids: structure, biosynthesis and physiological functions. Prog Lipid Res 1998;37:143–179.

103. Bhardwaj N, Friedman SM, Cole BC, Nisanian AJ. Dendritic cells are potent antigen-presenting cells for microbial superantigens. J Exp Med 1992;175:267–273.

104. Sieling PA, Jullien D, Dahlem M, et al. CD1 expression by dendritic cells in human leprosy lesions: correlation with effective host immunity. J Immunol 1999;162:1851–1858.

105. Stenger S, Hanson DA, Teitelbaum R, et al. An antimicrobial activity of cytolytic T cells mediated by granulysin. Science 1998;282:121–125.

106. Stenger S, Mazzaccaro RJ, Uyemura K, et al. Differential effects of cytolytic T cell subsets on intracellular infection. Science 1997;276:1684–1687.

107. Carroll KK, Guthrie N, Ravi K. Dolichol: function, metabolism, and accumulation in human tissues. Biochem Cell Biol 1992;70:382–384.

108. Brennan PJ, Besra GS. Structure, function and biogenesis of the mycobacterial cell wall. Biochem Soc Trans 1997;25:188–194.

109. Moody DB. Polyisoprenyl glycolipids as targets of CD1-mediated immune responses. Cell Mol Life Sci 2001;58:1461–1474.

110. Shinkai K, Locksley RM. CD1, tuberculosis, and the evolution of major histocompatibility complex molecules. J Exp Med 2000;191:907–914.

Index

From: *Infectious Disease: Innate Immunity*
Edited by: R. A. B. Ezekowitz and J. A. Hoffman © Humana Press Inc., Totowa, NJ